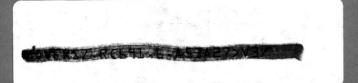

Date Due

	DISCARD		

BRODART, INC.　　　Cat. No. 23 233　　　Printed in U.S.A.

DES PLAINES, ILLINOIS　60016

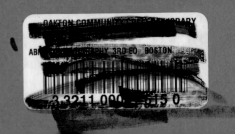

Abrams Angiography

Vascular and Interventional Radiology

Abrams Angiography

Vascular and Interventional Radiology

THIRD EDITION

HERBERT L. ABRAMS, M.D.
Editor

Philip H. Cook Professor of Radiology, Harvard Medical School;
Chairman of Radiology, Brigham and Women's Hospital and
Sidney Farber Cancer Institute, Boston

Volume III

Little, Brown and Company   Boston

TO MARILYN

Contents

Volume I

vii

Volume II

Volume III

V. The Extremities
SECTION 1. ANGIOGRAPHY OF THE
EXTREMITIES

VI. Interventional Techniques
SECTION 1. ANGIOPLASTY

SECTION 2. OCCLUSIVE AND
INFUSION TECHNIQUES

Notice

The indications and dosages of all drugs in this book have been recommended in the medical literature and conform to the practices of the general medical community. The medications described do not necessarily have specific approval by the Food and Drug Administration for use in the diseases and dosages for which they are recommended. The package insert for each drug should be consulted for use and dosage as approved by the FDA. Because standards for usage change, it is advisable to keep abreast of revised recommendations, particularly those concerning new drugs.

V

The Extremities

1. Angiography of the Extremities

Arteriography of the Patient with Previous Aortoiliac Surgery

ANDREW B. CRUMMY

The aging of our population and improvements in surgical and anesthetic technique have increased the number of patients undergoing surgery for disease of the abdominal aorta and iliac vessels. In addition, sufficient years have passed so that there are many patients who have recurrent symptoms or who have developed complications related to their aortoiliac surgery. Therefore, the number of patients who have had previous aortoiliac surgery and require arteriography is steadily increasing.

In patients with straightforward abdominal aortic and iliac artery disease, the problem can generally be assessed by a few pertinent questions and a simple physical examination. The diagnosis is seldom in doubt, and arteriography is done for staging. The arteriogram is used to demonstrate (1) the exact site of obstruction, (2) whether the distal vessels are satisfactory for anastomosis, and (3) whether the outflow vessels will allow sufficient flow to maintain patency. In the postoperative patient, detailed knowledge of the nature of previous vascular surgery and the current clinical problem is essential for the performance of an adequate examination [28].

Arteriographic Technique

The arteriographic technique for evaluation of the patient who has had previous aortoiliac surgery may differ significantly in several respects from the examination of the patient who has not had surgery. If either femoral artery is available for catheterization, this is the preferred route. As a practical matter, at least one of the distal anastomoses will have to be to an iliac artery. Generally, then, the ipsilateral groin will not have an incision. Arteriography is performed in the usual manner [6], with the positioning of the catheter varied according to the problem (Figs. 76-1, 76-2).

When use of the femoral route is precluded, our preference is for translumbar arteriography (Figs. 76-3–76-11). The puncture should be made in the aorta rather than the graft. Unless the patient has a graft that extends above the renal arteries, a very unusual circumstance, one is generally in good position if the entry is made at the L1 level. It is also useful to check the vascular clips that are invariably present and to make the entrance cephalad to the most proximal clip. Fluoroscopic control during the placement of the needle greatly simplifies this maneuver.

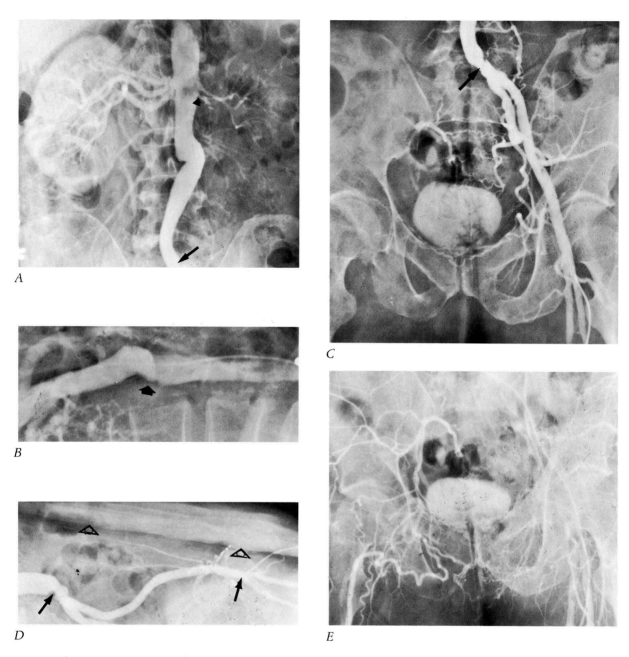

Figure 76-1. The patient had recurrence of claudication in the right lower extremity following placement of an aortic–bilateral common iliac graft. (A) An anteroposterior view of the graft, the right arm of which is obstructed. The arrowhead indicates an incidental left renal artery stenosis, and the solid arrow points to an irregularity of the left anastomosis. (B) Satisfactory appearance of the end-to-end aortic anastomosis (*arrow*). (C) Antegrade filling of the iliac system as well as opacification of cross-pelvic collaterals. The arrow identifies the anastomosis. (D) In lateral view, a large posterior plaque, not seen in the frontal view, is outlined at the anastomosis (*left arrow*). The open arrowheads indicate the interface between the bolus bags and the anterior aspect of the pelvis, and the right arrow points to the posterior origin of the profunda femoral artery, which is normal. (E) The right profunda femoral artery has now filled through collaterals and is the entire source of blood for that extremity.

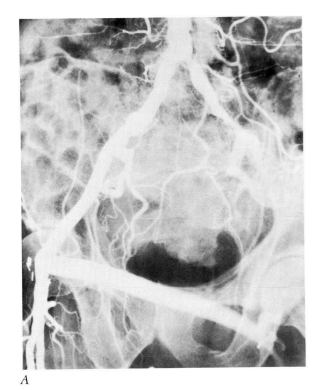

A

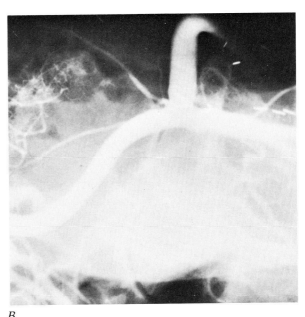

B

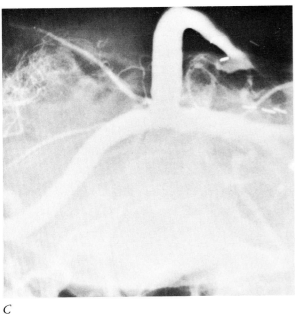

C

Figure 76-2. A femorofemoral graft was used to bypass the left iliac artery disease in an elderly patient who was not considered a candidate for an aortofemoral graft. Recurrent symptoms on the left prompted this examination. (A) The right common femoral artery has been entered below the graft. There is excellent filling of the distal aorta, pelvic vessels, collaterals, and graft. (B, C) Flow in graft gradually opacifies the left femoral artery. The anastomoses are best seen in lateral projection.

Our technique of translumbar puncture is similar to that discussed in Chapter 45. An 18-gauge, 22-cm Teflon sheath needle with four very distal side holes is used. Injection rates as rapid as 20 cc per second can be readily accommodated by this needle. Frequently, however, a slower injection rate is employed because obstruction is a major indication for these studies.

The sleeve is flexible, so it can be passed either distally or proximally, depending upon the par-ticular problem. In the presence of an open aortic bifurcation graft and with the need to study runoff vessels (i.e., the vessels distal to the inguinal ligament), distal placement of the tip is preferred because this will obviate loss of contrast into the visceral vessels. On the other hand, in the presence of severe proximal obstruction or occlusion, one must fill the collateral vessels, which for the most part are the high lumbar, intercostal, and superior mesenteric arteries. Such fill is best achieved by passing the catheter tip cephalad so that the injection is made into the distal thoracic aorta (Fig. 76-3) [31].

The direction of the catheter tip can usually be altered by manipulation of a 3-mm J guidewire [32]. On occasion, a tip deflector, such as that marketed by Cook, is useful. If puncture of the aorta is made with a relatively acute angle between the needle and the distal aorta, proximal

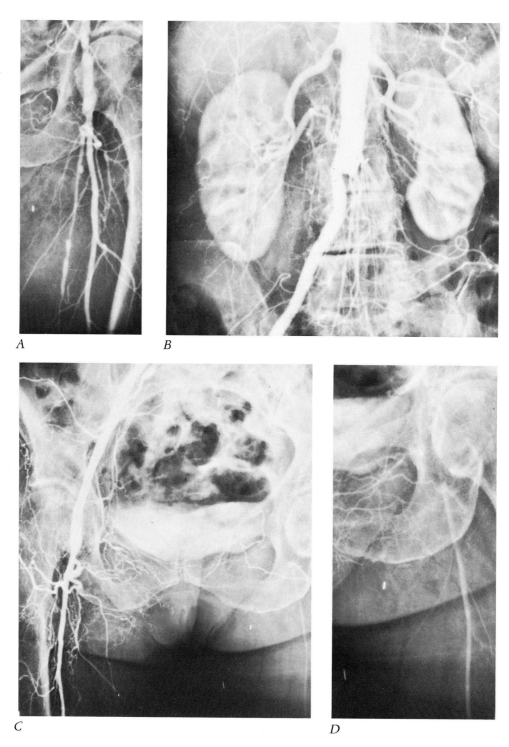

A

B

C

D

Figure 76-3. (A) The distal left ileofemoral system of a patient with bilateral lower extremity ischemia. There is significant obstruction in the common femoral artery just distal to the inguinal ligament and at its bifurcation. (B, C, and D) Symptoms recurred on the left, and reexamination showed that the right limb of the graft was normal. The left limb was obstructed, but flow through anterior pelvic collaterals gradually filled the left profunda femoral system. Presumably progression of disease in the common femoral artery resulted in thrombosis of the vessel and the graft. The loss of runoff caused retrograde propagation of thrombus to the graft bifurcation.

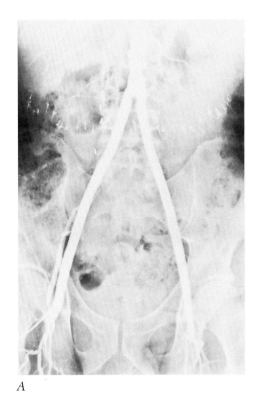
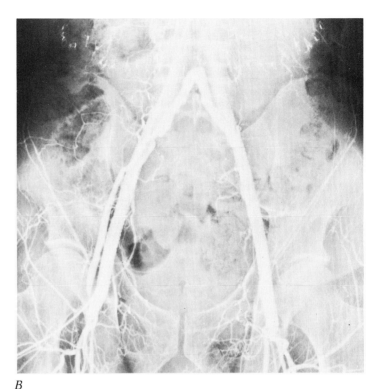

A   *B*

Figure 76-4. Arteriography of an aortofemoral graft performed through the right limb of the graft. (A) End-to-end aortic anastomosis and end-to-side femoral anastomoses. The graft is normal and provides excellent opacification of the femoral vessels. (B) Filling of the circumflex vessels and retrograde flow in the native external and common iliac systems.

passage of the tip is usual. Entry with the needle almost perpendicular to the aorta facilitates distal passage.

The use of the axillary brachial artery system is a reasonable alternative; as a matter of fact, it is the preferred approach of some angiographers for study of the abdominal aorta and pelvic vessels in lower extremity vascular disease. We find this a technically more difficult puncture, and the passage around an elongated, ectatic aortic arch may be time consuming. The upper extremity access is also the only approach that carries the risk of a cerebral vascular accident.

Only when a satisfactory alternative is not available do we use the graft for access (Fig. 76-4). We are reluctant to puncture grafts because of two problems unique to prostheses [12]. Synthetic material or vein does not have the muscular wall of an artery and therefore lacks the ability to contract and close the puncture site. Also, the neointima that lines prostheses can be easily stripped away from the wall, possibly resulting in obstruction or embolization.

If catheterization of a graft is required (e.g., to study the lower extremity vessels in the presence of an axillofemoral bypass), the use of a new Potts needle is recommended (Fig. 76-5). This will ensure a sharp tip and facilitate a single-wall puncture. The needle is passed slowly so that blood appears through the lumen of the obturator before the posterior wall is punctured. There is generally a considerable amount of perivascular fibrosis, and the use of a Teflon dilator is helpful in establishing a tract to the vessel. The dilator has the additional advantage of being sharply tapered, minimizing the possibility of intimal stripping.

A Teflon-coated 3-mm J guidewire facilitates smooth passage and minimizes the possibility of guidewire disruption of the neointima. Generally, if no problem is encountered at the puncture site, passage through the graft is problem-free. The smallest-diameter catheter that will deliver the required amount of contrast should be used. A 55-cm 5.3 French catheter will allow injection of 18 cc per second and is usually satisfactory. When the catheter is being moved, especially during removal, it is best to keep a guidewire in

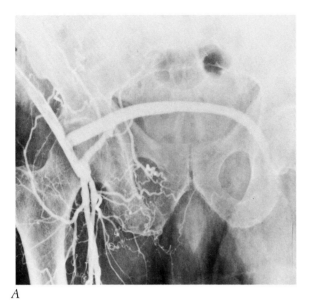
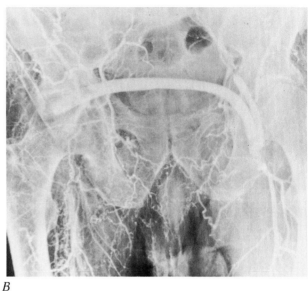

A   *B*

Figure 76-5. Right axillofemorofemoral graft performed because of bilateral lower extremity ischemia. Recurrent left-sided symptoms resulted in reexamination. (A) A catheter needle is in place in the distal axillary limb. There is an intraluminal filling defect representing thrombus in the proximal portion of the femoral limb, and the thrombus extends proximally and distally in the axillary limb. The proximal right femoral vessels are well filled. (B) Good opacification of the distal femoral limb and the left femoral system outlines a short segment of advanced disease just distal to the anastomosis. Note the retrograde filling of the common femoral and distal external iliac arteries as well as of the iliac circumflex vessel. Poor flow within the femoral limb of the graft was presumed to have resulted in thrombosis with retrograde propagation into the axillary portion.

place to prevent catheter disruption as it passes through the synthetic material.

After removal of the catheter, particular care must be given to achieving hemostasis. It is important that pressure on the puncture site not bring about complete occlusion of the graft because this may predispose to thrombosis. Also, great care must be exercised to avoid a hematoma because an infected hematoma may require removal of the prosthesis.

The choice of approach and filming sequence depends upon the patient's problems. As a general rule, relatively large volumes of contrast introduced at moderate injection rates (about 60 cc at 15–20 cc/second) are best used to fill vessels distal to obstruction as well as pseudoaneurysms and other spaces that may have small communications with the vascular tree. Moderate to slow filming rates are adequate (one per second × 15 or one per second × 10, then one every second × 5). The contrast is usually injected into the lower thoracic aorta. Biplane films of the suprarenal aorta, the graft including the proximal and distal anastomoses, and the runoff vessels should

be obtained. On occasion, particularly when the thrombosis is acute and collaterals are not fully developed, it may be difficult to fill the femoral vessels. The injection of 25 to 50 mg of Priscoline just prior to contrast injection may increase collateral flow and aid opacification of the runoff vessels [7]. Despite acute ischemia, which may be severe, reactive hyperemia may induce additional vasodilatation and is our preferred method [6]. A blood pressure cuff is placed around the thigh, inflated to above the systolic pressure for 7 minutes, and released just prior to the injection. During the vasoocclusive phase the patients may have some discomfort, but usually with reassurance they are willing to tolerate it.

Angiography suites are generally kept relatively cool for the comfort of the angiography team. In such circumstances, ischemic extremities may rapidly cool, with resultant vasoconstriction that will handicap the examination. This may be obviated by properly covering the extremities.

We are convinced that biplane filming is essential for adequate evaluation of these complex

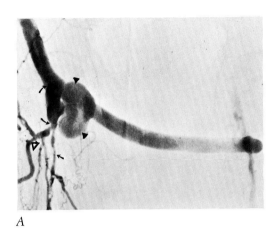
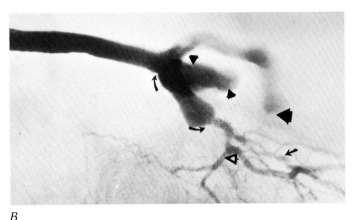

A   B

Figure 76-6. An elderly patient who had a previous axillobifemoral graft sought attention because of a groin mass, which he thought was an inguinal hernia. (A and B) Anteroposterior and lateral projections show the aortobifemoral graft with a pseudoaneurysm arising at the origin of the femoral limb. Both projections were necessary to define accurately the relationships of the pseudoaneurysm to the grafts. The solid arrowheads indicate the pseudoaneurysm. The curved arrows outline the endarterectomized portion of the common femoral and proximal profunda femoral arteries. The straight arrows point to the distal trunk of the profunda, which is severely involved with atherosclerosis. The open arrowheads identify the hypertrophied lateral femoral circumflex vessel, which is the main supply to the distal extremity. In (B), the large arrowhead points to the anastomosis of the graft to the left profunda artery. On the basis of this detailed pathoanatomic information, the surgeons were able to approach the graft in such a way that they could place one stitch to close the small leak that had occurred at the takeoff of the femoral arm.

problems (Fig. 76-6; see also Figs. 76-1, 76-2, 76-11). In areas such as the pelvis and proximal thigh, overlap of bilaterally symmetric arteries can be eliminated by angulation of the tube for simultaneous biplane filming or by obtaining both oblique projections with separate runs. Angulation of the tube will result in differences in the length of the beam path in tissue and cause unequal film exposure. This discrepancy can be overcome by using a water bolus on the anterior surface of the pelvis and thighs. Intravenous fluid bags are satisfactory for this purpose [6].

To reduce patient discomfort, we use lidocaine (injectable type), 2 mg per cubic centimeter mixed with the contrast agent. There is some controversy about its efficacy; however, our observations, which have been confirmed by others, are that the regimen is helpful [6, 13]. Nonionic contrast agents are expected to be introduced into the United States soon. The European experience suggests that they will eliminate much of the discomfort and increase patient safety [1].

Computerized fluoroscopy (CF), developed by Mistretta and associates at the University of Wisconsin, is a technique for real-time digital processing of x-ray transmission data from image-intensified videofluoroscopy systems [8, 22, 25, 29]. The signal from the iodine is logarithmically amplified and subtracted on-line by a small dedicated computer. Because amplification of the iodine signal is coupled with subtraction, satisfactory studies of the abdominal aorta and the pelvic vessels can be achieved by the intravenous injection of 60 cc of contrast agent (about 400 mg I/cc), delivered at the rate of 14 cc per second through a 2-cm, 16-gauge Angiocath in the basilic vein or a 5.3 French catheter in the superior vena cava. Exposures are made every 1.5 seconds as a bolus from the intravenous injection passes through the area. Motion interferes with subtraction, so the patient must remain immobile, and peristalsis should be suppressed by the intravenous administration of glucagon just prior to the study. Because the subtraction is done electronically, the images are available for immediate evaluation, and additional studies in other projections can be made as indicated. Moreover, the amount of subtraction can be varied so that some anatomic information can be left in the image to aid orientation.

With computerized fluoroscopy it is possible to detect aneurysms, false aneurysms (Fig. 76-7), and stenoses and to determine the patency of grafts (Figs. 76-8, 76-9). The information has been useful in the management of postoperative aortoiliac problems [29].

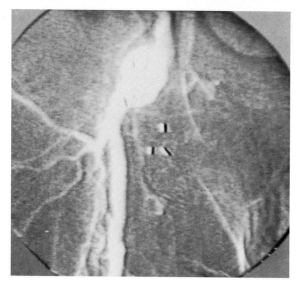

Figure 76-7. The patient was examined because of a right inguinal mass that developed after an aortobifemoral graft was placed. Computerized fluoroscopic (CF) intravenous videoarteriography was performed with the injection of 60 cc of contrast agent at the rate of 14 cc per second. A false aneurysm, located at the right femoral anastomosis of the graft, is seen. The information is sufficient to characterize the mass as a pseudoaneurysm. The lack of any constitutional symptoms, tenderness, or erythema suggested that the pseudoaneurysm was not infected.

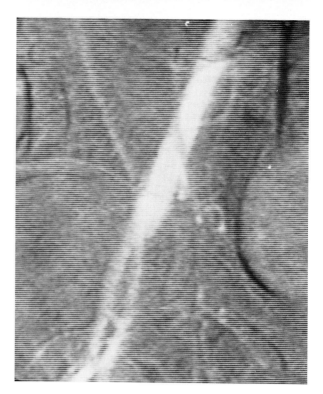

Figure 76-8. A computerized fluoroscopic intravenous video arteriogram following injection of 60 cc of contrast agent at the rate of 13 cc per second. The distal end of an aortofemoral graft can be seen. There is excellent filling of the superficial and profunda femoral arteries as well as of the iliac circumflex artery.

Figure 76-9. A computerized fluoroscopic intravenous video arteriogram following injection of 60 cc of contrast agent at the rate of 14 cc per second. (A) The donor end of a femorofemoral graft is shown, with good delineation of the external iliac and common femoral arteries. (B) The distal end of the graft is shown to be patent. The endarterectomized segment of the left common femoral artery has become aneurysmal. The profunda vessel and its lateral femoral circumflex branch are well delineated.

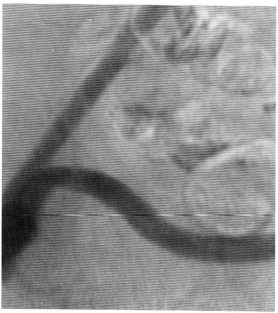

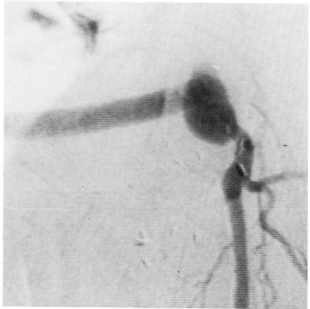

A

B

The intravenous videoarteriography technique of computerized fluoroscopy eliminates the risks associated with intraarterial catheterization. The major hazard is related to the intravascular administration of contrast agent, a risk common to both intravenous video studies and standard arteriography. The safety of the technique is such that outpatient arteriography is feasible, and this should result in a considerable reduction in costs. In addition, elimination of some of the risks of standard arteriography should allow broadening of the indications for arteriographic examination.

Postoperative Problems

IMMEDIATE PROBLEMS

Vascular problems immediately following aortoiliac surgery are generally related to technical errors that may result in thrombosis or hemorrhage. Graft thrombosis is usually secondary to an unsatisfactory anastomosis or poor distal outflow (runoff). Graft occlusion can also be due to obstruction secondary to dissection of intima that was inadequately reattached following endarterectomy, ordinarily at the site of or near the anastomosis [18]. Acute graft thrombosis can usually be diagnosed on the basis of clinical information, occasionally supplemented by simple Doppler ultrasound studies; as a rule arteriography is omitted. Significant bleeding—that is, an amount that would require reoperation—will be manifested clinically, and arteriography is not required [28]. However, if a patient is transferred from another institution because of graft failure in the immediate postoperative period, it is our practice to perform an arteriogram to define exactly the pathoanatomic situation. Similarly, arteriography is performed in a patient with postoperative bleeding if the clinical conditions permit.

LATE POSTOPERATIVE PROBLEMS

At times it is difficult to know whether a problem is related to a surgical misadventure or to progression of the underlying disease. For example, thrombosis of a limb of a graft could be due to a poor anastomosis or to advancement of the atherosclerotic process. It also may be impossible to know whether a pseudoaneurysm is a cause or the result of an infection. For the most part, what is primary is not important; rather, diagnosis of

the problem and delineation of the extent of the process and the involved anatomy are paramount for potential repair.

Graft Thrombosis

Graft thrombosis, which is more prevalent in patients with occlusive than with aneurysmal disease, may occur either abruptly or insidiously after a good initial result [5, 9]. The major cause is progression of the basic atherosclerotic process in the runoff vessels, although poor surgical technique may also be a factor (see Figs. 76-3, 76-5) [5]. In most circumstances, the profunda femoral artery provides sufficient flow for the graft to remain patent [23]. Therefore, it is essential that the profunda vessel be adequately evaluated, including its orifice, which is a common site of occlusive disease. Because the profunda orifice is posterior in relation to the common femoral artery, a lateral or oblique view must be obtained (see Fig. 76-1D).

The profunda artery may have main trunk obstruction as well as branch orifice stenosis distally (see Figs. 76-5, 76-6, 76-11) [15]. Because many of the lesions may be accessible to an extended endarterectomy, the entire profunda should be studied. Biplane views of the distal profunda artery have not been found to contribute useful information consistently, and we therefore obtain them only on the rare occasion when they appear to be necessary.

If both limbs of the graft are occluded, the thrombosis will extend proximally to the first branch vessels, usually a large pair of lumbar arteries or the renal arteries. Correction requires that any technical problems be rectified and any inadequacy of runoff corrected, or rethrombosis will occur. Removal of thrombus from the graft with a Fogarty catheter may be satisfactory. Otherwise, the graft will have to be replaced or a new bypass established, such as an axillofemoral or a femorofemoral bypass [9].

If one limb of the graft is open and thrombectomy fails, an iliofemoral or a femorofemoral bypass rather than replacement of the graft may be best. In these circumstances, assessment of the status of the patent graft limb is mandatory (see Fig. 76-1). If arteriography shows an obstruction of questionable hemodynamic significance, the pressure should be measured before and after reactive hyperemia. If there is a pressure gradient at rest or a gradient of more than 15 mm Hg after reactive hyperemia. it is unlikely that the graft will accommodate flow to both extremities; in such cases the gradient will have to be corrected or an alternative procedure done.

Progression of Disease

As previously discussed, progression of atherosclerotic disease may cause graft thrombosis (see Figs. 76-3–76-5) [9, 20]. On the other hand, the profunda femoral artery may provide runoff adequate to maintain patency, but distal disease may cause claudication, rest pain, or tissue necrosis [15]. Arteriography, which is useful for confirming the status of the graft and visualizing the vessels of the extremity, should be performed by injection of a large volume of contrast at the aortic bifurcation with filming of the extremity vessels.

After aortic–common iliac grafting, the internal and external iliac vessels fill in a normal antegrade manner (see Fig. 76-1). Following an end-to-end aortic anastomosis and an end-to-side external iliac or femoral anastomosis, the iliac system fills by retrograde flow in the external iliac artery as well as through collaterals (see Figs. 76-4, 76-11). With an end-to-end external iliac or femoral anastomosis, filling is largely retrograde through the profunda collaterals and antegrade through the lumbar collaterals. Because these vessels are perfused, their potential for aneurysm development persists (see Fig. 76-11). Aneurysms of these sites may be manifested in a variety of ways, including (1) by rupture, (2) as a mass, (3) through ureteral compression, and (4) by peripheral embolization.

Ultrasound may be helpful in delineating the size, shape, and location of a mass as well as its acoustic characteristics. The relationship of the mass to vessels in the pelvis may, however, be difficult to define. Computed tomography (CT) has an advantage in that it can show the uptake of contrast agent within the lumen of the aneurysm, but CT scans show only a cross section rather than the long axis of the vessel. Intravenous video CF angiography can show the vessel as well as the aneurysm, and while conventional arteriography affords better spatial resolution, such detailed resolution may not be necessary in all circumstances; conventional arteriography should be performed only if the additional detail is required.

Pseudoaneurysms and Infected Grafts

Because they may be cause or effect or exist independently, it is difficult to consider pseudoaneurysms and infected grafts separately. If blood extravasates slowly, a hematoma may form, providing some degree of tamponade. The outer layer of the hematoma may become fairly well organized and fibrotic, but the portion adjacent to the artery generally remains filled with liquid blood. Such a lesion is called a pseudoaneurysm because none of the layers of the vessel forms part of the hematoma wall, and the hematoma communicates with the vascular lumen.

False aneurysms, when present in a patient with a graft, are usually seen in the region of an anastomosis (see Figs. 76-6, 76-7, 76-11) [16]. They are the result of an insidious leak that remains occult until a mass is palpable or an associated complication such as an infection or a massive bleed occurs. Infection may disrupt the suture line, resulting in bleeding, and, depending upon the circumstances including the rate of hemorrhage, a false aneurysm may form or exsanguination may occur.

Infection in the area of a vascular prosthesis is a feared complication [11]. Szilagyi et al. [26] reported an incidence of 0.7 percent when the distal anastomoses were done through an abdominal incision, but the rate more than doubled to 1.6 percent when groin anastomoses were performed. Most infections are believed to be the result of contamination through the incision [30]. However, injury to the gastrointestinal tract and primary infection of an aneurysm at the time of surgery are also factors in graft infection [17, 24]. Hematogenous seeding secondary to bacteremia, whatever the cause, likewise plays a role in late infection. Pressure necrosis of the gastrointestinal tract from pulsations of the relatively rigid prosthesis or a pseudoaneurysm may result in an aortoenteric fistula.

The clinical manifestations of an infected graft or a pseudoaneurysm are in part related to the virulence of the organisms, the response of the host, and the location. In the groin, the classic signs of infection are tenderness and erythema; swelling may be seen early. If the skin breaks down, there may be extravasation of pus and some bleeding. The same process may occur in the abdomen, but early symptoms will be less likely, and thus diagnosis will be more difficult.

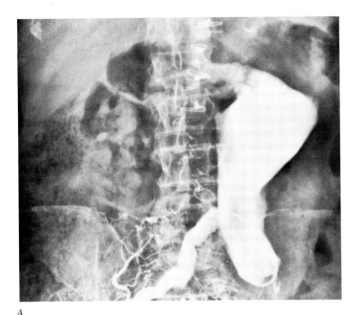

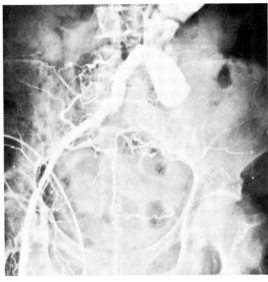

A

B

C

Figure 76-10. A patient who had had a well-functioning aortic–bilateral common iliac graft for a number of years noted pyrexia and malaise. At the time of admission, she was febrile and had an absent left femoral pulse; hematologic studies were compati-

ble with an infection. The diagnosis of an infected graft was made, and arteriography was undertaken to delineate the anatomy. (A and B) Right transfemoral aortogram shows marked extravasation of contrast agent into a huge paravascular pseudoaneurysm. The pseudoaneurysm extended from L2 inferiorly along the left limb of the graft to the midportion of the sacroiliac joint. There is excellent filling of the vessels in the right hemipelvis that course to the left as collaterals around the obstructed left graft limb (B). (C) Lateral projection shows that the pseudoaneurysm extends into the posterior paraspinal area. No further attempt to delineate the anatomy was made. The diagnosis was an infected graft with a large pseudoaneurysm and obstruction of the left limb. At surgery, the aortic and left iliac anastomoses were disrupted, and the blood was contained by the large infected pseudoaneurysm. The graft was removed, and the patient was observed. Because her extremities did not show evidence of additional ischemia, an extraanatomic bypass was not required.

DIAGNOSIS

Any patient with a vascular graft and fever should be suspected of having an infected graft. A film of the involved area showing gas bubbles in the region of the graft is diagnostic. Ultrasound and CT scan may show fluid collections in the paraprosthetic region. However, it may be difficult to distinguish a pseudoaneurysm from an abscess unless there is associated gas. In the presence of pyrexia, contamination must be presumed. A gallium scan demonstrating localization of the isotope in the paraprosthetic area is strongly suggestive of infection, especially if the localization is near a suture line [2, 4].

If attention is drawn to an uninfected graft because of bleeding, palpable mass, etc., arteriography may provide valuable information. Malposition or unusual contour of the graft may suggest abnormality, and contrast may opacify a pseudoaneurysm [6]. If surgery is contemplated, knowledge of the vascular anatomy is helpful in planning possible removal of the graft and any corrective surgery (Fig. 76-10, 76-11).

With a firm clinical diagnosis of an infected

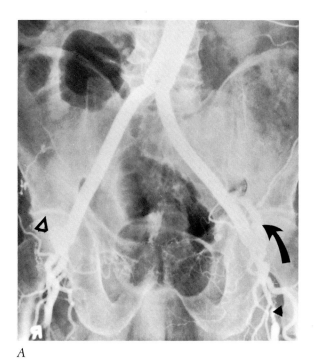

A

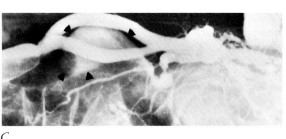

C

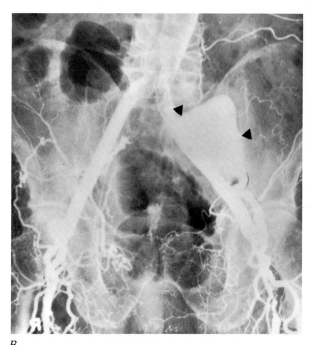

B

Figure 76-11. The 83-year-old patient had an aortobifemoral graft because of an abdominal aortic aneurysm 6 years previously. At that time, the right iliac artery was obstructed, and the left common iliac artery was aneurysmal. The iliac artery aneurysm was ligated proximally and distally and left in situ. The patient was seen at this time because of a palpable left pelvic mass. (A) A translumbar aortogram shows excellent filling of the aortobifemoral graft. The solid arrowhead points to distal profunda femoral artery obstruction. The open arrowhead shows a small pseudoaneurysm at the site of the anastomosis. The overall size of the pseudoaneurysm is best appreciated by combining both the anteroposterior (A and B) and lateral projections (C). The straight arrow points to retrograde flow in the left common femoral and external iliac arteries. In (B) and (C) frontal and lateral projections in a later phase show a large aneurysm of the left common iliac artery, which is outlined by the arrowheads. Note that the left limb of the graft is displaced anteriorly by the aneurysm. (C) was taken with the patient prone so that the contrast is layered in the dependent portion of the graft. For ease of viewing, the film is displayed as if the patient were supine. It was presumed that the left iliac artery sutures had deteriorated and that the vessel had recanalized with increase in size of the aneurysm. The patient was explored by an extraperitoneal approach; the aneurysm was exposed and again ligated proximally and distally and evacuated. The patient has done well.

graft, the primary role of arteriography is the definition of the vascular anatomy. Of particular importance is the state of the distal vessels, which determines the feasibility of the secondary repair. Demonstration of the presence and extent of a pseudoaneurysm is also helpful [11]. In a patient in whom the diagnosis is not clear, the demonstration of a pseudoaneurysm greatly enhances the possibility of an infected graft.

Aortoenteric Fistula and Paraprosthetic Enteric Fistula

Four years after aortic reconstructive surgery was initiated, the first aortoenteric fistula was reported [3, 10]. The major clinical manifestations of this potentially catastrophic complication are gastrointestinal bleeding and sepsis. These symptoms in any patient who has had previous aortic surgery must raise the possibility of an aortoenteric fistula [2].

The infrarenal aorta and the transverse part of the duodenum are juxtaposed, and it is necessary to interpose viable tissue between the duodenum and aortic suture line to prevent pressure necrosis of the bowel caused by the pulsations of the relatively rigid prosthesis. Damage to the bowel wall compromises its integrity, leading to contamination of the area with enteric bacteria. In the presence of such an infection, disruption of the anastomosis will almost surely ensue.

A frank, free communication of the vascular lumen and the bowel will produce rapid exsanguination. Fortunately, since the fistula is usually small and plugged with thrombus and other debris, bleeding is intermittent and generally not massive. There is little about the clinical circumstances except the history of prior aortic surgery and the combination of gastrointestinal bleeding and sepsis to suggest a fistula.

Barium studies are of little utility because the patients are likely to be in an age group in which many lesions with a potential for bleeding are found, necessitating that a lesion be proved responsible for the bleeding. An aortoenteric fistula can, of course, coexist with another source of bleeding. The presence of barium will handicap endoscopy, ultrasound, CT scanning, and arteriography.

Upper gastrointestinal endoscopy may identify many lesions and actually demonstrate the bleeding. On occasion, the gastrointestinal side of the fistula may be visualized. A major handicap to this approach is that manipulation of the duodenum may disrupt the precarious state of hemostasis existing in the fistula. Therefore, some recommend that endoscopy, if done, be carried out in the operating room with the patient prepared for surgery.

While ultrasound and CT scanning may suggest a pseudoaneurysm, these diagnostic modalities are generally not particularly helpful. Arteriography may demonstrate a false aneurysm or a paragraft extravasation of contrast agent, but unless the patient is bleeding profusely at the time of arteriography, the bleeding per se is unlikely to be identified. In a patient suspected of having a graft complication who is briskly bleeding, the risks of surgery without angiographic information are probably less than the risk of exsanguination because of delay.

A less common type of fistula, paraprosthetic

enteric, is caused by erosion of bowel remote from a suture line and is ordinarily without a false aneurysm [27]. A major predisposing factor is a graft that is too long, causing anterior bowing of the proximal portions of the iliac limbs with resultant pressure necrosis of the bowel. Under these circumstances, the manifestations of infection rather than bleeding are paramount [6]. The bleeding that occurs is the outcome of bowel necrosis and does not represent a communication with the vascular lumen through a disrupted suture line. Contamination of the area of necrosis with intestinal organisms is inevitable, and gallium scanning may be helpful in localizing inflammation in the region of the prosthesis.

The role of arteriography is preeminent in defining the vascular anatomy and the state of vessels that may be used for extraanatomic bypass.

Arteriovenous Fistulas

Arteriovenous fistulas are rare complications of aortoiliac surgery. They are generally recognized during surgery and immediately repaired, but they may also occur as a late complication, commonly manifested by (1) high-output cardiac failure, (2) distal ischemia, (3) a palpable mass, (4) bruit, and (5) thrill [19].

Arteriography is required to confirm the diagnosis and delineate the anatomy. Determination of the exact site of the fistula, the relationship of involved vessels, and the presence of potential collaterals is important. Large-volume injections with multiple projections and very rapid filming (up to six per second) are essential aspects of the examination.

Failure of Prosthetic Materials

Deterioration of prosthetic materials may be the source of clinical problems [14]. Aneurysmal dilatation of synthetic grafts, which may lead to rupture or loss of integrity of the anastomosis due to deterioration of the suture material, is a well-recognized problem, now greatly reduced by the use of new synthetics. Generally, the manifestations are those associated with true or false aneurysms of any cause, and the arteriographic approach is similar to that previously discussed.

ACKNOWLEDGMENT

I wish to acknowledge the assistance of William D. Turnipseed, M.D., Director of Perivascular Surgery, William S. Middleton Veterans Administration Hospital, Madison, Wisconsin, who reviewed the manuscript and made helpful suggestions.

References

1. Almén, T., Boijsen, E., and Lindell, S. E. Metrizamide in angiography: I. Femoral angiography. *Acta Radiol. [Diagn.]* (Stockh.) 18:33, 1977.
2. Bernard, V. M., and Kleinman, L. H. Aortoenteric Fistulas. In J. J. Bergan and J. S. T. Yao (eds.), *Surgery of the Aorta and Its Body Branches.* New York: Grune & Stratton, 1979. P. 591.
3. Brock, R. C. Aortic hemografting: A report of six successful cases. *Guys Hosp. Rep.* 102:204, 1953.
4. Causey, D. A., Fajman, W. A., Perdue, G. D., Sones, P. J., Tarcan, Y. A., and Leigh, T. F. Roentgenographic Diagnosis of Postoperative Synthetic Vascular Graft Infections. Presented at the American Roentgen Ray Society, April 21–25, 1980, Las Vegas.
5. Crawford, E. S., Manning, L. G., and Kelley, T. F. "Redo" surgery after operations for aneurysm and occlusion of the abdominal aorta. *Surgery* 81:41, 1977.
6. Crummy, A. B., Rankin, R. S., Turnipseed, W. D., and Berkoff, H. A. Biplane arteriography in ischemia of the lower extremity. *Radiology* 126:111, 1978.
7. Crummy, A. B., Sherry, J. J., and Ahlstrand, R. A. A technique for peripheral arteriography using talazoline. *Australas. Radiol.* 17:308, 1973.
8. Crummy, A. B., Strother, C. M., Sackett, J. F., Ergun, D. L., Shaw, C. G., Kruger, R. A., Mistretta, C. A., Turnipseed, W. D., Lieberman, R. P., Myerowitz, P. D., and Ruzicka, F. F. Computerized fluoroscopy: A digital subtraction technique for intravenous angiocardiography and arteriography. *AJR* 135:1131, 1980.
9. Downs, A. R. Management of Aortofemoral Graft Limb Occlusion. In J. J. Bergan and J. S. T. Yao (eds.), *Surgery of the Aorta and Its Body Branches.* New York: Grune & Stratton, 1979. P. 551.
10. Dubost, C., Allary, M., and Oeconomos, N. Resection of an aneurysm of the abdominal aorta: Reestablishment of the continuity by a preserved human arterial graft with result after five months. *Arch. Surg.* 64:405, 1952.
11. Ehrenfeld, W. K., Wilbur, B. G., Olcott, C. N., and Stoney, R. J. Autogenous tissue reconstruction in the management of infected prosthetic grafts. *Surgery* 85:82, 1979.
12. Eisenberg, R. L., Mani, R. L., and McDonald, E. J., Jr. The complication rate of catheter angiography by direct puncture through aortofemoral bypass grafts. *AJR* 126:814, 1976.
13. Gordon, I. J., and Westcott, J. L. Intra-arterial lidocaine: An effective analgesia for peripheral angiography. *Radiology* 124:43, 1977.
14. Greenhalgh, R. M., and Chir, M. Dilation and Stretching of Knitted Dacron Grafts Associated with Failure. In J. J. Bergan and J. S. T. Yao (eds.), *Surgery of the Aorta and Its Body Branches.* New York: Grune & Stratton, 1979. P. 621.
15. Hill, D. A., McGrath, M. A., Lord, R. S. A., and Tracy, G. D. The effect of superficial femoral artery occlusion on the outcome of aortofemoral bypass for intermittent claudication. *Surgery* 87:133, 1980.
16. Hollier, L. H., Batson, R. C., and Cohn, I., Jr. Femoral anastomotic aneurysms. *Ann. Surg.* 191:715, 1980.
17. Jarrett, F., Darling, R. C., Mundth, E. D., and Austen, W. G. Experience with infected aneurysms of the abdominal aorta. *Arch. Surg.* 110:1281, 1975.
18. Knudson, J. A., and Downs, A. R. Reoperation following failure of aortoiliofemoral arterial reconstruction. *Can. J. Surg.* 21:316, 1978.
19. Littooy, F. N., and Baker, W. H. Major Arteriovenous Fistulas of the Aortic Territory. In J. J. Bergan and J. S. T. Yao (eds.), *Surgery of the Aorta and Its Body Branches.* New York: Grune & Stratton, 1979. P. 605.
20. Malone, J. M., Goldstone, J., and Moore, W. S. Autogenous profundaplasty: The key to long-term patency in secondary repair of aortofemoral graft occlusion. *Ann. Surg.* 188:817, 1978.
21. Mani, R. L., and Costin, B. S. Catheter angiography through aortofemoral grafts: Prevention of catheter separation during withdrawal. *AJR* 128:328, 1977.
22. Mistretta, C. M., and Crummy, A. B. Digital Fluoroscopy. In C. M. Coulam, J. J. Erickson, F. D. Rollo, and A. E. James, Jr. (eds.), *The Physical Basis of Medical Imaging.* New York: Appleton-Century-Crofts, 1981. Pp. 107–122.
23. Okike, S., and Bernatz, P. E. The role of the deep femoral artery in revascularization of the lower extremity. *Mayo Clin. Proc.* 51:209, 1976.
24. Scher, L. A., Brener, B. J., Goldenkranz, R. J., Alpert, J., Brief, D. K., Parsonnet, V., and Tiro, A. C. Infected aneurysms of the abdominal aorta. *Arch. Surg.* 115:975, 1980.
25. Strother, C. M., Sackett, J. F., Crummy, A. B., et al. Clinical applications of computerized fluoroscopy. The extracranial carotid artery. *Radiology* 136:780, 1980.

26. Szilagyi, D. E., Smith, R. F., Elliott, J. P., and Vrandecic, M. P.   Infection in arterial reconstruction with synthetic grafts. *Ann. Surg.* 176: 321, 1972.

27. Thompson, W. M., Jackson, D. C., and Johnsrude, I. S.   Aortoenteric and paraprosthetic-enteric fistulas: Radiologic findings. *AJR* 127:235, 1976.

28. Thompson, W. M., Johnsrude, I. S., Jackson, D. C., Older, R. A., and Wechsler, A. S.   Late complications of abdominal aortic reconstructive surgery. *Ann. Surg.* 185:326, 1977.

29. Turnipseed, W. D., Crummy, A. B., Strother, C., Sackett, J., Ergun, D., Kruger, R., Mistretta, C., and Belzer, F. O.   IV Computerized Arteriography, a Technique for Visualizing the Peripheral Vascular System. Presented at the 34th Annual Meeting of the Society for Vascular Surgery, June 26–27, 1980, Chicago.

30. Veith, F. J.   Surgery of the Infected Aortic Graft. In J. J. Bergan, and J. S. T. Yao (eds.), *Surgery of the Aorta and Its Body Branches.* New York: Grune & Stratton, 1979. P. 521.

31. Vine, H. S., and Sacks, B. A.   Visualization of the distal arterial vessels in complete aortic occlusion. *AJR* 134:847, 1980.

32. White, R. I., Jr.   Angiography of the Abdominal Aorta and Its Branches. In R. I. White, Jr. (ed.), *Fundamentals of Vascular Radiology.* Philadelphia: Lea & Febiger, 1976. P. 53.

Femoral Arteriography

KLAUS M. BRON

Femoral arteriography is the most frequently performed vascular examination in the average hospital radiology department. This reflects the high incidence of obstructive peripheral vascular disease and the improved techniques of revascularization, both by surgery [121] and by percutaneous transluminal angioplasty [49, 137].

Screening patients with clinically suspected peripheral vascular disease by Doppler ultrasound [99] has eliminated the need to obtain arteriograms in those who fail to demonstrate any significant abnormality. Arteriography remains the most important technique for establishing the presence and anatomic extent of the intravascular and soft tissue disease process. For the vascular surgeon and the interventional angiographer, the arteriogram is the single most effective diagnostic test in the evaluation of the patient with vascular obstruction. The arteriogram provides the definitive information on which to base a recommendation for the best type of revascularization in a particular situation.

Arteriographic Anatomy

NORMAL ANATOMY

The description of the normal arterial anatomy and collateral circulation of the pelvis and lower extremities is derived from several standard texts [5, 37, 114], articles [41, 93], and my own arteriographic observations.

The common femoral artery is the continuation of the external iliac artery distal to the inguinal ligament (Fig. 77-1). The common femoral artery gives off a deep branch, the profunda femoris, medial to the neck of the femur. The continuation of the common femoral artery in the thigh is the superficial femoral artery, which runs medial and anterior to the femur.

The profunda femoris artery (Fig. 77-1) is the most significant branch of the common femoral artery because it serves as the main blood supply to the thigh muscles. It is the prime collateral vessel to the leg when the superficial femoral artery is occluded. The profunda femoris and superficial femoral arteries are nearly equal in caliber at their origins. The profunda femoris divides rapidly into several branches: the medial circumflex femoral, lateral circumflex femoral, perforating, and muscular branches (Fig. 77-1). The medial circumflex femoral artery divides into several branches, one or more of which anas-

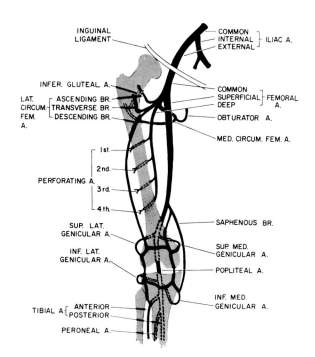

INGUINAL
LIGAMENT

COMMON
INTERNAL ⎤ ILIAC A.
EXTERNAL

INFER. GLUTEAL A.

LAT. ⎡ ASCENDING BR.
CIRCUM.⎤ TRANSVERSE BR.
FEM. ⎣ DESCENDING BR.
A.

COMMON
SUPERFICIAL ⎤ FEMORAL
DEEP ⎦ A.

OBTURATOR A.

MED. CIRCUM. FEM. A.

PERFORATING A.
1 st.
2nd.
3 rd.
4 th.

SUP. LAT.
GENICULAR A.

INF. LAT.
GENICULAR A.

SAPHENOUS BR.

SUP. MED.
GENICULAR A.

POPLITEAL A.

INF. MED.
GENICULAR A.

TIBIAL A. ⎡ ANTERIOR
⎣ POSTERIOR

PERONEAL A.

Figure 77-1. A composite drawing of the normal anatomy of the femoral artery, its branches, the distal runoff arteries, and the potential collateral vessels.

tomose with the obturator and internal pudendal branches of the internal iliac artery.

The lateral circumflex femoral artery (Fig. 77-1) divides into the ascending, transverse, and descending branches. These vessels anastomose with the superior and inferior gluteal branches of the internal iliac, the deep iliac circumflex branch of the external iliac, and the first perforating arteries. The medial and lateral circumflex femoral branches constitute important collateral pathways when the common and external iliac or common femoral arteries are occluded.

The four perforating branches of the profunda femoris artery descend caudally along the posteromedial aspect of the femur and obliquely penetrate the adductor magnus muscle to reach the back of the thigh. The terminal branches of these perforating arteries anastomose freely with the small muscular branches of the superficial femoral artery (see Fig. 77-4).

The superficial femoral artery functions primarily as a conduit to supply blood to the knee and calf areas. In the thigh it gives off some small muscular branches and the descending genicular or saphenous artery (Fig. 77-1). The superficial femoral artery lies medial to the femur and in the lower third of the thigh runs posteriorly to pass through the adductor canal. As it passes through

this tendinous hiatus in the adductor magnus muscle, the vessel becomes the popliteal artery.

The popliteal artery lies posterior in the intercondylar (popliteal) fossa (Fig. 77-1; see also Fig. 77-5) and continues across the knee joint to end in three terminal branches. The important anastomotic branches of the popliteal artery are the superior and inferior medial and lateral genicular vessels (Fig. 77-1; see also Fig. 77-31). The genicular branches join with descending branches of the lateral circumflex and the descending genicular branch of the superficial femoral artery to form collaterals around the knee when the popliteal artery is occluded.

The distal runoff arteries, the anterior and posterior tibial and peroneal, are the three terminal branches of the popliteal artery. These vessels supply blood to the several calf muscles. The anterior tibial artery runs anteriorly through the interosseous membrane between the tibia and the fibula (Fig. 77-1). It is the only major artery in the anterior muscle compartment of the lower leg and continues into the foot as the dorsalis pedis artery. The posterior tibial artery is the direct continuation of the popliteal artery. It supplies the muscles of the posterior compartment and is the nutrient artery to the tibia; it continues into the foot along the medial malleolus. The peroneal artery is the third terminal branch of the popliteal and lies between the anterior and posterior tibial arteries. It provides branches to the calf muscles and is the nutrient artery to the fibula.

COLLATERAL CIRCULATION

The collateral circulation when pelvic or lower extremity arteries are occluded involves the branches of the internal iliac artery (Fig. 77-2). This is part of the visceral collateral circulation. The external iliac artery, via its deep circumflex iliac and inferior epigastric branches, also contributes to the collateral circulation of the leg (Fig. 77-3). This is part of the parietal collateral circulation. The internal iliac artery divides into an anterior and a posterior portion. The obturator and internal pudendal arteries, which are branches of the anterior division of the internal iliac artery, anastomose with the medial circumflex femoral branches of the profunda femoris artery. The superior and inferior gluteal arteries, which are posterior division branches, anastomose with the lateral circumflex femoral artery. The branches of the internal iliac artery

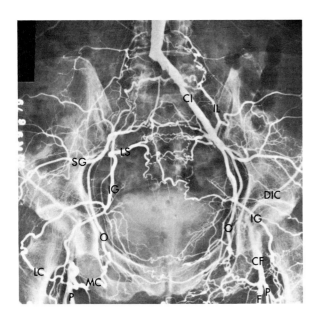

Figure 77-2. Multiple iliac artery occlusions with mainly visceral or left internal iliac branch artery collateral circulation reconstituting the right profunda femoris (*P*), and the left common femoral (*CF*), superficial femoral (*F*), and profunda femoris (*P*) arteries. The internal iliac branches that form the collaterals are the superior gluteal (*SG*), inferior gluteal (*IG*), obturator (*O*), lateral sacral (*LS*), and iliolumbar (*IL*). The profunda femoris (*P*) branches that complete the collateral circulation are the medial (*MC*) and lateral (*LC*) circumflex femoral arteries. The obturator (*O*) and lateral sacral (*LS*) arteries send branches across the pelvis to their counterparts on the contralateral side. *CI* = common iliac artery, *DIC* = deep iliac circumflex branch.

Figure 77-3. (A) Multiple iliac artery occlusions are shown with both visceral and parietal collateral circulation. The right collaterals are visceral, the branches of the internal iliac artery (see Fig. 77-2 for abbreviations). The left collaterals are mainly parietal. *IP* = internal pudendal. (B) The right common iliac and internal iliac arteries are patent, and the remaining major pelvic vessels are occluded except for the reconstituted left common femoral artery. The left parietal collateral circulation comprises a lumbar artery (*L*) anastomosing with the deep iliac circumflex branch of the external iliac artery. The left superficial femoral and profunda femoris arteries are patent. The left internal iliac artery branches reconstitute only minimally.

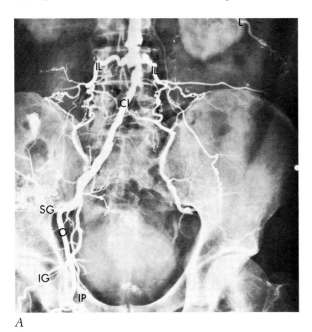

A

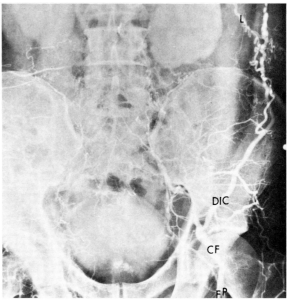

B

are all paired, but only the obturator, internal pudendal, and lateral sacral arteries anastomose transversely with their contralateral partners. The posterior division branches, superior and inferior gluteal arteries, anastomose only ipsilaterally.

The common and superficial femoral arteries are devoid of any branches that anastomose with the pelvic arteries. The profunda femoris artery, through its medial and lateral circumflex femoral branches, anastomoses extensively with the pelvic arteries. The profunda femoris artery also anastomoses freely with the popliteal artery branches, around the knee, via the descending lateral circumflex and the perforating branches. Thus, when the superficial femoral artery is occluded, the profunda femoris artery is the single most important vessel involved in the thigh collateral network between the pelvis and the lower leg (Fig. 77-4).

At the knee level, when the popliteal artery is occluded, collateral circulation develops to reconstitute the distal runoff arteries. This circulation largely comprises small, unnamed branches from the medial and lateral genicular, popliteal, superficial femoral, and profunda femoris arteries (Fig. 77-5). The level at which the popliteal artery is occluded helps to determine the source of the collaterals. More frequently at this site than elsewhere in the lower extremity, the collateral vessels are not particularly dilated and may not be very tortuous. Branches from the medial genicular arteries tend to reconstitute the posterior tibial artery, whereas the lateral genicular arteries reconstitute the anterior tibial artery.

At the ankle the peroneal artery may provide collateral circulation to both the anterior and posterior tibial arteries. When the posterior tibial artery is occluded at its origin or elsewhere in the calf, its continuation into the foot may nevertheless still be patent; reconstitution occurs via a collateral from the peroneal artery just above the ankle joint. The posterior and anterior tibial arteries may also contribute collaterals to each other just below the ankle joint (Fig. 77-6).

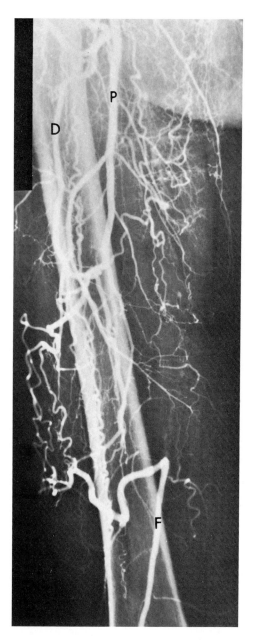

Figure 77-4. In the thigh, the profunda femoris artery (*P*) and its descending lateral circumflex branch (*D*) form the principal collateral circulation between the pelvis and the lower leg when the superficial femoral artery is occluded. The distal superficial femoral artery (*F*) is reconstituted via the collateral circulation.

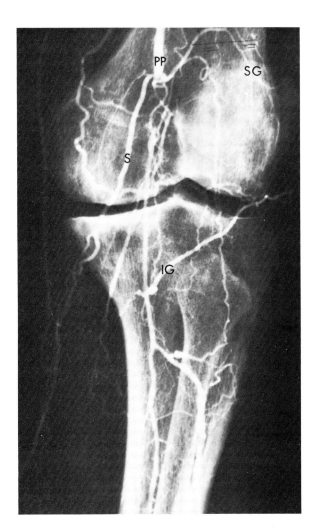

Figure 77-5. At the knee, in response to a segmental occlusion of the popliteal artery (*PP*) several collateral branches have developed: the lateral superior genicular (*SG*), the lateral inferior genicular (*IG*), and the sural (*S*). Other, unnamed collateral branches are also present.

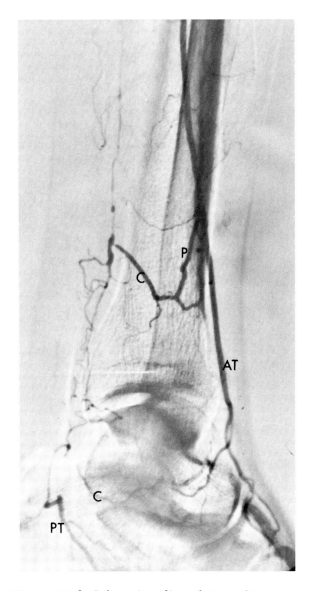

Figure 77-6. Subtraction film of the ankle in the oblique position demonstrates some of the unnamed collaterals (*C*) derived from the peroneal (*P*) and anterior tibial (*AT*) arteries. Only the distal posterior tibial artery (*PT*) reconstitutes via collateral circulation.

ANATOMIC ANOMALIES

The lower extremity arteries are essentially devoid of anomalies except for the distal runoff vessels. The two variations encountered most frequently at this level involve the peroneal and anterior tibial arteries. Normally, the peroneal artery is a branch of the common posterior tibial artery (see Fig. 77-1). However, as a variant, it may arise from a common branch with the anterior tibial artery (Fig. 77-7). This configuration, which is a mirror image of the normal anatomy, may be present unilaterally or bilaterally.

The other common variation relates to the origin of the anterior tibial artery. This vessel usually originates from the popliteal artery at the level of the interosseous notch between the tibia and the fibula. As a variant, this vessel may arise more cephalad, near the knee joint or even above it (Fig. 77-8). In rare instances the posterior tibial artery may be atrophic or nondeveloped, resulting in a two-vessel runoff.

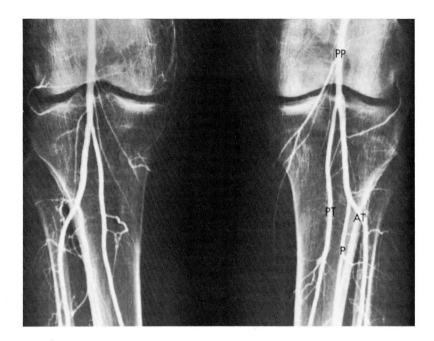

Figure 77-7. The origin of the distal runoff arteries is anomalous, bilaterally. Normally the posterior tibial (*PT*) and peroneal (*P*) arteries arise from a common trunk (see Fig. 77-1). In this anomaly there is a mirror image reversal of the normal, with the anterior tibial (*AT*) and peroneal arteries arising from a common trunk off the popliteal artery (*PP*).

Figure 77-8. The origin of the left anterior tibial artery (*AT*) is anomalous. The right anterior tibial artery arises normally at the proximal end of the interosseous membrane, whereas the left arises near the knee joint space. The posterior tibial (*PT*) and peroneal (*P*) arteries are normal bilaterally.

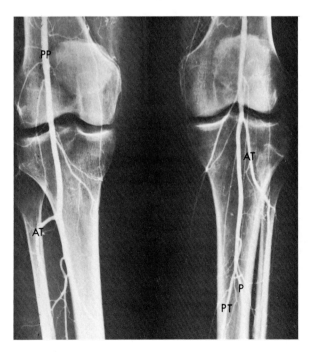

Technique

Percutaneous transfemoral catheterization is at present the method of choice for examining vascular disease of the aorta and lower extremities. Historically, translumbar aortography, introduced by dos Santos [29], was the technique first employed. In 1953, when Seldinger [107] described the ingeniously simple technique of percutaneous catheterization, most major centers abandoned the translumbar technique. A 1975 review [129] describes the evolution of the various catheters, techniques, and angiographic equipment that have been utilized in the examination of patients with obstructive peripheral vascular disease. The transfemoral catheter technique of arteriography facilitates examination of the aorta (for inflow disease) and permits serial filming of the pelvis, thigh, and runoff vessels in multiple views. These features are extremely important for complete evaluation of obstructive peripheral vascular disease.

PATIENT PREPARATION

All patients referred for arteriography should be examined by the angiographer in order (1) to evaluate the clinical need for the arteriogram, (2) to examine the patient's physical condition and palpate the lower extremity pulses, and (3) to obtain informed consent by explaining the procedure and its potential complications. A note is entered in the chart outlining the discussion of the procedure with the patient. In the general evaluation of the patient, associated conditions such as diabetes mellitus, hypertension, angina, blood dyscrasias, and previous allergic response to radiopaque contrast material should be assessed. In all patients, renal function must be determined prior to the procedure to ensure adequate contrast excretion—particularly in diabetic patients since renal failure may result from the injection of radiopaque contrast [128]. Adequate hydration prior to the procedure is important in order to prevent any untoward reaction from the renal excretion of the contrast material. If the patient is receiving anticoagulant therapy or has a bleeding tendency, the appropriate clotting studies should be performed and any deficiency corrected prior to angiography, to prevent postprocedure complications from hematomas or bleeding at the puncture site.

Premedication for the procedure usually comprises moderate analgesia with morphine or Demerol, and Vistaril or a barbiturate, in doses appropriate for the patient's age and weight. Rarely is general anesthesia required except in children. Injected radiopaque contrast material may cause transient nausea and vomiting. To prevent particle aspiration, all solid foods are restricted for 4 to 6 hours prior to the procedure. However, clear liquids are encouraged so the patient does not become dehydrated. In diabetics receiving insulin or oral hypoglycemic agents, the medication dosage is adjusted to take into account the reduced caloric intake. The appropriate anatomic region for arterial puncture, inguinal or axillary, is shaved and readied for catheterization.

PUNCTURE AND CATHETERIZATION

The arterial puncture site for catheterization is determined according to the clinically symptomatic area and the presence of an accessible pulse. Puncture of the femoral artery is preferred because of the artery's proximity to the aorta and lower extremities and its superficial location in the inguinal area. If both femoral artery pulses are palpable, the least symptomatic extremity is selected for catheterization. Thus one can avoid such potential postcatheterization problems as (1)

a hematoma at the puncture site that could interfere with a subsequent bypass graft or further compromise the circulation to a partially ischemic leg, or (2) the possibility that manual compression of the puncture site to prevent bleeding could induce further thrombosis of a partially compromised circulation.

When both femoral pulses are absent, the axillary artery, especially the left one, is a suitable site for percutaneous catheterization [15, 47]. An alternative is transbrachial catheterization, but catheterization in this location carries a higher risk of local complications. Direct needle puncture translumbar aortography is an alternative to percutaneous peripheral artery catheterization, and a variation of this technique uses a catheter [4, 103]. From personal experience I prefer the transaxillary to the translumbar approach when the femoral arteries are occluded. Direct needle puncture of the femoral artery with retrograde injection of contrast is another technique for demonstrating the lower extremity arteries. An 18-gauge needle can be inserted into the artery and attached to flexible tubing, which in turn is connected via a stopcock to the pressure injector. Instead of a needle, an 18-gauge Teflon sheath can be inserted into the femoral artery. Both femoral arteries can be used simultaneously if necessary, but often a forceful unilateral retrograde injection of 40 to 50 cc at 12 to 14 cc per second will cause enough contrast spillover at the aortic bifurcation to allow visualization of the opposite side. The major disadvantages of this technique are a lack of adequate contrast visualization of the abdominal aorta and the not infrequent need to catheterize both femoral arteries in order to study the circulation.

A previous endarterectomy of the iliac or femoral arteries is no contraindication to transfemoral catheterization. Most angiographers consider a pelvic prosthetic bypass graft a relative contraindication to transfemoral catheterization since it may lead to complications of thrombosis or local bleeding. When no other catheterization site is available, it may be necessary to puncture a graft. A 1976 report claims graft puncture to be a safe procedure [34], and another indicates how to avoid complications [81].

When catheterization is performed, sterile precautions are observed by the angiographer and his assistants. The previously shaved puncture site is cleansed with a suitable skin antiseptic solution (Betadine) and the area draped with sterile towels. The femoral artery is punctured below the inguinal ligament in order to avoid potential retroperitoneal or scrotal hematomas following the procedure. The femoral puncture site is approximately 1 to 2 cm below the inguinal skin crease, or below an imaginary line drawn between the anterior superior iliac spine and the pubic eminence. Local anesthesia at the puncture site is provided by the injection of 10 cc of 2 percent Xylocaine (lidocaine). It is important to infiltrate the femoral artery sheath on each side in order to minimize pain and avoid local arterial spasm.

A Seldinger-type needle is used to puncture the artery. The overlying skin is nicked with a scalpel blade to ease passage of the needle, and an attempt is made to skewer the artery by passing through both the anterior and posterior walls. The needle stylet is removed and the blunt cannula withdrawn until a strong, steady flow of blood spurts from the cannula. Frequently a slight popping sensation is felt as the blunt cannula is withdrawn, just before the steady backflow of blood is observed. The forceful spurt of blood indicates that the blunt cannula tip is free in the vessel lumen and well situated so that the guidewire can be inserted. Unless a strong spurt of blood is observed, no attempt should be made to pass the guidewire into the artery. It is very important that the guidewire move easily into the artery with a minimum of force; otherwise complications at the puncture site may occur. Passage of the guidewire through the pelvic arteries and aorta may be observed fluoroscopically, and the wire should be in the abdominal aorta before a catheter is introduced.

Guidewires are available in a variety of sizes, constructions, and coatings. The basic wire that has proved to be extremely effective in femoral arteriography is either a 0.035- or a 0.038-inch stainless wire with a fixed core, a 3-cm straight flexible tip, and a length of 145 cm. Some angiographers prefer J wires, or movable-core wires, but there seems to be no particular advantage to these wires in the routine situation.

A wide choice of catheters is commercially available for percutaneous transfemoral arteriography. Most angiographers base their selection on the principle of using a catheter with the smallest outer diameter that will deliver the desired amount of contrast without rupturing. The most popular catheters currently used for femoral arteriography are 6 or 7 French size and either polyethylene or Teflon in composition. There is a 1977 report [82] that a 5 French catheter may be equally effective and possibly

safer, since its smaller diameter causes less lumen obstruction. All these catheters are of the end-hole variety and may be either straight with side holes or pigtail-shaped with side holes. A tip occluder is usually used with the straight end-hole catheter [96]. The purpose of the tip occluder or pigtail shape is to ensure that the bulk of the injected contrast will exit via the catheter's side holes, rather than through the end hole. The contrast emerging from the side holes is more readily directed into the aortic branches. The usual length of the catheter used is 100 to 120 cm, since this is appropriate for the moving-tabletop technique of serial filming. After insertion of the catheter into the artery, it is regularly flushed during the procedure every 3 to 4 minutes with a heparinized saline solution to prevent clotting.

In elderly patients referred for examination, the iliac arteries are often tortuous and partially obstructed by arteriosclerotic lesions. It may, therefore, be impossible or extremely difficult to pass the guidewire retrograde through the iliac arteries into the abdominal aorta. In order to solve this problem a J guidewire [64] or J-shaped catheter [6] may be substituted for the straight guidewire in an attempt to traverse the sites of resistance. The J-shaped catheter offers the advantage of permitting the injection of a test dose of contrast material in the iliac artery and instant visualization of the extent and degree of obstruction fluoroscopically. This information allows the angiographer to decide whether, in the partially obstructed vessel, retrograde catheterization is possible from the particular femoral puncture site. When retrograde transfemoral catheterization is impossible, the examination is generally completed from the transaxillary approach.

The arteriography is concluded by withdrawing the catheter and applying digital pressure at the puncture site. Usually pressure applied for 5 to 15 minutes will be sufficient to prevent bleeding or hematoma formation at the puncture site. This is particularly important in hypertensive patients and in those who may have a coagulopathy. A pressure dressing is applied to the puncture site for 24 hours, and the patient is kept at bed rest for 3 to 4 hours following the procedure.

SERIAL FILMING EQUIPMENT

The femoral arteriogram, particularly in obstructive vascular disease, must demonstrate the anatomic integrity of the leg circulation from the aorta to the ankles. Over the years various pieces of angiographic equipment have been devised to demonstrate the physiologic circulation of injected contrast material as it flows from the aorta toward the ankles. To demonstrate the blood flow, various design configurations have been used in which either the patient, the x-ray tube, or the films are moved [129]. The shifts are made singly or in combination, in a sequential manner, as the injected contrast moves through the circulation. The earliest pieces of equipment all depended on manual power to supply movement. Film cassettes of varying size, x-ray tables of unique design, and tube stands of exceptional heights all have been proposed and given limited acceptance.

At present most angiographers use a system for femoral arteriography that employs an automatic serial film changer and a programmable moving tabletop with synchronized kilovoltage regulation [1]. The patient on the table moves over the film changer. The specific areas of interest—namely, the pelvis, thigh, knee, and runoff—are sequentially automatically filmed after a single injection of radiopaque contrast material.

EXAMINATION SEQUENCE, CONTRAST QUANTITY, INJECTION, AND FILM RATES

The diffuse nature of obstructive vascular disease makes it imperative that the abdominal aorta and its branches be examined as part of femoral arteriography. Thus potential inflow and the branch artery obstructions are certain to be visualized. When retrograde transfemoral catheterization is the method of approach, the catheter tip is positioned in the aorta at the T12–L1 interspace with the side holes opposite the renal arteries. Serial films are obtained in the anteroposterior and lateral positions, either simultaneously or successively. The lateral view often provides information not obvious in the anteroposterior view. Approximately 35 to 50 cc of methylglucamine diatrizoate 76 is injected at a flow rate of 20 to 25 cc per minute, in order to opacify the abdominal aorta. Films are obtained at a rate of two per second for 4 seconds, one per second for 3 seconds, and one every 2 seconds for 8 seconds. Variations from this basic filming rate are determined by a test injection of contrast into the aorta with fluoroscopic observation of its rate of clearance. If the contrast clearance is more rapid than normal, the filming rate is increased; conversely, if it is slower the rate is decreased.

For pelvic and lower extremity filming, the catheter is pulled down and positioned with the tip 4 cm above the aortic bifurcation, so that the side holes remain proximal to the bifurcation. The moving tabletop is programmed to stop serially and film the pelvic, thigh, knee, and runoff arteries. A single bolus of 60 to 70 cc of contrast, injected at a rate of 10 cc per second, is usually adequate to opacify the pelvic and leg arteries to the ankle. The contrast injection triggers the sequential filming and movement of the table. The film exposure rate is as follows: pelvis, one per second for 4 seconds; thigh, one per second for 3 seconds; knee, one per second for 4 seconds; and lower leg, one per second for 4 seconds. In some patients the pattern of their obstructive disease causes unequal circulation times between the two extremities. Then the standard filming sequence may fail to demonstrate adequately the anatomy of the two sides. In this event, the filming rate must be altered according to the observed flow and the nonvisualized circulation reexamined.

When transaxillary catheterization is required for femoral arteriography, the filming sequence is reversed. The pelvis and lower extremities are examined before the abdominal aorta. From this approach the catheter tip is positioned in the abdominal aorta at the L1–2 interspace, rather than the T12–L1 interspace, in order to maintain the side holes opposite the renal arteries. All the other technical factors of filming rate, table-movement program, contrast quantity, and injection rate are unchanged.

POSITIONING

The principle of filming vessels in more than one view is well established in obstructive disease of the cerebral, coronary, and visceral circulations but is less well observed in peripheral vascular disease. Views of vessels in different planes generally offer additional information about the contour and lumen. A lateral view of the infrarenal aorta, when an aneurysm or obstructive lesion (Fig. 77-9) is present, may demonstrate findings about the extent, location, and size of the lesion not available in the anteroposterior projection [35, 109, 120]. This is particularly important if bypass surgery is contemplated for a distal obstructive lesion. In that situation the severity of any inflow obstruction must be carefully assessed so that the blood flow is adequate to maintain graft patency.

Obstructive lesions in the pelvic arteries should also be viewed in more than one plane

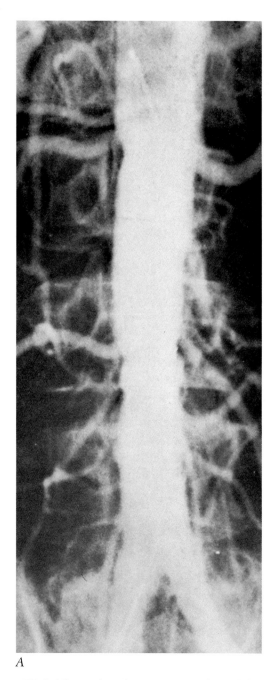

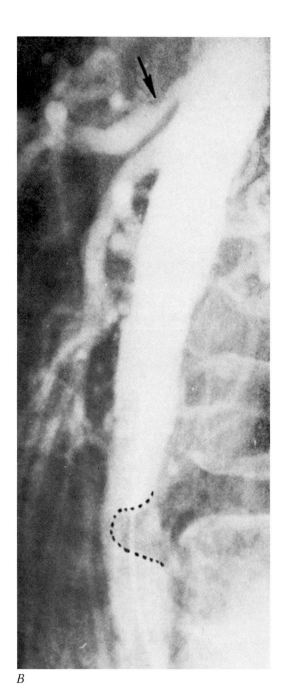

A

B

Figure 77-9. The patient has symptomatic peripheral vascular disease, a midline abdominal bruit, and diminished femoral artery pulses. (A) The anteroposterior view demonstrates only minimal arteriosclerotic changes of the abdominal aorta. (B) The lateral view reveals a large plaque extending into the lumen from the posterior wall (*dotted line*). This lesion causes inflow obstruction and was not appreciated in the anteroposterior view. There is also an associated celiac artery stenosis (*arrow*).

[108]. Unlike the aorta, in which the lateral view offers the best projection, the pelvic arteries are best studied in the oblique projection [87]. Initially a standard anteroposterior view of the pelvis should be obtained. If there is any suspicion of stenotic lesions in the iliac or common femoral arteries, the appropriate oblique view is filmed. It is not unusual that the anteroposterior view fails to separate the origins of the superficial and profunda femoris arteries at the bifurcation of the common femoral artery. An oblique view will separate the vessels and indicate the severity of any obstruction (Fig. 77-10). Similarly, the origin of the internal iliac artery may be inadequately

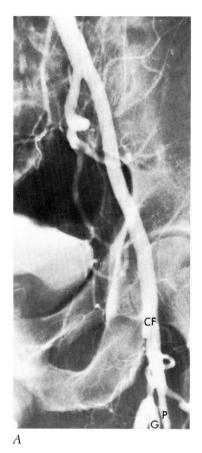
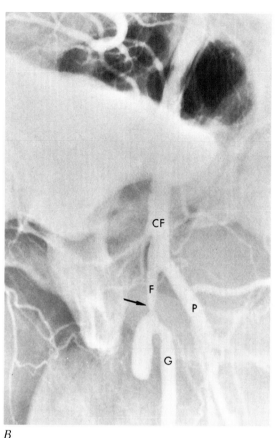

A   *B*

Figure 77-10. Left femoropopliteal bypass graft. (A) The anteroposterior view does not clearly demonstrate any abnormality at the bifurcation of the common femoral artery (*CF*) into the graft (*G*) and profunda femoris artery (*P*). (B) The right posterior oblique view distinctly separates the origin of the graft (*G*) and profunda femoris artery (*P*). There is a definite proximal stenosis (*arrow*) of the occluded superficial femoral artery (*F*).

visualized in the standard anteroposterior view and is better projected in the oblique (Fig. 77-11). Pelvic oblique views are valuable not only for the imaging of the native circulation but especially for evaluating bypass graft anastomoses (Figs. 77-12, 77-13). The particular oblique projection used depends on which vessel needs to be studied. The left posterior oblique position is best for assessing the right common femoral bifurcation (superficial and profunda femoris arteries) and the bifurcation of the left common iliac (internal and external iliac) arteries. The reverse oblique projection, the right posterior oblique, best demonstrates the bifurcations in the opposite vessels. Thus, the pelvic arteries are first studied in the anteroposterior projection, but if any doubt remains about an inadequately visualized focal obstruction or bifurcation, the appropriate oblique view is obtained.

In the evaluation of obstructive lesions of the femoral, popliteal, and runoff arteries, the anteroposterior view generally suffices. However, a recent report [24] indicates that it could be advantageous to obtain a simultaneous lateral view for better structural detail. A lateral view is very useful indeed in evaluating tumors and aneurysms in the thigh, knee, or calf area. At the ankle, the distal runoff arteries are best demonstrated when the feet are externally rotated, since this rotation separates the vessels and sometimes moves them away from the dense cortex.

PAIN CONSIDERATIONS

The injection of radiopaque contrast material during femoral arteriography is invariably painful for the patient. The perception of pain, of course, varies from patient to patient; some people find it excruciating whereas others merely complain of an annoyance. Nevertheless, the fact that the

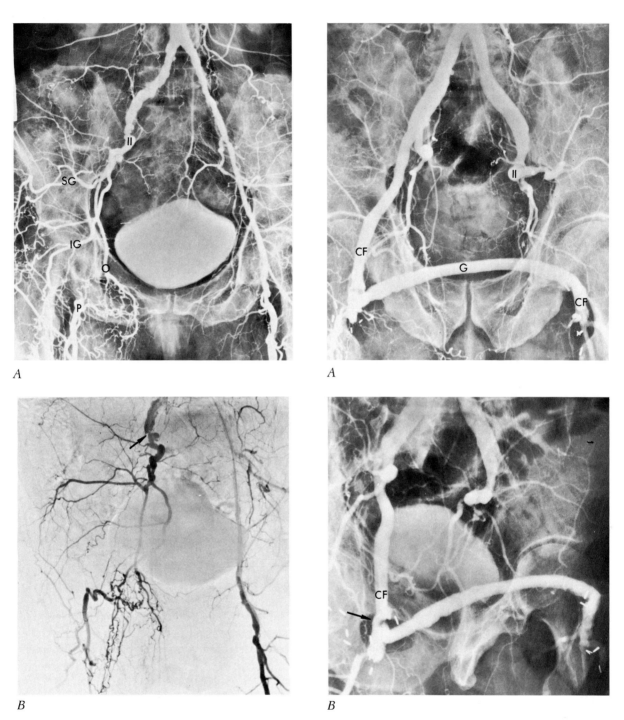

A

B

A

B

Figure 77-11. Occlusive right external iliac and common femoral disease and superficial femoral artery occlusion in the same patient as in Figure 77-4. Reconstitution of the profunda femoris artery *(P)* to provide circulation to the leg depends on the collateral branches of the internal iliac artery *(II)*. (A) The anteroposterior view shows arteriosclerotic changes at the origin of the internal iliac artery (see Fig. 77-2 for abbreviations). (B) The right posterior oblique view (subtraction) clearly shows the severe stenosis at the origin of the internal iliac artery *(arrow)*.

Figure 77-12. An extraanatomic femorofemoral bypass graft was created to provide a blood supply to an ischemic left leg. The ischemia was secondary to occlusion of the left external iliac artery and inadequate collaterals from the internal iliac artery *(II)*. (A) The anteroposterior view shows the patent graft *(G)* from the right to left common femoral artery *(CF)*. (B) The left posterior oblique view shows the severe stenosis *(arrow)* of the right common femoral artery *(CF)*. The stenosis was only questionable in the anteroposterior view.

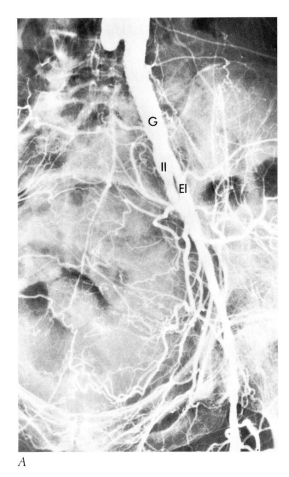

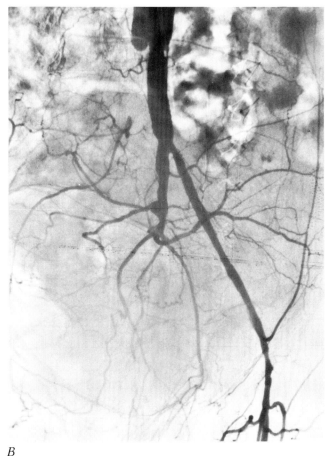

A   *B*

Figure 77-13. The right limb of an aortobiiliac bypass graft was occluded. A left-to-right femorofemoral bypass was contemplated to restore blood flow to the right leg. (A) Although the left graft limb (*G*) is patent, the bifurcation into the internal (*II*) and external (*EI*) arteries is overlapped and the vessel lumen size uncertain. (B) The right posterior oblique view (subtraction) shows the distal anastomosis and bifurcation to be normal.

majority of patients do experience a moderate to severe degree of pain has prompted a search for either an effective intraarterial anesthetic or a less painful contrast agent.

Several studies [1, 48, 50] have indicated that the intraarterial infusion of lidocaine is effective for diminishing the pain induced by the injection of radiopaque contrast material. The perception of decreased pain was reported both subjectively and objectively, in particular, apparently, when analgesic premedication was given in conjunction with the intraarterial lidocaine infusion. However, the effectiveness of lidocaine in relieving pain is not unchallenged. A 1978 report [33] indicates that lidocaine is totally ineffective as an intraarterial analgesic. According to this report, 22 patients were given no premedication but had lidocaine added to the injected contrast material. In 12 (55%) of these patients the pain was more

severe than when the contrast material alone was injected.

Research on contrast material indicates that hypertonicity appears to be important in inducing pain during intraarterial injection [79]. Conray in an isosmotic concentration has been shown to cause no pain when injected [33]. Similarly, the nonionic contrast material metrizamide is less painful during femoral arteriography than the ionic contrast agent Isopaque [3]. More investigation is required concerning both an effective, safe intraarterial analgesic and a nonionic contrast agent before any definite recommendations can be made for pain relief in femoral arteriography.

FLOW AUGMENTATION

In about 25 percent of all femoral arteriograms the popliteal and particularly the distal runoff ar-

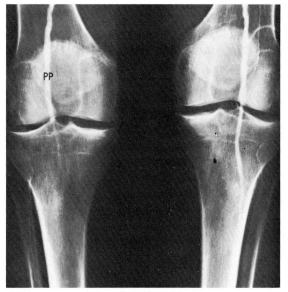

A

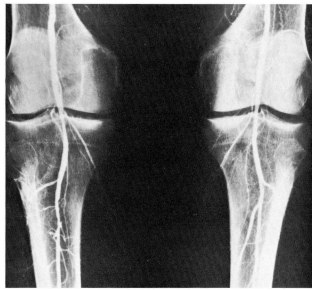

B

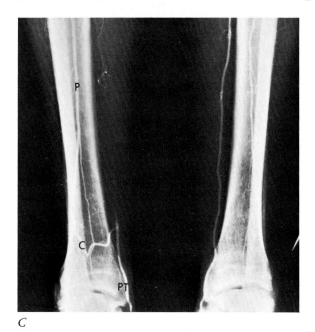

C

Figure 77-14. Combined lesion–occlusive peripheral vascular disease, involving the iliac and superficial femoral arteries, in the same patient as in Figure 77-2. (A) Initially the distal runoff arteries were not visualized; contrast demonstrated vessels only to the popliteal artery (*PP*) level at 11 seconds. (B) Following ischemic exercise the distal runoff vessels were seen at the knees and down to the ankles, at 7 seconds. The right posterior tibial artery is occluded. (C) The right posterior tibial artery (*PT*) reconstitutes at the ankle via a collateral (*C*) from the peroneal artery (*P*).

teries (tibial and peroneal) are inadequately visualized for anatomic delineation [65]. The poor contrast visualization results from delayed or diminished blood flow to the lower leg. The decreased circulation may have a variety of causes, such as diminished cardiac output, vasoconstriction, a previous aortic bypass graft, an abdominal aortic aneurysm, and ectatic calcified arteries. The presence of proximal obstruction in the aorta and iliac and superficial femoral arteries, and poor collateral circulation, merely compound the problem of diminished circulation.

The anatomic delineation of the distal runoff arteries is important to determine the extent of the obstructive disease and the potential feasibility of revascularization to the popliteal and, more distally, to the peroneal or tibial arteries. To circumvent the problem of poor or absent visualization of the runoff arteries, two techniques have been used effectively: reactive hyperemia [10, 127] and pharmacologic vasodilation [36, 63]. In both instances the blood flow to the popliteal artery and its branches is increased, augmenting the concentration of radiopaque contrast visualized in these vessels (Fig. 77-14). The pharmacologic drugs used for this purpose have been tolazoline hydrochloride (Priscoline) and bradykinin. In general, vasoactive drugs have proved less effective than reactive hyperemia for enhancing contrast visualization of the distal runoff arteries.

Reactive hyperemia is produced by ischemia alone or in conjunction with exercise. When ischemia is used, a blood pressure cuff is wrapped around the thigh and inflated to 150 mm Hg for 5 to 7 minutes. Exercise may be added to the ischemia by actively or passively flexing and extending the foot (approximately 80–100 times) while the blood pressure cuff is inflated around the thigh. The addition of exercise causes more profound ischemia and consequently more reactive hyperemia.

In either case, whether with exercise and ischemia or ischemia alone, the arteries are examined immediately after release of the blood pressure cuff. One leg or both simultaneously may be examined this way, depending on how adequately the distal runoff has been demonstrated previously. In a report of 55 patients [65] with obstructive peripheral vascular disease who were studied after reactive hyperemia, excellent contrast visualization of the tibial and peroneal arteries was achieved in 50 patients (91%). It is worth noting that reactive hyperemia is also useful for enhancing visualization of the iliac and femoral arteries when proximal vessel obstruction diminishes blood flow to these areas. Why leg muscle ischemia results in hyperemia is not clearly understood. Possible explanations for this phenomenon have included tissue anoxia, local carbon dioxide and lactic acid accumulation, the release of vasoactive polypeptides, and reduced venous pressure.

SPECIAL SITUATIONS

In specific instances because of the particular type of lesion being investigated, certain modifications in technique are necessary. Changes in the route of catheterization, the site of catheter placement, the amount and rate of contrast injected, and the filming rate may be necessary.

In patients with aortic thrombosis or previous aortobifemoral bifurcation grafts, the left axillary artery approach to the abdominal aorta is used [15, 47] rather than standard retrograde transfemoral catheterization. The patient with a peripheral artery aneurysm or an arteriovenous fistula will have an altered rate of blood flow at the site of interest. In this instance the catheter is introduced on the same side as the lesion, and a change in the amount, rate of contrast injection, and filming is required. Since the flow rate in an aneurysm is usually decreased, the injection and filming rates should be reduced. The reverse is true for an arteriovenous fistula. In both conditions, views in addition to the standard anteroposterior projection may be helpful in demonstrating the lesions.

When a peripheral bone or soft tissue tumor is suspected, the femoral artery of the symptomatic leg is catheterized to enhance the degree of contrast filling in any tumor vessels. The catheter tip is positioned in the external iliac artery rather than at the aortic bifurcation. Magnification views of the tumor are helpful and should be obtained in more than one projection.

Indications for Femoral Arteriography

The primary indications are vascular lesions and bone or soft tissue tumors of the lower extremities. The incidence of vascular lesions greatly exceeds that of tumors. The vascular lesions can be classified by etiology, namely, arteriosclerosis obliterans, emboli, aneurysms, thromboangiitis obliterans, arteriovenous fistula, arteriovenous malformation, trauma, graft, and spasm. Management of these lesions is chiefly surgical, either by endarterectomy, resection, or bypass graft. Preoperative arteriography is therefore required to define accurately the location and anatomic extent of the lesions [40, 52].

ARTERIOSCLEROSIS OBLITERANS

Arteriosclerotic obstructive lesions are by far the most common indications for aortofemoral arteriography. The etiology of these lesions is unknown, but hypercholesterolemia, dietary intake of saturated fatty acids, diabetes mellitus, heredity, obesity, cigarette smoking, and many other factors may exert an important influence. Arteriosclerotic lesions start as localized stenosing plaques affecting the intima or media that subsequently proceed to vessel occlusion [13]. These lesions in the lower extremities are most prevalent in the older patient, with a peak incidence in the 60s and 70s. It is not unusual to encounter symptomatic patients with arteriosclerosis in the 50s and occasionally even in the 40s, but below this age it is rare. The ratio of males to females studied for symptomatic arteriosclerotic peripheral vascular disease is approximately 4 to 1.

The symptoms and signs encountered reflect ischemia in the extremity as a result of arterial

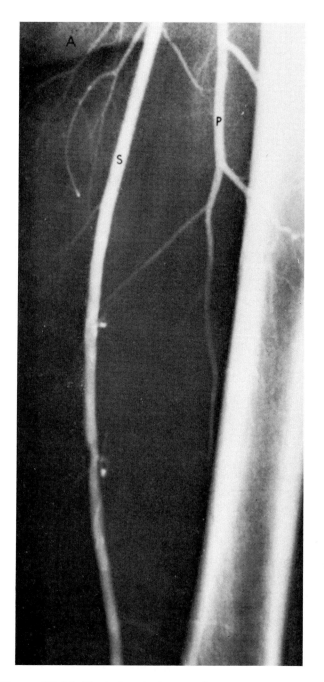
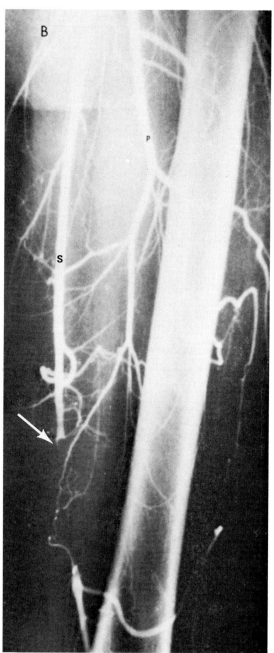

Figure 77-15. Typical early lesion of arteriosclerosis in the adductor canal region progressing from stenosis to occlusion. (A) Minimal segmental stenosis of the superficial femoral artery (S) at the tendinous hiatus in the adductor magnus muscle. (B) Progression to segmental occlusion (*arrow*) with reconstitution of the popliteal artery, mainly via profunda femoris artery (P) branches.

obstruction. The symptomatic patient is aware of progressive or acute intermittent claudication as the chief presenting complaint. This cramping pain occurs most often in the calf muscles and is induced by exercise (walking) and relieved by rest. The pain may also occur in the thigh and buttock, depending on the site of the vascular obstruction. Pain at rest or nocturnal cramps are evidence of more severe disease and indicate a poor prognosis and possible imminent gangrene. The strength of the peripheral pulses is the physical finding of most significance in this disease. The pulses must be palpated and both sides compared from the aorta to the feet. The

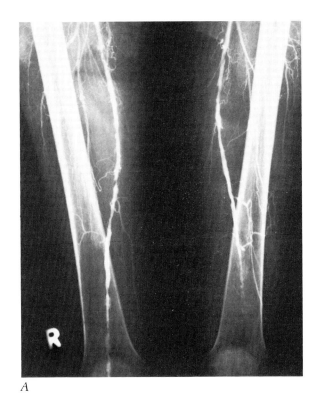

A

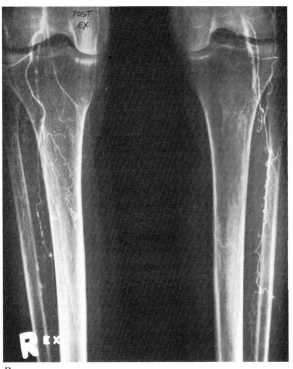

B

Figure 77-16. Adult onset of diabetes mellitus, with gangrenous toe changes in the left foot and associated occlusive arterial disease in the pelvis, thigh, and runoff vessels (same patient as in Fig. 77-3). (A) There are severe diffuse segmental stenoses in both superficial femoral arteries. The proximal left popliteal artery is not visualized. (B) The lack of any runoff arteries was seen only after ischemic exercise when vessel filling was maximal. The right and left popliteal arteries are occluded. There is minimal collateral artery filling, and none of the distal runoff arteries reconstitute because of the severity of the disease.

absence of a pulse usually indicates a proximal obstruction. In some cases, collateral circulation secondary to an occlusion may be adequate to induce a weak pulse. Audible bruits, a palpable thrill, hair loss, temperature and color changes, and the degree of venous filling are other important physical findings in evaluating the extent of vascular insufficiency.

The diffuse nature of the arteriosclerotic process leads ultimately to multiple sites of obstruction. However, arteriographic investigation has shown that most occlusive lesions are segmental [51]. One of the most common sites of disease initially is the adductor canal portion of the superficial femoral artery (Fig. 77-15). The continuous mechanical trauma to the vessel as it passes through the tendinous hiatus is generally credited with the early and frequent stenosis and occlusion at this site [51, 77]. In terms of decreasing frequency, obstruction occurs in the superficial femoral artery, the distal runoff vessels, and the popliteal artery. Various occlusive

patterns [51] encountered in the lower extremities have been described, but they have limited prognostic significance because there is such marked variability in the site and degree of disease.

The pattern of arteriosclerosis obliterans in the lower extremities is affected by diabetes mellitus. Especially in the runoff arteries, diabetic patients have a higher incidence of lesions and a more severe degree of obstruction than do nondiabetics [51]. Also, two-thirds of combined lesions of the femoral, popliteal, and runoff arteries occur in diabetic patients (Fig. 77-16). The profunda femoris artery likewise shows the effects of diabetes; this vessel is rarely obstructed, but if stenosis or occlusion occurs it is almost exclusively in diabetic patients.

In the evaluation of lower extremity occlusive vascular disease, the factor determining the suitability for revascularization is the condition of the inflow arteries (aorta and iliac vessels) and the distal runoff arteries (the terminal branches of the

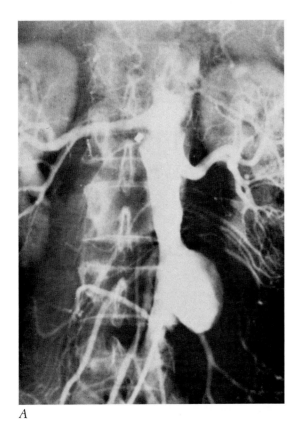

A

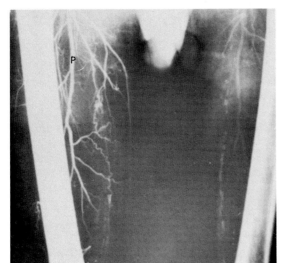

C

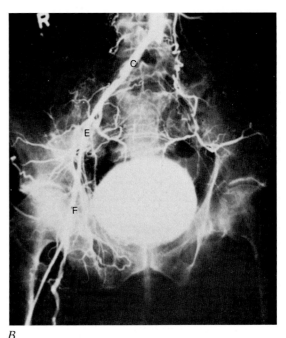

B

Figure 77-17. Severe symptoms of peripheral vascular insufficiency particularly marked in the left leg. There is combined inflow obstruction with iliac artery occlusive lesions and an unsuspected aortic aneurysm. (A) The saccular aortic aneurysm is seen opposite the third lumbar vertebra. (B) The left common iliac, external iliac, and left common femoral arteries are occluded. A few left internal iliac artery branches reconstitute from the iliolumbar collateral vessel. The right common (*C*) and external (*E*) iliac arteries are patent, along with the common femoral artery (*F*). (C) In the thigh, the right profunda femoris artery (*P*) is patent and fills rapidly. The corresponding vessel on the left is poorly visualized; it was reconstituted by only the few internal iliac artery branches. Note the bilateral occlusions of the superficial femoral arteries and the calcifications in the walls of these vessels.

popliteal below the knee). In my own series of 100 consecutive symptomatic patients with arteriographically demonstrated stenosis or occlusion of the superficial femoral, popliteal, or distal runoff arteries, 57 had associated common or external iliac artery obstruction. The iliac artery lesions encountered included a discrete stenosis or occlusion in 34 patients, diffuse arteriosclerosis in 21, and aneurysms in 10. In the same series, 62 patients had associated arteriosclerotic disease of the infrarenal abdominal aorta; of these, 32 had diffuse arteriosclerosis involving the entire aortic circumference, 18 had arteriosclerosis primarily involving the posterior wall, 9 had aneurysms, 4 had marked narrowing above the bifurcation, and 1 had a discrete aortic stenosis (Fig. 77-17). A reported series in the literature [52] confirms these observations. In that study of 321 extremities, 74 percent of the occlusions occurred as combined lesions whereas 26 percent were isolated or involved only a single leg artery. In 27 percent of the occlusions there was associated obstructive aortoiliac disease.

The incidence of associated aortic branch artery obstruction was analyzed in my series; 55 patients had stenosis or occlusion of one or more branch arteries. Obstructive lesions at the splanchnic artery origins (the celiac, superior, and inferior mesenteric) were determined in the 100 patients from the lateral aortogram film. The renal artery lesions were best seen in the anteroposterior view. Lesions of multiple visceral vessels occurred in 26 patients and bilateral renal artery involvement in 8. Blood pressure measurements consistent with hypertension were obtained in 44 patients.

The combination of aortic arteriosclerosis and iliac artery disease was noted to occur in 36 patients. This is less than the frequency of involvement of either area alone. The arteriosclerotic process does not necessarily affect all vessels simultaneously; thus, skipped areas of uninvolved vessels are common.

An interesting observation concerns the greater degree of involvement of the posterior aortic wall by arteriosclerosis compared with the anterior and lateral walls. Explanations for this finding may be that the lumbar artery origins fix the aorta at these sites, or perhaps that the intervertebral disks or osteophytic spurs impinge on the aortic lumen. Any such condition might cause disturbances in the laminar blood flow, which could damage the aortic wall and predispose that portion to arteriosclerosis. Occasionally lesions of the aorta are evident only in the lateral view because the obstructive process extends from the anterior or the posterior wall, without affecting the lateral walls in the supine position.

In 8 of 100 patients a unique appearance of the aorta was observed and referred to as the "hourglass" deformity. The indentations of the aorta roughly correspond to the level of the intervertebral disks. The blood flow through this portion of the aorta is markedly delayed, probably because of a loss of elasticity of the aortic wall.

There is also a form of arteriosclerosis that is ectatic rather than constricting. The precise nature of this change is uncertain except that the medial coat of the artery has lost its elastic lamina and the intima is less involved. The vessel may assume the appearance of a string of aneurysms, and the rate of blood flow through the artery is sharply reduced. This appearance is most often seen in the superficial femoral arteries but has also been observed in the common iliac and common femoral arteries.

REVASCULARIZATION

Surgical revascularization is an attempt to restore adequate blood flow to an ischemic extremity in order to relieve clinical symptoms or prevent subsequent gangrene and amputation [25, 121]. Revascularization employs two surgical techniques, endarterectomy and bypass grafting; the latter is the more common [8, 27]. Endarterectomy is usually limited to segmental occlusions of the aorta and the iliac arteries but may be extended to segmental occlusions of the superficial femoral and proximal popliteal arteries. When endarterectomy is used in the aorta, extreme care must be taken not to embolize atheromatous debris into the renal arteries [123]. Bypass grafts consist either of natural material such as autologous vein or of artificial woven Dacron or Gore-Tex. The natural vein grafts are preferable since their patency rate is higher than that of artificial grafts. Recently there has been renewed interest in percutaneous transluminal angioplasty as a nonsurgical technique for restoring blood flow in obstructed pelvic and extremity arteries [49, 137]. This technique, first described by Dotter [31] in 1964, received a technologic boost by the development of an effective balloon catheter. The technique is limited at present to segmental stenoses of the pelvic and leg arteries and to segmental occlusions of 5 cm or less in the superficial femoral or proximal popliteal arteries (Fig. 77-18). It has been estimated that these indications limit the applicability of the technique to approximately 25 to 30 percent of all patients with clinically symptomatic peripheral vascular disease.

Surgical revascularization of bilateral aortoiliac occlusions is best accomplished by introduction of an aortobifemoral Dacron graft, rather than by endarterectomy [58]. It has been shown that even for unilateral aortoiliac occlusive disease a bilateral bifurcation graft is preferable to a unilateral one. In a 1973 study of 5-year patency rates, only 52 percent of unilateral grafts remained patent whereas 78 percent of the bilateral bifurcation grafts were patent [75]. The main reasons for bypass graft failures are progression of the arteriosclerotic process distal to the graft, changes

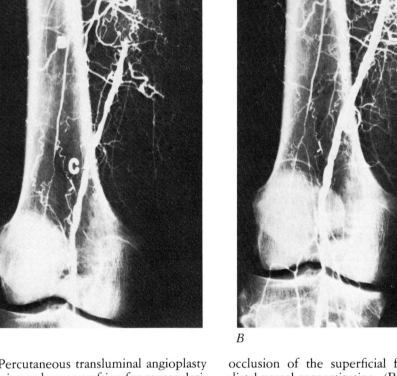

A

B

Figure 77-18. Percutaneous transluminal angioplasty offers an alternative to bypass grafting for revascularization in symptomatic vascular occlusive disease. (A) The prerecanalization study shows a 4-cm segmental occlusion of the superficial femoral artery (*F*) and distal vessel reconstitution. (B) After balloon dilation the postrecanalization study shows restoration of luminal continuity.

at the anastomosis (false aneurysm, stricture, or infection) (Fig. 77-19; see also Fig. 77-10), and problems with the graft itself (incorrect caliber and length or kinks) [18, 117]. The late failure rate of either unilateral or bilateral aortic bifurcation grafts ranges from 10 to 28 percent [92].

Extraanatomic grafts—namely, femorofemoral crossover (see Fig. 77-12) and axillofemoral bypasses—are used mainly when one limb of an aortic bifurcation graft is occluded [14, 22]. The crossover femorofemoral bypass graft was originally introduced for the poor-surgical-risk patient with unilateral iliac artery occlusion [126]. Because of its low operative risk, technical simplicity, and high graft patency rate, this procedure is favored when one limb of a bifurcation graft is occluded. A "steal phenomenon" may occur in the donor limb after a femorofemoral bypass if a significant stenosis is present in the proximal iliac artery of the donor limb [125].

In ischemic disease of the leg, the indications [101] for bypass grafting are (1) limb salvage as an alternative to amputation and (2) relief of severe claudication interfering with occupation or limiting activities in retirees. A femoropopliteal graft (Fig. 77-20) is the most popular for alleviating ischemic symptoms, but if necessary femorotibial or femoroperoneal bypass grafts can be performed as alternatives. The femoropopliteal graft carries a lower complication rate than the other types of distal grafts [102]. The choice of a femoropopliteal bypass graft depends on

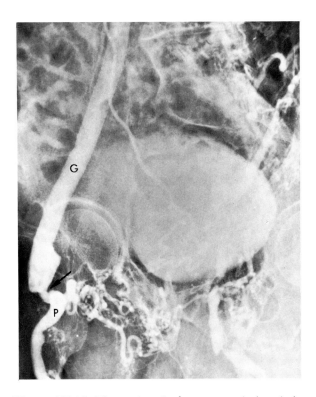

Figure 77-19. The patient had recurrent ischemic leg symptoms after an aortobifemoral graft (*G*). In the right posterior oblique view, a right distal anastomotic aneurysm and stenosis (*arrow*) at the origin of the profunda femoris artery (*P*) are evident. The right superficial femoral artery is occluded. The left limb of the bifurcation graft is occluded.

patency of the popliteal artery and one distal branch, preferably a tibial artery [101].

The alternative distal grafts (femorotibial and femoroperoneal) are mainly limb salvage procedures performed in order to avoid amputation. Both these grafts have higher rates of complications than a femoropopliteal graft [53]. Resorting to one of the more distal grafts is warranted only when the popliteal artery is occluded and a patent tibial or peroneal artery is demonstrated angiographically (Fig. 77-21). Diabetes mellitus influences the severity of obstructive disease in the distal runoff arteries. The incidence of distal runoff artery occlusion, tibial and peroneal, is higher in diabetic patients than in those with only uncomplicated arteriosclerosis. The weight of evidence [53, 102] indicates that bypass grafts to the small-caliber runoff arteries preserve limb function and offer an alternative to amputation. Thus it is imperative that angiography clearly de-

lineate the anatomic features of the distal runoff arteries down to the ankles.

EMBOLI

Embolic obstruction, like thrombosis, may produce partial or complete arterial occlusion. Emboli are a common cause of acute arterial occlusion, and the diagnosis is usually inferred from the clinical history [26, 131]. Atrial fibrillation, recurrent cardiac arrhythmias, myocardial infarction with mural thrombus, and bacterial endocarditis are the most common systemic conditions that predispose to peripheral arterial emboli. There is reason to believe that the incidence of embolic occlusion may be increasing as a result of improved cardiac care, an aging population, and more extensive use of prosthetic heart valves. Aortic aneurysms and atheromatous plaques may also cause embolization if a clot or plaque fragment breaks off and lodges distally. Ulcerated atheromatous plaques, moreover, may shower cholesterol emboli into the small arteries of the leg, causing occlusion [21]. Emboli may obstruct a normal vessel but more frequently obstruct an already compromised arteriosclerotic artery. Newer techniques for managing emboli have increased the limb-salvage rate and decreased the need for amputation. The mortality from arterial emboli remains high because of the seriousness of the predisposing cardiac disease that is nearly always present [122].

The leg arteries, and specifically the superficial femoral artery, are the vessels most often occluded by emboli. In a series [122] of 203 embolectomies, 75 percent of the emboli lodged in the lower extremities, with 42 percent of these in the femoral artery. Additional vessels embolically occluded were as follows: iliac, 19 percent; popliteal, 14 percent; posterior tibial, 1 percent; and anterior tibial, 0.5 percent. The source of emboli in this series was mainly cardiac (78%); cardiovascular surgery accounted for 7 percent, and in 10 percent no etiology was established.

The success of therapy for acute embolic occlusion depends on the rapid recognition of the clinical problem and location of the obstruction. Arteriography is the most effective diagnostic procedure for confirming the clinical diagnosis, the extent of the occlusion, the degree of collateral circulation, and the condition of the distal circulation. The arteriographic appearance of embolic occlusion is fairly typical; a proximal

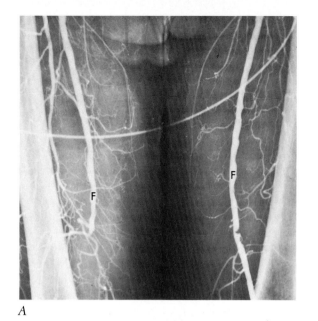

A

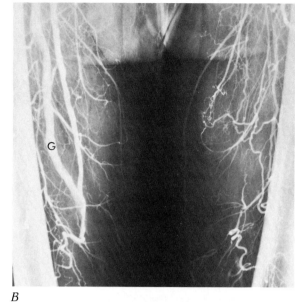

B

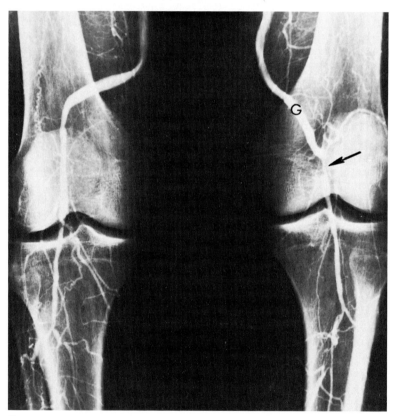

C

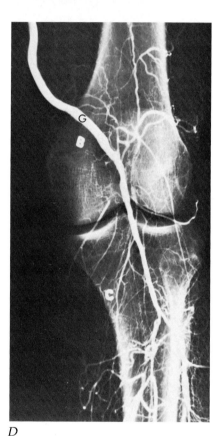

D

Figure 77-20. Typical problems of progressive arteriosclerotic peripheral ischemic disease and the complications of revascularization. (A) In September, 1978, the patient was studied for right calf claudication. There was segmental occlusion of the right distal superficial femoral artery (F). The left distal superficial femoral artery (F) had a severe segmental stenosis. (B) In March, 1979, the patient was reexamined for left calf claudication. A right femoropopliteal bypass (vein) graft (G) was patent. The left superficial femoral artery was totally occluded. (C) In January, 1980, there were recurrent ischemic symptoms in the left leg. A left femoropopliteal bypass (Gore-Tex) was patent but stenosed (*arrow*) at the distal anastomosis. The stenosis was probably secondary to fibrosis. The right femoropopliteal graft was patent. (D) The left graft (G) anastomotic stenosis was transluminally dilated with a balloon catheter. The lumen was restored to normal caliber, but by the following day the entire left femoropopliteal graft was thrombosed. A leg amputation was ultimately required.

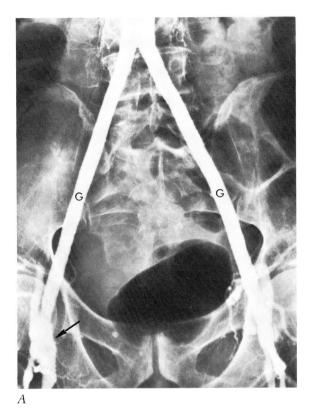
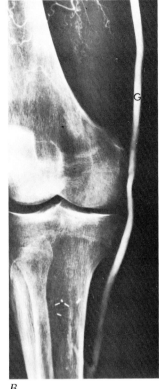
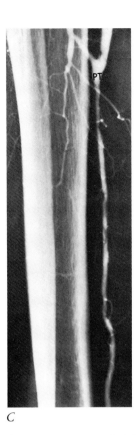

A *B* *C*

Figure 77-21. Multiple grafts may be required to restore adequate circulation in diffuse obstructive peripheral vascular disease. (A) An aortobifemoral bypass graft (*G*) was required because of bilateral common iliac artery occlusions. A right distal anastomotic aneurysm is evident (*arrow*). (B) In addition the patient had occlusion of the right superficial femoral and popliteal arteries. A femoroposterior tibial bypass graft (*G*) was created. (C) The posterior tibial artery (*PT*) was the only patent distal runoff artery. The arterial lumen was diffusely irregular because of arteriosclerotic changes.

curved margin reflects the nonopaque embolus protruding into the contrast-filled lumen (Fig. 77-22). In acute occlusion there is usually little, if any, collateral circulation evident, but this circumstance depends on the time interval between the occlusion and the arteriographic study.

Embolectomy, the treatment for embolic occlusion, should be performed as soon as possible after the diagnosis is established [76, 111]. The limb-amputation rate is proportional to the time delay between acute occlusion and embolectomy. In two 1970s reports [39, 122], when embolectomy was performed within 24 hours, the amputation rate ranged from 0.1 to 4.4 percent, whereas after 24 hours the amputation rate ranged from 4.3 to 19.4 percent. It has been suggested that the longer the delay before embolectomy, the greater are the chances of thrombosis distal to the primary site of acute occlusion [80]. Embolectomy is now generally performed by the Fogarty technique using a balloon catheter

[38]. The procedure can be performed under local anesthesia in the poor-surgical-risk patient and is both technically simple and effective. Following embolectomy in patients who survive, the limb-salvage rate has been reported as high as 93 and 95 percent in two series of 163 and 300 patients, respectively [39, 122].

ANEURYSMS

Primary aneurysms of the lower extremity arteries are generally caused by arteriosclerosis obliterans [2]. Secondary or acquired aneurysms may be caused by trauma, a bypass graft, mycotic infection, or a kinked vessel. Arteriosclerotic aneurysms in the lower extremity primarily involve the popliteal artery; the superficial femoral and the distal runoff arteries are rarely involved with primary aneurysms, but acquired aneurysms are not infrequent in these vessels.

A primary popliteal artery aneurysm presents

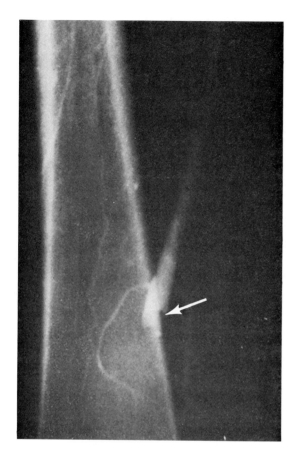

Figure 77-22. Atrial fibrillation and acute insufficiency due to an embolus in the right leg of a 62-year-old man. Note the smooth, curved, concave edge at the point of occlusion (*arrow*) and the minimal distal collateral circulation.

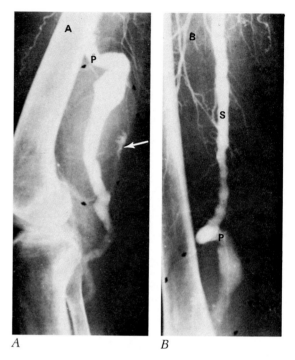

A   *B*

Figure 77-23. (A) Lateral view of a popliteal artery (*P*) aneurysm with amorphous (*arrow*) and rimlike (*arrowheads*) calcification. Note displacement of the surrounding vessels and lack of contrast filling of the aneurysm. (B) The aneurysm in the anteroposterior view demonstrates the ectatic superficial femoral artery (*S*) and the extremely slow blood flow through the area.

clinically as a palpable mass behind the knee that usually does not pulsate because the lumen is clot-filled [42, 135]. The presence of pain depends on how rapidly the aneurysm expands or on the occurrence of wall dissection. In my experience most such lesions have been calcified, and both rimlike and amorphous patterns have been observed (Fig. 77-23). Slightly less than half the aneurysms encountered in my studies occurred bilaterally, although one side was usually more prominent than the other. The aneurysms studied were all saccular in type and usually filled with clot; thus little or no contrast entered the lumen (Fig. 77-24). It is important to assess the arterial patency distal to the aneurysm. The size of the aneurysm was best appreciated from the rim calcification, if present, or by displacement of the surrounding arteries. Venous displacement with clinical symptoms of thrombophlebitis has

been reported secondary to popliteal artery aneurysms [110]. In nearly every case of popliteal aneurysm in my series the superficial femoral artery proximal to the aneurysm was ectatic, and numerous small aneurysmal dilations were noted (see Fig. 77-23). The blood flow was slow through the ectatic superficial femoral artery and further delayed through the aneurysm. Thus, more contrast and a slower film rate than normal were needed to demonstrate these lesions. A lateral view of the aneurysm was usually obtained and often provided more information about the lesion than the standard anteroposterior view. In three patients with bilateral popliteal aneurysms, multiple aneurysms were noted involving the common femoral or iliac arteries or the aorta.

Superficial femoral artery aneurysms were rarely encountered. These lesions when seen were either saccular or fusiform, clot-filled, and usually unilateral. In contrast to the popliteal and superficial femoral artery aneurysms, the common femoral artery aneurysms in my studies

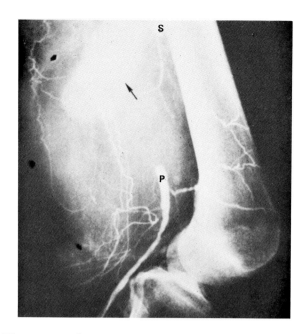

Figure 77-24. A popliteal artery aneurysm with segmental occlusion of the distal superficial femoral (*S*) and popliteal (*P*) arteries. The saccular aneurysm (*arrowheads*) is much larger, although mostly clot filled, than the small fraction that contains contrast material (*arrow*).

were usually fusiform. Anastomotic aneurysms at the common femoral artery, secondary to a prosthetic graft, were usually saccular. The majority of common iliac artery aneurysms were extensions of fusiform infrarenal abdominal aortic aneurysms, but a few discrete saccular lesions occurred. The external iliac artery is rarely the site of a primary aneurysm.

Traumatic aneurysms (see Fig. 77-26) are usually false aneurysms or pulsating hematomas and are the result of arterial laceration. This is usually secondary to accidental penetrating injury, but occasionally iatrogenic laceration due to surgery causes an aneurysm. Traumatic aneurysms may be associated with a traumatic arteriovenous fistula.

THROMBOANGIITIS OBLITERANS

Buerger's disease or thromboangiitis obliterans [16] is a form of progressive arterial occlusive disease that characteristically occurs in young males. Symptoms are usually confined to the feet or lower legs. Pain at rest, mostly a burning sensation, is the main clinical feature. This is in contrast to exercise-induced intermittent claudica-

tion noted in arteriosclerosis obliterans. The rest pain is most often excessive when compared to the visible features of ischemia, and this element, too, is characteristic. Other findings are an association with smoking, involvement of the upper extremities, and recurrent thrombophlebitis. Intimal thickening with an inflammatory cell response and preservation of the media are associated with Buerger's disease [88].

Not all pathologists consider this pathologic lesion unique. Investigators have questioned the existence of thromboangiitis obliterans as a distinct disease entity [130]. In the literature, reports of specific arteriographic findings associated with this entity by some authors are denied by others [115]. I have been unable personally to verify any specific arteriographic findings to confirm the clinically suspected diagnosis of Buerger's disease. In my patients there was occlusion of one or more distal runoff arteries with collateral circulation. The angiographic findings were indistinguishable from those observed with occlusion due to arteriosclerosis obliterans. Perhaps the only significant arteriographic feature in these patients was little or no evidence of any arteriosclerotic changes in the larger, more proximal arteries. However, considering that the patients were mainly young adults, this was not unexpected.

ARTERIOVENOUS FISTULA

An arteriovenous fistula is an abnormal "short circuit" between an adjacent artery and a vein that is either acquired or congenital in origin. Clinicians have long been fascinated by the lesion because of its pathophysiologic features. In the next section of this chapter the congenital variety of arteriovenous malformations is considered.

The acquired fistulas almost always involve penetrating trauma from gunshot, stab wounds, shrapnel particles, or fracture fragments. Gunshot and stab wounds account for about 50 percent of the lesions in most civilian reports [32, 57]. Less common causes are steel or glass splinters, iatrogenic injury in pelvic surgery [46] or intervertebral disk surgery, balloon thrombectomy [45], and percutaneous arterial catheterization [118]. An essential element for the development of a fistula is that the vascular injury occur at a site where the artery and vein are in close proximity [23]. Most acquired fistulas occur in the extremities, since adjacent arteries and veins are relatively close to the surface. The lower extremities are more frequently involved in both civilian and war injury–acquired fistulas, and the femoral artery is the single vessel most often affected [56, 57]. At the fistula site there may be a localized, pulsatile soft tissue mass, but a palpable thrill, an audible bruit, and venous dilation indicate the diagnosis. In chronic fistulas, severe limb edema and pain may be evident.

The local features and systemic hemodynamic consequences of arteriovenous fistulas have been investigated in elegant work by Holman [59–61]. The pathophysiology of fistulas results from the excessive shunting of blood from the arterial to the venous circulation. There is marked increase in venous return to the heart, with consequent increased cardiac output, rapid pulse rate, and widened pulse pressure. The development of these systemic manifestations depends on the size of the fistulous communication. In turn, the size of the fistula depends on the size of the artery involved and the length of time the fistula has been present. Thus, a small fistula will probably not be hemodynamically significant while a large fistula may result in congestive heart failure. The permanent or transient closure of an arteriovenous fistula causes an immediate, dramatic bradycardia. This is called Branham's sign [11] and is diagnostically useful, since temporary digital compression of the fistula elicits bradycardia. The therapy for acquired arteriovenous fistulas is surgical closure in order to reverse the deleterious hemodynamic changes.

While nuclear studies [54] and ultrasound [113] have shown promise in the evaluation of arteriovenous fistulas, arteriography is essential if surgical intervention is contemplated. The information obtained by this technique will demonstrate (1) the size and number of feeding arteries, (2) the collateral circulation, (3) the venous circulation distal to the fistula, (4) a possible aneurysm, and (5) the arterial circulation distal to the fistula. In general, acquired fistulas (Fig. 77-25) have a single feeding arterial branch that is markedly dilated. However, in multiple fragment injuries, several arterial feeders may be present. The multiple channels may be revealed only after one or more have been ligated in an attempt to ablate the fistula. The venous channels distal to the fistula become dilated because of the increased blood flow and direct exposure to arterial pressure. As competence of the venous valves becomes impaired on account of the increased blood flow, retrograde venous flow may occur. A false aneurysm may form as a result of the initial

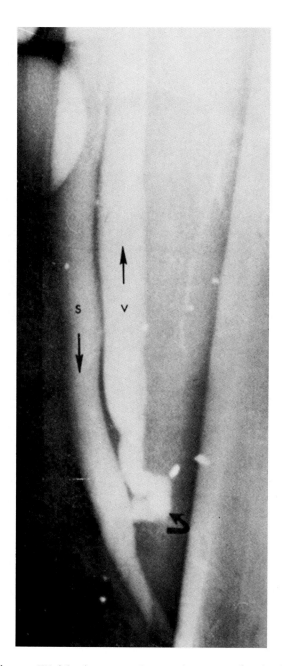

Figure 77-25. A traumatic arteriovenous fistula developed many years after the original injury by shrapnel fragments. Observe the immediate contrast filling of the dilated vein (*V*) through the shunt (*curved arrow*) from the dilated superficial femoral artery (*S*). Note that the artery returns to normal caliber distal to the shunt.

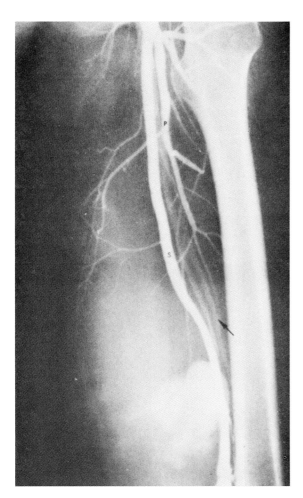

Figure 77-26. An acute traumatic arteriovenous fistula and false aneurysm caused by a stab wound. There is immediate venous filling (*arrow*) from the superficial femoral artery (*S*). Note that both the superficial femoral and profunda femoris (*P*) arteries are normal in caliber. There is contrast extravasation into the thigh in a false aneurysm with displacement and narrowing of the superficial femoral artery.

arterial injury if there is extravasation of blood (Fig. 77-26).

The arteriographic technique employed with fistulas must be altered to compensate for the rapid blood flow. Thus, approximately 1.5 times the usual amount of contrast is injected as close to the fistulous site as possible, and the filming rate is increased so that two to three films per second are obtained for 4 to 5 seconds.

ARTERIOVENOUS MALFORMATION

Although congenital fistulas, like the acquired kind, may occur in any organ, the majority are

located in the extremities [124]. Congenital arteriovenous fistulas have been described by a confusing variety of names (*hemangioma simplex, angioma cavernosum, port-wine mark, cirsoid aneurysm, congenital arteriovenous aneurysm,* and *racemose aneurysm*). Descriptive as these terms are, the underlying and unifying pathologic defect in this entity is the anomalous development of the primitive vascular system. During early embryologic development future arteries and veins are poorly differentiated and normally communicate with each other. The potential for persistence of the communications exists, and at a more mature stage this persistence is abnormal. Hence this probably accounts for the clinical varieties of congenital fistulas designated as cirsoid aneurysms, arteriovenous malformations, or cavernous hemangiomas.

To understand the clinical and arteriographic manifestations of these congenital lesions, a few simple facts of development must be kept in mind. Wollard [134], in his study of the embryology of the vascular system of the limb, discovered three stages of development: the stage of undifferentiated capillary network, the retiform stage (consisting of large plexiform vessels communicating between a central artery and a cardinal vein), and the stage at which mature vascular stems appear after the primitive elements disappear. Arrested development or maldevelopment at any of these stages probably accounts for the various forms of such lesions.

Szilagyi et al. [116] suggest a classification of these lesions based on a correlation of their clinical and angiographic changes with the stages of embryologic development. Thus, a simple cavernous hemangioma (Fig. 77-27) represents arrested development at the capillary network stage. The microfistulous and macrofistulous arteriovenous aneurysms are due to arrest at the retiform stage. Anomalous mature vascular channels result from maldevelopment at the stage of gross differentiation.

The terms *microfistula* and *macrofistula* designate whether the abnormal arteriovenous communication can be demonstrated by arteriography; only the macrofistulas are detectable by this technique. In any single patient a combination of hemangiomatous, microfistulous, and macrofistulous communications may be present because the different stages of embryologic development overlap.

Arteriography is very helpful for evaluation of these lesions even though the clinical diagnosis

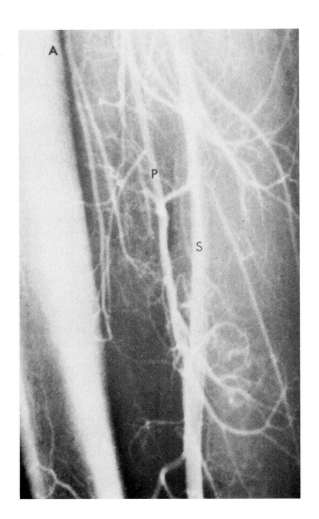

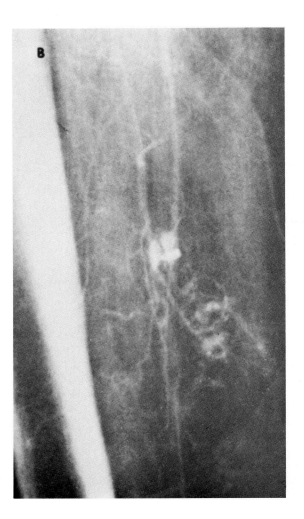

Figure 77-27. A congenital arteriovenous malformation of the capillary type with a biopsy diagnosis of cavernous hemangioma. (A) The lesion in the thigh receives its blood supply from the profunda femoris (P) and superficial femoral (S) arteries. Both vessels are normal in caliber. (B) Localized dilated contrast-filled spaces are observed late in the arterial phase, and no premature venous filling occurs.

may be quite obvious. Physical findings of a soft tissue swelling, with or without pigmentation, limb enlargement, prominent venous swelling, bruit, tenderness, and spontaneous bleeding, are all characteristic. Unlike acquired arteriovenous fistulas, the congenital variety seldom cause systemic hemodynamic changes. Arteriography is important to (1) define the site and extent of the arterial supply, (2) assess the feasibility of surgical extirpation, and (3) help establish the adequacy of surgical resection. The common arteriographic feature in all these lesions is venous filling that is earlier than normal. The arterial vessels are not always dilated, but the veins usually are distended and complex. The lesions may be appreciated best in the venous or capillary phase of the injection (Fig. 77-28).

The therapy for congenital fistulas mainly has been surgical [43], but permanent success resulting in a preserved, functioning extremity has been very limited. The lack of success stems from the multiple-source blood supply to the lesions. In the management of patients, there usually have been repeated attempts to eradicate the lesion by successive ligation of the feeding arteries. This finally results in the alternative of limb amputation or recurrence of the lesion.

Attempts to find suitable therapeutic alternatives to surgery for congenital fistulas have been mainly experimental, utilizing transcatheter arterial embolization [136] and electrocoagulation [44]. In one clinical report [112] of transcatheter embolization, Gelfoam was successfully used to occlude two arteriovenous fistulas, one acquired

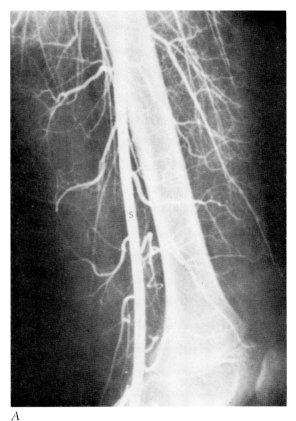

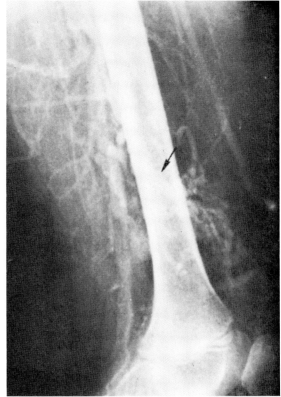

A

B

Figure 77-28. A congenital arteriovenous malformation of the venous type with a previous attempted excisional biopsy. (A) The superficial femoral artery (*S*) is not dilated, but its branches are more numerous than normal. Profunda femoris artery branches also supply the lesion. (B) In the venous phase the venous character of the lesion is evident from the numerous dilated, tortuous vessels observed (*arrow*).

and the other congenital. I have attempted occlusion of a congenital fistula in the thigh of a child by means of a tissue adhesive (cyanoacrylate). This lesion had recurred after previous surgical ligation. The embolization was successful initially, but the lesion recurred at a more distal site in approximately 2 years.

TRAUMA

Traumatic arterial injury of the pelvis and lower extremities, unless promptly recognized, can cause severe hemorrhage or ischemia and thus carries a high risk of death or loss of limb [17]. In the civilian population pelvic fracture is the major form of trauma responsible for massive extraperitoneal hemorrhage. It is generally impossible to distinguish clinically whether the source of bleeding is arterial or venous [90], but the former is less responsive to fluid replacement. Inability to identify the bleeding source [12, 97] causes the threat of fatal hemorrhage after pelvic

trauma. Surgical exploration has been the traditional technique used in attempts to establish the bleeding site, but it is usually unsuccessful in the presence of massive hemorrhage [98]. If the tamponading effect of hemorrhage is disturbed by surgical exploration, fatal hemorrhage and intraperitoneal rupture may be reactivated [83]. Even when successful, surgical exploration may result in sepsis. Surgical ligation of the internal iliac artery, whether or not the bleeding site is identified, has been the accepted way to manage massive pelvic hemorrhage [12, 55] despite these shortcomings. Blind ligation, without an established definite site of bleeding, is essentially a last-chance form of therapy. Its success has been variable [91, 100] because the proximal ligation leaves numerous pelvic arterial collaterals free to rebleed.

Arteriography offers an alternative to surgery for both the diagnosis and management of massive pelvic hemorrhage [83, 104]. The arteriogram can reveal the site of contrast extravasation

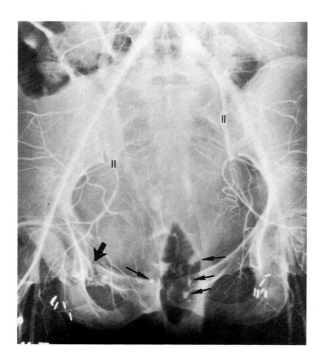

Figure 77-29. Massive hemorrhage resulting from acute traumatic injury to the pelvis. The arteriogram demonstrated contrast extravasation (*arrows*) originating from several internal iliac artery (*II*) branches, bilaterally. Note the fractured right superior pubic ramus (*thick arrow*) and the mass effect of the hemorrhage causing cephalad bowel displacement.

and thus help to identify the individual vessels that are bleeding (Fig. 77-29). Further, by studying the contralateral internal iliac artery, one can identify the potential collaterals. With this information, the bleeding may be managed by surgical ligation of the appropriate arteries, by percutaneous transcatheter embolization [83], or by balloon catheter tamponade [104]. Thus, arteriography should be used early in the evaluation of traumatic pelvic hemorrhage to diminish the mortality and morbidity of prolonged and massive hemorrhage.

Arterial injury, such as laceration or contusion of the lower extremity vessels, is common especially following penetrating or blunt injuries secondary to bullets (Fig. 77-30), stab wounds, or fractures. Before the Korean War, the usual treatment for severe arterial injury in an extremity was vessel ligation and limb amputation [28]. The intent was to preserve life even if the extremity had to be sacrificed. Experience with arterial reconstruction during the Korean War, subsequently confirmed by civilian experience, has established this procedure as the treatment of choice for traumatic arterial injury.

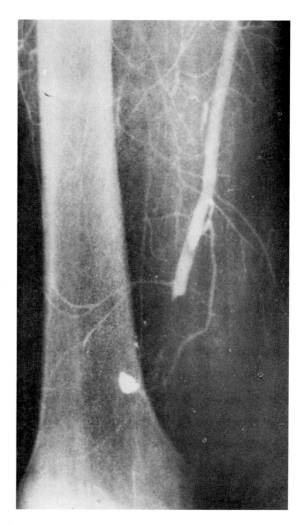

Figure 77-30. Acute traumatic injury with occlusion of the distal superficial femoral artery due to a bullet fragment. Note the lack of contrast extravasation, probably because of vessel spasm. Note also the early collateral vessel formation.

Arteries near the surface, fixed in position or adjacent to bone, in general are the ones most readily injured by the common mechanisms of trauma, namely, penetrating or blunt injury [68]. The distal superficial femoral artery is often the site of injury after fracture of the femur because of the vessel's proximity to the bone and its relatively fixed position in the adductor canal. Signs of arterial injury may not be evident at first, but ischemic symptoms may develop after the acute injury (Fig. 77-31). Another frequently damaged vessel is the popliteal artery, behind the knee. Because the muscles of this region hold the artery fixed in position, a posterior dislocation of the knee may injure the vessel. The anterior tibial artery, similarly, is easily injured as it passes

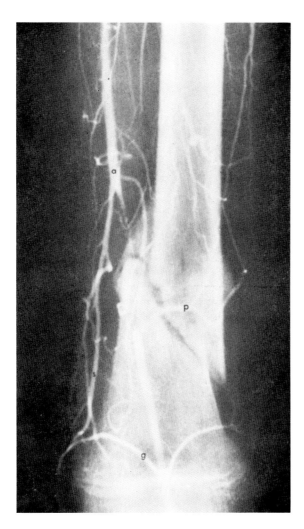

Figure 77-31. A late posttrauma arteriogram to evaluate the extent of arterial injury. The fractured femur has caused segmental occlusion of the superficial femoral artery (*a*). The collateral circulation is composed of the profunda femoris (*p*), the saphenous branch (*s*), and the medial superior genicular (*g*) arteries.

through the interosseous membrane when the proximal tibia is fractured. The close approximation of the anterior tibial artery and bone in the distal portion of the leg makes this another site where the artery is readily injured.

Traumatic injury of the popliteal artery, while clinically similar to injury of the superficial femoral artery, differs from the latter in its response to surgical repair. Surgical repair of the injured popliteal artery more frequently results in amputation than repair of the superficial femoral artery [66]. Furthermore, penetrating injury to the popliteal artery has a better limb-salvage rate than does blunt injury.

The clinical diagnosis of arterial injury in the lower extremities depends on recognizing the signs of acute ischemia distal to the traumatized site. The signs and symptoms are pain, blanched skin, coldness to touch, loss of cutaneous sensation, absent motor function, and absent or faint arterial pulses. These findings usually are sufficient to give a strong suggestion of the diagnosis. An arteriogram may be necessary to confirm and to pinpoint the lesion prior to surgical repair, providing definitive therapy is not unduly delayed. Since arterial spasm can mimic the clinical and arteriographic findings of severe arterial trauma, the diagnosis must be established by surgical exploration [95].

The mechanism of arterial injury in the extremity vessels, regardless of cause, is postulated to involve either (1) overstretching, without transection, or (2) transection. An experimental trauma study [9] has indicated that the intima ruptures before either the medial or the adventitial layer. Arterial contusion may occur without transection and form an intramural hematoma, or the intima may dissect and form a flap. Transection of the wall generally results from penetrating injury by either a fractured bone fragment or an external object.

All the potential mechanisms of arterial injury cause partial or complete vessel obstruction, and this threatens viability of the extremity. The *ischemic time* refers to the time elapsed before definitive repair of the arterial injury is attempted. It is a well-recognized fact that the longer the ischemic time, the greater the likelihood that arterial reconstruction will fail, necessitating amputation [89]. Chances of developing muscle contracture or atrophy are similarly increased. Ischemic times or delay before arterial reconstruction of more than 6 to 12 hours has been said to be critical [28, 67, 89]. However, the length of the ischemic time may be relative since additional factors such as the degree of associated soft tissue damage and the development of collateral circulation can influence the result. The techniques of surgical reconstruction for arterial injury include primary end-to-end anastomosis, patch grafts, and bypass grafts.

SPASM

Arterial spasm unrelated to severe arterial injury is a well-recognized entity in arteriography that may occur during or after the procedure [132]. It may be a response to the arterial trauma of catheterization, irritation of the vessel wall by the

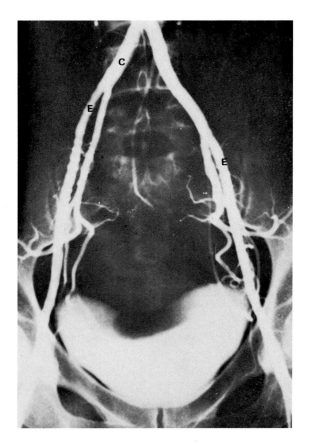

Figure 77-32. The typical appearance of standing waves in both external iliac arteries (E). The beaded pattern is more pronounced on the right. The common (C) and internal iliac arteries are normal.

radiopaque contrast material, or a combination of both. Spasm is most often encountered in small-diameter vessels with a prominent muscle coat. Children and young adults are more prone to develop arterial spasm than older individuals, for the latter may have fibrosis of the medial coat [78]. This phenomenon is demonstrated arteriographically as a localized narrowing of the artery with delayed blood flow distal to the site of spasm.

A distinctive arteriographic wave pattern (Fig. 77-32) has occasionally been observed in the superficial femoral, popliteal, pelvic, mesenteric, and other arteries throughout the body [74]. Various descriptive terms have been applied to this appearance, including *standing waves, stationary arterial waves, beading, crenation, bamboo pattern,* and *string of pearls.* The phenomenon is not associated with any known pathologic process in the vessel at the site of the change. Fibrous dysplasia, a specific pathologic entity, has an ar-

teriographic appearance very similar to that of standing waves, but the two entities generally do not affect the same vessels. Standing waves appear arteriographically in a pattern generally more uniform and regular than is fibrous dysplasia. More significant, on subsequent angiograms the standing-wave pattern usually disappears spontaneously.

The mechanism causing the arterial standing-wave pattern has been debated. Theander [119] observed that these arterial waves were noted in areas of decreased arterial flow—proximal to an occlusion or a severe tortuosity, for example. Other authors implicate arterial spasm [69, 78], while some claim that purely physical factors such as pressure waves [94] are responsible. Another hypothesis accounts for both the physical and biologic mechanisms previously assumed and stresses the flow-pulse factor [74].

TUMORS

The tumors encountered in the lower extremity can be classified as tumors primary in bone, tumors primary in soft tissue, and metastatic lesions. Under the categories of bone and soft tissue tumors, malignant as well as benign lesions should be considered. This chapter is confined mainly to malignant lesions because, in general, the benign tumors are avascular. Metastatic lesions may be subdivided into bone and soft tissue masses.

The demonstration of some of these lesions by arteriography is well documented, and the importance of this technique now is well respected [30, 70, 84, 105]. The effectiveness of arteriography depends on the histologic nature of the lesion because the technique merely reflects certain characteristic vascular changes in the various pathologic entities. Although the ultimate diagnosis in all tumors depends on histologic examination of the tissue, arteriography provides very significant information helpful in the management of these lesions. It aids in distinguishing benign from malignant lesions, determines the extent of the lesion and the best site for biopsy, identifies the vessels providing the tumor's blood supply, suggests a definite histologic cell type at times, and also may reveal a hidden, unsuspected metastasis.

The usual arteriographic finding of malignant tumors is increased vascularity consisting of tortuous, irregular vessels that do not gradually diminish in diameter (Fig. 77-33). The ves-

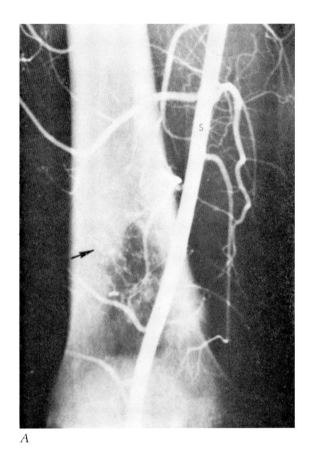

A

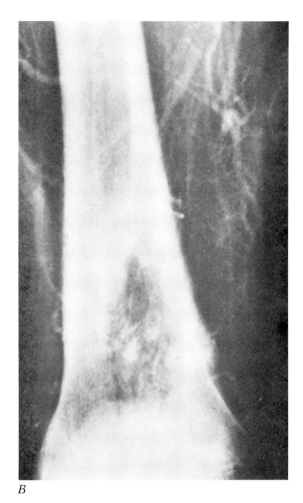

B

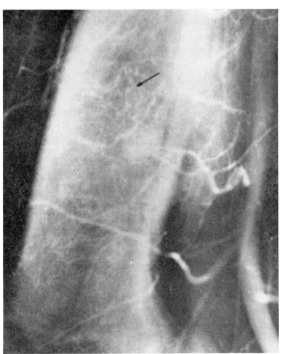

C

Figure 77-33. An osteogenic sarcoma of the femur. (A) The arterial phase demonstrates tumor vessels (*arrow*) in the area of the lytic bone lesion. The superficial femoral artery (*S*) is the main source of blood supply to the tumor. (B) There is early venous filling and a faint suggestion of tumor stain in the area of the lytic bone lesion. Note the periosteal elevation along the medial aspect of the femur. (C) The lateral view demonstrates the extent of the lesion and the chaotic pattern of the tumor vessels (*arrow*).

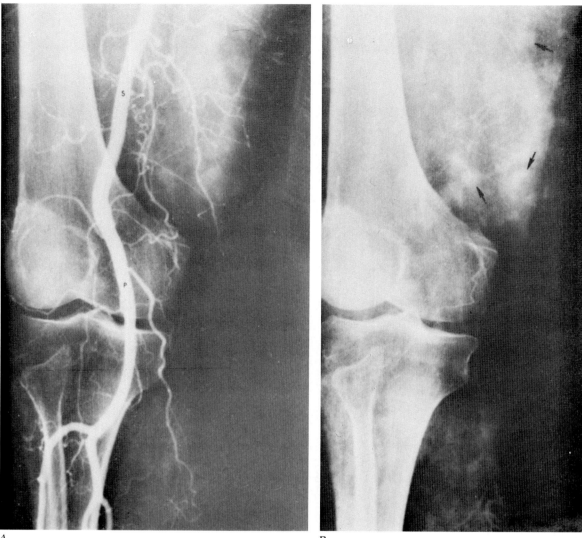

A

B

Figure 77-34. A malignant melanoma involving the lower leg, thigh, and inguinal nodes. (A) The superficial femoral artery (*S*) demonstrates numerous branches that supply multiple discrete melanomatous nodules in the soft tissues. (B) In the capillary phase these nodules are hypervascular and vary in size (*arrows*). *P* = popliteal continuation of superficial femoral artery.

sels may have altered diameters and appear to be beaded. Tumor stain or blush may be present, and the vascular pattern has an overall disorganized or chaotic appearance. Lakes of contrast filling due to dilated vascular spaces and early venous filling due to fine arteriovenous shunts may be observed.

Unfortunately, all malignant lesions of bone and soft tissue do not exhibit this pattern. Even when malignant neoplasms do show this pattern, they may demonstrate only some of its features and then only to a varying degree. Furthermore,

malignant tumors of the same histologic type do not necessarily exhibit the same arteriographic pattern (Figs. 77-34, 77-35). The well-recognized fact that there are variations in tumor growth and in the degree of histologic differentiation may account for the arteriographic variations demonstrated. Arteriographic interpretation also is complicated by benign tumors [85] and chronic inflammatory lesions [19], which occasionally may simulate the arteriographic appearance of a malignant tumor. Thus, although arteriography has its limitations, it is still a worthwhile diagnos-

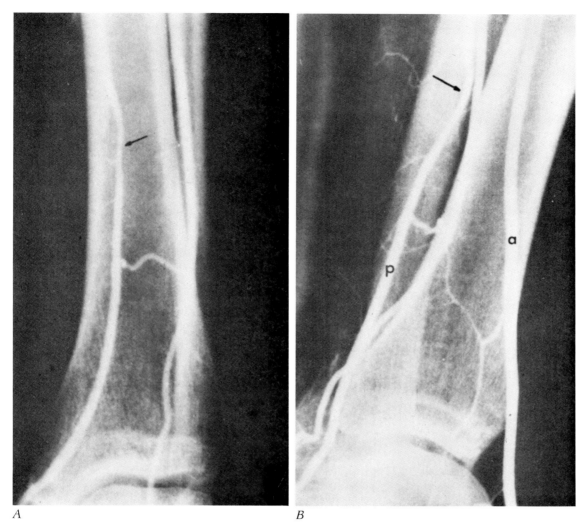

A   *B*

Figure 77-35. A malignant melanoma involving the foot and lower leg. (A) Anteroposterior view demonstrates a focal narrowing (*arrow*) of the posterior tibial artery. (B) Lateral view confirms this narrowing (*arrow*) of the artery (*p*) and shows localized displace- ment of the vessel. Tumor encasement of the vessel by a melanomatous lesion causes the narrowing. Unlike the malignant melanoma in Figure 77-34, this lesion is not hypervascular. Note the normal anterior tibial artery (*a*).

---

tic adjunct in the evaluation of lower extremity tumors.

From my own experience and that reported in the literature, a few generalizations concerning the arteriographic findings in specific lesions are apparent. Most osteogenic sarcomas [72] display areas of increased vascularity (see Fig. 77-33) dispersed in relatively avascular zones, which help to identify these lesions. Chondrosarcomas [73] vary greatly in their degree of vascularity and cover a spectrum from avascular to highly vascular malignancies. They sometimes show characteristic scalloped or wavy vessels. In the soft tissue

malignancies of the lower extremity, the degree of vascularity has been said to serve as an index to the degree of their malignancy [30, 70]. Fibrosarcomas [71], like chondrosarcomas, vary markedly in the degree of their vascularity, but the more vascular tumors are highly malignant. Liposarcomas (Fig. 77-36), rhabdomyosarcomas (Fig. 77-37), and synovial sarcomas may be quite vascular, but nothing characteristic distinguishes these lesions from one another [70]. Metastatic lesions [106] to bone or soft tissue usually display the same characteristics as the primary lesion. Thus, secondary lesions from the kidney (Fig.

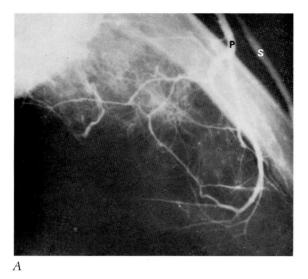

A

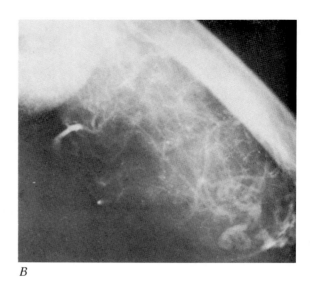

B

Figure 77-36. A liposarcoma of the thigh forming a large, firm soft tissue mass. (A) The tumor is moderately vascular, supplied by branches of the profunda femoris artery (*P*) but not by the superficial femoral artery (*S*). Irregular fine tumor vessels and areas of tumor stain are evident. (B) There is early venous filling, and the veins are dilated and tortuous. The tumor was moderately well circumscribed.

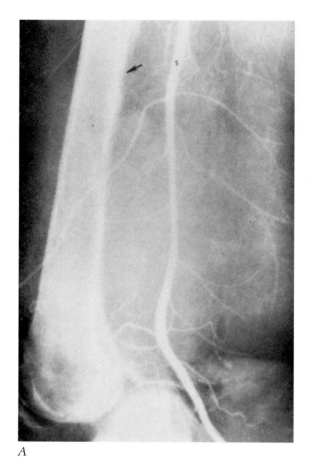

A

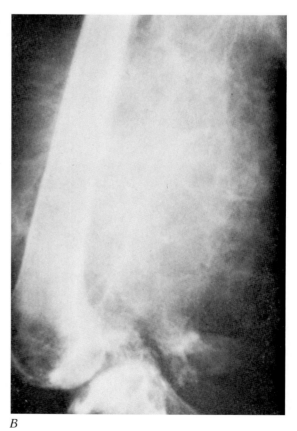

B

Figure 77-37. A rhabdomyosarcoma of the distal thigh, causing a large soft tissue mass and bone involvement. (A) The arterial phase demonstrates a relatively hypovascular mass around which are stretched branches of the superficial femoral artery (*S*). The superficial femoral artery is compressed and displaced by the mass. There is cortical erosion (*arrow*) of the femur due to the tumor. (B) In the venous phase the chaotic nature of the vascularity is best appreciated, even though no distinct early venous filling is seen. A diffuse and uneven tumor stain is seen in different parts of the tumor.

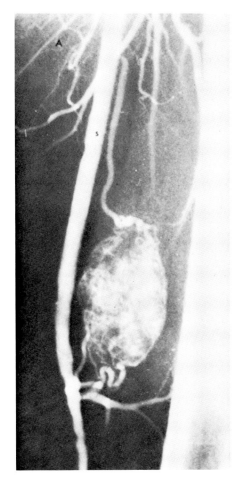
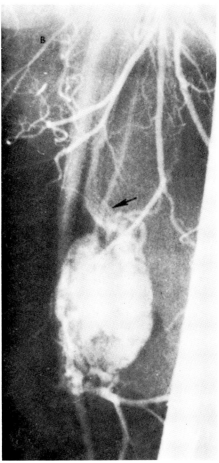

Figure 77-38. A metastasis from a renal cell carcinoma, clinically unsuspected, detected incidentally during arteriography for peripheral vascular disease. (A) The circumscribed hypervascular area derives its blood supply from the superficial femoral artery (*S*). The metastasis typically reflects the appearance of a primary renal cell carcinoma. (B) Tumor stain and early venous filling (*arrow*) are evident.

77-38) and thyroid might be expected to be notably vascular because the primary lesions are hypervascular.

References

1. Agee, O. F., and Kaude, J. Arteriography of the pelvis and lower extremities with moving table technique. *AJR* 107:860, 1969.
2. Allen, E. V., Barker, N. W., and Hines, E. A. *Peripheral Vascular Diseases* (3rd ed.). Philadelphia: Saunders, 1962.
3. Almén, T., Boijsen, E., and Lindell, S. E. Metrizamide in angiography: I. Femoral angiography. *Acta Radiol.* [*Diagn.*] (Stockh.) 18:33, 1977.
4. Amplatz, K. Translumbar catheterization of the abdominal aorta. *Radiology* 81:927, 1963.
5. Anson, B. J. (ed.). *Morris' Human Anatomy* (12th ed.). New York: Blakiston, Div. of McGraw-Hill, 1966.
6. Baum, S., and Abrams, H. L. A J-shaped catheter for retrograde catheterization of tortuous vessels. *Radiology* 83:436, 1964.
7. Beall, A. C., Diethrich, E. B., Morris, G. C., and DeBakey, M. E. Surgical management of vascular trauma. *Surg. Clin. North Am.* 46:1001, 1966.
8. Bell, J. W. Surgical treatment of chronic occlusion of the terminal aorta. *Am. Surg.* 38:481, 1972.
9. Bergan, F. Traumatic intimal rupture of the popliteal artery with acute ischemia of the limb in cases with supracondylar fractures of the

femur. *J. Cardiovasc. Surg.* (Torino) 4:300, 1963.

10. Boijsen, E., and Dahn, I. Femoral angiography during maximal blood flow. *Acta Radiol. [Diagn.]* (Stockh.) 3:543, 1965.

11. Branham, H. H. Aneurismal varix of the femoral artery and vein following a gunshot wound. *Int. J. Surg.* 3:250, 1890.

12. Braunstein, P. W., Skudder, P. A., McCarroll, J. R., Musolino, A., and Wade, P. A. Concealed hemorrhage due to pelvic fracture. *J. Trauma* 4:832, 1964.

13. Brest, A. N., and Moyer, J. H. (eds.). *Atherosclerotic Vascular Disease.* New York: Appleton-Century-Crofts, 1967.

14. Brief, D. K., Alpert, J., and Parsonnet, V. Crossover femorofemoral grafts. A reappraisal. *Arch. Surg.* 105:889, 1972.

15. Bron, K. M. Selective visceral and total abdominal arteriography via the left axillary artery in the older age group. *AJR* 97:432, 1966.

16. Buerger, L. *The Circulatory Disturbances of the Extremities, Including Gangrene, Vasomotor and Trophic Disorders.* Philadelphia: Saunders, 1924.

17. Byström, J., Dencker, H., Jäderling, J., and Meurling, S. Ligation of the internal iliac artery to arrest massive haemorrhage following pelvic fracture. *Acta Chir. Scand.* 134:199, 1968.

18. Christensen, R. D., and Bernatz, P. E. Anastomotic aneurysms involving the femoral artery. *Mayo Clin. Proc.* 47:313, 1972.

19. Cockshott, W. P., and Evans, K. T. The place of soft tissue arteriography. *Br. J. Radiol.* 37:367, 1964.

20. Conkle, D. M., Richie, R. E., Sawyers, J. L., and Scott, H. W., Jr. Surgical treatment of popliteal artery injuries. *Arch. Surg.* 110:1351, 1975.

21. Crane, C. Atherothrombotic embolism to lower extremities in arteriosclerosis. *Arch. Surg.* 94:96, 1967.

22. Crawford, F. A., Sethi, G. K., Scott, S. M., and Takaro, T. Femorofemoral grafts for unilateral occlusion of aortic bifurcation grafts. *Surgery* 77:150, 1975.

23. Creech, O., Jr., Gantt, J., and Wren, H. Traumatic arteriovenous fistula at unusual sites. *Ann. Surg.* 161:908, 1965.

24. Crummy, A. B., Rankin, R. S., Palzkill, B., Holmes, K. A., Orme, D. L., and Graham, N. Lower extremity arteriography: Biplane technique. *Appl. Radiol.* 9:51, 1980.

25. Darling, R. C. Peripheral arterial surgery. *N. Engl. J. Med.* 280:26, 1969.

26. Darling, R. C., Austen, W. G., and Linton, R. R. Arterial embolism. *Surg. Gynecol. Obstet.* 124:106, 1967.

27. DeBakey, M. E., Crawford, E. S., Cooley, D. A., and Morris, G. C. Surgical considerations of occlusive disease of the abdominal aorta and iliac and femoral arteries: Analysis of 803 cases. *Ann. Surg.* 148:306, 1958.

28. DeBakey, M. E., and Simeone, F. A. Battle injuries of the arteries in World War II. An analysis of 2471 cases. *Ann. Surg.* 123:534, 1946.

29. dos Santos, R. Technique de l'aortographie. *J. Int. Chir.* 2:609, 1937.

30. dos Santos, R. Arteriography in bone tumours. *J. Bone Joint Surg.* [Br.] 32:17, 1950.

31. Dotter, C. T., and Judkins, M. P. Transluminal treatment of arteriosclerotic obstruction: Description of a new technic and a preliminary report of its application. *Circulation* 30:654, 1964.

32. Dry, L. R., Conn, J. H., Chavez, C. M., and Hardy, J. D. Arteriovenous fistula: An analysis of fifty-eight cases. *Am. Surg.* 38:154, 1972.

33. Eisenberg, R. L., Mani, R. L., and Hedgcock, M. W. Pain associated with peripheral angiography: Is lidocaine effective? *Radiology* 127:109, 1978.

34. Eisenberg, R. L., Mani, R. L., and McDonald, E. J. The complication rate of catheter angiography by direct puncture through aortofemoral bypass grafts. *AJR* 126:814, 1976.

35. Eisenman, J. I., and O'Loughlin, B. J. Value of lateral abdominal aortography. *AJR* 112:586, 1971.

36. Erikson, U. Peripheral arteriography during bradykinin induced vasodilation. *Acta Radiol. [Diagn.]* (Stockh.) 3:193, 1965.

37. Figge, F. H. J., and Hild, W. J. (eds.). *Sobotta/ Figge Atlas of Human Anatomy* (9th ed.). Baltimore: Urban & Schwarzenberg, 1977.

38. Fogarty, T. J., Cranley, J. J., Krause, R. J., Strasser, E. S., and Hafner, C. D. A method for extraction of arterial emboli and thrombi. *Surg. Gynecol. Obstet.* 116:241, 1963.

39. Fogarty, T. J., Daily, P. O., Shumway, N. E., and Krippaehne, W. Experience with balloon catheter technic for arterial embolectomy. *Am. J. Surg.* 122:231, 1971.

40. Foster, J. H. Arteriography: Cornerstone of vascular surgery. *Arch. Surg.* 109:605, 1974.

41. Friedenberg, M. J., and Perez, C. A. Collateral circulation in aorto-ilio-femoral occlusive disease: As demonstrated by a unilateral percutaneous common femoral artery needle injection. *AJR* 94:145, 1958.

42. Friesen, G., Ivins, J. C., and Janes, J. M. Popliteal aneurysms. *Surgery* 51:90, 1962.

43. Fry, W. J. Surgical considerations in congenital arteriovenous fistula. *Surg. Clin. North Am.* 54:165, 1974.

44. Gardner, A. M. N., and Stewart, I. A. The treatment of arteriovenous malformation by endarterial electrocoagulation. *Br. J. Surg.* 59:146, 1972.

45. Gaspard, D. J., and Gaspar, M. R. Arteriove-

nous fistula after Fogarty catheter thrombectomy. *Arch. Surg.* 105:90, 1972.

46. Gaylis, H., Levine, E., Van Dongen, L. G. R., and Katz, I. Arteriovenous fistulas after gynecologic operations. *Surg. Gynecol. Obstet.* 137:655, 1973.

47. Glenn, J. H. Abdominal aorta catheterization via the left axillary artery. *Radiology* 115:227, 1975.

48. Gordon, I. J., and Westcott, J. L. Intraarterial lidocaine. An effective analgesic for peripheral angiography. *Radiology* 124:43, 1977.

49. Grüntzig, A., and Kumpe, D. A. Technique of percutaneous transluminal angioplasty with the Grüntzig balloon catheter. *AJR* 132:547, 1979.

50. Guthaner, D. F., Silverman, J. F., Hayden, W. G., and Wexler, L. Intraarterial analgesia in peripheral arteriography. *AJR* 128:737, 1977.

51. Haimovici, H., Shapiro, J. H., and Jacobson, H. G. Serial femoral arteriography in occlusive disease: Clinical-roentgenologic considerations with a new classification of occlusive patterns. *AJR* 83:1042, 1960.

52. Haimovici, H., and Steinman, C. Aortoiliac angiographic patterns associated with femoropopliteal occlusive disease: Significance in reconstructive arterial surgery. *Surgery* 65:232, 1969.

53. Hallin, R. W. Femoropopliteal versus femorotibial bypass grafting for lower extremity revascularization. *Am. Surg.* 42:522, 1976.

54. Handa, J., Handa, H., Torizuka, K., Hamamoto, K., and Kousaka, T. Radioisotopic study of arteriovenous anomalies. *AJR* 115:751, 1972.

55. Hauser, C. W., and Perry, J. F., Jr. Control of massive hemorrhage from pelvic fractures by hypogastric artery ligation. *Surg. Gynecol. Obstet.* 121:313, 1965.

56. Hewitt, R. L., and Collins, D. J. Acute arteriovenous fistulas in war injuries. *Ann. Surg.* 169:447, 1969.

57. Hewitt, R. L., Smith, A. D., and Drapanas, T. Acute traumatic arteriovenous fistulas. *J. Trauma* 13:901, 1973.

58. Hobson, R. W., II, Rich, N. M., and Fedde, C. W. Surgical management of high aortoiliac occlusion. *Am. Surg.* 41:271, 1975.

59. Holman, E. The physiology of an arteriovenous fistula. *Arch. Surg.* 7:64, 1923.

60. Holman, E. *Abnormal Arteriovenous Communications: Peripheral and Intracardiac; Acquired and Congenital* (2nd ed.). Springfield, Ill.: Thomas, 1968.

61. Holman, E. Reflections on arteriovenous fistulas. *Ann. Thorac. Surg.* 11:176, 1971.

62. Hughes, C. W. Acute vascular trauma in Korean War casualties: An analysis of 180 cases. *Surg. Gynecol. Obstet.* 99:91, 1954.

63. Jacobs, J. B., and Hanafee, W. N. The use of

Priscoline in peripheral arteriography. *Radiology* 88:957, 1967.

64. Judkins, M. P., Kidd, H. J., Frische, L. H., and Dotter, C. T. Lumen following safety J-guide for catheterization of tortuous vessels. *Radiology* 88:1127, 1967.

65. Kahn, P. C., Boyer, D. N., Moran, J. M., and Callow, A. D. Reactive hyperemia in lower extremity arteriography: An evaluation. *Radiology* 90:975, 1968.

66. Kelly, G. L., and Eiseman, B. Civilian vascular injuries. *J. Trauma* 15:507, 1975.

67. Kirkup, J. R. Major arterial injury complicating fracture of the femoral shaft. *J. Bone Joint Surg.* [Br.] 45:337, 1963.

68. Klingensmith, W., Oles, P., and Martinez, H. Fractures with associated blood vessel injury. *Am. J. Surg.* 110:849, 1965.

69. Köhler, R. Regular alternating changes in arterial width in lower limb angiograms. *Acta Radiol.* [*Diagn.*] (Stockh.) 3:529, 1965.

70. Lagergren, C., and Lindbom, Å. Angiography of peripheral tumors. *Radiology* 79:371, 1962.

71. Lagergren, C., Lindbom, Å., and Söderberg, G. Vascularization of fibromatous and fibrosarcomatous tumors: Histopathologic, microangiographic and angiographic studies. *Acta Radiol.* (Stockh.) 53:1, 1960.

72. Lagergren, C., Lindbom, Å., and Söderberg, G. The blood vessels of osteogenic sarcomas: Histologic, angiographic and microangiographic studies. *Acta Radiol.* (Stockh.) 55:161, 1961.

73. Lagergren, C., Lindbom, Å., and Söderberg, G. The blood vessels of chondrosarcomas. *Acta Radiol.* (Stockh.) 55:321, 1961.

74. Lehrer, H. The physiology of angiographic arterial waves. *Radiology* 89:11, 1967.

75. Levinson, S. A., Levinson, H. J., Halloran, L. G., Brooks, J. W., Davis, R. J., Wolf, J. S., Lee, H. M., and Hume, D. M. Limited indications for unilateral aortofemoral or iliofemoral vascular grafts. *Arch. Surg.* 107:791, 1973.

76. Levy, J. F., and Butcher, H. R., Jr. Arterial emboli: An analysis of 125 patients. *Surgery* 68:968, 1970.

77. Lindbom, Å. Arteriosclerosis and arterial thrombosis in the lower limb: A roentgenological study. *Acta Radiol.* [*Suppl.*] (Stockh.) 80:1, 1950.

78. Lindbom, Å. Arterial spasm caused by puncture and catheterization: An arteriographic study of patients not suffering from arterial disease. *Acta Radiol.* (Stockh.) 47:449, 1957.

79. Lindgren, P., Saltzman, G. F., and Törnell, G. Vascular effects of metrizoate compounds, Isopaque Na and Isopaque Na/Ca/Mg. *Acta Radiol.* [*Suppl.*] (Stockh.) 270:44, 1967.

80. Linton, R. R. Peripheral arterial embolism: A discussion of the postembolic vascular changes

and their relation to the restoration of circulation in peripheral embolism. *N. Engl. J. Med.* 224:189, 1941.

81. Mani, R. L., and Costin, B. S. Catheter angiography through aortofemoral grafts: Prevention of catheter separation during withdrawal. *AJR* 128:328, 1977.

82. Mani, R. L., Helms, C. A., and Eisenberg, R. L. Use of a 5 French catheter with multiple side holes in abdominal aortography. *Radiology* 123:233, 1977.

83. Margolies, M. N., Ring, E. J., Waltman, A. C., Kerr, W. S., Jr., and Baum, S. Arteriography in the management of hemorrhage from pelvic fractures. *N. Engl. J. Med.* 287:317, 1972.

84. Margulis, A. R. Arteriography of tumors: Difficulties in interpretation and the need for magnification. *Radiol. Clin. North Am.* 2:543, 1964.

85. Margulis, A. R., and Murphy, T. O. Arteriography in neoplasms of extremities. *AJR* 80:330, 1958.

86. Mavor, G. E. The pattern of occlusion in atheroma of the lower limb arteries. The correlation of clinical and arteriographic findings. *Br. J. Surg.* 43:352, 1956.

87. McDonald, E. J., Jr., Malone, J. M., Eisenberg, R. L., and Mani, R. L. Arteriographic evaluation of the femoral bifurcation: Value of the ipsilateral anterior oblique projection. *AJR* 127:955, 1976.

88. McKusick, V. A., Harris, W. S., Ottesen, O. E., Goodman, R. M., Shelley, W. M., and Bloodwell, R. D. Buerger's disease: A distinct clinical and pathologic entity. *J.A.M.A.* 181:5, 1962.

89. Miller, H. H., and Welch, C. S. Quantitative studies on the time factor in arterial injuries. *Ann. Surg.* 130:428, 1949.

90. Miller, W. E. Massive hemorrhage in fractures of the pelvis. *South. Med. J.* 56:933, 1963.

91. Motsay, G. J., Manlove, C., and Perry, J. F. Major venous injury with pelvic fracture. *J. Trauma* 9:343, 1969.

92. Mozersky, D. J., Sumner, D. S., and Strandness, D. E. Long term results of reconstructive aortoiliac surgery. *Am. J. Surg.* 123:503, 1972.

93. Muller, R. F., and Figley, M. M. The arteries of the abdomen, pelvis, and thigh: I. Normal roentgenographic anatomy; II. Collateral circulation in obstructive arterial disease. *AJR* 77:296, 1957.

94. New, P. F. J. Arterial stationary waves. *AJR* 97:488, 1966.

95. Nolan, B., and McQuillan, W. M. Acute traumatic limb ischaemia. *Br. J. Surg.* 52:559, 1965.

96. Olin, T. *Studies in Angiographic Technique.* Lund: Hakan Ohlssons Boktryckeri, 1963.

97. Peltier, L. F. Complications associated with fractures of the pelvis. *J. Bone Joint Surg.* [Am.] 47:1060, 1965.

98. Quinby, W. C., Jr. Pelvic fractures with hemorrhage. *N. Engl. J. Med.* 284:668, 1971.

99. Raines, J. K., Darling, R. C., Buth, J., Brewster, D. C., and Austin, W. G. Vascular laboratory criteria for the management of peripheral vascular disease of the lower extremities. *Surgery* 79:21, 1976.

100. Ravitch, M. M. Hypogastric artery ligation in acute pelvic trauma. *Surgery* 56:601, 1964.

101. Reichle, F. A., and Tyson, R. R. Bypasses to tibial or popliteal arteries in severely ischemic lower extremities: Comparison of long-term results in 233 patients. *Ann. Surg.* 176:315, 1972.

102. Reichle, F. A., and Tyson, R. R. Comparison of long-term results of 364 femoropopliteal or femorotibial bypasses for revascularization of severely ischemic lower extremities. *Ann. Surg.* 182:449, 1975.

103. Riddervold, H. O., and Seale, D. L. Translumbar aortography with Teflon catheters. *Acta Radiol.* [*Diagn.*] (Stockh.) 12:619, 1972.

104. Ring, E. J., Athanasoulis, C., Waltman, A. C., Margolies, M. N., and Baum, S. Arteriographic management of hemorrhage following pelvic fracture. *Radiology* 109:65, 1973.

105. Rosenberg, J. C. The value of arteriography in the treatment of soft tissue tumors of the extremities. *Int. Surg.* 41:405, 1964.

106. Schobinger, R. The arteriographic picture of metastatic bone disease. *Cancer* 11:1264, 1958.

107. Seldinger, S. I. Catheter replacement of the needle in percutaneous arteriography: A new technique. *Acta Radiol.* (Stockh.) 39:368, 1953.

108. Sethi, G. K., Scott, S. M., and Takaro, T. Multiple angiography for more precise evaluation of aortoiliac disease. *Surgery* 78:154, 1975.

109. Simon, H., and Fairbank, J. T. Biplane translumbar aortography for evaluation of peripheral vascular disease. *Am. J. Surg.* 133:447, 1977.

110. Sprayregen, S. Popliteal vein displacement by popliteal artery aneurysm. Report of 2 cases. *AJR* 132:838, 1979.

111. Stallone, R. J., Blaisdell, F. W., Cafferata, H. T., and Levin, S. M. Analysis of morbidity and mortality from arterial embolectomy. *Surgery* 65:207, 1969.

112. Stanley, R. J., and Cubillo, E. Nonsurgical treatment of arteriovenous malformations of the trunk and limbs by transcatheter arterial embolization. *Radiology* 115:609, 1975.

113. Stephenson, H. E., Jr., and Lichti, E. L. Application of the Doppler Ultrasonic Flowmeter in the surgical treatment of arteriovenous fistula. *Am. Surg.* 37:537, 1971.

114. Strandness, D. E., Jr. (ed.). *Collateral Circulation in Clinical Surgery.* Philadelphia: Saunders, 1969.

115. Szilagyi, D. E., DeRusso, F. J., and Elliot, J. P. Thromboangiitis obliterans: Clinicoangiographic correlations. *Arch. Surg.* 88:824, 1964.

116. Szilagyi, D. E., Elliott, J. P., DeRusso, F. J., and Smith, R. F. Peripheral congenital arteriovenous fistulas. *Surgery* 57:61, 1965.

117. Szilagyi, D. E., Smith, R. F., Elliott, J. P., Hageman, J. H., and Dall'Olmo, C. A. Anastomotic aneurysms after vascular reconstruction: Problems of incidence, etiology, and treatment. *Surgery* 78:800, 1975.

118. Thadani, U., and Pratt, A. E. Profunda femoral arteriovenous fistula after percutaneous arterial and venous catheterization. *Br. Heart J.* 33:803, 1971.

119. Theander, G. Arteriographic demonstration of stationary arterial waves. *Acta Radiol.* (Stockh.) 53:417, 1960.

120. Thomas, M. L., and Andress, M. R. Value of oblique projections in translumbar aortography. *AJR* 116:187, 1972.

121. Thompson, J. E., and Garrett, W. V. Peripheral-arterial surgery. *N. Engl. J. Med.* 302:491, 1980.

122. Thompson, J. E., Sigler, L., Runt, P. S., Austin, D. J., and Patman, R. D. Arterial embolectomy: A 20 year experience with 163 cases. *Surgery* 67:212, 1970.

123. Thurlbeck, W. M., and Castleman, B. Atheromatous emboli to the kidneys after aortic surgery. *N. Engl. J. Med.* 257:442, 1957.

124. Tice, D. A., Clauss, R. H., Keirle, A. M., and Reed, G. E. Congenital arteriovenous fistulae of the extremities: Observations concerning treatment. *Arch. Surg.* 86:130, 1963.

125. Trimble, I. R., Stonesifer, G. L., Jr., Wilgis, E. F. S., and Montague, A. C. Criteria for femorofemoral bypass from clinical and hemodynamic studies. *Ann. Surg.* 175:985, 1972.

126. Vetto, R. M. The treatment of unilateral iliac artery obstruction with a transabdominal, subcutaneous, femorofemoral graft. *Surgery* 52:342, 1962.

127. Wahren, J., Cronestrand, R., and Juhlin-Dannfelt, A. Leg blood flow during exercise in patients with occlusion of the iliac artery: Pre- and postoperative studies. *Scand. J. Clin. Lab. Invest.* 32:257, 1963.

128. Weinrauch, L. A., Robertson, W. S., and D'Elia, J. A. Contrast media–induced acute renal failure. *J.A.M.A.* 239:2018, 1978.

129. Wendth, A. J., Jr. Peripheral arteriography. An overview of its origin and present status. *CRC Crit. Rev. Diagn. Imaging* 6:369, 1975.

130. Wessler, S., Ming, S. C., Gurewich, V., and Freiman, D. G. A critical evaluation of thromboangiitis obliterans: The case against Buerger's disease. *N. Engl. J. Med.* 262:1149, 1960.

131. Weston, T. S. Arterial embolism of the lower limbs. *Australas. Radiol.* 11:354, 1967.

132. Wickbom, I., and Bartley, O. Arterial "spasm" in peripheral arteriography using the catheter method. *Acta Radiol.* (Stockh.) 47:433, 1957.

133. Widrich, W. C., Singer, R. J., and Robbins, A. H. The use of intra-arterial lidocaine to control pain due to aortofemoral arteriography. *Radiology* 124:37, 1977.

134. Woollard, H. H. The development of the principal arterial stems in the forelimb of the pig. *Contrib. Embryol.* 14:139, 1922.

135. Wychulis, A. R., Spittell, J. A., Jr., and Wallace, R. B. Popliteal aneurysms. *Surgery* 68:942, 1970.

136. Zannetti, P. H., and Sherman, F. E. Experimental evaluation of a tissue adhesive as an agent for the treatment of aneurysms and arteriovenous anomalies. *J. Neurosurg.* 36:72, 1972.

137. Zeitler, E., Grüntzig, A., and Schoop, W. (eds.). *Percutaneous Vascular Recanalization: Technique, Applications, Clinical Results.* New York: Springer, 1978.

Venography of the Lower Extremities

KEITH RABINOV
SVEN PAULIN

The popularity of venography of the lower extremities has waxed and waned since this procedure was first described by Berberich and Hirsch in 1923 [24]. The primary reason has been that shortcomings in technique gave rise to unreliable appearances and thus to inaccurate interpretations. There has also been concern over possible complications of the procedure itself.

Improvements in the understanding of the dynamics of flow of venous blood and of contrast material in the veins of the lower extremities, however, have led to the development of reliable techniques. It is thus possible to define more precisely the parameters of the normal venogram and to identify the abnormal findings with certainty. The accuracy of interpretation has so greatly improved that venography is now considered the standard against which other methods of diagnosis of venous thrombosis are measured.

The use of more dilute contrast materials has reduced the incidence of postvenography discomfort or thrombosis. Nonionic contrast materials hold further promise in this regard.

Newer, noninvasive tests are increasingly used for the diagnosis of deep vein thrombosis. Although they do not achieve the same high degree of diagnostic accuracy, they can be used to screen for the presence of deep vein thrombosis under certain circumstances, as in subgroups of patients at high risk. Any current discussion of the practice of venography must therefore pay attention to these methods as well. The complementary use of these tests in sequence with the phlebogram may be especially helpful for efficient patient management and to further the understanding of the natural history of deep vein thrombosis, its local sequelae such as the postthrombotic syndrome and venous ulcer, and its most serious complication, pulmonary embolism.

Venous Anatomy

With regard to phlebographic anatomy and functional considerations, the veins of the lower extremity may be classified as follows: the deep veins including the main trunks and muscle veins, the superficial veins, and the perforating veins (Figs. 78-1–78-4).

The *deep veins* are enclosed by the deep fascia, together with the muscles that surround and support them except at the ankle, where they are embedded in fat. The plantar venous arch is the

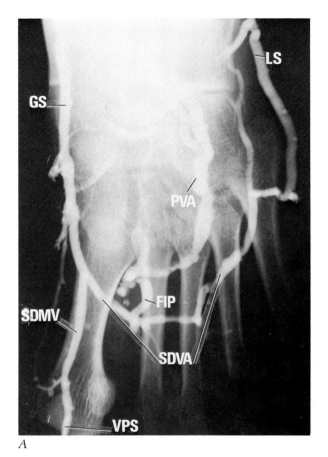

A

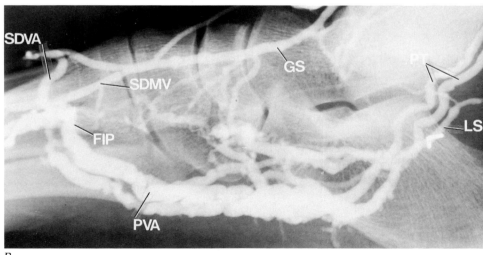

B

Figure 78-1. Venograms of the foot to show the normal pathways of opacification following injection into the superficial dorsal metatarsal vein of the great toe. (A) Anteroposterior view. (B) Lateral view. *FIP* = First intermetatarsal perforating vein; *GS* = greater saphenous vein; *LS* = lesser saphenous vein; *PT* = posterior tibial veins; *PVA* = plantar venous arch; *SDMV* = superficial dorsal metatarsal vein; *SDVA* = superficial dorsal venous arch; *VPS* = venipuncture site.

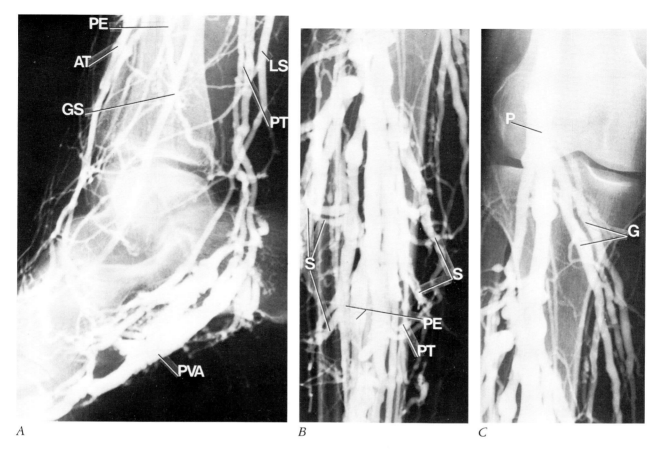

A   *B*   *C*

Figure 78-2. Normal venogram, representative spot films. (A) Lateral view of the foot and ankle. The anterior tibial veins are the proximal continuation of the dorsal veins of the foot, and the posterior tibial veins are the proximal continuation of the plantar veins. The peroneal veins have their origin at the ankle. Anteroposterior views of the calf (B) and knee (C). The deep axial veins and the muscle veins are spindle-shaped. *AT* = Anterior tibial veins; *G* = gastrocnemius muscle veins; *GS* = greater saphenous vein; *LS* = lesser saphenous vein; *PE* = peroneal veins; *P* = popliteal vein; *PT* = posterior tibial veins; *PVA* = plantar venous arch; *S* = soleal muscle veins.

largest deep vein of the foot, often reaching 1 cm in diameter (see Fig. 78-1). This arch splits in two in its posterior part, continuing as the lateral plantar veins, which are joined by smaller medial plantar veins below the medial malleolus [18, 52]. In the calf, three main deep trunks accompany their respective arteries (see Fig. 78-3). These trunks are generally paired, though occasionally single, and are connected to one another by intercommunicating veins. The posterior tibial veins are the direct continuation of the junction of the lateral and medial plantar veins of the foot, while the anterior tibial veins are the proximal continuation of the dorsal foot veins (see Fig. 78-2A). The peroneal veins arise from multiple tributaries at the ankle. These deep trunks merge in the upper third of the calf to form the popliteal vein, which is commonly single but which may be paired in up to 20 percent of normal cases.

The muscle veins of the calf are enclosed within the muscle bellies themselves. Multiple pairs of soleus muscle veins both medially and laterally empty into the posterior tibial or peroneal veins below the popliteal fossa (see Fig. 78-3). A great arch vein of the soleus muscle, connecting at both its upper and lower ends to the posterior tibial veins, is sometimes present. The gastrocnemius veins are somewhat variable, but usually there are two pairs of large medial veins and two pairs of smaller lateral veins, which empty into the popliteal vein above the knee joint.

The superficial femoral vein is often single, though it may be paired or partly paired (see Figs.

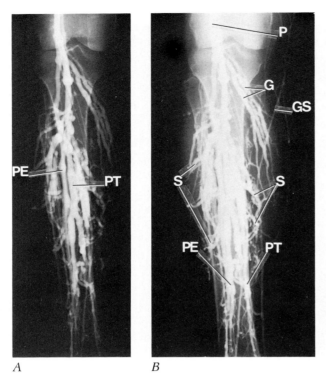

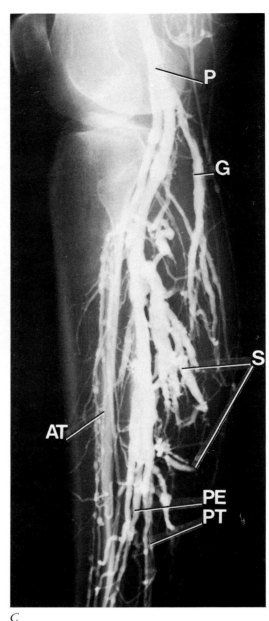

Figure 78-3. Normal venogram of the leg. Same patient as in Figure 78-2. Anteroposterior stereoscopic radiographs with darker (A) and lighter (B) technique. (C) Lateral view. The deep axial veins of the calf are paired. The soleal veins join the posterior tibial and peroneal veins in the calf. The gastrocnemius veins drain into the popliteal vein above the knee joint. Abbreviations as in Figure 78-2.

78-4, 78-16). The profunda femoris vein drains primarily the thigh muscles, but in 50 percent of instances it has a large communication with the popliteal vein or the femoral vein in the adductor canal [109].

The pelvic veins, including the external iliac vein, internal iliac vein, and common iliac vein, are practically always single channels (see Fig. 78-4B, C).

The *superficial veins,* consisting of the long and short saphenous trunks and their tributaries and arcades (see Fig. 78-27), lie in the subcutaneous tissues external to the deep fascia. They begin in the foot where the superficial dorsal metatarsal veins converge to form the superficial dorsal venous arch (see Fig. 78-1). The medial and lateral extremities of this arch continue proximally as the trunks of the greater and lesser saphenous veins respectively.

The short saphenous trunk passes behind the lateral malleolus and upward along the midline of the posterior aspect of the calf to join the popliteal vein. Alternatively, it may terminate in some instances in the femoral vein, the long saphenous vein, or a deep vein of the calf. A single tributary is commonly present, joining the short saphenous trunk at the popliteal fossa.

The long saphenous trunk passes anterior to the medial malleolus, posteromedial to the medial femoral condyle, to empty into the femoral vein at the groin together with several other tributaries [52, 71]. It usually has two tributaries in the thigh and two in the calf. Multiple arcades

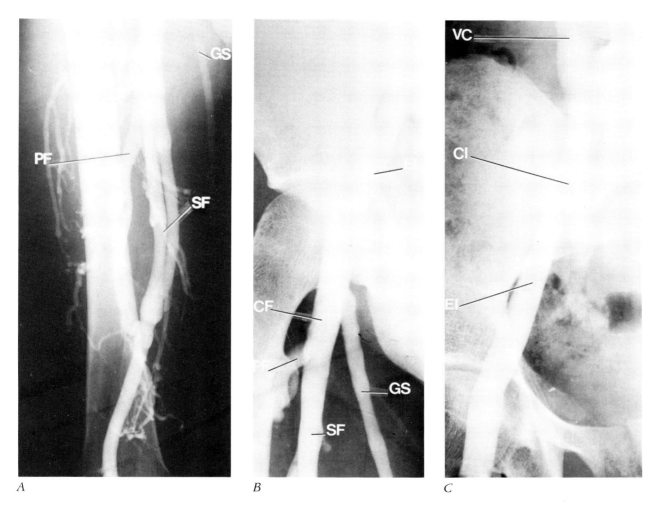

A   *B*   *C*

Figure 78-4. Normal venogram. Same patient as in Figures 78-2 and 78-3. (A) Anteroposterior radiograph of the thigh. Anteroposterior spot films of the groin (B) and pelvis (C). *CF* = Common femoral vein; *CI* = common iliac vein; *EI* = external iliac vein; *GS* = greater saphenous vein; *PF* = profunda femoris vein; *SF* = superficial femoral vein; *VC* = inferior vena cava.

(commonly three) join the greater and lesser saphenous systems. Accessory saphenous veins may also be present.

Other superficial veins may bypass the saphenous veins to drain more proximally into gluteal veins or veins of the lower abdomen [71].

The *perforating veins* penetrate through the deep fascia to connect the deep veins with the superficial veins. They are present at all levels of the lower extremity from the foot to the groin (see Fig. 78-27) and their number has been estimated to be at least 90 in each leg [71].

Multiple perforating veins connect the superficial dorsal venous arch of the foot with the plantar venous arch [52]. Some of these are also present along the medial and lateral aspects of the foot. A very large one is constantly present in the proximal first intermetatarsal space (see Fig. 78-1).

At the level of the ankle and calf, there are direct perforating veins associated with each of the paired deep trunks and indirect perforating veins associated with some of the muscle veins. Some of these perforating veins, such as the posttibial perforating vein (Boyd's vein), and perforating veins associated with the gastrocnemius veins are known to be important collaterals when the main deep trunks are obstructed [71].

In the thigh, perforating veins join the long saphenous vein or, more commonly, one of its tributaries, with the femoral vein in the region of Hunter's canal [50, 52] (see Figs. 78-27, 78-29).

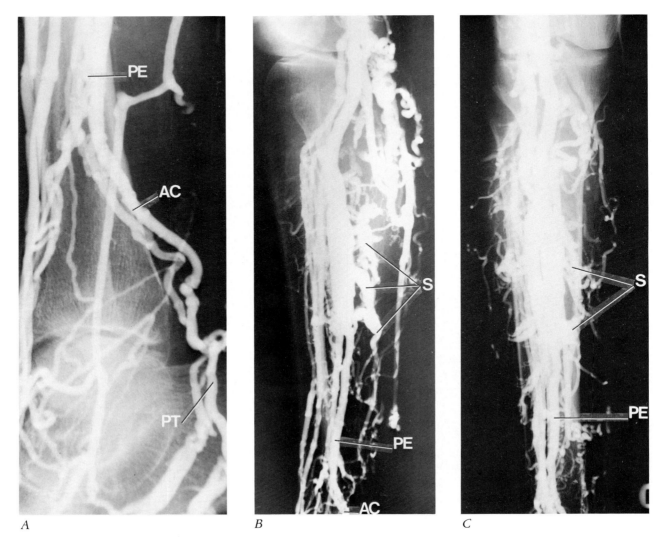

A   *B*   *C*

Figure 78-5. Anomalous entry of the posterior tibial veins into the peroneal veins in the ankle. (A) Lateral view of the foot and ankle. Lateral (B) and anteroposterior (C) views of the calf. Note that the posterior tibial veins are absent in the calf above the ankle and that the peroneal veins are larger than normal (com-pare with Figure 78-3). The soleal muscle veins in the medial part of the calf opacify normally. *AC* = Anomalous connection between the posterior tibial and peroneal veins; *PE* = peroneal veins; *PT* = posterior tibial veins; *S* = soleal muscle veins.

The entrance of the lesser saphenous vein into the popliteal vein and that of the greater saphenous vein into the femoral vein at the groin are the highest perforating veins of each of these systems.

Valves are normally present in all superficial, perforating, and deep veins of the lower extremity except for the perforating veins in the foot, which are ordinarily without valves [71]. The valves are oriented in such a way as to direct blood flow from the superficial veins to the deep veins, and centrally toward the heart. Valves are located closer to each other, the more distal the vein [71]. Even veins as small as 0.15 mm contain valves [143]. The number of vein valves is quite variable [50]. According to a detailed study [143], there are 9 to 11 valves in the anterior tibial veins, 9 to 19 in the posterior tibial veins, 7 in the peroneal veins, 1 in the popliteal vein, and 3 in the superficial femoral vein. The external iliac vein contains valves in only 25 percent of instances. The common iliac vein rarely has valves.

Variations in venous topography are common. One of these most frequently encountered in the deep veins is the joining of the posterior tibial veins with the peroneal veins, which are then larger than usual (Fig. 78-5).

Dynamics of Venous Blood Flow

The deep veins have very little smooth muscle in their walls [101]. They therefore constitute a passive reservoir, the diameter of each deep vein being determined by internal and external pressures and flow. The superficial veins, on the other hand, contain smooth muscle and respond to temperature and direct stimuli [101, 143].

The deep veins of the lower extremity can be characterized as "capacity vessels"; i.e., they can accommodate widely varying volumes of blood in response to minimal changes in pressure [101]. At low pressures the veins are partly collapsed into an elliptical cross-sectional configuration [143]. Even small increases (15 mm Hg) in venous transmural pressure may cause them to distend to a circular cross-sectional configuration. Such increases in pressure easily occur upon assumption of the upright position.

At rest, local venous pressures are primarily hydrostatic, corresponding to the vertical height of a column of blood to the level of the atrium [141, 143]. Intravascular measurements have shown the venous pressure at the ankle in the recumbent position to be 7 to 16 mm Hg, and in the standing position, 78 to 92 mm Hg [120]. The pressures in the deep and superficial systems are about equal, since the valves are open, leaving the superficial and deep venous systems in free communication with each other. Small local pressure gradients are sufficient to open some of the many valves existing throughout the venous system and to close others so that regurgitant flow is prevented and blood flow is gently directed centrally. This central flow is also influenced by a small but more or less continuous dynamic pressure transmitted through the capillaries and small venules from the arterial side, as well as by pulsatile movements of the immediately adjacent arteries. Changes in the intrathoracic pressure

impart a phasic quality to the venous return. Both respiratory movements and the diastolic-suction effect of the right ventricle contribute to the venous return toward the heart.

Postural changes of the body greatly influence venous pressure and flow. For example, elevation of the leg above the horizontal in a recumbent person causes a passive emptying of the veins and rapid shift of blood toward the heart. On the other hand, as much as 250 to 350 cc of blood may shift into the veins of each lower extremity when the upright position is assumed [101, 143]. As already noted, venous pressure at the ankle rises appreciably with assumption of the upright position.

With muscle contraction, the dynamics of venous return are quite different from those at rest. Thus, with contraction of the leg muscles, blood is impelled centrally by a series of reciprocating musculovenous pumps in the foot, calf, and thigh [15, 16, 52, 100]. The best known of these is in the calf, consisting of the intramuscular veins (gastrocnemius and soleus veins), which perform like bellows, and the intermuscular veins (anterior and posterior tibial veins and peroneal veins). These veins, particularly the intramuscular veins, are markedly compressed by the contracting muscles, the veins and muscles together constituting a "peripheral heart." The pressures within the muscles may rise as high as 250 mm Hg during contraction [99], augmenting the local venous pressure by up to 100 mm Hg [16]. A single maximal calf contraction in the upright subject may eject 50 to 75 cc of blood proximally out of the leg [100]. During relaxation of the muscles, the deep veins refill with blood from more distal deep veins as well as with blood sucked in from superficial veins. Repetition of this action results in a drop of pressure in the deep veins in the normal subject to less than half the preexisting hydrostatic pressure [101].

The venous drainage of the skin and subcutaneous tissues of the ankle region occurs directly through the perforating veins into the deep veins (see Fig. 78-27). Above this level, venous blood from these superficial structures ascends through the superficial veins, entering the deep veins higher up [50].

The venous valves not only direct the venous flow centrally but also serve to interrupt the venous column of blood above them, preventing reflux and limiting the venous pressure under conditions such as activity or coughing [101].

Dynamics of Venous Contrast Filling in the Normal Venogram

The physical properties of water-soluble radiopaque contrast materials differ significantly from those of blood. In 1943 Kjellberg [94] pointed out that layering of contrast material beneath blood frequently occurs in the venous system. Factors that determine the degree of layering include the specific weight (specific weight of contrast material for phlebography is approximately 1.3 compared with 1.05 for that of blood), the viscosity of contrast material, the rate of injection, the velocity of the bloodstream, and the caliber and position of the vessels. The limited injection rates that can be accomplished through the small needles used for peripheral injection are insufficient for complete mixing with the large blood volume of the venous compartment. In the supine position the injectate streams in a central direction rather quickly, and predominantly through the dependent venous pathways. Application of flow-reducing measures—tourniquets, inflatable pneumatic cuffs, or the Valsalva maneuver—in an effort to delay the contrast runoff will also distend the leg veins, and such conditions of slow flow will further enhance the layering of the heavy contrast material. Kjellberg warned against misinterpreting as clots the apparent vascular filling defects that may be caused by this incomplete mixing and layering. In experimental models as well as clinical phlebographic studies he showed that complete filling of a vessel's lumen was not accomplished until a vertical position was reached. He also noted that nonopaque blood may "percolate" upward through the heavy opaque contrast stream at the site of merging veins, giving the impression of well-demarcated filling defects. Similar observations were made by Swart and Dingendorf [144] and Fox and Hugh [53].

Because of these factors, complete and reliable filling of the entire venous system of the lower extremity in the supine position is a very difficult if not impossible task. Elaborate techniques using ankle tourniquet, pneumatic thigh cuffs, patient exercise, or power injection have been suggested [38, 113, 115, 118] but they have not gained wide acceptance, partly because of their technical complexity.

Although suggested earlier by Lindblom [96], the performance of phlebography in the predominantly upright position was evaluated in great detail and popularized in 1954 by Greitz [64], who noted that the reliability of venous opacification was greatly improved when the phlebogram was obtained in this position. Under such circumstances, the peripherally injected contrast medium will, because of gravity, remain in the dependent parts for many minutes. Although the contrast material itself is continuously diluted and propelled centrally by the blood flow through the resting extremity, this process occurs so slowly that continuous injection through the peripherally placed needle will result in increasing filling of the distended veins from below upward.

The contrast material injected into a superficial vein of the foot will freely enter the deep veins of the foot and leg. The use of a tourniquet at the ankle not only is unnecessary but may actually interfere with the normal filling of the anterior tibial veins and the gastrocnemius veins. It is also important that the leg be relaxed and non-weight-bearing so that the contrast material can enter the veins within the deep fascial compartment. Muscle contraction, even as slight as that induced by weight bearing, may compress the deep veins enough to prevent their opacification.

The dorsal metatarsal vein at the base of the great toe is the preferred site of injection since this vein gives direct access to the entire superficial and deep venous system of the foot from which all the superficial and deep veins higher up will fill (see Fig. 78-1).

Contrast medium ascends through the various veins in orderly fashion at about the same rate. The top of the opaque column in the superficial veins may be slightly ahead of that in the deep veins at any given moment. The anterior tibial veins empty earlier than the other veins, possibly because of their relatively smaller size. The muscle veins in the calf fill primarily from below via deep or superficial veins, though there may be some reflux downward from above. Active or passive emptying of these veins prior to the procedure is not necessary in order to fill them, nor is the use of cuffs or tourniquets. The gastrocnemius veins are usually the last veins to fill entirely, often completing filling in their upper portions after the superficial femoral vein is well opacified at the groin. Gastrocnemius vein filling may be absent when the superficial veins have been removed surgically, since this eliminates the source of flow from which they normally fill. In such circumstances the state of these veins cannot be determined venographically.

Opacification of the deep femoral vein may present an exception since significant filling from below occurs in only approximately 50 percent of cases. This is explained by the lack of large communications between the deep femoral vein and the popliteal or distal superficial femoral vein in such instances [104]. The deep femoral vein can usually be filled from above downward to at least the first or second valve by means of the Valsalva maneuver.

Standard Technique of Venography

Many different techniques have been described for the performance of venography of the lower extremities. The method described here [122] is based upon our own experience but includes also many important observations made by previous authors [9, 48, 64, 65, 68]. Paying attention to the known dynamics of venous blood flow and to the properties of contrast material, this technique is designed to produce optimal filling of the veins [155], to reduce the generation of artifacts, and, if the latter are unavoidable, to allow their proper recognition.

The examination is performed with the patient in the semiupright position (30–45 degrees) (Fig. 78-6). The patient stands on a box or rotating platform [67] with the other foot so that the injected leg is non-weight-bearing and completely relaxed. A 23-gauge scalp vein needle or a plastic cannula [61] is placed in a superficial vein of the foot, preferably in the superficial dorsal metatarsal vein of the great toe. Such a small-caliber needle or cannula is preferred since it easily enters the thick-walled movable subcutaneous veins of the foot and yet its small lumen is adequate to permit high enough injection rate of the contrast materials now in use. The foot veins are ordinarily adequately distended and brought into prominence by the patient's semiupright position and a tourniquet is placed temporarily at the ankle.

Any edema fluid can be massaged away if the veins should be obscured. Spontaneously contracted veins or those that are spastic following a puncture may be brought out successfully by wrapping the foot in a warm towel or by gently

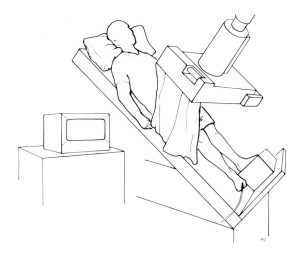

Figure 78-6. Patient undergoing phlebographic examination of the lower extremity. The leg being examined is not weight-bearing. No tourniquet is used. The venous puncture is performed near the base of the great toe, and the injection is monitored under fluoroscopy.

slapping the overlying skin, since these veins tend to dilate in response to such direct stimuli or heat.

Any approved and marketed radiopaque water-soluble contrast agent containing approximately 20 percent iodine is suitable in most instances. Higher concentrations are unnecessary and produce a greater incidence of undesirable side effects. Lower concentrations often result in unsatisfactory studies and may make fluoroscopic control difficult, especially if the legs are muscular or heavy. The contrast materials now recommended for venography are less viscous than those previously used (which contained 28% iodine), and they tend to be carried away with the bloodstream more rapidly. For this reason, and also to shorten the length of time the contrast material is in contact with the endothelium, the injection should be completed as quickly as possible. The injection is therefore done by hand rather than by drip infusion as recommended by Kirschner et al. [93]. Power injectors are not used because of the potential danger of extravasation occurring.

The injection is performed under fluoroscopic monitoring at a rate of 0.5 to 1.0 cc per second. Abnormal flow patterns and localized filling defects can be immediately recognized. The amount of contrast material necessary for complete opacification of the veins is determined by direct fluoroscopic observation, usually 125 to 150 cc for each leg. The injection site should be observed fluoroscopically and visually in order that any extravasation can be recognized at once. Each segment of the venous system from the foot to the groin is recorded on spot films in various projections so that optimal display of the venous pathways is accomplished without overlapping (see Figs. 78-2, 78-4). Gentle palpation can be helpful to achieve complete opacification in local areas of imperfect filling. For the best radiographic detail, a small focal-spot tube (0.6 mm) and an automatic phototimer are used.

After completion of filling in all areas, the injection rate used during spot filming is slowed and radiographs are taken with an overhead tube at 40 inches target–film distance and Bucky film tray (see Fig. 78-3). Films measuring 7 by 17 inches are adequate for most patients. In the calf, anteroposterior stereoscopic views using lighter-and-darker technique are taken for the optimal demonstration of the superficial as well as the deep veins. A single lateral film of the same area is added.

An anteroposterior film of the thigh follows (see Fig. 78-4A). After completion of radiographic exposures the examiner immediately returns to the fluoroscopic mode for further evaluation of the upper femoral and iliac veins, in which flow defects are common at the sites of large-vein confluence. Here the patient is requested to perform a Valsalva maneuver and at the same time to press the foot down against the support of the examiner's hand as though to stand on the toes. By this combined maneuver the contrast material is propelled proximally and also fills the upper portion of the profunda vein in retrograde fashion down to at least the first valve (see Fig. 78-4B). Similarly, partial reflux filling of the internal iliac vein can be accomplished. Reactivation of a calf pump without a Valsalva maneuver will usually demonstrate the common iliac vein and portions of the lower vena cava as well (see Fig. 78-4C). The entire procedure can ordinarily be completed in approximately 5 minutes.

In the presence of deep vein thrombosis, any active efforts on the patient's part have to be omitted entirely because of the potential risk of embolization. Instead, the upper portions can be demonstrated by quickly returning the table to the horizontal plane and elevating the leg, to drain the contrast centrally, recording the iliac veins by spot films or large radiographs appropriately timed. Improved opacification of the iliac

veins by elevation of the leg while the table is still 30 degrees semiupright has been reported by Rampton and Armstrong [123]. Similar results have been obtained by placing the patient in the horizontal prone position [109]. In general, efforts are always made to demonstrate the venous structures as high as the inferior vena cava.

At the end of the examination, with the patient returned to the horizontal position, any residual contrast material detectable on fluoroscopy should be emptied from the leg either by elevation or by gentle massage or exercise. If thrombi are present in the leg veins, only passive drainage should be carried out.

The routine performance of the examination does not require the use of a tourniquet or cuff during the injection. The need for such devices is obviated by the semiupright position, in which the large volume of contrast injected easily distends and fills the entire venous system. Their use may, however, be called for under certain circumstances—as in the presence of extensive deep vein thrombosis where the contrast flow is diverted into the superficial veins exclusively, rendering the deep system completely unopacified. The tourniquet may be effective in some instances in forcing some contrast material to enter the deep veins. When such extensive flow diversions are present, it may be necessary to continue the rapid injection of contrast material during filming in order to demonstrate the collateral venous pathways.

An alternative method to overcome difficulties in filling of the deep veins in the presence of thrombosis is a maneuver described by Bergvall [25]. The patient is returned to the horizontal position and the leg is *injected* while elevated approximately 30 degrees instead of being dependent. The improved filling probably results from the fact that any liquid blood has been drained by this maneuver, allowing easier entrance of the contrast material into the deep compartment (Fig. 78-7).

A tourniquet may also be helpful in reducing abundant contrast filling of extensive varicose veins that may obscure the important events in the deep system. Here the tourniquet may be used during the initial part of the injection. An alternative method is to wrap the leg with an Ace bandage.

In any event, since the use of a tourniquet promotes stasis in the foot veins [146], increases the risk of extravasation, and renders the examination more uncomfortable, we recommend its

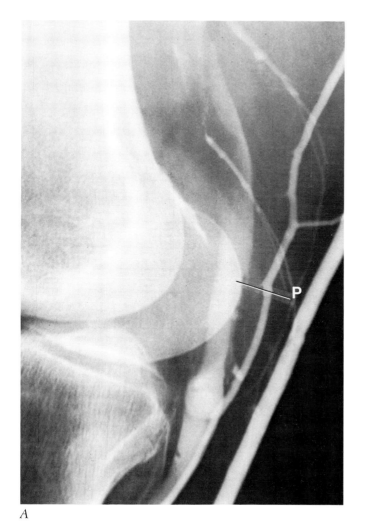
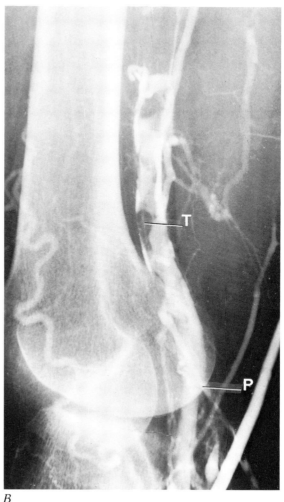

A   *B*

Figure 78-7. Venogram illustrating the effect of the Bergvall maneuver. (A) Lateral view of the popliteal vein (*P*) with the injection performed in the standard semiupright position. The popliteal vein is partly opacified, and a filling defect in the veins might be suspected. (B) Reinjection with the table horizontal and leg elevated 30 degrees, according to Bergvall, shows greatly improved opacification of the popliteal vein (*P*). The thrombus (*T*) is now much more clearly defined.

application sparingly and only under carefully controlled conditions.

The phlebographic technique here described, which makes use of the semiupright patient position and large volumes of contrast material, renders conclusive findings in the great majority of cases. It is rarely necessary to perform more proximal punctures in the popliteal or femoral veins to delineate the central extension of venous thrombosis.

In the rare event that percutaneous puncture of a peripheral foot vein proves to be unsuccessful, a higher-positioned superficial vein on the foot or the ankle may have to be used. In such instances it is advisable to direct the puncture distally so as to direct the contrast flow into the periphery. Only on very rare occasions is venous cutdown or intraosseous injection needed.

The Normal Venogram

A normal venogram as the result of the phlebographic technique just described is defined as follows (see Figs. 78-2–78-4):

1. Contrast filling has occurred in the normal fashion.

2. All deep and superficial veins are opacified except for the profunda femoris vein, which is demonstrated in only 50 percent of instances.
3. All veins are normal in appearance and free of filling defects.

On the radiographic films the veins are easily recognizable, and their topographic relationship to the osseous and soft tissue structures of the leg permit their easy anatomic identification [66].

In general, the lumina of contrast-filled normal veins are smoothly delineated, but they may be gently undulated or even slightly beaded. They may vary in shape and form. Thus the three paired deep main trunks are usually spindle-shaped or fusiform. The muscle veins are also fusiform, but they are shorter than the main trunks. Among the three paired trunks, the anterior tibial veins are the smallest, whereas either the posterior tibial veins or the peroneal veins may be the largest. The communicating veins are often slightly wavy or curved and tend to have a larger diameter closer to their junction with the deep veins. They are often single but may be paired and may enter the deep veins obliquely or perpendicularly. The superficial veins are generally smaller in caliber than the deep veins. They have parallel walls and thus a structure that appears more tubular or "straw-shaped."

Valves are ordinarily present and visible throughout the venous system. The valve leaflets are readily recognized in profile. The sinuses behind the valve leaflets are also usually quite evident. They may become more prominent with the performance of the Valsalva maneuver.

The veins are likely to vary in caliber according to the size and activity of the extremity (Fig. 78-8). The muscle veins, for example, vary greatly in caliber with the mass of muscle that they subserve; they may therefore be capacious and saccular in the muscular athletic calf. On the other hand, they may be very small and sparsely filled in elderly patients. Further, with prolonged bed rest or extended use of elastic stockings or Ace bandages, the veins generally diminish in caliber throughout the extremity and may become quite attenuated.

The diagnosis of a normal venogram constitutes information that strongly influences the patient's clinical management. Only a complete and high-quality phlebogram can exclude thrombosis with the required degree of certainty. Any significant deviation from the normal appearance must be regarded as pathologic unless it can be

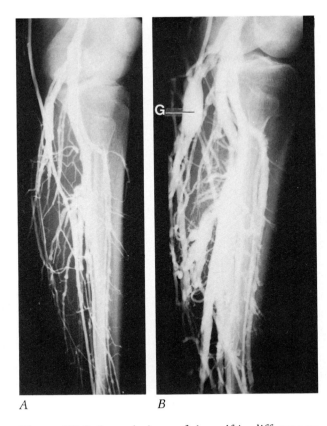

A   *B*

Figure 78-8. Lateral views of the calf in different patients to show the variation in the size of veins in the calves of normal patients. (A) Slender leg of young woman. (B) Large muscular calf of athletic male. Note the large saccular gastrocnemius veins (*G*).

explained by an unavoidable fault in technique, prior surgery, etc.

Pitfalls in Performance and Interpretation

Although the standard technique aims at the optimal and most complete opacification of the venous system, in reality this ideal cannot be accomplished in all instances. Limiting circumstances are frequently related to the condition of the patient: inadvertent muscle contractions, inability to cooperate, illness so severe that the venogram must be obtained in bed, etc. Known artifacts may be expected under these circumstances and can be readily recognized. Familiarity with the most common of these artifacts is important since they may closely simulate the radiologic signs of venous thrombosis [10, 122, 149].

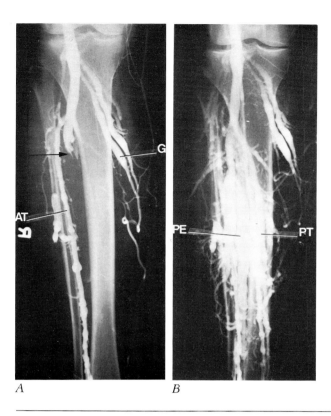

A   *B*

Figure 78-9. Artifactual nonopacification of the posterior tibial and peroneal veins caused by the combined use of the tourniquet in the weight-bearing patient. (A) Anteroposterior view of the leg with the patient weight-bearing and a tourniquet applied at the ankle. The posterior tibial and peroneal veins are not opacified and appear to end just below the entrance of the anterior tibial veins (*arrow*). Contrast material ascends through the anterior tibial and gastrocnemius veins. (B) Reinjection performed immediately afterward but with the patient bearing no weight on the leg and with the tourniquet removed. The appearance of the venogram is normal. *AT* = Anterior tibial veins; *G* = gastrocnemius veins; *PE* = peroneal veins; *PT* = posterior tibial veins.

Figure 78-10. Artifactual nonopacification of the anterior tibial veins (*AT*) caused by compression of these veins against the tibia by the tourniquet (*TQ*). (A) Lateral view of the ankle during injection with the tourniquet in place. The anterior tibial vein is compressed against the tibia and fails to opacify. (B) Upon reinjection with the tourniquet removed, the anterior tibial veins opacify normally.

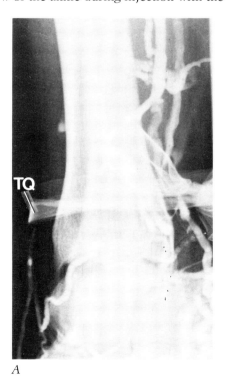

A

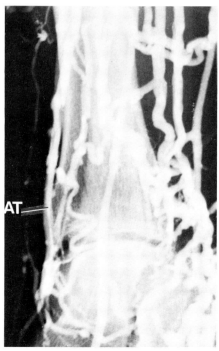

B

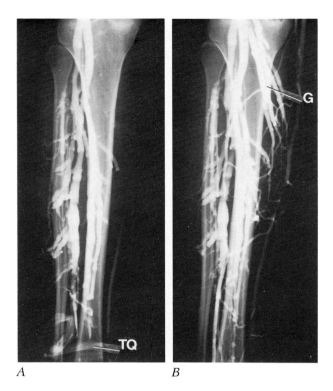

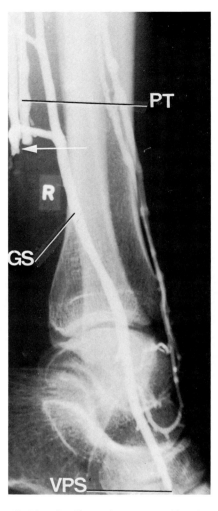

Figure 78-11. Artifactual nonopacification of the gastrocnemius veins (*G*) caused by the tourniquet (*TQ*). (A) Anteroposterior view of the leg with the tourniquet applied at the ankle during the injection. The tourniquet has occluded the superficial veins that normally drain into the gastrocnemius veins, preventing their opacification. (B) Reinjection performed immediately afterward with the tourniquet removed. The gastrocnemius veins now opacify normally.

Figure 78-12. Artifactual nonopacification of the distal parts of the posterior tibial veins produced by injection into the greater saphenous vein in the proximal part of the foot. The usual routes of access of the contrast material into the deep plantar veins are bypassed, and retrograde flow into them may be prevented by valves in the saphenous vein. The posterior tibial veins appear to end, simulating venous occlusion (*arrow*). Reinjection distally in the foot in such instances will result in normal opacification of the plantar venous arch and posterior tibial veins. *GS* = Greater saphenous vein; *PT* = posterior tibial veins; *VPS* = venipuncture site.

It is well established that contraction of the calf muscles results in compression of the deep veins, thus causing incomplete filling during phlebography. Not generally appreciated, however, is the fact that weight bearing, such as occurs in a standing or semiupright position, may also cause incomplete filling of the deep veins as well as flow diversions of contrast material and apparent abrupt endings of veins [122]. The combination of weight bearing and tourniquet may have a particularly detrimental effect upon venous opacification, resulting in very restricted venous filling and bizarre appearances that may simulate all the signs of deep vein thrombosis (Fig. 78-9). Pseudoobstruction of the popliteal vein due to compression by tensed muscles in the popliteal fossa has been described [12] but is unlikely to occur with the technique described herein since the leg is relaxed.

A tourniquet, most commonly placed at the ankle to direct the contrast material preferentially into the deep system, compresses not only the superficial venous pathways but also the anterior tibial veins by squeezing them against the bony structures and thus preventing their filling (Fig. 78-10). A tourniquet may also prevent filling of the gastrocnemius veins by compressing the

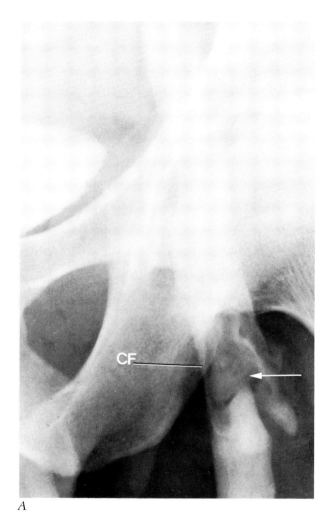

A

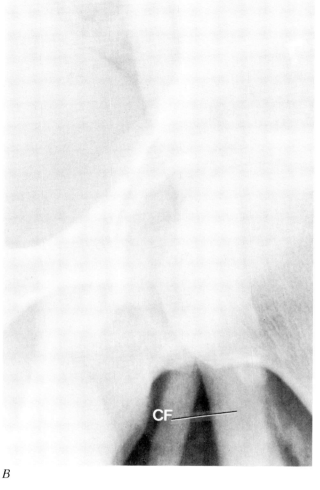

B

Figure 78-13. Flow defect caused by the entry of unopacified blood from the profunda vein into the common femoral vein (*CF*). (A) Anteroposterior spot film showing flow defect (*arrow*). (B) Repeat film immediately afterward with Valsalva maneuver showing the common femoral vein to be normal.

superficial veins that drain into them from the lower calf (Fig. 78-11).

Injection performed more proximally than the ideal site at the base of the large toe may result in incomplete filling of the distal veins. For example, needle placement along the medial aspect of the proximal foot may cause the contrast material to bypass the deep veins in the foot and ankle and to progress directly upward into the superficial system or anterior tibial veins to the level of the midcalf (Fig. 78-12). Proximal injections along the lateral aspect of the foot may direct the contrast material into the lesser saphenous system, again causing nonfilling of the deep veins in the foot and distal calf. Such appearances may simulate those of deep vein thrombosis.

Artifactual filling defects may be due to in-

complete mixing and separation of flow between the unopacified blood and contrast medium. These are seen most commonly at the junctions of large veins such as the entrance of the profunda femoris vein into the common femoral vein (Fig. 78-13) and at the entrance of the internal iliac vein into the common iliac vein. Irregular opacification simulating local filling defects may also occur in deep calf veins shortly after calf contraction; conversely, central filling defects may be seen in superficial varicose veins in the presence of valvular incompetence [10]. All these filling defects tend to be inconstant and changing in appearance. Fluoroscopic observation and the use of multiple spot films are necessary to avoid diagnostic errors.

Finally, it may be emphasized that the use of

insufficient volume of contrast material will increase the frequency with which mixing and flow-induced artifacts will occur. Hence, the use of relatively large volumes of contrast medium, as suggested for complete and reliable phlebographic examination, is urged.

Complications of Venography

Immediate side effects or symptoms associated with the injection of the usual contrast materials include urticaria, nausea, metallic taste, and sensation of warmth. Cramplike pain occurring in the foot and calf during the injection is probably related to the hyperosmolar contrast material, which has to be injected in large quantities.

Systemic reactions to contrast materials in conjunction with the performance of venography of the lower extremities are similar to those reported in other types of radiologic contrast examinations and are uncommon [20, 39].

Pulmonary embolism produced by the performance of phlebography is very rare. Albrechtsson and Olsson [4] reported two cases of nonfatal pulmonary emboli arising from postphlebographic thrombosis. The possibility that the procedure will dislodge preexisting fresh thrombi must be considered but also appears to be extremely rare. We have recorded two patients with clinical signs and symptoms and pulmonary radionuclide scan evidence of pulmonary embolism within an hour following phlebography (see Fig. 78-21). Obviously it is advisable to avoid any active or passive maneuvers such as muscle exercise or vigorous massage of the leg during venography if deep vein thrombosis is present.

Delayed side effects may follow the performance of venography of the lower extremities. Pain, tenderness, and erythema in the ankle or lower calf, the so-called postphlebographic syndrome, occurred in 24 percent of patients in whom the phlebogram was obtained with 60 percent contrast material [26]. The incidence of these symptoms was reduced to 7.5 percent with the use of 45 percent contrast material. Bettmann et al. [27] noted that the development of this syndrome did not necessarily correlate with the subsequent development of postphlebographic thrombosis, which has been reported to occur in an incidence of 2.7, 26, 33, and 48 percent with the injection of 60 percent contrast material [4,

5, 20, 27]. The frequency of postphlebographic thrombosis was reduced from 26 to 9 percent (3% deep and 6% superficial) by the substitution of 45 percent contrast material [27]. These complications are therefore believed to be strongly related to the concentration and composition of the injected contrast material. Arndt et al. [13] reported a decreased incidence of complications with the infusion of heparin into the leg veins immediately before and after the venogram was obtained. The prophylactic use of heparin in the prevention of postvenographic thrombosis is controversial. A thorough discussion of this matter can be found in a 1979 dissertation by Olsson [117].

Postvenographic thrombosis appears generally to be a self-limited process, provoked by the irritating nature of the hyperosmolar contrast material. It responds favorably to symptomatic treatment in most instances, though occasionally the symptoms may be severe enough to require anticoagulation. Recent reports of phlebography performed with metrizamide, a nonionic contrast material of significantly lower osmolarity, indicate a marked reduction of immediate or delayed patient discomfort and the complete absence of abnormal radioactive fibrinogen uptake tests in follow-up examinations [6]. Obviously, the use of such modern radiographic contrast agents will reduce these unpleasant side effects significantly, if not eliminate them completely.

Another rare but serious consequence to phlebography is necrosis of the skin and subcutaneous tissue at the site of injection. This complication occurs when contrast material extravasates because of either faulty position of the needle or increased venous pressure, which may accompany deep vein thrombosis or the use of the tourniquet. A greatly reduced incidence of extravasation has been reported with the use of a small, flexible Teflon cannula in place of the needle [61]. At least nine cases of severe complications associated with contrast extravasation have been reported [39, 60, 62, 137]. Eight of these nine cases have been associated with use of the tourniquet. Preexisting arterial disease or chronic venous insufficiency predisposes the tissues to the development of this complication.

Gangrene of the toes was reported by Thomas [146] in two cases, apparently caused by trapping of the contrast material in the foot veins rather than by extravasation. In one case deep vein thrombosis was present, and in the other there was a venous anomaly in conjunction with a hemangioma. In both instances reduced venous flow, compounded by the use of the tourniquet, may have contributed to this complication.

For patients with a history of previous serious reaction to contrast material, iodine sensitivity, allergies, or the presence of renal failure, a relative contraindication exists and the expected benefit of the examination should be reassessed in the light of these circumstances.

The Abnormal Venogram

The major clinical reasons for venography are to search for thrombus in patients suspected of having acute deep vein thrombosis or pulmonary embolism, to demonstrate the location of incompetent perforating veins in the presence of varicose veins, and to evaluate the venous system in the presence of chronic venous insufficiency.

Acute Deep Vein Thrombosis

The optimal practice of venography in the diagnosis of deep vein thrombosis requires that the radiologist be familiar not only with the radiologic aspects of this disease but also with its natural history, clinical manifestations, pathology, and therapy, and the relationship to its most serious complication, pulmonary embolism. With such background knowledge, the radiologist may appropriately integrate use of venography with the practice of newer noninvasive methods available for the diagnosis and follow-up of deep vein thrombosis.

The basic pathologic process in deep vein thrombosis is the bland clotting of blood within the deep veins, resulting in thrombi that may vary in size from microscopic to massive and forming a cast of the entire venous system of the extremity. It is estimated that there are 2.5 million cases of acute deep vein thrombosis each year in the United States [133].

Thrombi tend to start behind valve cusps [129]. They grow circumferentially and longitudinally by accretion, forming successive layers of platelet-fibrin and red-cell thrombus. The attachment of the thrombi is fibrinous and exists at first only at the site of origin, a major

portion of the thrombus being unattached. Later, additional attachments may develop, with invasion of fibrocytes and capillaries from the venous epithelium into the clot. This is, however, not a universal occurrence, and not infrequently, as serum is squeezed out and the aging clot contracts, its surface is pulled away from the vein wall. This retraction, together with the thrombolytic activity of the endothelium, may keep the thrombus attachment quite restricted (see Fig. 78-25B).

If the thrombus is large enough to obstruct the flow in the vein, it may also extend in retrograde fashion. Under such conditions, the thrombus is considered to consist of a body attached to the vein wall, a tail growing against the blood flow toward the periphery, and a thrombus head that propagates centrally toward the inferior vena cava and right heart (see Fig. 78-25B). It is from this head that potential pulmonary emboli may become detached.

Radiologic Signs of Acute Deep Vein Thrombosis

All phlebographic manifestations of deep vein thrombosis are related to the presence of the thrombus itself or to the changes in blood flow that are caused by it. No radiologic phlebographic signs have been described that indicate inflammation in the vein wall either preceding or following the thrombosis.

Conclusive evidence of deep vein thrombosis consists in the direct demonstration of a constant filling defect or defects in veins (Figs. 78-14–78-18) representing the actual thrombus [29, 99, 122, 157]. Filling defects should be confirmed in more than one view. They may be present in veins at any level of the extremity from the foot [63, 100] to the inferior vena cava.

Highly suggestive of, but not conclusive for, the diagnosis of deep vein thrombosis are ending of the opaque column in a vein, failure to opacify a vein or veins, and abnormal diversion of contrast flow (Figs. 78-19–78-22). The last two signs often appear together. Nonopacification of the calf veins usually indicates extension of the thrombotic process to involve the popliteal or higher veins [114]. The combination of intraluminal clot and inflammation and edema at

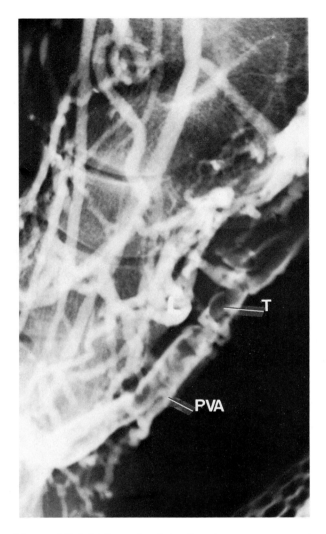

Figure 78-14. Thrombosis in the plantar venous arch. Lateral view of the foot. The plantar venous arch is the second most common site of deep vein thrombosis. *PVA* = Plantar venous arch; *T* = thrombus.

These veins are also rather densely opacified during venography because they transport the contrast material exclusively and in a relatively less dilute state than usual. The communicating veins may also be quite dilated, so that their valves become incompetent and the flow through them is reversed. Entry of this unopacified blood into the superficial veins may cause streaming or "knothole" defects in the opacified superficial veins (Fig. 78-23).

Although the indirect signs of ending of the opaque column, nonopacification, and flow diversion are highly suggestive of deep vein thrombosis, they can occasionally be caused by marked leg edema, cellulitis, muscle rupture, hematoma, or periarticular cysts, and the diagnosis of deep vein thrombosis is justified only after exclusion of these conditions. Most common is muscle rupture with hematoma. The usual history is that of a sudden acute pain in the calf during effort, with marked painful swelling beginning immediately and then increasing over the next few hours. Within a week to 10 days, bluish yellow discoloration may appear in the calf or ankle, caused by degradation products of the hematoma leaking through the fascia. In our experience, patients with these hematomas frequently develop the complication of venous thrombosis in the injured area. If the basic process is deep vein thrombosis rather than muscle rupture with hematoma, the swelling and tenderness usually do not appear until several days after the injury.

The phlebographic signs of hematoma may vary from a minimal spreading of the veins to displacement and compression of veins, extensive flow diversion and nonfilling, and ending of the opaque column in veins. No venous thrombi, however, will be visible in the uncomplicated case of muscle rupture. Veins tend to fill in normal fashion but to empty quickly because of compression caused by the hematoma (Fig. 78-24). The phlebographic abnormalities may be minimal, far out of proportion to the clinical signs and symptoms. The opposite situation may exist in deep vein thrombosis where phlebography may show extensive thrombotic changes in comparison with the minimal clinical findings.

If total nonopacification of the deep veins occurs initially, further attempts should be made to demonstrate the deep veins as previously described, preferably using the Bergvall maneuver, or the tourniquet under carefully controlled circumstances.

the attachment sites to the endothelium may raise the pressure in the inelastic deep fascial compartment to a level above the venous pressure outside it and prevent the contrast material from entering the deep veins within this space. According to Brodelius et al. [30], this occurs in up to 80 percent of instances of extensive acute deep vein thrombosis. Under these circumstances, the superficial veins tend to be dilated and the flow through them is rapid since they carry an increased share of the venous return from the leg.

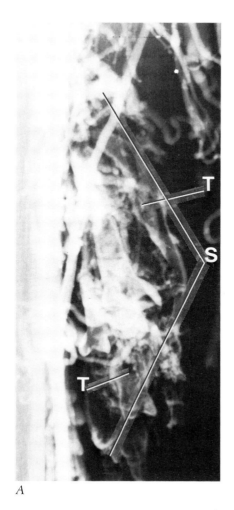

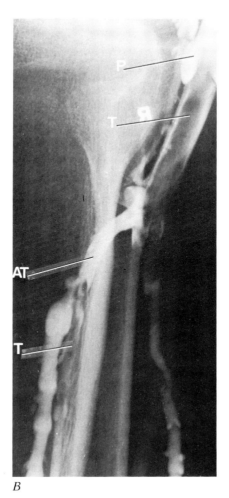

A   *B*

Figure 78-15. Thrombi in the calf veins. (A) Thrombi in the soleal muscle veins. Lateral view of the calf. The calf veins are the most common site of deep vein thrombosis. Thrombi arising in the calf veins may at-tain large size. (B) Spread of venous thrombosis from the calf to the popliteal vein in another patient. *AT* = Anterior tibial veins; *S* = soleal muscle veins with thrombi; *T* = thrombi; *P* = popliteal vein.

Venography is a reliable test for confirming or excluding deep vein thrombosis. Demonstration of the actual thrombus makes the diagnosis certain. A properly obtained normal venogram showing none of the signs just described excludes deep vein thrombosis for practical clinical purposes [155]. Since anticoagulation therapy is effective in controlling the thrombotic process in most patients [42, 132, 135], it is ordinarily not necessary to demonstrate the entire extent of the thrombotic process or its additional presence in other locations once the presence of thrombus has been demonstrated in the deep veins or identified in the form of an embolus in the pulmonary arteries. It is more important to show clearly the total extent of the thrombotic process when venous interruption or thrombectomy is considered because of nonadherent clot constituting a likely source of pulmonary embolism [31], or when there is contraindication to, or complication or failure of, anticoagulation.

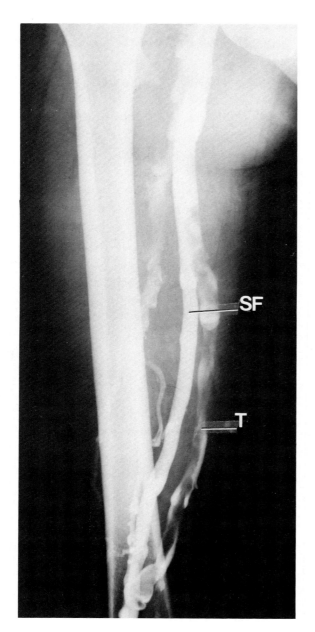

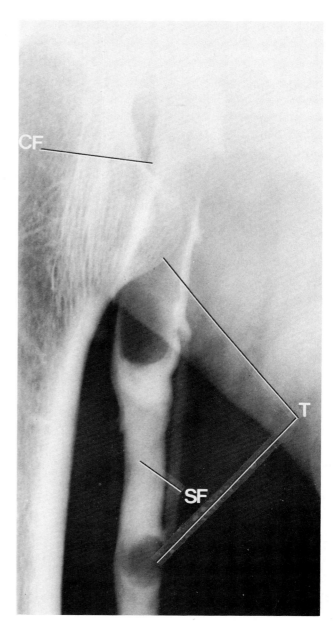

Figure 78-16. Thrombosis in one channel of a partially duplicated superficial femoral vein. The other channel is normal. Preservation of flow through the patent channel or around incompletely occluding thrombi (see Fig. 78-26) readily explains the false-negative or indeterminate results of the impedance phlebogram in such cases. *SF* = Superficial femoral vein, normal channel; *T* = thrombosed channel of superficial femoral vein.

Figure 78-17. Thrombi in the upper femoral vein. Anteroposterior spot film of upper femoral region. The more proximal larger thrombus appears to have only a small area of attachment to the vein wall. *CF* = Common femoral vein; *SF* = superficial femoral vein; *T* = thrombi.

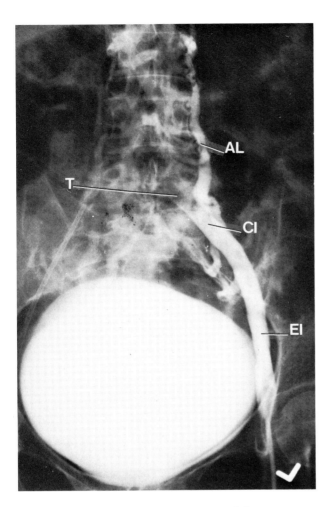

Figure 78-18. Thrombotic occlusion of the upper part of the common femoral vein with collateral flow through the ascending lumbar vein. Anteroposterior view of the iliac area. The occlusion was demonstrated on spot films of the area during standard lower limb venography but is better visualized on this catheter injection into the femoral vein. The patient presented with chronic swelling in the calf and thigh. *AL* = Ascending lumbar vein; *CI* = common iliac vein; *EI* = external iliac vein; *T* = thrombus.

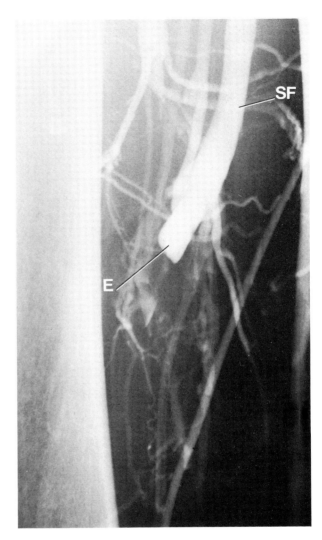

Figure 78-19. Abrupt ending of the opaque column (*E*) in a vein. Anteroposterior view of the superficial femoral vein (*SF*) showing that the opaque column ends in a downward direction. Occluded veins may also appear to end in an upward direction (see also Figs. 78-18, 78-20B). This sign indicates occlusion of the vein if it has not been produced by a failure of technique (see Fig. 78-12).

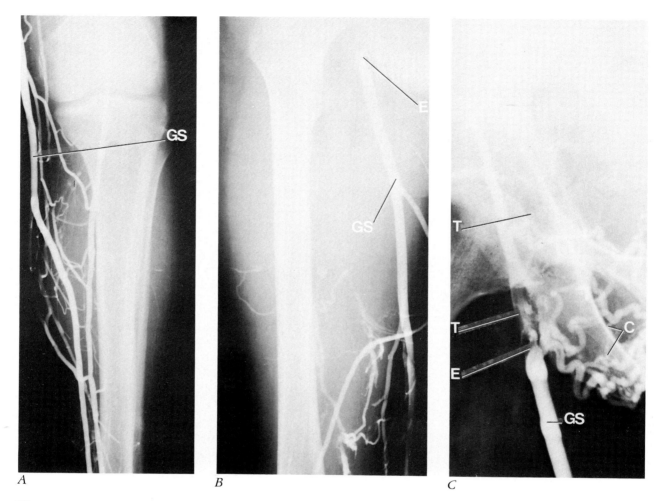

Figure 78-20. Failure of the deep veins to opacify and extensive diversion of flow in a patient with widespread acute deep vein thrombosis. Anteroposterior views of the leg (A), thigh (B), and pelvis (C). There is practically no opacification in the deep veins in any of these areas. Contrast material ascends exclusively through the superficial veins, which are densely opacified and slightly dilated. Collateral flow is evident in the pubic region. A small thrombus is visible in the upper end of the greater saphenous vein, and a large thrombus can be faintly seen in the external iliac vein. C = Collateral veins at pubic region; GS = greater saphenous vein; T = thrombus; E = ending of the opaque column in the saphenous vein.

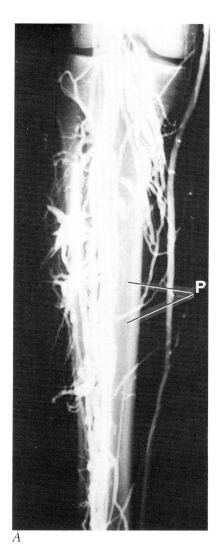 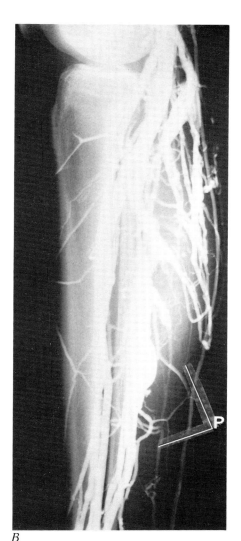

A   *B*

Figure 78-21. Thrombosis of the posterior tibial veins. Anteroposterior (A) and lateral (B) views of the leg. The posterior tibial veins (*P*) are unopacified. Small thrombi were seen in the proximal part of the peroneal veins and soleal muscle veins. Note that the soleal muscle veins in the medial part of the calf are not opacified (compare with Fig. 78-5). This patient suffered a pulmonary embolus within minutes following performance of the phlebogram.

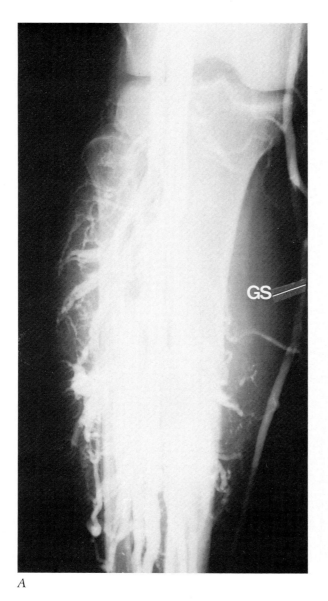

A

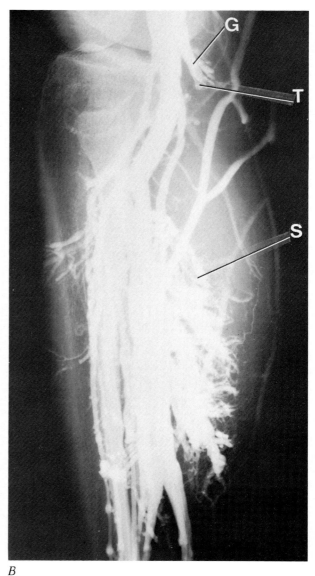

B

Figure 78-22. Thrombosis of the gastrocnemius veins. Anteroposterior (A) and lateral (B) views of the calf. Marked swelling in the proximal calf displaces the greater saphenous vein (*GS*) medially and the soleal muscle veins (*S*) downward. Small amounts of thrombus (*T*) are present in the stumps of the gastrocnemius veins (*G*), which are otherwise unopacified. Compare with Figures 78-11 and 78-24.

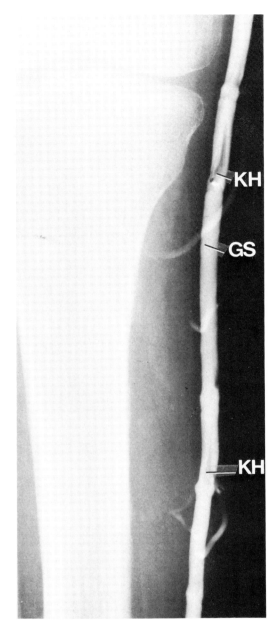

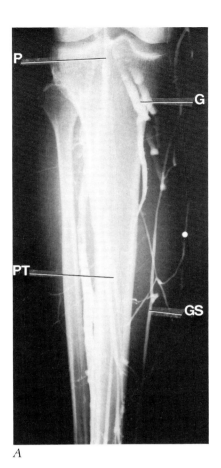

A

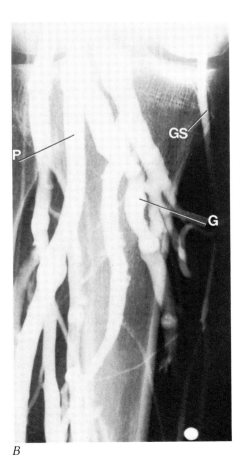

B

Figure 78-23. Flow defects caused by entry of un-opacified blood from the deep veins into the greater saphenous vein (*GS*), so-called knotholes (*KH*). An-teroposterior view of the upper calf. Note non-opacification of the deep veins and dense contrast material in the dilated greater saphenous vein.

Figure 78-24. Phlebographic appearance of muscle ▶ hematoma. (A) Anteroposterior view of the leg. There is marked soft tissue swelling displacing and compress-ing the veins. The BB is at the site of greatest clinical swelling. (B) Earlier spot film of the upper calf shows that the veins filled much better earlier in the exam-ination but have emptied quickly because of compres-sion. No thrombi are seen. *G* = Gastrocnemius veins; *GS* = greater saphenous vein; *P* = popliteal vein; *PT* = posterior tibial veins.

Phlebographic Changes Related to the Age of the Thrombosis

Correlation between phlebographic and clinical findings to establish venographic criteria for age of a thrombotic process must necessarily be inconsistent, because the process is often asymptomatic for a varying number of days initially. More precise determination of onset can be accomplished by the prospective use of the radioactive fibrinogen uptake test. When used in combination with phlebography, this test has helped to assess more accurately the natural history of deep vein thrombosis. Sequential veno-

graphic studies [73] have shown that within 10 days to 2 weeks the abnormal flow pattern induced by deep vein thrombosis will return toward normal, with at least some contrast material entering the deep calf veins. Total nonopacification of the deep veins in the calf does not usually persist permanently. From the appearance of the thrombotic process, it can be deduced that initial nonvisualization during the acute stages of the process was not necessarily caused by total thrombosis but was probably related to raised pressure within the deep calf compartment. Permanent occlusion of the femoral and iliac veins is much more frequent.

The fate of a vein containing thrombus on an initial examination is variable. The vein may re-

---

Figure 78-25. Morphologic changes in the appearance of thrombus according to age. Anteroposterior views of the superficial femoral veins in two different patients. (A) Fresh thrombus (*T*) almost entirely filling the lumen of the vein. A thin layer of contrast material (*CM*) almost completely separates the thrombus from the vein wall. (B) Aging thrombus (*T*) showing early stages of retraction. The thrombus has shrunk and is separated from the vein wall except for attachments at several locations (*arrows*). The layer of contrast material (*CM*) between the thrombus and the vein wall is much wider. The margins of the thrombus have an undulating contour. Venography was performed 1 month following gastric resection with complicated postoperative course. The impedance phlebogram was abnormal.

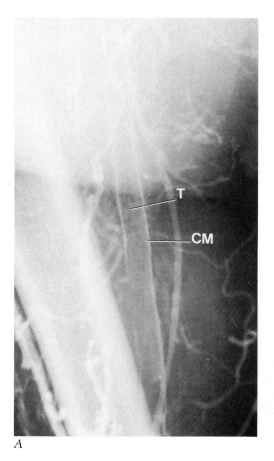

A

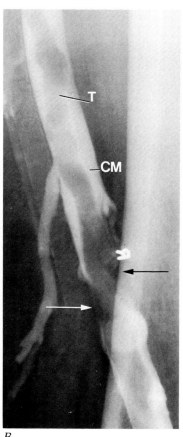

B

turn to an entirely normal appearance with complete resorption of the clot, it may become completely occluded, or it may recanalize (see Figs. 78-32, 78-33) [147]. These changes can take place over a varying period of time of many days, weeks, or months. Recanalization of originally totally or partially occluded veins occurs as a rule within 6 months but may not be complete for up to 4 years [72]. In general, resorption of thrombus in the peripheral veins is much slower than in the pulmonary arteries. Thrombolytic therapy increases the rate of resorption but appears to be less effective the later it is initiated after the onset of symptoms.

Phlebographic assessment of the age of the thrombus is possible to a certain degree by paying attention to certain morphologic appearances [147]. Fresh clots are characterized by having a small area of attachment to the vein wall, usually behind a valve [76], but otherwise being separated from the vein wall and having a smooth "turgid" appearance. They are surrounded by a thin layer of contrast agent filling the space between the thrombus and the adjacent vein wall (Fig. 78-25A). Within 48 hours the thrombus may show increasing adherence to the vein wall, causing the separating contrast layer at the areas of fixation to disappear. Finally, these adhesions may result in obliteration of the entire internal circumference, with complete occlusion of the vein. On the other hand, thrombi may lose fluid content, shrinking and retracting within a few days to a more irregular contour and allowing increased width of the surrounding contrast layer (Fig. 78-25B).

Etiology and Incidence of Deep Vein Thrombosis

Although further knowledge concerning the clotting process continues to accumulate [107, 129], the pathogenesis of deep vein thrombosis is still believed to be multifactorial and to involve the basic triad described by Virchow in 1856: slowing of the venous blood flow, injury to the intima, and increased coagulability of the blood itself. Some individuals in the general population appear to be particularly prone to repeated episodes of deep vein thrombosis without obvious cause.

On the other hand, certain conditions such as malignancy, obesity, and increasing age are known to predispose to the development of deep vein thrombosis [107]. Other recognized provoking factors are trauma, surgery, prolonged immobilization, status postmyocardial infarction, congestive failure, use of the contraceptive pill, etc. Gjöres [57] estimated that in 18 percent of a series of 303 patients the thrombosis had apparently arisen as a primary spontaneous event. The results of several workers [40, 77, 88, 91, 136, 139] agree that deep vein thrombosis occurs in 25 to 30 percent of patients undergoing abdominal surgery and in 40 to 60 percent of patients with fracture or surgery of the hip or upper femur or undergoing knee surgery. In nonsurgical conditions, the incidence of deep vein thrombosis varies from less than 1 percent among users of the contraceptive pill to 17 to 30 percent of patients with myocardial infarction or in coronary care units [88, 103]. At extremely high risk are elderly patients with fracture of the femur or myocardial infarction, in whom the incidence of deep vein thrombosis may be as high as 75 to 85 percent [86, 103, 130]. In general, deep vein thrombosis is slightly more common in the left leg than in the right leg, possibly because of compression of the left iliac vein by the right iliac artery.

Clinical studies have shown the thombotic process to be bilateral in approximately 30 percent of patients [33, 88], and a recent randomized autopsy study of patients who died in the hospital has shown the process to be bilateral in approximately 85 percent [76]. According to Wheeler and Patwardhan [153], deep vein thrombosis "exists on a wide spectrum of severity ranging from the extremely common but relatively benign calf vein thrombosis to the less common but more dangerous femoral or iliac vein thrombosis." The results of the pioneering studies performed by Rössle [126] on postmortem examinations lead to the general opinion that deep vein thrombosis begins most commonly in the venous sinuses of the calf muscles, especially the soleal sinusoids (see Fig. 78-15A). From here they may extend into the posterior tibial and peroneal veins and above to the popliteal veins (see Fig. 78-15B). The first large phlebographic series performed by Bauer [22] supported this concept, as have more recent postmortem examinations [75, 76, 130], venographic studies [33, 90, 113, 138], and isotope tests [8, 90]. The fate of such initial calf vein thrombi may vary significantly. In 30 to 35 percent of patients they lyse within 72 hours, and in another 50 percent they persist but remain localized to the calf [90]. In only 20 to 30 percent of instances does proximal propagation occur into the larger veins of the thigh [88, 90, 112].

The original site of deep vein thrombosis may, however, be found in other locations such as the iliofemoral segments [105]. This site is particularly common in patients who have had local trauma or surgery to the thigh or hip [139]. Under these circumstances, extension of the thrombosis in the peripheral direction may also occur. Still, the latter type of deep vein thrombosis progression is less frequent, according to Schmitt [127], who analyzed phlebograms obtained in general patient data using morphologic criteria for recent and older thrombi. Schmitt concluded that local factors determined the primary site of origin, but in their absence, simultaneous or consecutive development of thrombi

may occur at different sites. Sevitt [129, 130] has shown by dissection studies that thrombosis can begin at various places in the leg and describes six main primary sites of origin. These findings have been confirmed by Havig [76]. The data presented in these papers are in basic agreement that the calf veins are the most common site of deep vein thrombosis, with a progressively diminishing incidence in the popliteal, femoral, and iliac veins. The profunda femoris vein is involved in approximately 17 percent of instances [76]. However, it is rarely the sole site of deep vein thrombosis, being associated with thrombosis of the iliac veins in 63 percent of instances and thrombosis of more peripheral veins in 85 percent [76].

As already noted, the thrombotic process is a common and benign disease [88]. Its course tends to be self-limited in the majority of in-

Figure 78-26. Thrombosis of the greater saphenous vein (*GS*) extending into the common femoral vein (*CF*). (A) Anteroposterior radiograph of the calf. (B) Anteroposterior spot film of the groin region. The thrombus (*T*) in the greater saphenous vein extended from the midcalf level through the thigh to the saphenofemoral junction. The impedance phlebogram was reported as equivocal.

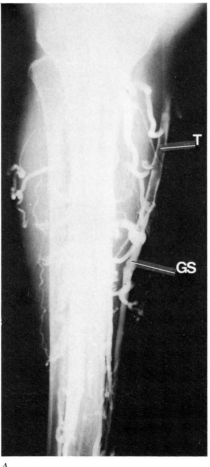

A

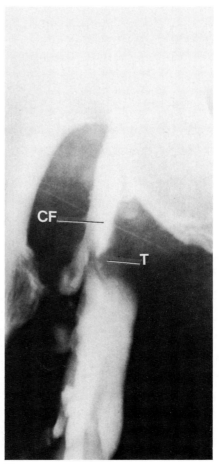

B

stances. It is estimated that in more than half of the cases the condition is undiagnosed and untreated and apparently resolves spontaneously. The tendency to be a clinically silent process, with objective signs and symptoms manifest in only 50 percent of occurrences [90, 107], can be explained by the fact that the clotting process during thrombus formation is bland and noninflammatory [129]. Evidence has been brought forward that inflammation does not precede and cause the thrombosis [76, 129]; rather, the formation of the thrombus irritates the vein wall and adjacent tissue, causing secondary inflammation, which, in turn, accounts for the presence of clinical signs and symptoms. It is therefore appropriate to use the term *deep vein thrombosis* rather than *thrombophlebitis* [142], since the latter term implies that inflammation is a primary cause of the process.

The local clinical signs and symptoms of deep vein thrombosis are the result of obstruction or inflammation produced by the thrombus [107, 114]. Inflammation occurs at the site of origin or of subsequent adherence of the thrombus to the endothelium of the vein. Fresh thrombi may have a very limited attachment, so that a large portion of the clot has no direct contact with the vein wall. Further, venous blood may flow around such thrombi with relatively little interference (Fig. 78-26) or may ascend through collateral pathways (see Fig. 78-16). These circumstances explain why there may be minimal or no signs and symptoms even in the presence of extensive fresh vein thrombosis. They also explain why the signs and symptoms occurring in conjunction with deep vein thrombosis are nonspecific and may simulate those of other common conditions: cellulitis, arthritis, muscle rupture, soft tissue hematoma. Indeed, sensitivity and specificity of the clinical signs of deep vein thrombosis are very low, approximately 50 percent, giving rise to the general statement that deep vein thrombosis may be both a greatly overdiagnosed and a greatly underdiagnosed condition [78].

Venography in Pulmonary Embolism

The diagnosis of pulmonary embolism relies heavily on the use of chest x-ray films, radionuclide scans, and pulmonary angiography. Since, however, pulmonary embolism is not a disease process itself, but rather a complication of deep vein thrombosis, the use of venography might be indicated to search for sites of potential emboli. Browse and Thomas [33] have shown that pulmonary emboli arise from deep vein thrombosis in all sites in proportion to their incidence. Consequently, these authors state that because the calf veins are the most common site of deep vein thrombosis, they are also the most common site of origin for pulmonary emboli. Kakkar et al. [90] reported no clinical evidence of pulmonary embolism in patients who, with radioactive fibrinogen scanning, showed thrombosis limited to the calf, but they observed a 44 percent incidence of pulmonary embolism when the thrombosis extended to the popliteal and femoral veins. However, using phlebography for diagnosis and localization of deep vein thrombosis, Moreno-Cabral et al. [106] found an incidence of pulmonary embolism of 66 percent following popliteal vein thrombosis and 33 percent following tibial vein thrombosis. The diagnosis of pulmonary embolism was based on abnormal findings on radionuclide scans and thus included cases that were clinically silent. A dissection study of the lower extremity venous tree and pulmonary arteries by Havig [76] showed that in 25 percent of patients with serious pulmonary emboli and in 45 percent of patients with not serious pulmonary emboli, the emboli arose from the calf veins. Obviously such variations in the reported incidence and site of origin of pulmonary emboli may be explained by the different methods used to detect both deep vein thrombosis and pulmonary embolism rather than reflect a true difference in the occurrence of these events.

There are an estimated 500,000 cases of pulmonary embolism and 50,000 cases of fatal pulmonary embolism in the United States annually [107]. Although it is known that 85 to 95 percent of pulmonary emboli arise from leg veins [107, 133], only about half of the patients have any prior symptoms or clinical evidence of venous thrombosis in the legs [33, 55, 78, 90, 128]. Indeed, Kakkar [89] states that 80 percent of pulmonary emboli arise without any premonitory signs in the legs. This circumstance explains why deep vein thrombosis is often not diagnosed until pulmonary embolism has occurred. The diagnostic dilemma is compounded by the fact that pulmonary embolism itself may be clinically silent in a great number of instances [32, 106].

According to Hirsch [78], and Browse and Thomas [33], venography demonstrates the presence of thrombus in the veins of the lower extremities in 70 percent of patients with pulmonary embolism. Browse et al. [32] found that the less specific fibrinogen uptake test can be positive in 85 percent of patients with pulmonary embolism. Negative results from these tests suggest that the emboli may have originated from another source, but one has to consider the possibility that the negative finding merely indicates that the thrombi have already been entirely cleared from the extremity.

Superficial Vein Thrombosis

Thrombosis is a relatively common occurrence in superficial veins, especially in varicose veins. In the majority of instances, the thrombotic process is restricted to the superficial veins, though Hafner et al. [74] reported a 17 percent incidence of deep vein thrombosis in association with superficial vein thrombosis. Our own experience in a small ongoing series of patients who appear with definite clinical signs and symptoms and phlebographic findings of superficial vein thrombosis is in agreement with their data. Accompanying deep vein thrombosis is most commonly limited to the calf. However, superficial vein thrombosis may propagate directly into the saphenofemoral or saphenopopliteal junctions [50, 58, 59, 74, 86] (Fig. 78-26). Pulmonary embolism in association with superficial vein thrombosis has been reported in approximately 10 percent of instances [87, 158]. Serious embolism arising from isolated superficial vein thrombosis is reported to be uncommon [82, 107]. However, thrombi in dilated superficial veins may be large; indeed, fatal emboli from isolated superficial vein sources have been reported [58, 119].

For these reasons, it is recommended that superficial vein thrombosis not be taken lightly. Conservative treatment may suffice if the process is present only peripherally. Many surgeons, however, recommend saphenous ligation and removal of thrombosed varicosities, especially if the process extends above the knee [3, 50, 82, 87].

Diagnostic Strategy in Deep Vein Thrombosis

Whenever the presence of deep vein thrombosis is suspected, the clinician must realize that he is faced with a disease process that is symptomatic in only half the cases, and even then its signs and symptoms are nonspecific and mimicked with equal frequency by other entities. Further, the thrombotic process is benign and self-limited in the great majority of instances but carries the potential risk of serious or even fatal consequences. On the one hand, there is danger that significant disease may be undiagnosed and untreated. On the other hand, lengthy and expensive treatment which itself has the potential for serious complications may be inappropriately administered.

A number of useful objective tests have been developed to assist or improve the clinically difficult and insecure diagnosis of lower limb thrombosis [116, 121]. Among these, radiographic contrast phlebography must still be considered the gold standard because of its ability to demonstrate practically the entire venous system from the foot to the inferior vena cava. It demonstrates both the main channels and most tributaries and provides the fullest delineation of the extent of thrombosis in the living patient. Its performance requires only standard radiologic equipment. It yields immediate results, revealing the thrombus itself, thereby providing a high degree of certainty of diagnosis and at the same time some indication of the age of the thrombotic process. No additional tests are required. The accuracy of venography is estimated to be approximately 95 percent, probably approaching 100 percent when extensive large thrombus formations in the most serious locations are considered.

On the other hand, venography is invasive and at times uncomfortable, and it is associated with unavoidable radiation exposure. It may have complications, though these can be reduced to a minimum by scrupulous technique and the use of suitable contrast agents, as mentioned previously. Because of its complexity and cost, phlebography is not ideal either as a screening test or for sequential monitoring.

For these reasons, integration of a variety of newer noninvasive techniques into the diagnostic workup for deep vein thrombosis must be considered. Impedance plethysmography and phleborheography are able to detect different patterns of changes in venous blood volume in normal and abnormal extremities, while the Doppler ultrasound method records changes in the velocity of venous blood flow [21, 44, 152, 153]. Radionuclide venography [47] illustrates the pathways followed by ^{99m}Tc microspheres injected into a peripheral foot vein.

These methods have in common the ability to detect abnormalities in venous blood flow that are due to thrombotic occlusion of the major venous pathways in the popliteal, femoral, and iliac regions. In this respect they have an accuracy of 85 to 90 percent. However, they are generally regarded as being much less reliable in evaluation of the calf veins. Further, they are not specific for thrombosis since similar changes in the mechanics of venous blood flow may be caused by congestive heart failure, extensive leg edema, local soft tissue masses, and limited arterial inflow into the extremity.

A negative test result in any of these methods excludes deep vein thrombosis in the large proximal venous channels with an accuracy of approximately 90 percent. False-negative results are explained by the occasional failure of even large thrombi to cause enough obstruction of flow to be detected [49] (see Figs. 78-16, 78-26).

Thermography detects and records increased heat emission that may be caused by deep vein thrombosis or other pathologic processes. It can also show shift of blood from the deep veins to the superficial veins. Although the temperature elevation itself is nonspecific, the anatomically based patterns of involvement that can be shown by thermography may be more significant [124].

The radioactive fibrinogen uptake test is based on the incorporation of ^{125}I fibrinogen into actively forming thrombus, where it can be detected and localized by external scanning with a probe. It is an extremely useful research tool and is particularly well suited to prospective surveillance of patients in the postoperative state or in other high-risk medical situations [88]. It also provides a way to follow the course of a known localized thrombus since the distribution of the radioactive material can be mapped sequentially over 7 to 10 days. A shortcoming of this method, probably explaining its limited use for clinical diagnosis in general, is its very high sensitivity in the calf but lowered sensitivity above the mid-thigh level because of background activity. Further, it shows only actively forming clots and does not detect thrombi that were present before the test was performed. Radioactive fibrinogen will also accumulate locally in areas of recent surgery, trauma, or inflammation and therefore is of limited specificity. Final results of the test are not available for 24 to 48 hours, though the substitution of ^{99m}Tc plasmin is likely to make this technique faster [117]. Another practical shortcoming lies in the high sensitivity of the test to early thrombus formation, which is likely to be of little clinical significance in the majority of such occurrences.

In view of the wide variety of conditions that predispose to the development of deep vein thrombosis, the subtleties of existing diagnostic criteria, and the variety of methods available, it is impractical to propose a single rigid diagnostic protocol. Decisions regarding the use of the phlebogram or its substitution by, or use in combination with, these alternative less invasive tests will be guided by considerations that relate either to the location of the thrombotic process or to the particular clinical setting.

Determination of deep vein thrombosis localization and extension is of considerable importance because it can identify situations of lesser or greater clinical seriousness. While deep vein thrombosis in the calf veins is the most common occurrence—these veins are involved in 80 to 95 percent of instances [33, 76, 138]—serious complications are relatively infrequent. In fact, the importance of diagnosing calf vein thrombosis has been questioned [153]. Proximal extension does take place in about 20 percent of instances but can usually be detected by a noninvasive method such as the ^{125}I fibrinogen scan. However, calf vein thrombosis cannot be dismissed completely since it can be a source of pulmonary emboli, as mentioned previously [33]. While emboli arising from calf veins are usually clinically silent [32], pulmonary emboli arising from the calf veins may be large enough to be clinically serious [76, 106]. Arguments for and against anticoagulation treatment for calf vein thrombi should be based on the degree of local symptomatology as well as the size, site, and extent of thrombi [88]. These details are most accurately obtained by phlebography, which is, in fact, the only really practical method in general clinical use today that can provide the necessary information regarding deep vein thrombosis in the calf veins.

On the other hand, if deep vein thrombosis is suspected in the popliteal-femoral-iliac area, which is the case in approximately 50 percent of instances [33, 76, 138], a screening test such as impedance phlebography or Doppler ultrasound may be recommended. If the test is negative, main channel deep vein thrombosis is probably not present, but if clinical suspicion of deep vein thrombosis persists, sequential monitoring with screening tests should be considered. Because false-positive results occur, it is considered advisable to obtain a confirmatory contrast venogram before long-term anticoagulation is undertaken [92]. As confidence in the noninvasive methods has increased with experience, however, the institution of anticoagulation treatment without obligatory confirmation with a venogram has become accepted in some centers [156].

Recommendations for substituting noninvasive tests for venography can also be made in certain subgroups of patients. For example, patients at high risk but without clinical symptoms may be managed under continuous sequential testing with noninvasive screening techniques in an effort to detect the early manifestations of deep vein thrombosis before anticoagulation therapy is started. An alternative solution to the problem as it exists in high-risk patients is to administer prophylactic treatment using either low-dose anticoagulation or mechanical devices that accomplish rhythmic emptying of the calf veins [88]. With the use of such measures, venous thrombosis and thromboembolism are believed to be preventable diseases in the majority of instances [54, 55, 79, 112, 128].

It is reasonable to assume that combinations of screening techniques may play an increasingly larger role in the diagnosis of deep vein thrombosis and the management of patients suffering from this condition, thus limiting the need for the costly and invasive phlebogram to cases in which it can employ its diagnostic potentialities with an optimum yield [80, 85, 108, 117, 140].

Varicose Veins

Varicose veins have been reported to exist in as many as 4 percent of the adult population [154]. They may be a purely cosmetic problem in some patients but cause marked discomfort in others. Varicose veins may be associated with serious and incapacitating complications such as hemorrhage, thrombosis, eczema, or ulceration and may thus constitute a health care problem of considerable magnitude.

Varicose veins are dilated, elongated, and tortuous and have lost their valvular competence. It is useful to classify them as primary or secondary.

Primary varicose veins are those in which the abnormalities are limited to the superficial veins or to the superficial and perforating veins, the deep venous system being normal. Primary varicose veins are also referred to as saphenous dysfunction. The cause of the local venous dilatations is unknown [51, 131]. It does not reside in the valves since these are anatomically intact in the varicose veins themselves as well as in the incompetent perforating veins with which they are commonly associated [41, 51, 56]. Rather, primary dilatation of the veins and valve seats appears more likely to result in valvular incompetence [7, 41, 51, 97]. Degenerative changes may, however, occur later in the valves, leading at times to their complete disappearance [41]. Although the initiating cause for the venous dilatation is not clear, conditions of abnormal wall weakness, increased distending forces, general wear and tear, multiple small arteriovenous fistulas, etc., have been implicated. In rare instances, a specific predisposing factor can be identified, such as a large congenital or traumatic arteriovenous fistula, a congenital anomaly of the veins themselves, or congenital absence of valves. Once initiated, the development of varicosis tends to be a progressive process, and the incidence and severity increase with age.

Secondary varicose veins are those that are caused by insufficient deep and perforating veins as a result of previous deep vein thrombosis. They are part of the postthrombotic syndrome, which is dealt with in greater detail in a later section.

As noted in the section on anatomy, the long and short saphenous systems lie upon the deep fascia. The single exception is the upper portion of the short saphenous trunk, which is partly invested by the deep fascia and is thus rarely palpable or visible even when it is varicose [50, 71]. The trunks of the long and short saphenous veins are covered by the deep layer of superficial fascia, while their tributaries and arcades are located external to this layer and are thus unsupported by it [52].

Among the large number of perforating veins in the lower extremity there are relatively few that, because of their location and frequent incompetence, have reached clinical recognition (Fig. 78-27). These are found at fairly constant sites [50, 71]. Probably the most important are two perforating veins on the medial aspect of the ankle and lower third of the leg (Fig. 78-28; see also Fig. 78-30A). These connect the superficial posterior arch vein with the posterior tibial veins of the deep system. Laterally and posteriorly, at the junction of the lower and middle thirds of the calf is found the lateral perforating vein, which connects the posterolateral tributary of the lesser saphenous vein with the peroneal veins. Slightly higher, a midcalf perforating vein, present in only 25 percent of instances, drains into the soleal

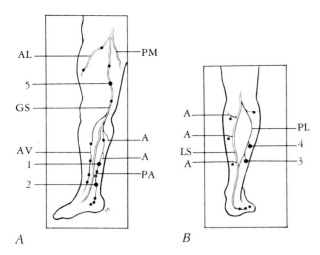

A   *B*

Figure 78-27. Diagrammatic illustration of the superficial veins and most common sites of perforating veins, represented by the smaller dots. (A) Anterior view. (B) Posterior view. The locations of some of the clinically most significant perforating veins are indicated by the larger dots; i.e., the upper (*1*) and middle (*2*) internal perforating veins, the external (*3*) and midcalf (*4*) perforating veins, and the perforating vein in Hunter's canal (*5*). The greater saphenous vein (*GS*) has an anterolateral (*AL*) and a posteromedial (*PM*) tributary in the thigh and two tributaries in the calf—the anterior vein (*AV*) of the leg and the posterior arch vein (*PA*). The lesser saphenous vein has a single posterolateral tributary (*PL*). Multiple arcades join the posterior arch vein with the trunk of the lesser saphenous vein (*LS*). Note that the perforating veins usually join the tributaries and arcades (*A*) rather than the main saphenous trunks. (After Dodd and Cockett [50] and Fegan [52].)

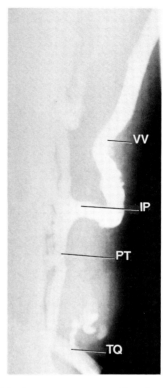

Figure 78-28. Incompetent perforating vein in the calf of a patient with primary varicose veins. The incompetent perforating vein (*IP*) is dilated and smooth in contour. The varicose superficial vein (*VV*) has been opacified by outward flow of contrast material from the posterior tibial vein (*PT*) above the tourniquet (*TQ*). The posterior tibial vein is normal.

sinusoids. The perforating veins at the lower calf level are especially well developed since, as previously noted, they normally carry the venous return from the superficial tissues of the foot and ankle directly into the deep veins [50]. It is incompetence of these perforating veins, most commonly the medial ones, that cause the so-called blowout syndrome described by Cockett and Jones [37]. Other perforating veins in the calf that when incompetent are clinically significant include the posttibial perforating vein (Boyd's vein), which exits between the heads of the gastrocnemius muscles approximately 6 to 10 cm below the knee [71], and other indirect musculocutaneous perforating veins that connect with the soleal or gastrocnemius veins on the posterior aspect of the calf [52].

Clinically most important, in the thigh, are the hunterian perforating veins, which connect a

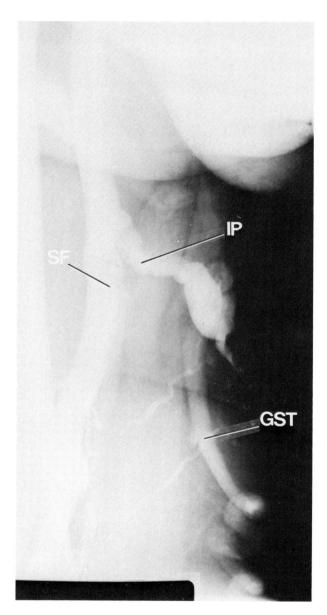

Figure 78-29. Incompetent perforating vein in the thigh in another patient with primary varicose veins. Anteroposterior radiograph of the thigh. A varicose tributary of the greater saphenous vein has been opacified by outward flow of contrast material from the superficial femoral vein above the tourniquet. The superficial femoral vein is normal. This perforating vein is in the midthigh, somewhat higher than the usual hunterian perforating veins. *GST* = Greater saphenous tributary; *IP* = incompetent perforating vein; *SF* = superficial femoral vein.

tributary of the long saphenous vein with the superficial femoral vein in the region of the adductor canal (Fig. 78-29; see also Fig. 78-27).

Finally, the upper terminations of the long and short saphenous trunks at the groin and in the popliteal fossa represent the highest perforating vein of each of these systems, and both are frequent, important sites of incompetence.

In general, perforating veins connect with the tributaries and arcades of the superficial system rather than with the saphenous main trunks.

Under normal conditions the perforating veins each contain valves that are oriented in such a way as to allow blood flow only from the superficial veins to the deep veins. Flow studies by Bjordal [28] have shown that, in the presence of primary varicose veins, the blood flow through the incompetent perforating veins occurs predominantly in the normal direction; i.e., from the superficial veins into the deep veins. There is, however, at times intermittent flow outward from the deep veins in conjunction with muscle contraction. This differs from the flow pattern in secondary varicosities, where the deep system is abnormal and where blood flow through the incompetent perforating veins is predominantly reversed.

Two different sequences of development of flow abnormalities associated with primary varicose veins have been described [7, 36, 43]. The theory of descending sequential incompetence (centrifugal theory) postulates that reflux downward into the saphenous veins is the primary event, causing progressive distal dilatation of the superficial veins and eventually of the perforating veins [28, 99]. The centripetal theory, on the other hand, proposes that reflux through incompetent perforating veins is the initial defect, causing progressive dilatation of the veins upward in the central direction, with ultimate incompetence at the saphenofemoral junction [52]. It is conceivable that the dilatation may commence at any site or sites in the superficial or perforating veins and spread progressively to involve other areas. In any event, once gross incompetence of the upper end of the saphenous vein has occurred, a circular flow pattern of relatively large magnitude may be established, characterized by downward flow through the saphenous veins, through the perforating veins, and into the deep veins, adding considerably to the load of the muscle pumps of the leg [28].

When saphenous incompetence is present, it most commonly affects the long saphenous vein

(Fig. 78-30). The lesser saphenous vein is incompetent in only 10 to 14 percent of instances [50, 125]. The deep venous trunks and muscle veins may occasionally be varicose [14, 65] (Fig. 78-31).

PHLEBOGRAPHIC TECHNIQUE

The phlebographic technique used in the examination of varicose veins and incompetence of perforating veins is based on our own experience and on the observation of others [68, 148]. It differs from the standard technique already described [122] in that the first 50 to 60 cc of contrast material is injected at the usual site with a tourniquet in place at the ankle in order to direct all the contrast material into the deep veins. Sites of ulceration should be avoided in securing the tourniquet, which should be tight enough to prevent filling of the superficial veins but not so tight that it occludes the deep veins. Under these circumstances, the superficial veins can fill only when contrast material leaks out into them through the incompetent perforating veins above the tourniquet. These should be sought for carefully under fluoroscopy, especially at the sites of predilection referred to previously. The location of any incompetent perforating veins is marked on the skin of the patient's leg, to facilitate their subsequent identification at surgery. The tourniquet is moved progressively higher as leaks through the incompetent perforating veins are noted, so as to locate the next higher site of incompetence. This sequential procedure should be continued up to the midthigh level in order to include potential incompetent perforating veins in the region of Hunter's canal. If no gross incompetence is seen, the patient is instructed to perform a Valsalva maneuver or to contract the leg muscles in an attempt to force contrast material from the deep veins into the superficial veins. After completion of this portion of the examination, the tourniquet is removed and additional contrast material injected to complete contrast filling of the entire venous system as described previously in the standard technique. At this time, additional varicosities unrelated to perforating vein incompetence may opacify from below. Varicosities in the groin associated with reflux into incompetent saphenous tributaries at the oval fossa may then also become apparent.

Descending venography, performed in the recumbent patient by injection directly into the femoral vein simultaneously with performance of the Valsalva maneuver, has been described as a test for reflux down the femoral vein or down the long saphenous vein [69]. However, in our experience this technique is rarely necessary.

PHLEBOGRAPHIC FINDINGS

The radiologic appearances of varicose veins are similar in both primary and secondary varicosities. Some of the largest varicose veins described are of the primary type, being due to retrograde saphenous reflux. Varicosities can be present at any level in the groin, thigh, or calf. Typical varicose changes have also been described in the foot [19]. The dilatation of the superficial veins may be regional or focal, with the dilated segment merging abruptly with a segment of normal caliber. The saphenous trunks themselves are often less dilated in comparison with the tributaries and arcades, which tend to become markedly tortuous and dilated and which most commonly represent the varicosities that are clinically palpable and visible [41] (see Figs. 78-29, 78-30A). The less marked involvement of the major trunks can be explained by the fact that they are protected by the deep layer of superficial fascia. Also, as noted previously, the perforating veins most frequently connect with the tributaries and arcades rather than with the main trunks. Thus, the pressure and flow of outward reflux through the incompetent perforating veins is exerted primarily into the tributaries and arcades. The saphenous trunks, however, can become greatly dilated (see Fig. 78-30B,C). When the long saphenous trunk itself is involved, it is often twisted into a typical spiral configuration and shows peculiar eccentric dilatations below the valves [41].

Incompetent perforating veins can be demonstrated in relation to varicose veins in a high percentage of instances [151]. Usually only one or two—occasionally three—sites of incompetence are demonstrated. Incompetent perforating veins (see Figs. 78-28–78-30A) appear dilated and tortuous but smooth-walled, though they may occasionally show the irregular appearance of recanalization. Small amounts of contrast material can pass from the deep system into the superficial veins; this is of no clinical significance if it occurs through normal-appearing perforating veins. Intact valves are usually visible in such perforating veins. Occasionally, the contrast material will flow rapidly out of the leg, sometimes with

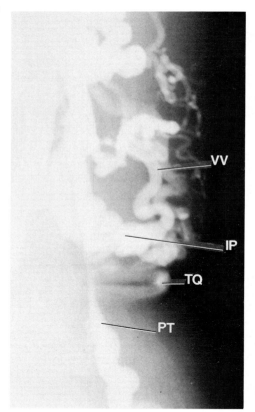

A

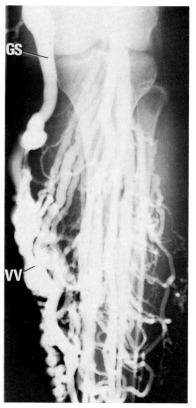

B

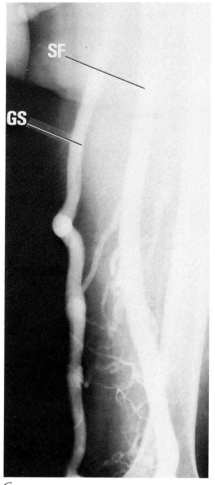

C

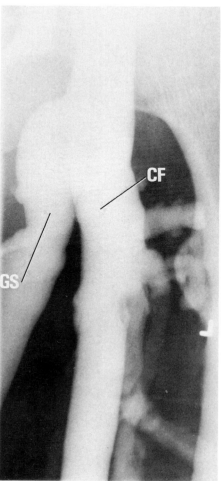

D

1912

noticeable pulsatile flow. This is probably the result of arteriovenous shunting.

At the end of the examination, the leg is actively exercised to propel the contrast material out of the veins. At this time it may be noted that the superficial and deep veins do not empty in the normal fashion. The reason is that the contrast material is repeatedly passed back and forth between the dilated superficial veins and the deep veins, through incompetent perforating veins. The degree of retention can be used as an indicator of the degree of functional abnormality in the presence of either varicose veins or chronic venous insufficiency.

Many varicose veins that are obvious on clinical examination do not opacify during venography, perhaps because they constitute capacious spaces with relatively limited avenues of blood, resulting in a slow mixing and exchange of blood and contrast material. The phlebographic demonstration of known varicosities is, however, less important than the documentation and localization of abnormally functioning incompetent perforating veins.

There is a strong tendency for varicosities to recur after operation. Indeed, it is not uncommon to encounter recurrence rates of 15 to 22 percent or even higher if radical extirpation of the abnormal veins is not done [70, 95, 97, 145]. Strong evidence exists [51, 70, 110] that recurrences are usually the result of failure to identify and remove all sources of venous incompetence. This possibility favors the performance of phlebography for meticulous preoperative identification. Frequent sites of residual incompetence are tributaries at the groin, perforating veins in the calf, the saphenopopliteal junction,

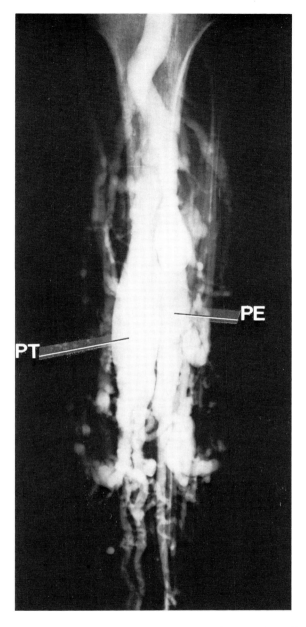

◄ **Figure 78-30.** Incompetent perforating veins and dilated greater saphenous trunk in a patient with primary varicose veins. (A) Lateral view spot film of the lower calf. The contrast material has leaked out from the normal deep veins through paired incompetent perforating veins leading into varicose superficial veins. Anteroposterior radiographs of the leg (B) and thigh (C). The greater saphenous trunk is dilated and tortuous. (D) Anteroposterior spot film of the groin. Saphenofemoral incompetence can be inferred from the greatly dilated bulbous appearance of the upper end of the saphenous vein where it joins the femoral vein. The superficial femoral vein is normal. *CF* = Common femoral vein; *GS* = greater saphenous vein; *IP* = incompetent perforating veins; *PT* = posterior tibial vein; *SF* = superficial femoral vein; *TQ* = tourniquet; *VV* = varicose superficial veins.

Figure 78-31. Varicose deep veins believed to be primary in origin. There are also varicosities of the superficial system, and a single incompetent perforating vein was present medially and one laterally in the low calf. The posterior tibial (*PT*) and peroneal (*PE*) veins are greatly dilated.

etc. Varicose veins may also gradually return postoperatively simply as a progression of the basic disease process itself.

Chronic Venous Insufficiency; Venous Ulcer; Postthrombotic Syndrome

Permanent damage in the veins after healing of acute deep vein thrombosis may result in late sequelae of edema, induration, eczema, secondary varicose veins, and ulceration of the leg, referred to collectively as the postthrombotic syndrome. According to Bauer [23], ulcers developed in 20 percent of patients within 5 years following a bout of deep vein thrombosis, in 52

percent within 10 years, and in 79 percent at a later date. Bauer also noted that heparin is effective prophylaxis against the development of this syndrome.

The syndrome is estimated to exist in 1 to 2 percent of the general population and to affect approximately a million persons in the United States alone [72, 81, 98, 154]. Since only about 50 percent of patients with acute deep vein thrombosis have any signs or symptoms, it is not surprising that a history of previous deep vein thrombosis can be obtained in only about half of the patients with the postthrombotic syndrome [2, 43]. If complicated by significant proximal venous flow impairment, symptoms of venous claudication may occur in addition to the other clinical findings described [111]. In accordance with the incidence of deep vein thrombosis, the

---

Figure 78-32. Postthrombotic changes with chronic venous insufficiency and secondary varicose veins. Anteroposterior views of the calf (A) and thigh (B). The varicosities of the superficial veins are similar in appearance to primary varicosities. However, many of the deep veins of the calf are occluded. The superficial femoral vein in the thigh is smaller than usual, is irregular in contour, and contains webs. No valves are seen. These appearances are due to recanalization following thrombosis. The flow is predominantly in the superficial veins, which are dilated and more densely opacified than normal. *GS* = Greater saphenous vein; *PF* = profunda femoris vein; *SF* = superficial femoral vein; *VV* = varicose veins; *W* = web.

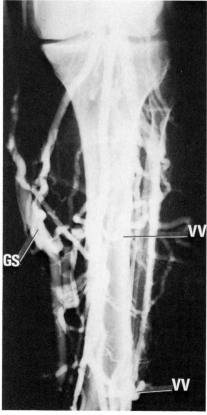

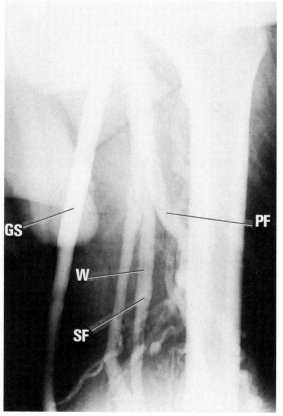

A   B

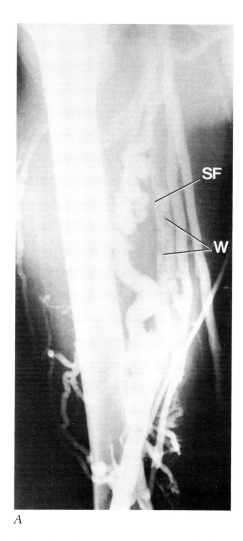

A

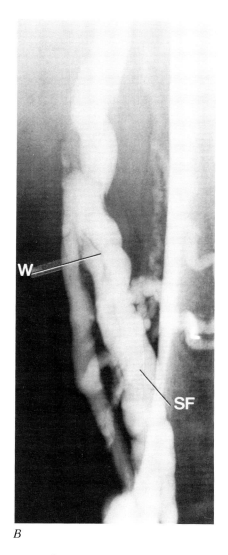

B

Figure 78-33. Postthrombotic appearance of deep veins. Anteroposterior views of the thigh in two patients. (A) The superficial femoral vein is narrower than normal and exhibits numerous internal webs. An irregularly dilated varicose vein is seen lateral to it. (B) The superficial femoral vein is irregularly dilated, and some webs or synechiae can be seen within it. Recanalized veins are fibrosed and most commonly remain narrowed, as in (A). They may become dilated, as in this case, if the elastic tissue has been destroyed [76]. *SF* = Superficial femoral vein; *W* = webs.

syndrome is more common in the left leg than in the right.

In the past, venous ulcers have been thought always to be due to the postthrombotic state. However, it is now believed that in about half the instances such ulcers occur as a complication of primary incompetence of perforating veins [72]. Long-standing gross incompetence of the saphenous veins, which may cause incompetence of perforating veins [28], may also result in venous ulcer [81, 134].

Although in 90 percent of instances venous

ulcer can be shown to be related to incompetence of the superficial or deep venous system, in approximately 10 percent of patients indistinguishable changes may be caused by conditions other than venous disease, including arterial occlusion, chronic infection, and trauma [72].

The term *chronic venous insufficiency* refers to all chronic conditions in which the venous return is impaired because of abnormal function of the venous-muscular pump [83]. A serious consequence of the malfunctioning venous structures is the development of ambulatory venous hypertension [100]. Whereas local resting venous pressure is essentially the same in the normal person and in the patient with chronic venous insufficiency, under conditions of exercise the venous pressure in the normal leg is reduced by the action of the muscle pump but remains unchanged or even increases in the presence of venous dysfunction. In advanced cases of venous insufficiency, pressure rises comparable to systolic arterial pressures generated in the deep muscle veins during calf muscle contraction [15, 17] can be exerted directly outward through the incompetent perforating veins into the tributaries and arcades, causing the blowout syndrome [37, 50]. Similar high pressures are developed in these veins in association with coughing and straining when venous valve incompetence exists in the saphenous trunks [34]. The transmission of high venous pressures into the delicate subcutaneous veins results in stasis, leakage of protein and cells, focal venous thrombosis, fibrosis, and ultimately tissue necrosis and ulceration [17, 50]. Opening of arteriovenous shunts with resultant anoxia, and lymphatic obstruction, may also contribute to these tissue changes [11].

Venography performed to evaluate the extremity for the postthrombotic syndrome is carried out as described in the previous section for varicose veins. As already noted, the phlebographic appearance and location of incompetent perforating veins and of superficial varicosities in the postthrombotic state are indistinguishable from those in uncomplicated varicose veins (Fig. 78-32A). However, in the chronic postthrombotic state, the contrast material often flows preferentially through the superficial veins (Fig. 78-32B). Some authors are of the opinion that venous ulcers are practically always due to incompetent perforating veins [14, 50, 72]. Phlebography is able to demonstrate surgically proved incompetent perforating veins with an accuracy of approximately 80 to 90 percent [148, 151]. These veins may be directly under the ulcer itself or may be located nearby.

When the syndrome has resulted from previous deep vein thrombosis, the appearance of the deep venous system may show corresponding residual abnormalities [65, 83] (Figs. 78-32, 78-33). The degree of abnormality in the venographic appearance will not necessarily correlate strongly with the clinical severity of symptoms [2, 102]. Abnormal changes may include narrowing or occlusion of the veins. There may be opacification of fewer veins than normal or there may be pro-

fusion of collateral superficial or deep veins. Recanalized veins have irregular margins and bizarre-appearing or multichanneled lumina with webs [76] (Figs. 78-32B, 78-33). These veins are generally reduced in caliber in accordance with the fibrotic thickening of their walls. They may appear valveless on the phlebogram, but autopsy studies have shown that the valves are usually substantially unaffected [76]. Such veins may subsequently become dilated (Fig. 78-33B), probably on account of loss of their elastic tissue.

Use of Venography in Varicose Veins and in Chronic Venous Insufficiency

The diagnosis of these conditions depends to a large degree on a thorough clinical examination, and there is no uniform agreement on the need for venography. Some authors [72] believe that it is rarely indicated; others regard it as both very helpful and reliable [35, 46, 148, 151]. Most investigators would agree that venography is indicated at least in the workup of extensive recurrent varicosities. We are of the opinion that venography provides pertinent and important information and that it should be performed prior to initial surgery for extensive varicose veins or treatment of chronic venous insufficiency. It provides a map of the superficial trunks, tributaries, and arcades, to identify the site of any incompetent perforating veins, and to show the condition of the deep veins. Such information when combined with the clinical findings provides a baseline for a complete surgical treatment of all varicosities and any abnormal dilated connections with the deep venous system. Further, by demonstrating whether or not the deep veins are involved, it allows more accurate prognosis and appropriate recommendations for supportive therapy to be determined. For example, if abnormalities are limited to the superficial and perforating veins, careful ligation and removal of these veins will result in a high rate of cure. On the other hand, if the deep venous system has become insufficient because of previous deep vein thrombosis, damage is permanent and surgery is much less effective. A combination of surgery and continued supportive therapy (e.g., elastic stockings) must then be carried out on a permanent basis [45, 72]. Varicose veins secondary to previous deep vein thrombosis may contribute to stasis and may be removed if desired [46, 51, 102] since there is practically always patency of some deep veins except during the first 2 to 3 months following acute deep vein thrombosis [68].

Other methods exist that may be used not only to evaluate the venous system in the presence of varicose veins or chronic venous insufficiency but also to predict which patients may develop these abnormalities. Such methods are manometry [2], plethysmography [84], and photoplethysmography [1], as well as Doppler ultrasound and thermography.

References

1. Abramowitz, H. B., Queral, L. A., Flinn, W. R., Nora, P. F., Peterson, L. K., Bergan, J. J., and Yao, J. S. T. The use of photoplethysmography in the assessment of venous insufficiency: A comparison to venous pressure measurements. *Surgery* 86:434, 1979.
2. Abramowitz, I. The post-phlebitic syndrome—a critical assessment of diagnostic parameters. *S. Afr. J. Surg.* 10:153, 1972.
3. Agrifoglio, G. The Surgical Treatment of Varicose Veins: A Method Practiced in Italy. In J. T. Hobbs (ed.), *The Treatment of Venous Disorders: A Comprehensive Review of Current Practice in the Management of Varicose Veins and the Post-thrombotic Syndrome.* Philadelphia: Lippincott, 1977.
4. Albrechtsson, U., and Olsson, C. G. Thrombotic side-effects of lower limb phlebography. *Lancet* 1:723, 1976.
5. Albrechtsson, U., and Olsson, C. G. Thrombosis after phlebography: A comparison of two contrast media. *Cardiovasc. Radiol.* 2:9, 1979.
6. Albrechtsson, U., and Olsson, C. G. Thrombosis following phlebography with ionic and non-ionic contrast media. *Acta Radiol. [Diagn.]* (Stockh.) 20:46, 1979.
7. Alexander, C. J. The theoretical basis of varicose vein formation. *Med. J. Aust.* 1:258, 1972.
8. Allenby, F., and Jeyasingh, K. The site of origin of venous thrombosis. *Am. Heart J.* 89:123, 1975.
9. Almén, T., and Nylander, G. Serial phlebography of the normal lower leg during muscular contraction and relaxation. *Acta Radiol.* (Stockh.) 57:264, 1962.
10. Almén, T., and Nylander, G. False signs of thrombosis in lower leg phlebography. *Acta Radiol. [Diagn.]* (Stockh.) 2:345, 1964.
11. Antal, S. C., and Reiss, R. Post-thrombotic leg ulcer and its surgical treatment. *Am. J. Surg.* 131:710, 1976.
12. Arkoff, R. S., Gilfillan, R. S., and Burhenne, H. J. A simple method for lower extremity phlebography—pseudo-obstruction of the popliteal vein. *Radiology* 90:66, 1968.
13. Arndt, R. D., Grollman, J. H., Gomes, A. S., and Bos, C. J. The heparin flush: An aid in preventing post-venography thrombophlebitis. *Radiology* 130:249, 1979.
14. Arnoldi, C. C. A comparison between the phlebographic picture as seen in dynamic intraosseous phlebography and the clinical signs and symptoms of chronic venous insufficiency. *J. Cardiovasc. Surg.* (Torino) 2:184, 1961.
15. Arnoldi, C. C. On the conditions for the venous return from the lower leg in healthy subjects and in patients with chronic venous insufficiency. *Angiology* 17:153, 1966.
16. Arnoldi, C. C., Greitz, T., and Linderholm, H. Variations in cross sectional area and pressure in the veins of the normal human leg during rhythmic muscular exercise. *Acta Chir. Scand.* 132:507, 1966.
17. Arnoldi, C. C., and Linderholm, H. On the pathogenesis of the venous leg ulcer. *Acta Chir. Scand.* 134:427, 1968.
18. Askar, O., and Aly, S. A. The veins of the foot: Surgical anatomy and its relation to disorders of the venous return from the foot. *J. Cardiovasc. Surg.* (Torino) 16:53, 1975.
19. Askar, O., Kassem, K. A., and Aly, S. A. A clinico-radiological study of the "varicose foot." *J. Cardiovasc. Surg.* (Torino) 16:71, 1975.
20. Athanasoulis, C. A. Phlebography for the Diagnosis of Deep Leg Vein Thrombosis. In J. Fratantoni and S. Wessler (eds.), *Prophylactic Therapy of Deep Vein Thrombosis and Pulmonary Embolism.* Bethesda, Md.: National Institutes of Health, 1975.
21. Barnes, R. W. Doppler Ultrasonic Diagnosis of Venous Disease. In E. F. Bernstein (ed.), *Noninvasive Diagnostic Techniques in Vascular Disease.* St. Louis: Mosby, 1978.
22. Bauer, G. A venographic study of thromboembolic problems. *Acta Chir. Scand.* 84 [Suppl. 61], 1940.
23. Bauer, G. A roentgenological and clinical study of the sequels of thrombosis. *Acta Chir. Scand.* 86 [Suppl. 74], 1942.
24. Berberich, J., and Hirsch, S. Die rontgenographische Darstellung der Arterien und Venen im lebenden Menschen. *Klin. Wochenschr.* 2:2226, 1923.
25. Bergvall, U. Phlebography in acute deep venous thrombosis of the lower extremity. A comparison between centripetal ascending and descending phlebography. *Acta Radiol. [Diagn.]* (Stockh.) 11:148, 1971.

26. Bettmann, M. A., and Paulin, S.   Leg phlebography: The incidence, nature and modification of undesirable side effects. *Radiology* 122:101, 1977.

27. Bettmann, M. A., Salzman, E. W., Rosenthal, D., Clagett, P., Davies, G., Nebesar, R., Rabinov, K., Ploetz, J., and Skillman, J.   Reduction of venous thrombosis complicating phlebography. *AJR* 134:1169, 1980.

28. Bjordal, R. I.   Haemodynamic Studies of Varicose Veins and the Post-thrombotic Syndrome. In J. T. Hobbs (ed.), *The Treatment of Venous Disorders: A Comprehensive Review of Current Practice in the Management of Varicose Veins and the Post-thrombotic Syndrome.* Philadelphia: Lippincott, 1977.

29. Borgström, S., Greitz, T., van der Linden, W., Molin, J., and Rudics, I.   Ascending phlebography in fresh thrombosis of the lower limb. *AJR* 94:207, 1965.

30. Brodelius, Å., Lörinc, P., and Nylander, G.   Phlebographic techniques in the diagnosis of acute deep venous thrombosis of the lower limb. *AJR* 111:794, 1971.

31. Browse, N. L.   Personal views on published facts. What should I do about deep vein thrombosis and pulmonary embolism? *Ann. R. Coll. Surg. Engl.* 59:138, 1977.

32. Browse, N. L., Clemenson, G., and Croft, D. N.   Fibrinogen-detectable thrombosis in the legs and pulmonary embolism. *Br. Med. J.* 1:603, 1974.

33. Browse, N. L., and Thomas, M. L.   Source of non-lethal pulmonary emboli. *Lancet* 1:258, 1974.

34. Burkitt, D. P.   Varicose veins: Facts and fantasy. *Arch. Surg.* 111:1327, 1976.

35. Burnand, K., O'Donnell, T., Thomas, M. L., and Browse, N. L.   Relation between post-phlebitic changes in the deep veins and results of surgical treatment of venous ulcers. *Lancet* 1:936, 1976.

36. Chant, A. D. B., Jones, H. O., Townsend, J. C. F., and Williams, J. E.   Radiological demonstration of the relationship between calf varices and sapheno-femoral incompetence. *Clin. Radiol.* 23:519, 1972.

37. Cockett, F. B., and Jones, D. E.   The ankle blow-out syndrome. A new approach to the varicose ulcer problem. *Lancet* 1:17, 1953.

38. Coel, M. N.   Adequacy of lower limb venous opacification: Comparison of supine and upright phlebography. *AJR* 134:163, 1980.

39. Coel, M. N., and Dodge, W.   Complication rate with supine phlebography. *AJR* 131:821, 1978.

40. Cohen, S. H., Ehrlich, G. E., Kauffman, M. S., and Cope, C.   Thrombophlebitis following knee surgery. *J. Bone Joint Surg.* 55A:106, 1973.

41. Cotton, L. T.   Varicose veins: Gross anatomy and development. *Br. J. Surg.* 48:589, 1961.

42. Crane, C.   Venous interruption for pulmonary embolism: Present status. *Prog. Cardiovasc. Dis.* 17:329, 1975.

43. Crane, C.   The surgery of varicose veins. *Surg. Clin. North Am.* 59:737, 1979.

44. Cranley, J. J.   Diagnosis of Deep Venous Thrombosis of the Lower Extremity by Phleborheography. In E. F. Bernstein (ed.), *Noninvasive Diagnostic Techniques in Vascular Disease.* St. Louis: Mosby, 1978.

45. Cranley, J. J.   Discussion of Post-phlebitic Syndrome. In J. J. Bergan and J. S. T. Yao (eds.), *Venous Problems.* Chicago: Year Book, 1978. Pp. 406–407.

46. Dale, W. A.   The swollen leg. *Curr. Probl. Surg.* 1–66, Sept. 1973.

47. Dean, R. H.   Radionuclide Venography and Simultaneous Lung Scanning: Evaluation of Clinical Application. In E. F. Bernstein (ed.), *Noninvasive Diagnostic Techniques in Vascular Disease.* St. Louis: Mosby, 1978.

48. DeWeese, J. A., and Rogoff, S. M.   Functional ascending phlebography of the lower extremity by serial long film technique: Evaluation of anatomic and functional detail in 62 extremities. *AJR* 81:841, 1959.

49. Dmochowski, J. R., Adams, D. F., and Couch, N. P.   Impedance measurement in the diagnosis of deep venous thrombosis. *Arch. Surg.* 104:170, 1972.

50. Dodd, H., and Cockett, F. B.   *The Pathology and Surgery of the Veins of the Lower Limb* (2nd ed.). New York: Churchill Livingstone, 1976.

51. Edwards, E. A.   Varicose veins and venous stasis. *Bol. Assoc. Med. P.R.* 49:49, 1957.

52. Fegan, G.   *Varicose Veins.* Springfield, Ill.: Thomas, 1967.

53. Fox, J. A., and Hugh, A. E.   Some physical factors in arteriography. *Clin. Radiol.* 15:183, 1964.

54. Gallus, A. S.   Venous Thromboembolism: Incidence and Clinical Risk Factors. In J. L. Madden and M. Hume (eds.), *Venous Thromboembolism: Prevention and Treatment.* New York: Appleton-Century-Crofts, 1976.

55. Gallus, A. S., Hirsh, J., Hull, R., and van Aken, W. G.   Diagnosis of venous thromboembolism. *Semin. Thromb. Hemostas.* 2:203, 1976.

56. Girdwood, W.   Do thrombosis and recanalization precede dilatation of calf-communicator veins? *S. Afr. Med. J.* 39:969, 1965.

57. Gjöres, J. E.   The incidence of venous thrombosis and its sequelae in certain districts of Sweden. *Acta Chir. Scand.* [Suppl.] 206:1, 1956.

58. Gjöres, J. E.   Surgical therapy of ascending thrombophlebitis in the saphenous system. *Angiology* 13:241, 1962.

59. Glover, W. J., Vaughn, A. M., Annan, C. M., and Caserta, J. A.   Venous thrombectomy in

the management of acute venous thrombosis of the saphenous system. *Am. J. Surg.* 93:798, 1957.

60. Gordon, I. J. Evaluation of suspected deep venous thrombosis in the arteriosclerotic patient. *AJR* 131:531, 1978.
61. Gothlin, J. The comparative frequency of extravasal injection at phlebography with steel and plastic cannula. *Clin. Radiol.* 23:183, 1972.
62. Gothlin, J., and Hallböök, T. Skin necrosis following extravasal injection of contrast medium at phlebography. *Radiologe* 11:161, 1971.
63. Gothlin, J., and Zurbriggen, S. Frequency of thrombosis and post-thrombotic conditions of the foot at phlebography. *Acta Radiol.* [*Diagn.*] (Stockh.) 16:107, 1975.
64. Greitz, T. The technique of ascending phlebography of the lower extremity. *Acta Radiol.* (Stockh.) 42:421, 1954.
65. Greitz, T. Ascending phlebography in venous insufficiency. *Acta Radiol.* (Stockh.) 44:145, 1955.
66. Greitz, T. Phlebography of the normal leg. *Acta Radiol.* (Stockh.) 44:1, 1955.
67. Grollman, J. H., Jr., and Straede, P. D. Rotating platform for ascending phlebography. *AJR* 129:941, 1977.
68. Gullmo, Å. On the technique of phlebography of the lower limb. *Acta Radiol.* (Stockh.) 46:603, 1956.
69. Gullmo, Å. The phlebographic Trendelenburg test. *Br. J. Radiol.* 36:812, 1963.
70. Haeger, K. Is non-radical surgery for varicose veins justifiable? *Vasa* 4:403, 1975.
71. Haeger, K. The Anatomy of the Veins of the Leg. In J. T. Hobbs (ed.), *The Treatment of Venous Disorders: A Comprehensive Review of Current Practice in the Management of Varicose Veins and the Post-thrombotic Syndrome.* Philadelphia: Lippincott, 1977.
72. Haeger, K. Leg Ulcers. In J. T. Hobbs (ed.), *The Treatment of Venous Disorders: A Comprehensive Review of Current Practice in the Management of Varicose Veins and the Post-thrombotic Syndrome.* Philadelphia: Lippincott, 1977.
73. Haeger, K., and Nylander, G. Acute phlebography. *Triangle* 8:18, 1967.
74. Hafner, C. D., Cranley, J. J., Krause, R. J., and Strasser, E. S. A method of managing superficial thrombophlebitis. *Surgery* 55:201, 1964.
75. Havig, Ö. Pathogenese der tiefen Venenthrombose—eine post-mortem Studie. *Vasa* 3:135, 1974.
76. Havig, Ö. Deep vein thrombosis and pulmonary embolism. *Acta Chir. Scand.* [Suppl.] 478:1, 1977.
77. Heatley, R. V., Morgan, A., Hughes, L. E., and Okwonga, W. Preoperative or postoperative deep-vein thrombosis? *Lancet* 1:437, 1976.

78. Hirsh, J. Deep vein thrombosis and pulmonary embolism. (Audio-cassette.) *Audio-Digest Foundation—Internal Medicine* 23:5, 1976.
79. Hirsh, J., and Genton, E. Low-dose Heparin Prophylaxis for Venous Thromboembolism. In J. Fratantoni and S. Wessler (eds.), *Prophylactic Therapy of Deep Vein Thrombosis and Pulmonary Embolism.* Bethesda, Md.: National Institutes of Health, 1975.
80. Hirsh, J., and Hull, R. Comparative value of tests for the diagnosis of venous thrombosis. *World J. Surg.* 2:27, 1978.
81. Hobbs, J. T. The Post-thrombotic Syndrome. In J. T. Hobbs (ed.), *The Treatment of Venous Disorders: A Comprehensive Review of Current Practice in the Management of Varicose Veins and the Post-thrombotic Syndrome.* Philadelphia: Lippincott, 1977.
82. Hobbs, J. T. Superficial Thrombophlebitis. In J. T. Hobbs (ed.), *The Treatment of Venous Disorders: A Comprehensive Review of Current Practice in the Management of Varicose Veins and the Post-thrombotic Syndrome.* Philadelphia: Lippincott, 1977.
83. Hojensgard, I. C. Phlebography in chronic venous insufficiency of the lower extremity. *Acta Radiol.* (Stockh.) 32:375, 1949.
84. Holm, J., Nilsson, N. J., Schersten, T., and Sivertsson, R. Elective surgery for varicose veins: A simple method for evaluation of the patients. *J. Cardiovasc. Surg.* (Torino) 15:565, 1974.
85. Hull, R., Hirsh, J., Sackett, D. L., Powers, P., Turpie, A. G. G., and Walker, I. Combined use of leg scanning and impedance plethysmography in suspected venous thrombosis. An alternative to venography. *N. Engl. J. Med.* 296:1497, 1977.
86. Hume, M., Sevitt, S., and Thomas, D. P. *Venous Thrombosis and Pulmonary Embolism.* Cambridge, Mass.: Harvard University Press, 1970.
87. Husni, E. Discussion. In J. J. Bergan and J. S. T. Yao (eds.), *Venous Problems.* Chicago: Year Book, 1978. Pp. 104–105.
88. Kakkar, V. V. Fibrinogen uptake test for detection of deep vein thrombosis—a review of current practice. *Semin. Nucl. Med.* 7:229, 1977.
89. Kakkar, V. V. The prevention of acute pulmonary embolism. *Br. J. Hosp. Med.* 18:32, 1977.
90. Kakkar, V. V., Flanc, C., Howe, C. T., and Clarke, M. B. Natural history of post-operative deep-vein thrombosis. *Lancet* 2:230, 1969.
91. Kaushal, S. P., Galante, J. O., McKenna, R., and Bachmann, F. Complications following total knee replacement. *Clin. Orthop.* 121:181, 1976.
92. Kiil, J., and Moller, J. C. Ultrasound and clinical diagnosis of deep vein thrombosis of the leg. *Acta Radiol.* [*Diagn.*] (Stockh.) 20:292, 1979.
93. Kirschner, L. P., Twigg, H., and Farkas, J. Drip infusion venography. *Radiology* 96:413, 1970.

94. Kjellberg, S. R. Die Mischungs- und Strömungsverhältnisse von wasserlöslichen Kontrastmitteln bei Gefäss- und Herzuntersuchungen. *Acta Radiol.* (Stockh.) 24:433, 1943.

95. Larson, R. H., Lofgren, E. P., Myers, T. T., and Lofgren, K. A. Long-term results after vein surgery. Study of 1,000 cases after 10 years. *Mayo Clin. Proc.* 49:114, 1974.

96. Lindblom, K. Phlebographische Untersuchung des Unterschenkels bei Kontrastinjektion in eine subkutane Vene. *Acta Radiol.* (Stockh.) 22:288, 1941.

97. Lofgren, K. A. Varicose veins. Their symptoms, complications, and management. *Postgrad. Med.* 65:131, 1979.

98. Lofgren, K. A., and Lofgren, E. P. Extensive ulcerations in the postphlebitic leg. *Surg. Clin. North Am.* 49:1033, 1969.

99. Ludbrook, J. Aspects of Venous Function in the Lower Limbs. Springfield, Ill.: Thomas, 1966.

100. Ludbrook, J. *The Analysis of the Venous System.* Bern: Huber, 1972.

101. Ludbrook, J. Applied Physiology of the Veins. In H. Dodd and F. B. Cockett (eds.), *The Pathology and Surgery of the Veins of the Lower Limb* (2nd ed.). New York: Churchill Livingstone, 1976.

102. Luke, J. C. Evaluation of the deep veins following previous thrombophlebitis. *Arch. Surg.* 61:787, 1950.

103. Maurer, B. J., Wray, R., and Shillingford, J. P. Frequency of venous thrombosis after myocardial infarction. *Lancet* 2:1385, 1971.

104. Mavor, G. E., and Galloway, J. M. D. Collaterals of the deep venous circulation of the lower limb. *Surg. Gynecol. Obstet.* 125:561, 1967.

105. Mavor, G. E., and Galloway, J. M. D. The iliofemoral venous segment as a source of pulmonary emboli. *Lancet* 1:871, 1967.

106. Moreno-Cabral, R., Kistner, R. L., and Nordyke, R. A. Importance of calf vein thrombophlebitis. *Surgery* 80:735, 1976.

107. Moser, K. M. Pulmonary embolism. *Am. Rev. Respir. Dis.* 115:829, 1977.

108. Moser, K. M., Brach, B. B., and Dolan, G. F. Clinically suspected deep venous thrombosis of the lower extremities. A comparison of venography, impedance plethysmography, and radiolabeled fibrinogen. *J.A.M.A.* 237:2195, 1977.

109. Mulvey, R. B. Ascending phlebography and iliac vein opacification. *Radiology* 97:51, 1970.

110. Nabatoff, R. A. Technique for operation upon recurrent varicose veins. *Surg. Gynecol. Obstet.* 143:463, 1976.

111. Negus, D. The post-thrombotic syndrome. *Ann. R. Coll. Surg. Engl.* 47:92, 1970.

112. Nicolaides, A. N., Dupont, P. A., Desai, S., Lewis, J. D., Douglas, J. N., Dodsworth, H., Fourides, G., Luck, R. J., and Jamieson, C. W. Small doses of subcutaneous sodium heparin in preventing deep venous thrombosis after major surgery. *Lancet* 2:890, 1972.

113. Nicolaides, A. N., Kakkar, V. V., Field, E. S., and Renney, J. T. G. The origin of deep vein thrombosis: A venographic study. *Br. J. Radiol.* 44:653, 1971.

114. Nylander, G., and Olivecrona, H. The phlebographic pattern of acute leg thrombosis within a defined urban population. *Acta Chir. Scand.* 142:505, 1976.

115. O'Dell, C. W., and Coel, M. N. Continuous injection supine phlebography. *J. Can. Assoc. Radiol.* 27:186, 1976.

116. O'Donnell, J. A., Lipp, J., and Hobson, R. W., II. New methods of testing for deep venous thrombosis. *Am. Surg.* 44:121, 1978.

117. Olsson, C. G. On the Diagnosis of Deep Vein Thrombosis (thesis). Lund: University of Lund, 1979.

118. Pavlov, H., MacMoran, J. W., Funch, R. B., Bernhard, R. A., and D'Orazio, E. A. Simplified outpatient lower extremity venography. *Radiology* 126:525, 1978.

119. Petropoulos, P., Enderli, J. B., Hadji, H., and Hahnloser, P. Die Gefahr der Lungenembolie bei der isolierten Thrombose der V. saphena magna. *Helv. Chir. Acta* 44:797, 1977.

120. Pollack, A. A., and Wood, E. H. Venous pressure in the saphenous vein at the ankle in man during exercise and change in posture. *J. Appl. Physiol.* 1:649, 1949.

121. Pollak, E. W. The choice of test for diagnosis of venous thrombosis. *Vasc. Surg.* 11:219, 1977.

122. Rabinov, K., and Paulin, S. Roentgen diagnosis of venous thrombosis in the leg. *Arch. Surg.* 104:134, 1972.

123. Rampton, J. B., and Armstrong, J. D., Jr. Bilateral venography of the lower extremities. *Radiology* 123:802, 1977.

124. Ritchie, W. G. M., Lapayowker, M. S., and Soulen, R. L. Thermographic diagnosis of deep venous thrombosis: Anatomically based diagnostic criteria. *Radiology* 132:321, 1979.

125. Rivlin, S. The surgical cure of primary varicose veins. *Br. J. Surg.* 62:913, 1975.

126. Rössle, R. Über die Bedeutung und Entstehung der Wadenvenen thrombosen. *Virchows Arch.* [*Pathol. Anat.*] 300:180, 1937.

127. Schmitt, H. E. *Aszendierende Phlebographie der tiefen Venenthrombose.* Bern: Huber, 1977.

128. Sevitt, S. Diagnosis and management of massive pulmonary embolism. *Proc. R. Soc. Med.* 61:143, 1968.

129. Sevitt, S. Pathology and Pathogenesis of Deep Vein Thrombi. In J. J. Bergan and J. S. T. Yao (eds.), *Venous Problems.* Chicago: Year Book, 1978.

130. Sevitt, S., and Gallagher, N. Venous throm-

bosis and pulmonary embolism—a clinical pathological study in injured and burned patients. *Br. J. Surg.* 48:475, 1961.

131. Shepherd, J. T.   Reflex Control of the Venous System. In J. J. Bergan and J. S. T. Yao (eds.), *Venous Problems.* Chicago: Year Book, 1978.

132. Sherry, S.   Therapy of Deep Vein Thrombosis and Pulmonary Embolism: Medical Approach. In J. Fratantoni and S. Wessler (eds.), *Prophylactic Therapy of Deep Vein Thrombosis and Pulmonary Embolism.* Bethesda, Md.: National Institutes of Health, 1975.

133. Sherry, S.   The problem of thromboembolic disease. *Semin. Nucl. Med.* 7:205, 1977.

134. Sigg, K.   Treatment of Varicose Veins by Injection-Sclerotherapy: A Method Practiced in Switzerland. In J. T. Hobbs (ed.), *The Treatment of Venous Disorders: A Comprehensive Review of Current Practice in the Management of Varicose Veins and the Post-thrombotic Syndrome.* Philadelphia: Lippincott, 1977.

135. Silver, D., and Sabiston, D. C.   The role of vena caval interruption in the management of pulmonary embolism. *Surgery* 77:1, 1975.

136. Smyrnis, S. A., Kolios, A. S., and Agnantis, J. K.   Deep-vein thrombosis in patients with fracture of the upper part of the femur. A phlebographic study. *Br. J. Surg.* 60:447, 1973.

137. Spigos, D. G., Thane, T. T., and Capek, V.   Skin necrosis following extravasation during peripheral phlebography. *Radiology* 123:605, 1977.

138. Stamatakis, J. D., Kakkar, V. V., Lawrence, D., and Bentley, P. G.   The origin of thrombi in the deep veins of the lower limb: A venographic study. *Br. J. Surg.* 65:449, 1978.

139. Stamatakis, J. D., Kakkar, V. V., Sagar, S., Lawrence, D., Nairn, D., and Bentley, P. G.   Femoral vein thrombosis and total hip replacement. *Br. Med. J.* 2:223, 1977.

140. Strandness, D. E., Jr.   Invasive and noninvasive techniques in the detection and evaluation of acute venous thrombosis. *Vasc. Surg.* 11:205, 1977.

141. Strandness, D. E., Jr.   Applied Venous Physiology in Normal Subjects and Venous Insufficiency. In J. J. Bergan and J. S. T. Yao (eds.), *Venous Problems.* Chicago: Year Book, 1978.

142. Strandness, D. E., Jr., Ward, K., and Krugmire, R., Jr.   The present status of acute deep venous thrombosis. *Surg. Gynecol. Obstet.* 145:433, 1977.

143. Sumner, D. S.   The Hemodynamics and Pathophysiology of Venous Disease. In R. B. Rutherford (ed.), *Vascular Surgery.* Philadelphia: Saunders, 1977.

144. Swart, B., and Dingendorf, W.   Experimenteller Beitrag zur optimalen Gefässdarstellung. *ROEFO* 97:637, 1962.

145. Tailored treatment for varicose veins (editorial). *Br. Med. J.* 1:593, 1975.

146. Thomas, M. L.   Gangrene following peripheral phlebography of the legs. *Br. J. Radiol.* 43:528, 1970.

147. Thomas, M. L., and McAllister, V.   The radiological progression of deep venous thrombus. *Radiology* 99:37, 1971.

148. Thomas, M. L., McAllister, V., Rose, D. H., and Tonge, K.   A simplified technique of phlebography for the localisation of incompetent perforating veins of the legs. *Clin. Radiol.* 23:486, 1972.

149. Thomas, M. L., McAllister, V., and Tonge, K.   The radiological appearances of deep venous thrombus. *Clin. Radiol.* 22:495, 1971.

150. Thomas, M. L., and O'Dwyer, J. A.   A phlebographic study of the incidence and significance of venous thrombosis in the foot. *AJR* 130:751, 1978.

151. Townsend, J., Jones, H., and Williams, J. E.   Detection of incompetent perforating veins by venography at operation. *Br. Med. J.* 3:583, 1967.

152. Wheeler, H. B.   Impedance Phlebography: The Diagnosis of Venous Thrombosis by Occlusive Impedance Plethysmography. In E. F. Bernstein (ed.), *Noninvasive Diagnostic Techniques in Vascular Disease.* St. Louis: Mosby, 1978.

153. Wheeler, H. B., and Patwardhan, N. A.   Evaluation of Venous Thrombosis by Impedance Plethysmography. In J. L. Madden and M. Hume (eds.), *Venous Thrombosis: Prevention and Treatment.* New York: Appleton-Century-Crofts, 1976.

154. Widmer, L. K., Mall, T., and Martin, H.   Epidemiology and Socio-medical Importance of Peripheral Venous Disease. In J. T. Hobbs (ed.), *The Treatment of Venous Disorders: A Comprehensive Review of Current Practice in the Management of Varicose Veins and the Post-thrombotic Syndrome.* Philadelphia: Lippincott, 1977.

155. Williams, W. J.   Venography. *Circulation* 47:220, 1973.

156. Young, A. E., Henderson, B. A., Phillips, D. A., and Couch, N. P.   Impedance plethysmography: Its limitations as a substitute for phlebography. *Cardiovasc. Radiol.* 1:233, 1978.

157. Zachrisson, B. E., and Jansen, Hj.   Phlebographic signs in fresh postoperative venous thrombosis of the lower extremity. *Acta Radiol. [Diagn.]* (Stockh.) 14:82, 1973.

158. Zollinger, R. W.   Superficial thrombophlebitis. *Surg. Gynecol. Obstet.* 124:1077, 1967.

Arteriography of the Upper Extremities

DAVID SUTTON

Examination Techniques

PERCUTANEOUS NEEDLE PUNCTURE

This technique was at one time fairly widely used, but in the last 10 years it has been almost completely replaced by catheter techniques. However, direct needle puncture is still used occasionally, when technical difficulties prevent successful catheterization.

Subclavian Artery Puncture

The subclavian artery is usually punctured at the root of the neck. The needle is inserted downward and inward just behind the midpoint of the clavicle. The patient lies with the head slightly extended and turned away from the site of the puncture. In some thin patients, the artery can be easily palpated. In others it may be difficult to feel. In these latter cases, the needle point is usually aimed at the first rib. This can be aided by using control films with markers.

The subclavian artery can also be punctured below the clavicle, particularly in thin patients. In this case, the needle is inserted upward and medially toward the artery as it comes over the first rib.

Axillary Artery Puncture

Occasionally in very thin people, the axillary artery can be very easily felt below the clavicle and can be readily punctured. In most cases, however, the artery is punctured in the axilla. The patient lies supine with the arm abducted and the elbow bent. The artery is then located by palpation of the axilla (except in very obese patients, the artery is usually identified without difficulty). A retrograde puncture is then made.

Brachial Artery Puncture

The brachial artery is commonly punctured just above the elbow, where it is most readily palpable. Sometimes it is punctured at a higher level, in the upper third of the arm. The brachial artery is more liable to spasm than the subclavian and axillary arteries, and therefore it is now little used.

CATHETER TECHNIQUES

In recent years catheter techniques have been further refined by the use of small-gauge thin-walled catheters. These catheters are usually of 5 French outside diameter and are undoubtedly safer than the 7 French or 8 French catheters that were used in the past. The Judkins headhunter catheters were at one time widely used for upper limb catheterization. We now routinely use the soft-walled Mani-type catheters, which are less traumatic to the intima in difficult catheterizations and are less likely to develop clot around their tips.

Transfemoral Catheterization

The catheters are passed from the femoral artery up into the aortic arch and then maneuvered with the use of appropriate guidewires into either subclavian artery. The catheter tip can then be sited in the subclavian, axillary, or brachial artery at a level appropriate to the particular examination.

Transaxillary Catheterization

This technique is less commonly used, but it can be useful in some cases. The catheter is usually passed retrogradely so that its tip lies in the axillary artery or the subclavian artery.

COMPLICATIONS

Local Hematoma

This complication can be particularly troublesome after arterial puncture in areas like the axilla, in which the tissues are lax. Staal et al. [11] have reported on two patients with severe nerve compression from large hematomas in the axilla after axillary catheterization.

The possibility of hematoma formation has been reduced by the use of a smaller catheter (4 French or 5 French) and by the use of a small needle for introducing the catheter.

After the investigation is finished and the needle or catheter withdrawn, firm pressure should be applied over the puncture site for at least 5 minutes or until all oozing has stopped. The puncture hole should be inspected some hours after the examination and then 24 hours later. The patient should be warned to report any further oozing or swelling.

False Aneurysm Formation

This complication is a danger with arterial puncture or catheterization at any site. Preventive measures are similar to those described for hematoma formation. A false aneurysm is essentially a pulsating hematoma, which has developed a capsule, communicating with an arterial lumen. If such a false aneurysm develops, surgical intervention is required to oversew the leaking point in the artery.

Subintimal Injection

This complication may occur whenever a needle with a long point has its tip partly in the arterial wall. The danger can be obviated by using needles with short, sharp bevels. Also, if there is any doubt about the needle tip's being correctly sited in the arterial lumen, small test doses of contrast material should be injected and filmed, or the contrast bolus should be observed on an image intensifier.

Subintimal injection can also occur when the catheter is passed retrogradely and the intima of the artery is damaged and elevated by either the guidewire or the tip of the catheter. Resistance to the passage of the guidewire or catheter usually is felt when this occurs; again, screening of small test doses should minimize the danger of a major subintimal injection. Fortunately, small subintimal catheter lesions are usually harmless. Since the catheter is usually advanced against the direction of blood flow, once the tip is removed from the intima, the normal blood flow will flatten out the elevated intima.

Perivascular Injection

This complication usually occurs with simple needle puncture, and it is more likely to happen when the worker is inexperienced. The precautions described for subintimal injection should be observed. If there is any doubt as to whether the needle point is correctly sited in the lumen, a small test dose should be screened or filmed.

Damage to Nerve Roots

This complication has been recorded after subclavian and axillary artery punctures. The damage results either from direct needle trauma to the nerve or from compression of the nerve by large hematomas.

Arteriovenous Fistula Formation

This complication is a theoretical danger of arteriography at any site because the arteries are close to the veins at most sites of puncture. In practice, however, the complication is a very rare one. We have encountered it only in regard to the vertebral artery. It appears to be more likely to occur with smaller arteries, and it has been recorded after brachial artery puncture.

Arterial Thrombosis

We have not encountered an example of iatrogenic thrombosis in the upper limb, but it is always a danger of arterial puncture at any site. The thrombosis may be a further complication of subintimal stripping. Or it may result from damage to, and elevation of, an atheromatous plaque by a traumatic puncture of the artery. Other cases of arterial thrombosis have been ascribed to stripping of clot from a catheter tip as the tip is withdrawn through the arterial wall.

If thrombosis and an ischemic limb occur immediately after an arterial catheterization or injection, local surgery to remove the clot may be indicated. The surgery should be undertaken if conservative measures have failed to restore circulation and pulses within a few hours. In the two cases of thrombosis in the femoral artery that we have encountered, the obstructive clot was quite localized (1 or 2 inches long) and was easily removed.

Catheter Clot Embolus

The formation of clot on the tips of catheters with peripheral embolus is a theoretical danger in all catheter procedures. It is less likely to happen when the smaller catheters are used and when the procedure is carried out rapidly and skillfully.

In catheterization of the upper limb, there may be difficulty at the apex of the subclavian curve and there is danger of traumatizing the vertebral origin. If injections have to be made from this area, care should be taken not to allow an excessive dose of contrast medium to enter the vertebral artery. It is also wise to use a contrast medium, such as Urografin 310, which is less toxic to nervous tissue.

Pneumothorax

Pneumothorax may be a complication of subclavian puncture at the root of the neck, where the artery is close to the apex of the lung. We have encountered this complication three times in about 100 direct punctures. In all our cases, the lung reexpanded rapidly, and there were no sequelae.

Allergic Reactions

Patients with a known history of severe allergy should be investigated by intravascular injection only when the examination is absolutely essential and then only after every medical precaution to avoid a severe reaction has been taken. This subject is discussed in detail in Chapter 4.

Hypotension

Although hypotension can occur after any arteriographic procedure, it is more common after major contrast injections into large arteries, such as the aorta, than after peripheral arteriography. Severe hypotension is particularly dangerous in patients with generalized arterial disease, because it can initiate thrombosis in a severely stenosed artery. It is a complication that should be carefully watched for, and, if it occurs, immediate measures should be taken to restore blood pressure to normal levels.

ANESTHESIA

Angiography of the upper limb can be readily performed under local anesthesia. After premedication about 1 hour before the examination, most patients tolerate the procedure quite well. General anesthesia may be necessary for the occasional very nervous patient or for children.

When it is desired to show good detail of the digital vessels (e.g., in the investigation of Raynaud's phenomenon), a general anesthesia may also be required. The digital vessels normally fill poorly under local anesthesia but dilate well under general anesthesia. Dilatation of the peripheral vessels can also be achieved by lidocaine block of the sympathetic fibers around the axillary artery. The angiogram can then be performed without general anesthesia. Vasodilatation of the hand can also be achieved by local warming. With temperatures of 33° C, there is usually good filling of the digital vessels [10].

APPARATUS

Most of the special serial filming machines used in angiography are unsuitable for serial angiography of the whole of the upper limb although they may be quite suitable for serial angiography of specific areas. It may be necessary, therefore, to improvise to deal with particular problems. We usually use a Schönander cut-film changer for specific areas of the upper limb, with the patient's arm positioned at a right angle to the body. Thus, if the hand is to be investigated, it is placed over the serial changer. Single film, local views of the upper arm are obtained by using a separate tube or by separate injections. The localization of the needle or catheter point is confirmed by single local films or by screening with an image intensifier.

CONTRAST MEDIA

For the upper limb, lower concentrations of contrast media are advisable. We prefer to use

Urografin 310, particularly if injections are being made in the first part of the subclavian artery, where some of the contrast media may go up the vertebral or ascending cervical artery, which may supply the cord. Chapter 3 discusses the contrast media in general use. For most purposes, 15 cc of contrast media is adequate. It can be injected by hand in about 2 seconds. If arteriovenous shunting occurs, the amount can be increased. The quantity depends on the degree of shunt.

Arteriographic Anatomy

NORMAL ANATOMY

The left subclavian artery arises directly from the aortic arch and passes upward in the thorax to the root of the neck. There it arches laterally across the front of the cervical pleura and behind the scalenus anticus muscle. The right subclavian artery arises from the innominate artery and pursues a similar course on the right side. The first part of each artery lies in the thorax, and the second part lies behind the scalenus anticus muscle. The third part extends downward and laterally from the lateral border of the scalenus anticus muscle to the outer borders of the first rib. Each subclavian artery rests on the upper surface of the first rib and lies in front of the lowest trunk of the brachial plexus.

The first main branch of the subclavian artery is the vertebral artery, which arises from the medial aspect of the first part of the subclavian artery, near its termination. Particularly on the left side, however, the vertebral artery may arise at a more proximal level. The thyrocervical trunk arises just distal to the vertebral artery; it gives off the inferior thyroid, transverse cervical, and suprascapular arteries.

The internal mammary artery arises from the lower margin of the subclavian artery, directly below the origin of the thyrocervical trunk. The costocervical trunk arises from the second part of the subclavian artery on the right side and from the first part of the subclavian artery on the left side.

The axillary artery is the direct continuation of the subclavian artery; it begins at the outer border of the first rib. It passes downward and laterally to the lower border of the teres major muscle, where it becomes the brachial artery. Its main branches are the superior thoracic, acromiothoracic, lateral thoracic, subcapsular, posterior circumflex, humeral, and anterior circumflex humeral arteries.

The brachial artery originates at the lateral border of the teres major muscle and ends in the cubital fossa, opposite the neck of the radius. The main branches are the profunda brachii artery, the ulnar collateral artery, and the supratrochlear artery. There are also some smaller muscular branches.

The radial artery arises from the termination of the brachial artery and is the smaller of its two terminal branches. It begins opposite the neck of the radius and ends in the palm of the hand by anastomosing with the deep branch of the ulnar artery to form the deep palmar arch. It gives off the radial recurrent artery and muscular and other small branches. At the wrist, it gives off the posterior carpal arch before terminating in the hand in the princeps pollicis artery and the deep palmar arch.

The ulnar artery is the other terminal branch of the brachial artery. It gives off the ulnar recurrent arteries, the common and anterior interosseous arteries, and muscular branches before anastomosing with the branches of the radial artery to form the superficial and deep palmar arches.

There is considerable variation in the distribution of the arteries of the hand. The common variations are described in the standard anatomic textbooks. Edwards [2] describes the possible variations in the organization of the arteries in the hand and digits. In most cases, however, the digital arteries follow a standard pattern [2]. The palmar digital arteries arise from the convex side of the superficial palmar arch. Each of the palmar digital arteries to the interdigital clefts is joined before it divides by a palmar metacarpal branch from the deep palmar arch.

The deep palmar arch gives off the palmar metacarpal arteries, which join the palmar digital arteries. Either the superficial arch or the deep palmar arch may be absent. The thumb is supplied by the princeps pollicis artery, which is given off by the radial artery as it enters the palm. The princeps pollicis artery divides into the palmar digital arteries, which anastomose with the dorsal digital arteries. The radialis indicis artery arises near the origin of the princeps pollicis artery and supplies the radial side of the index finger.

The posterior carpal arch lies on the back of the carpus and is formed by the union of the posterior carpal branches of the radial and ulnar arteries. It gives off the three dorsal metacarpal arteries.

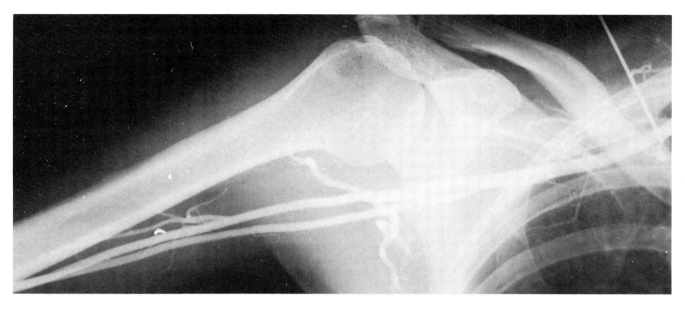

Figure 79-1. Bifurcation of the axillary artery into the radial artery and the ulnar artery.

CONGENITAL ANOMALIES

The right subclavian artery arises from the distal part of the aortic arch in rather more than 1 percent of cases and then passes upward behind the esophagus to reach the apex of the right lung. The left vertebral artery arises directly from the aortic arch instead of from the left subclavian artery in about 5 percent of cases.

Rarely, the axillary artery divides into the radial and ulnar arteries and there is no brachial artery (Fig. 79-1). More commonly (though still rarely), the radial and ulnar arteries arise from a high bifurcation of the brachial artery in the upper arm, or the brachial artery bifurcates at a lower level than usual [5]. These anomalies are of some importance when arteriography is attempted by brachial or axillary puncture.

Either the radial or the ulnar artery may be absent. It is then replaced by branches of its fellow or by an interosseous artery.

Vascular Lesions

ANEURYSMS

Congenital Aneurysms

Congenital aneurysms are exceptionally rare. In our material, we have seen only two examples of small, unsuspected aneurysms, both demonstrated as chance findings. One aneurysm arose from the brachial artery and the other from the axillary artery; both were saccular and about 5 mm in diameter. They resembled the berry aneurysms seen in the intracranial circulation. Although these aneurysms were probably of congenital origin, the possibility of their association with unrecalled trauma cannot be excluded.

Mycotic Aneurysms

Mycotic aneurysms are encountered more frequently, usually in the peripheral vessels of the forearm and hand. Most of our cases have been associated with bacterial endocarditis. Figure 79-2 shows such an aneurysm. These lesions tend to grow quite rapidly, and they require urgent treatment.

Syphilitic Aneurysms

In the upper limb, syphilitic aneurysms are rare and are becoming increasingly so. We have encountered specific aneurysms of the subclavian and axillary arteries but not of the more peripheral vessels.

Poststenotic Aneurysms

Poststenotic aneurysms are not infrequent in the subclavian artery in association with cervical rib or some other thoracic outlet syndrome. These aneurysms are usually small and fusiform, but occasionally they are very large. They may also be a source of peripheral emboli from clot within the lumen, and they usually require surgical inter-

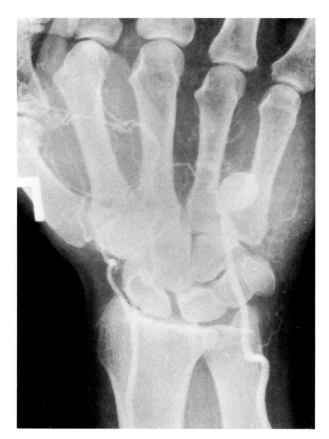

Figure 79-2. Mycotic aneurysm of the palm.

vention. The arterial stenosis may also be associated with vascular insufficiency and peripheral emboli.

Traumatic Aneurysms

Traumatic aneurysms may occur anywhere in the arterial tree of the upper limb. Such aneurysms are usually pseudoaneurysms (i.e., a tear in the arterial wall has permitted an encapsulated effusion of blood pulsating in continuity with the intraarterial blood). We have seen several examples of such false aneurysms involving the first or second part of the right subclavian artery after injuries to the chest in car accidents. Figure 79-3 illustrates such a case. Traumatic aneurysms also may be encountered elsewhere in the limb (Fig. 79-4).

Dissecting Aneurysms

Dissecting aneurysms of the aorta can involve the subclavian arteries, but it is very unusual for them to extend outside the thorax. Arteriectasis is a generalized fusiform dilatation of major arteries. The vessels are usually irregular and atheromatous and may show localized saccular dilatation. Figure 79-5 illustrates such a case, in a patient who had bilateral large axillary aneurysms and an associated thoracic outlet syndrome.

ANGIOMAS

Angiomatous malformations are not uncommon in the upper limb; they usually involve the peripheral vessels in the hand although occasion-

Figure 79-3. Traumatic aneurysm of the subclavian artery due to a crush injury of the chest in an automobile accident. (A) Preoperative angiogram. (B) Postoperative arteriogram after replacement by a Dacron graft.

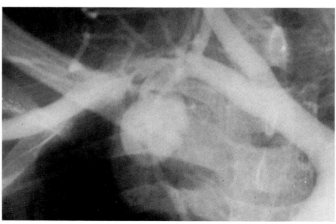

A

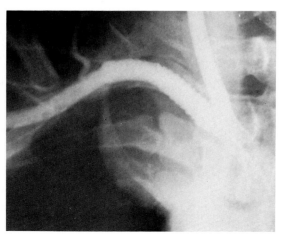

B

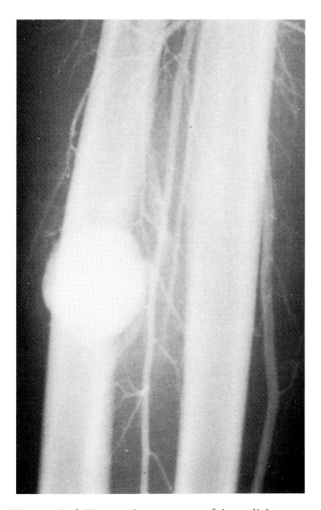

Figure 79-4. Traumatic aneurysm of the radial artery.

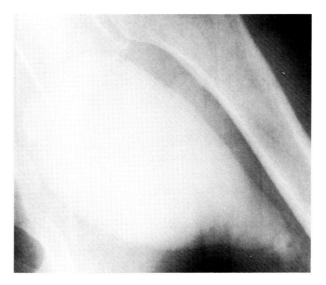

Figure 79-5. Giant poststenotic aneurysm of the axillary and brachial arteries associated with fusiform dilatation of the subclavian artery.

ally they are more proximal. The type that consists of direct arteriovenous communications at the arteriolar level is well shown by angiography (Fig. 79-6). They are very difficult to treat surgically because only a complete excision will cure the lesion. In most cases, proximal ligation is merely palliative because the angioma tends to recur rapidly from a collateral circulation. One of our patients, who had all the brachial, ulnar, and radial arteries tied, still had an angioma that filled very well at an angiogram performed a year later.

If direct surgery is to be attempted in these cases, first-class angiography showing all the feeding and drainage vessels is necessary. Rapid serial films are also required because of the rapid shunting of blood through the lesion. When the shunt is large, the dosage of contrast medium may have to be increased considerably to show the anatomy clearly. Some angiomas arise more distally in the circulation and are at the capillary

level. These are more difficult to demonstrate by angiography than are direct arteriovenous communications although small areas of shunting can be demonstrated occasionally (Fig. 79-7). When the lesion is largely venous, angiography is not very helpful, and venous varices are better demonstrated by venography.

ARTERIOVENOUS FISTULAS

In clinical practice, most of the arteriovenous fistulas encountered are of traumatic origin. As elsewhere in the body, the rupture of a diseased artery into a vein may be one cause, although it is extremely rare in the upper limbs. Arteriography itself has been cited as a cause of traumatic arteriovenous fistula. In our experience, this risk is rather unlikely unless small arteries are punctured. We have seen two examples after vertebral artery puncture but none elsewhere in the circulatory system. Arteriovenous fistula has been described at other centers after arteriography of the upper limb when the brachial artery has been punctured at the elbow.

Angiography of an arteriovenous fistula will usually require rapid serial filming and increased doses of contrast medium. It is very important that the angiographic studies clearly show the site of the fistula because it is notoriously difficult to demonstrate at surgery, when the surgeon is dealing with a mass of small, hypertrophied arteries and arterialized veins. In several of our

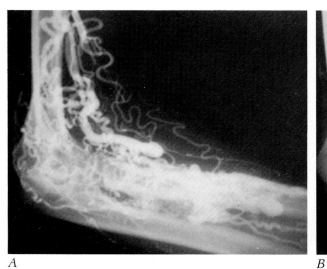
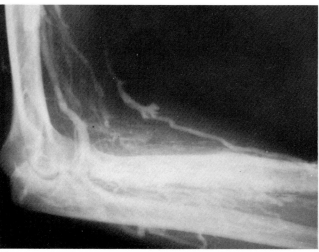

A   *B*

Figure 79-6. Angioma around the elbow (serial filming). (A) Early film. Multiple tortuous and dilated vascular channels are apparent, and there is premature venous opacification. (B) Later film. Draining veins are now better defined.

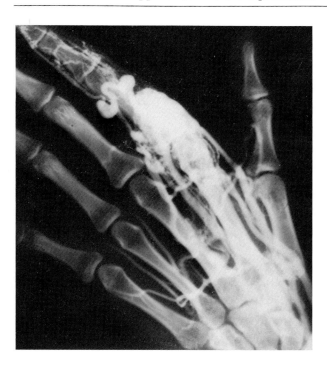

Figure 79-7. Angioma of the index finger.

cases, successful surgery has been possible only after adequate angiography clearly localized the site of the lesion.

EMBOLUS

Embolus to the upper limb is seen most commonly in patients with atrial fibrillation and is derived from intraatrial clot. Mitral stenosis is the commonest predisposing cause. Less common causes of peripheral embolus are intraventricular clot after myocardial infarction and paradoxical embolus from systemic venous thrombosis. Small peripheral emboli may occur from the poststenotic aneurysms associated with the scalenus anticus syndrome or from clot formation at the site of arterial compression.

These peripheral emboli usually affect the digital arteries and can give rise to digital gangrene. The larger emboli seen in mitral stenosis and atrial fibrillation usually involve a major vessel, and the brachial bifurcation is the commonest site. Such brachial emboli have a fairly good prognosis, and most of them respond to conservative treatment (Fig. 79-8).

STENOSES AND THROMBOSES

Arterial stenoses and thromboses are usually caused by atheroma and are particularly common in the lower limbs of males. Atheromatous irregularity of the major arteries to the upper limbs

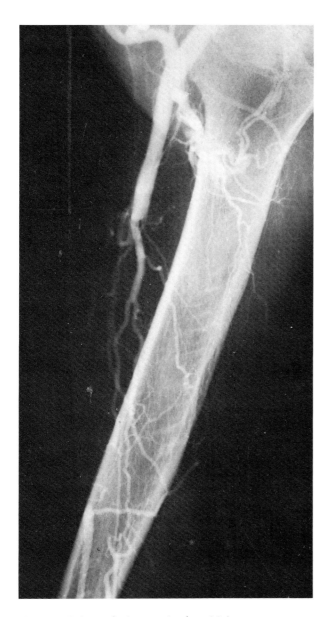

Figure 79-8. Embolus to the brachial artery.

Figure 79-9. Atheromatous stenosis of the axillary artery.

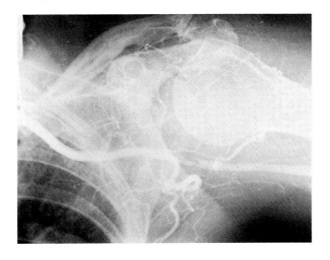

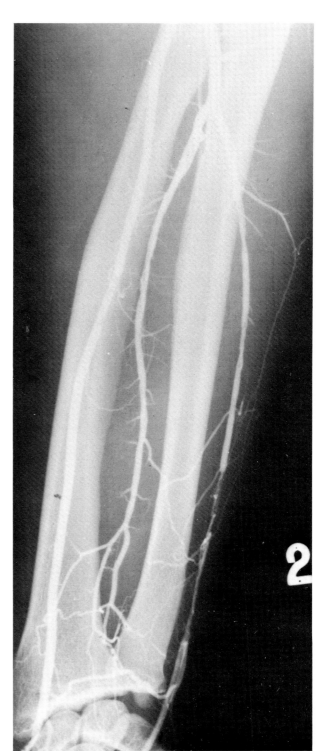

Figure 79-10. Stenoses of the ulnar artery. The patient was a young professional tennis player whose hand became numb and white during prolonged rallies but was normal during moderate activity.

is frequently demonstrated at angiography, but frank atheromatous stenoses and thromboses are less common than they are in the lower limbs (Fig. 79-9). Furthermore, the collateral circulation in the upper limbs is extremely good, and even when a thrombosis occurs, the symptoms are less marked than they would be in the lower limbs. Because the symptoms of major lesions are often slight and therefore are often not diagnosed, the true incidence of such lesions may be underestimated. Diagnostic symptoms are more likely to occur in someone who performs heavy manual labor or in an athlete who calls upon the arm to do more work than is normal. Peripheral stenotic lesions in the forearm may produce severe symptoms in such individuals (Fig. 79-10).

Stenoses or thromboses of the subclavian artery can also occur as a result of compression in a thoracic outlet syndrome. These lesions also cause poststenotic aneurysm or give rise to local thrombosis and clot formation, with the detachment of peripheral emboli. Raynaud's phenomenon may also result from such compression by a cervical rib or a fibrous or muscular band. Axillary thrombosis has been caused by chronic pressure on the axillary artery by a crutch in patients with an amputated or a paralyzed leg (see Fig. 79-5).

Another rare cause of arterial thrombosis in the upper limb is generalized blood disease (e.g., polycythemia). With the increased use of oral contraceptives, thrombosis from no apparent cause may also be encountered in women. An unusual cause encountered in our cases but not documented in the literature is fibromuscular hyperplasia (Fig. 79-11).

Atheromatous thrombosis of the subclavian artery may occur in the thorax, and the first part of the left subclavian artery is usually involved. In these cases, the left vertebral artery may act as a collateral vessel to the arm. The reverse flow in the vertebral artery in such a condition is usually referred to as subclavian steal, on the assumption that blood is being "stolen" from the brain.

On the right side, innominate occlusions or occlusion of the origin of the right subclavian artery may give rise to a similar syndrome. Such patients may present with symptoms suggesting cerebrovascular insufficiency or with low blood pressure in one arm. The low blood pressure is frequently less marked than would be expected (20–40 mm Hg) owing to the excellent collateral circulation.

Occlusion of the subclavian artery in the thorax may also occur as an acute lesion in association with dissecting aneurysms or, more insidiously, with Takayasu's syndrome or in nonspecific arteritis (Fig. 79-12).

Thromboses of Digital Vessels
Emboli can be a cause of such occlusions, but in many other cases the lesions are probably due to local atheroma of the peripheral vessels. Buerger's disease rarely affects the hands, but we

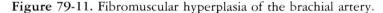

Figure 79-11. Fibromuscular hyperplasia of the brachial artery.

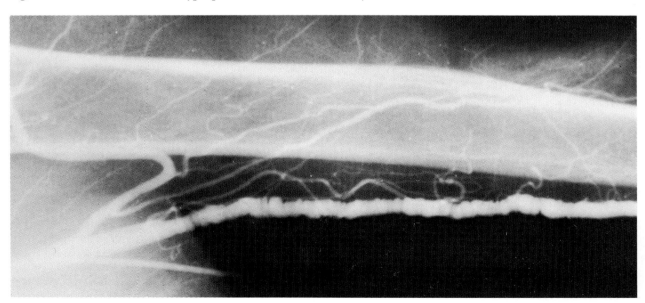

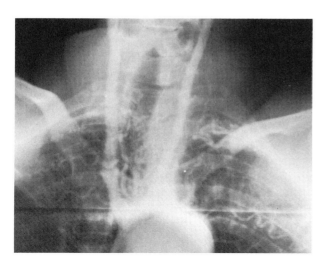

Figure 79-12. Bilateral thromboses of the subclavian arteries due to arteritis. Note the collateral circulation.

have encountered cases in which it has. In most cases of ischemia of the fingers in which angiography demonstrates a local occlusion (Fig. 79-13), the etiology is never clearly established but is assumed to be atheromatous. Rarer causes of peripheral occlusions, such as cryoagglutination, must be excluded.

RAYNAUD'S PHENOMENON

In this common condition, the hands are unusually sensitive to cold, and blanching of the hands occurs very rapidly on exposure to low temperatures. This phenomenon is thought to be due to peripheral arterial spasm, and in most cases it seems to be a functional condition. The so-called physiologic, functional, or primary Raynaud's phenomenon has to be differentiated from similar changes that may be secondary to organic dis-

Figure 79-13. Digital thromboses in two different patients.

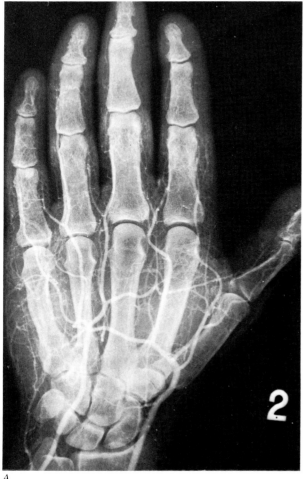

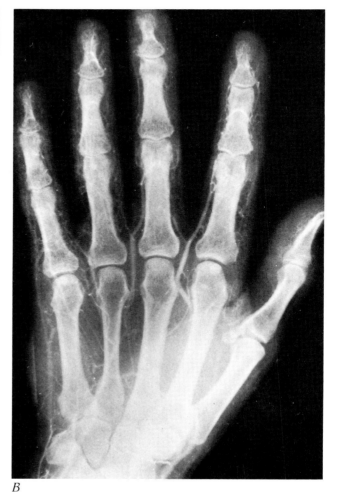

A   B

Table 79-1. Causes of Digital Ischemia
and Raynaud's Phenomenon

Lesions of major vessels (often with small vessel emboli)
  Atheroma
  Takayasu's disease
  Nonspecific arteritis
  African idiopathic aortitis
  Thoracic inlet syndrome
  Buerger's disease
  Fibromuscular hyperplasia
Collagen disorders
  Scleroderma
  Disseminated lupus erythematosus
  Rheumatoid arthritis
  Polyarteritis nodosa
  Polymyalgia rheumatica
Blood disorders
  Polycythemia
  Sickle cell disease
  Cryoagglutination
  Oral contraceptives–related
  Polyvinylchloride poisoning
Specific conditions
  Raynaud's phenomenon (spastic type)
  Vibrating tools–related
  Ergotism

ease. Most of the organic lesions are discussed elsewhere in the chapter; they include the thoracic outlet syndromes and atheromatous stenoses. Angiography will help to demonstrate or exclude organic lesions in the proximal or distal vessels.

Table 79-1 lists the many causes of secondary Raynaud's phenomenon and of digital ischemia.

Nail Dystrophies

Strickland and Urquhart [12] studied the digital vessels by angiography in patients with Raynaud's phenomenon and associated nail changes. They found a poor correlation with organic arterial disease and suggested that spasm might play a part in the nutritional changes because organic vascular change could not be consistently demonstrated.

SPASM

Acute spasm of peripheral arteries may result from direct trauma. Supracondylar fractures with damage to the brachial artery can give rise to acute spasm, which may then cause ischemic fibrosis of muscles in the forearm (Volkmann's ischemic contracture). The diagnosis is usually suspected on clinical grounds although arteriography is occasionally used to confirm it.

Ergotism

Ergotism is a rare cause of peripheral vascular spasm. Most of the cases now encountered are secondary to overdosage with ergotamine tartrate, which is used for the treatment of migraine. The overdose is usually self-administered, and in this respect suppositories are particularly dangerous. The lower limbs are usually affected, but spasm may occur in the arms. In seven cases reviewed by Allen et al. [1], the lower limbs were affected in all the cases and the upper limbs were affected in two cases. The angiographic appearances are characteristic and include a sudden narrowing of the major arteries (e.g., the common femoral or axillary arteries). The main arteries then continue as fine, smooth-walled vessels to the periphery. In the only two cases we have encountered, the femoral arteries were patent but resembled narrow threads only 2 to 3 mm in diameter [13].

Thoracic Outlet Syndromes

Thoracic outlet syndromes are discussed in detail in Chapter 44. In such cases, the blood supply to the upper limbs is obstructed (usually unilaterally), and the patient complains of pain, tingling, and numbness. Angiography is essential to the diagnosis and to the choice of treatment.

Tumors

Arteriography of the upper limb is occasionally helpful in the diagnosis and differential diagnosis of tumors of bone or soft tissues. Thus, os-

Figure 79-14. Malignant tumor of the clavicle (secondary renal cell carcinoma).

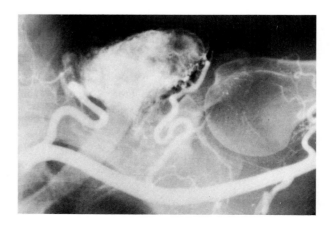

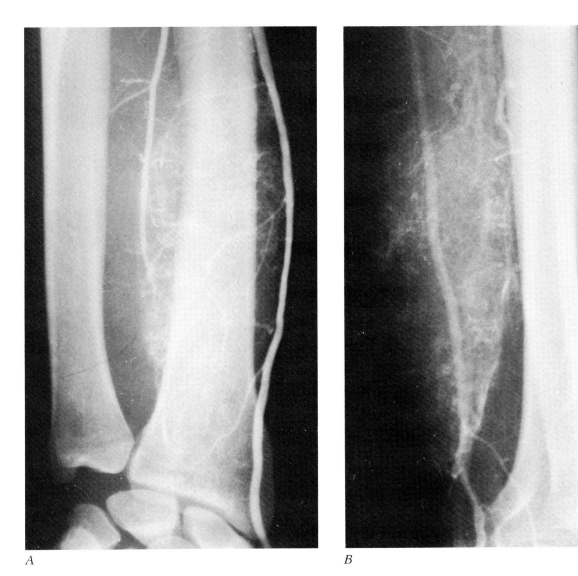

A   *B*

Figure 79-15. Malignant tumor of the forearm (histologically, rhabdomyosarcoma). (A) Anteroposterior view. (B) Lateral view.

teogenic sarcoma will show the typical pattern of a malignant tumor: arteriovenous shunts and hypervascularity in the tumor area. The differential diagnosis of bone tumors by angiography is discussed in other chapters. It should be noted that the angiogram may supply valuable evidence in confirming the diagnosis of malignant bone tumor and in showing its extent in the soft tissues. The same is true of the diagnosis of lumps in soft tissues in which clinical differentiation between sarcoma and benign conditions, such as hematoma or cyst, is difficult. Figures 79-14 and 79-15 show examples of different types of bone

and soft tissue tumors in the upper torso that are well shown by angiography.

Inflammatory and Other Disorders

Laws et al. [8] investigated 67 patients with rheumatoid arthritis and various other conditions by upper limb angiography. Rheumatoid arthritis was present in 42 patients. Three patients had polyarteritis, and most of the others were considered to have primary Raynaud's phenomenon. These workers found that in rheumatoid arthritis, occlusions occurred in one or more digital vessels in two-thirds of the patients. They also found that hyperemia occurred near bony erosions and in areas of synovial proliferations in 22 of 37 patients. In the three patients with polyarteritis, the main findings were multiple occlusions affecting vessels distal to the palmar arch and, frequently, a network of irregular, tortuous vessels replacing the occluded ones.

Embolization and Therapeutic Angiography

Embolization of angiomas, arteriovenous fistula, and vascular tumor can be performed in the arm as elsewhere in the body. The principles are discussed in Chapter 91. In the arm, particular care is necessary to use a superselective technique involving only the major supplying vessels and to avoid the entry of emboli into normal vessels and, especially, the vertebral artery or the ascending cervical artery.

References

1. Allen, E., Barker, N. W., and Hines, E. A., Jr. *Peripheral Vascular Disease.* Philadelphia: Saunders, 1962.
2. Edwards, E. A. Organization of the small arteries of the hands and digits. *Am. J. Surg.* 99:837, 1960.
3. Glazer, G., Myers, K. A., and Davies, E. R. Ergot poisoning. *Postgrad. Med. J.* 42:562, 1966.
4. Hink, V. C., Judkins, M. P., and Paxton, H. D. Simplified selective femorocerebral angiography. *Radiology* 89:1048, 1967.
5. Keller, F. S., Rösch, J., Dotter, C. T., and Porter, J. M. Proximal origin of radial artery. Potential pitfalls in hand angiography. *AJR* 134:109, 1980.
6. Kramer, R. A., Hecker, S. P., and Lewis, B. I. Ergotism. Report of a case studied arteriographically. *Radiology* 84:308, 1965.
7. Lang, E. K. Arteriographic diagnosis of the thoracic outlet syndrome. *Radiology* 84:296, 1965.
8. Laws, J. W., Lillie, J. G., and Scott, J. T. Arteriographic appearances in rheumatoid arthritis and other disorders. *Br. J. Radiol.* 36:477, 1963.
9. McCormack, J. J., Cauldwell, E. W., and Anson, B. J. Brachial and antebrachial arterial patterns of study of 750 extremities. *Surg. Gynecol. Obstet.* 96:44, 1953.
10. Rösch, J., Antonovic, R., and Parker, J. M. The importance of temperature in angiography of the hand. *Radiology* 123:323, 1977.
11. Staal, A., van Voorthuisen, A. E., and van Dijk, L. M. Neurological complications following arterial catheterisation by the axillary approach. *Br. J. Radiol.* 39:115, 1966.
12. Strickland, B., and Urquhart, W. Digital arteriography, with reference to nail dystrophy. *Br. J. Radiol.* 36:465, 1963.
13. Sutton, D., and Preston, B. J. Angiography in peripheral ischaemia due to ergotism. Report of two cases. *Br. J. Radiol.* 43:776, 1970.

Angiography of Bones, Joints, and Soft Tissues

CHARLES J. TEGTMEYER

Establishing the exact diagnosis of certain bone and soft tissue tumors remains one of the most perplexing problems in medicine. Often, there is considerable delay in the diagnosis because specific clinical symptoms are lacking. The radiologic examination is a critical step in the diagnosis of these lesions. However, because bone continually reacts to local and systemic changes in its environment by either removing or laying down mineralized matrix, the changes depicted on plain radiographs may be misleading and very difficult to interpret.

The pathologist plays a crucial role in the diagnosis of these lesions. Because these tumors are relatively uncommon, however, most pathologists do not have the opportunity to examine many bone and soft tissue tumors. The problem is further complicated because much of the biopsy material submitted for examination is inadequate: either the biopsy site is inappropriate or the biopsy specimen does not accurately represent the lesion. It has been repeatedly emphasized that close cooperation among the radiologist, pathologist, and surgeon is necessary to arrive at a correct diagnosis in these difficult lesions.

Although angiography is a well-established procedure in the evaluation of other neoplasms, it has not gained wide acceptance in the diagnosis of bone tumors—perhaps because the angiographic pattern does not always allow an exact diagnosis to be made. This is, however, also the case for the clinical, histologic, and other radiographic examinations of these lesions.

If the limitations of angiography are understood and the procedure is used properly in conjunction with other diagnostic studies, angiography can play a valuable role in the diagnosis of bone and soft tissue lesions.

Vascular Anatomy

A knowledge of the vascular anatomy is necessary to understand the findings made at angiography. Current knowledge of the vascular supply of the bones is based on the observations of Doan [12], Drinker et al. [14], Tilling [72], and Trueta [73].

The long bones have three sources of arterial blood: (1) nutrient arteries supplying the diaphysis and epiphysis, (2) the periosteal and perichondrial arteries, and (3) the metaphyseal and epiphyseal vascular systems. The nutrient

1937

arteries enter the diaphysis to supply the medullary cavity. There are extensive anastomoses between the nutrient arteries and the metaphyseal vessels. The nutrient arteries also anastomose with the rich periosteal blood supply, which perforates the compact bone to enter the haversian system. Branches from the vascular supply of the surrounding muscles and tendons also perforate the bone to supply the epiphyseal and metaphyseal portions of the bone. Although the epiphyseal and metaphyseal systems are separate, they anastomose with each other across the epiphyseal cartilage except for a short period of time during the development of the femoral head in the child. The venous drainage of the long bones is similar in distribution to the arterial blood supply.

Enlarged arteries are often seen coursing through the muscles and other soft tissues surrounding the tumors. These vessels supply the soft tissue tumors and feed the periosteal and perichondrial arteries that constitute the main blood supply in most bone lesions [86]. Depending on the location of the lesion, the metaphyseal and epiphyseal vessels may also contribute to the vascular supply of the tumor. The nutrient artery usually does not contribute a significant, angiographically visible blood supply to the tumor. If the tumor breaks out of the bone, the vessels supplying the surrounding tissue feed the tumor.

Technique

The percutaneous Seldinger technique is employed to introduce the catheter into the vascular tree. The angiographic demonstration of bone and soft tissue tumors is markedly improved when the catheter is directed with the arterial flow in the antegrade position [28]. Catheters with the appropriate shape are then used to select the major vessels supplying the region of the tumor.

The pelvis and upper thigh are studied using 5.0 or 6.5 French catheters. The contralateral femoral artery is used to approach these lesions. Either the aortic bifurcation or the common iliac artery is injected. The catheter is deflected over the aortic bifurcation with a Cook tip deflector to enter the ipsilateral common iliac artery. With this angiographic run as a map, the catheter is placed selectively in the major vessel supplying the tumor or as close to this vessel as possible.

As with all angiographic studies, the contrast medium should be injected as near the lesion as is feasible. Selective injections are then made into the vessels supplying the tumor, usually the internal or distal external iliac artery. Filling of the adjacent overlying vessels is thereby eliminated, aiding in the interpretation of the angiograms. This is a particularly necessary step in the pelvis. Injections are also repeated in different projections to delineate the entire extent of the tumor. If entry into the upper thigh is desired, a tight J-shaped guidewire can be passed into the common femoral or superficial femoral artery and the catheter advanced over the wire.

Lesions in the distal lower extremity are usually studied by entering the ipsilateral common femoral artery with an antegrade puncture. The antegrade puncture is easier to perform if a large sponge pad or blanket roll is placed under the patient's buttocks to hyperextend the hips. The small catheters used (5 French) can be easily advanced into the popliteal artery.

For lesions of the upper extremity, the femoral approach is ordinarily employed. A 5.2 or 6.5 French Cook HIH catheter can usually be advanced over a tight J-shaped guidewire into the brachial artery. The axillary approach can also be utilized. This approach makes it easy to select the branches of the subclavian and axillary arteries. A 5 French catheter with a small C-shaped curve at the tip is used.

Visualization of both the arterial and venous circulations is desirable in all cases since the venous phase of the arteriogram often provides extremely valuable information. The radiographs should be obtained initially at two films per second for 3 seconds, then one film per second for 10 seconds followed by films every 2 seconds for a total of 26 seconds. After the first run, the angiographic program can be tailored to the circulation of the individual lesion.

Depending on the size of the patient, 5 to 12 cc of contrast material is injected per second for 4 to 5 seconds. The average injection rate into the common iliac artery is 8 to 10 cc per second for a total of 40 cc of contrast material. The axillary and popliteal arteries require 7 to 8 cc per second for a total of 30 to 40 cc of contrast material.

Subtraction radiographs are extremely valuable in bone and soft tissue tumors. By eliminating the superimposed bones and the tumoral calcifications, they permit a more thorough evaluation of the vascular pattern. When the diagnosis is in doubt, magnification radiographs may also be helpful since they can enhance the visualization of tiny vessels.

Pharmacoangiography is important for the enhancement of bone and soft tissue tumors. Ekelund et al. [16] compared the effects of a vasoconstrictor (angiotensin) and a vasodilator (tolazoline) in 18 patients with bone and soft tissue tumors and concluded that angiotensin was more effective. Angiotensin is administered by diluting 10 to 15 mg in 10 cc of normal saline and injecting it slowly through the catheter at a rate of 5 cc per second. The angiogram is repeated 15 to 45 seconds later.

Many investigators [28, 35], however, feel that tolazoline (Priscoline) is more effective. A total of 25 to 50 mg of Priscoline is diluted in 10 cc of normal saline and infused slowly through the catheter. The amount depends on the size of the patient and the area studied. An injection of Renografin-76 is made 30 seconds later with the catheter in the antegrade position, with its tip as close to the lesion as possible. Subsequent contrast injections can be supplemented by 12.5 mg of Priscoline before each angiographic run.

Several points must be borne in mind when pharmacoangiography is employed. It is important to obtain a standard angiographic run before augmenting the angiography with vasoactive drugs. If a retrograde injection is performed, increasing the injection rate produces reflux into proximal vessels and does not improve the quality of the angiogram. Since Priscoline increases the intravascular volume and decreases the circulation time, a higher injection rate and a higher total volume are required [28].

Angiographic Appearance

The evaluation of the arteriogram is based on visualization of the entire circulation throughout the lesion. The arteries supplying the tumor need to be adequately opacified, and the film program should be long enough to visualize the capillary phase and the venous drainage.

MALIGNANT TUMORS

The angiographic picture of malignancy is a composite of several of the following factors:

1. Neovascularity.
2. Pooling or laking of contrast material.
3. Tumor stain or blush.

4. Encasement and occlusion of vessels.
5. Extension of the tumor outside the bone.
6. Displacement of vessels.
7. Arteriovenous shunts.
8. Large abnormal draining veins.
9. Tumor invasion of veins.
10. Abnormal course of veins.

Neovascularity
The term *neovascularity* or *pathologic vessel* has been defined by Strickland [70] as a vessel that is "deployed seemingly without purpose, keeps to no set course and shows no progressive diminution in calibre." Histologically, such a tumor vessel is a primitive vascular channel often consisting only of an endothelial layer surrounded by a connective tissue sheath. Hence its irregularly irregular course and caliber.

The presence of neovascularity is the single most important finding upon which the differentiation between benign and malignant is based [77]. Abnormal vascularity, however, may also be present in certain benign lesions [75], including giant cell tumors, aneurysmal bone cysts, osteoblastomas, and Paget's disease. Benign nerve sheath tumors and certain hemangiomas may also exhibit abnormal vascularity. Fortunately, most of these lesions can be differentiated by their clinical and plain film appearances.

Pooling or Laking of Contrast Material
Ill-defined accumulation of contrast material may be seen in a malignant lesion. These patchy accumulations of contrast material have been described as pooling or laking of contrast material. This appearance results from neovascular vessels that end their haphazard journey in amorphous spaces within necrotic tissue [70]. These amorphous spaces often retain contrast material well into the venous phase of the arteriogram. This angiographic finding is another expression of the abnormal vascularity seen in tumors and is a reliable sign of malignancy.

Tumor Stain or Blush
Diffuse staining of the tumor by contrast material is a nonspecific finding. The presence of a tumor blush by itself does not indicate malignancy. There is a small group of benign bone lesions that have a tendency to retain contrast material: giant cell tumors, aneurysmal bone cysts, osteoid osteomas, and osteoblastomas. This finding, however, is of great value in assessing the size of the

tumor, and it may indicate that the tumor has broken out of the bone.

Encasement and Occlusion
Encasement or occlusion of vessels is seen in malignant tumors. While atherosclerosis may also cause stenoses and occlusions of vessels, an abrupt termination of an otherwise normal artery in the area of a bone or soft tissue tumor is a frequent indicator of malignancy.

Tumor Extension
Extension of the tumor outside the confines of the bone is a reliable sign of malignancy. This sign is not seen in benign hypervascular lesions unless a fracture is present. Fractures occasionally cause bizarre-appearing hypervascularity [31]. Angiography, however, does not always define the complete intraosseous extent of the tumor, and skip metastases within the bone are not always seen [31].

Displacement of Vessels
The displacement of vessels is an indication of the anatomic extent of the tumor. This is important if a radical local resection is contemplated because the surgeon will know he will have to deal with these vessels. The degree of vascularity is also important in the preoperative assessment because it gives some indication of the blood loss to be expected.

Arteriovenous Shunts
Early opacification of the veins draining the tumor is an expression of rapid blood flow through the tumor. The presence of opacified veins during the arterial phase of the arteriogram indicates arteriovenous shunting and the presence of an abnormal microcirculation. This is not, however, a specific sign of malignancy.

Presence of Large Abnormal Draining Veins
Large abnormal draining veins are also seen in hypervascular lesions. These veins often encircle the tumors and are helpful in defining their extent. The identification of these major venous drainage pathways is important in order to facilitate early ligation and prevent tumor embolization during surgery [31].

Tumor Invasion of Veins
Direct invasion of the veins by the tumor may sometimes be seen. When present, this is a sign of malignancy.

Abnormal Course of Veins
Strickland [70] described another venous sign of malignancy: the presence of straight veins coursing at right angles to the normal flow of venous blood. This finding is more frequent in metastatic tumors than in primary lesions.

DIFFERENTIATION BETWEEN BENIGN AND MALIGNANT TUMORS

It must be remembered that the angiographic picture of malignancy is a composite of signs, all of which will not be present in any one tumor. Nevertheless, more than one sign of malignancy is usually present in a given tumor. Strickland [70] found angiographic evidence of malignancy in all but 2 of the 33 malignant bone tumors he examined. Voegeli and Uehlinger [77] examined 100 bone tumors with angiography and concluded that use of angiographic studies as a supplement to standard radiography increased the diagnostic accuracy in differentiating a benign from a malignant lesion by approximately 25 percent.

If the definitive angiographic signs of malignancy are present, it can be reasonably assumed that the lesion is malignant. The converse is *not* true, since a small number of malignant tumors, especially those that do not breach the cortex [68], fail to demonstrate any of the angiographic signs of malignancy. Therefore, a normal arteriogram does not entirely rule out a malignancy.

Benign bone neoplasms usually do not deviate from the normal angiographic appearance. The vessels may be displaced by the bulk of the tumor, and in some instances a tumor stain or blush and hyperemia are present. It is important to remember that a tumor stain or blush is not a specific sign of malignancy.

Furthermore, one often cannot distinguish among the individual types of bone tumors using the angiographic picture alone. This is not surprising considering the difficult diagnostic problem bone tumors cause the plain film radiographer, pathologist, and clinician.

Arteriography is of considerable assistance in distinguishing between benign and malignant bone tumors. In addition, angiography provides reliable information as to the extent of bone and soft tissue lesions. It accurately demonstrates the soft tissue extension of bone tumors [87]. It also defines the most suitable site for biopsy because the highly vascularized areas within a particular tumor correspond to its most malignant areas.

The necrotic areas within the tumor appear as avascular spaces, which can be avoided when the biopsy site is chosen.

Inflammatory Lesions of Bones

OSTEOMYELITIS

The invading organism may attack the bone directly from an infected wound, a penetrating injury, or a contaminated fracture or may gain access by hematogenous spread from a distant infection. Hematogenic osteomyelitis is the most common form and is predominantly a disease of infants and children. The most frequent infecting organism is *Staphylococcus aureus*, less commonly *Streptococcus*, and least commonly other organisms.

The plain film radiologic findings are well known. The primary locus of osteomyelitis in children is the metaphysis. Early changes are first noted in the soft tissue. The changes in the bone usually take 2 weeks to develop, and then small osteolytic areas appear in the metaphysis. Periosteal elevation occurs as the infection spreads and new bone is laid down. At this stage the infection often mimics neoplastic lesions. If treatment is delayed, the changes of chronic osteomyelitis will ensue.

The angiographic picture of osteomyelitis parallels the progress of inflammatory changes. These changes are seen first in the surrounding soft tissue and later in the bone. Hyperemia is observed, and the arteries and veins appear more numerous and are dilated. Rapid circulation is noted throughout the area of infection. The arteries are tortuous but have regular lumina and show none of the variations in caliber that characterize pathologic vessels [38]. The small contrast-filled vascular lakes often seen in malignancy are not present [26].

Chronic osteomyelitis is usually accompanied by a normal angiographic picture although occasionally hyperemia is seen.

BRODIE'S ABSCESS

Brodie's abscess, an often painful lesion usually found near the end of a long bone, frequently presents as a round or oval radiolucent area with a sclerotic rim. It has a radiographic appearance similar to that of an osteoid osteoma, but angiography can easily differentiate the lesions since Brodie's abscess is avascular [47, 86], while osteoid osteoma is highly vascular [47, 54].

Bone Tumors of Cartilaginous Origin

BENIGN TUMORS

Chondroblastoma

Chondroblastoma or Codman's tumor is a rare benign tumor of cartilaginous origin with a predilection for the epiphyses. The lesion usually occurs in the second decade of life and is more common in males than in females, with a ratio of 2 to 1.

Roentgenographically, the lesion appears as a radiolucent defect involving the epiphysis, and a thin sclerotic margin is often present. The lesion originates in the epiphysis but may enlarge and involve the metaphysis (Fig. 80-1A).

Experience with the angiographic patterns of chondroblastoma is limited. Yaghmai [86] reported the angiographic findings in five cases. The arteries supplying the lesions arose from the surrounding soft tissue, and his cases exhibited a low degree of vascularity with a faint tumor stain. We have obtained an angiogram of one completely avascular chondroblastoma. However, chondroblastomas may exhibit hypervascularity [64]. The vessels supplying the lesion may be extremely tortuous, but they appear to taper normally (Fig. 80-1B, C) and do not have the irregularly irregular course of malignancy.

The plain film differential diagnosis of chondroblastomas includes giant cell tumors. Angiographically, however, the entities are easily separated. The giant cell tumor has intense hypervascularity and a prolonged intense blush that is not seen in chondroblastomas.

Chondromyxoid Fibroma

Chrondromyxoid fibroma is a benign bone tumor, apparently derived from cartilage-forming connective tissue, that contains chondroid, myxoid, and fibrous elements. It occurs predominantly in the lower limb but may occur elsewhere, including the flat bones. While it may be found at any age, its peak incidence is in the second and third decades.

The radiographs usually suggest a benign process. In the long bones, the lesion is likely to be eccentrically situated in the metaphysis. It is visualized as a sharply outlined radiolucent defect,

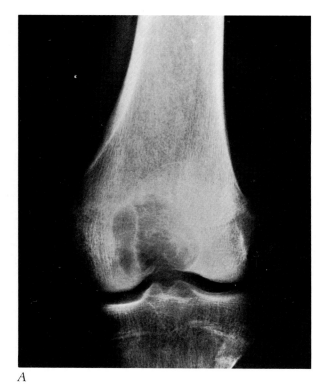

A

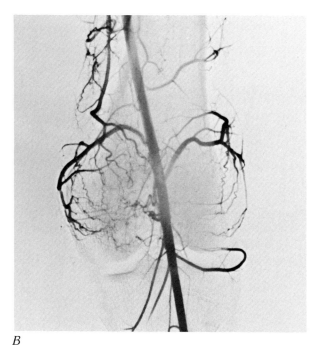

B

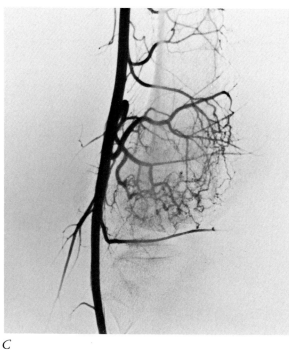

C

Figure 80-1. Chondroblastoma of the distal femur in a 14-year-old boy with a 6-month history of knee pain. (A) The plain film demonstrates a well-demarcated destructive lesion involving the epiphysis and distal metaphysis. (B) The subtraction film of the arteriogram demonstrates increased vascularity in the area of the tumor. Branches of the genicular arteries supply the tumor. (C) The lateral subtraction film shows the marked tortuosity of the vessels supplying the tumor.

which thins the cortex and which may contain trabeculae. Angiographically, the lesion is avascular and has a benign appearance [86].

Osteochondroma

The osteochondroma is the most common benign neoplasm of bone. It is a cartilage-capped bony protuberance composed of osseous and chondroid elements. The lesion is usually located at the metaphysis, particularly in the long bones around the knee. It can, however, involve any bone that develops from cartilage.

Vascular complications resulting from osteochondromas are not rare, particularly in the area of the knee. Because of their size and location, osteochondromas may damage the popliteal artery or vein. Both thrombosis [27] and pseudoaneurysms [23] have been reported in the popliteal artery. Angiography reveals that osteochondromas, because of their size, may displace vessels. The tumor, however, does not

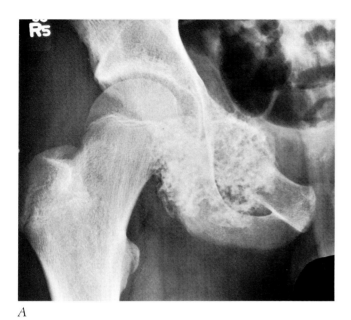

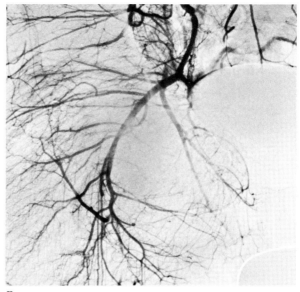

A

B

Figure 80-2. Osteochondroma of the pubic bone in a 15-year-old boy with a slowly enlarging mass. (A) A well-defined lesion containing extensive irregular calcification is present in the pubic bone. (B) The normal-appearing vessels are displaced by the lesion. No hypervascularity or neovascularity is present.

Figure 80-3. A low-grade chondrosarcoma of the pubic bone in a 61-year-old man. The lesion has been present for 9 years. (A) A huge mass arises from the pubic ramus near the symphysis. It contains amorphous calcification. (B) The hypovascular lesion displaces the surrounding normal vessels.

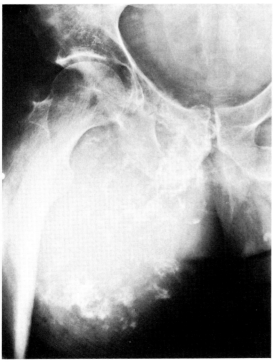

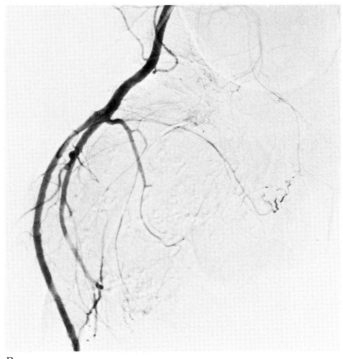

A

B

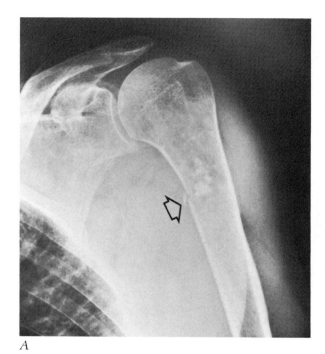

A

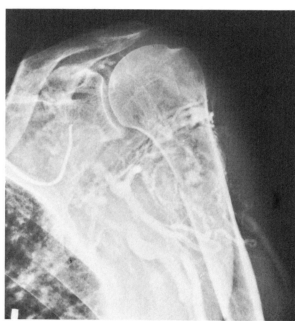

C

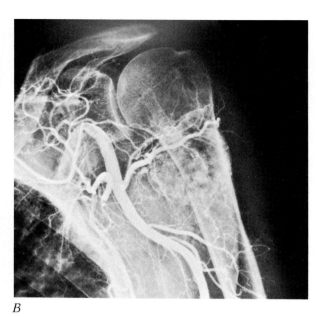

B

Figure 80-4. Chondrosarcoma of the humerus in a 73-year-old man. The patient related his shoulder pain to a fall on his left shoulder 7 weeks previously. (A) An ill-defined lytic defect containing flocculent calcification is present in the humerus. A pathologic fracture is seen (*arrow*). (B) The arteriogram exhibits abnormal vascularity and a tumor blush. The neoplasm extends into the surrounding soft tissue. (C) The pooling of contrast material within the tumor persists into the venous phase. Abnormal veins are seen draining the lesion.

MALIGNANT TUMORS

Chondrosarcoma
Chondrosarcoma is a malignant bone tumor of cartilaginous origin, arising either in bone (primary type) or from a preexisting cartilaginous lesion (secondary type). Central chondrosarcomas arise in the interior of the bone. Peripheral chondrosarcoma develops on the surface of the bone as a protruding mass. Chondrosarcoma is the second most common primary malignant bone tumor, if myeloma is excluded. The lesions usually occur in the fourth, fifth, and sixth decades of life; when the tumor occurs in childhood, it carries a grave prognosis.

Peripheral chondrosarcoma presents a distinct appearance radiographically. It is usually a large lobulated mass projecting from a flat or long bone. It is invariably calcified.

Central chondrosarcomas are more difficult to diagnose because they often present as benign-appearing radiolucent defects in the bone that

exhibit hypervascularity or abnormal vessels [84] (Fig. 80-2).

Enchondroma
An enchondroma is a benign cartilaginous neoplasm located within the medullary cavity of a bone. It is poorly vascularized and reveals no abnormal vessels [69].

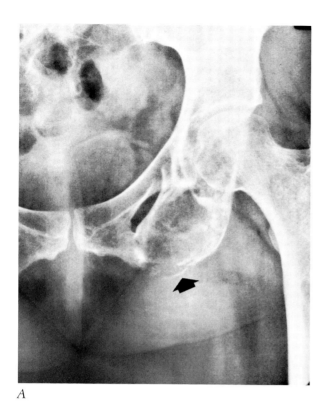

A

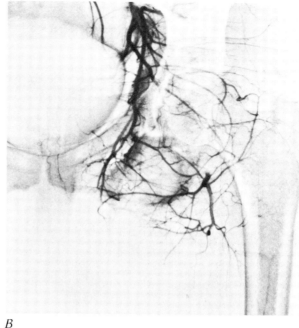

B

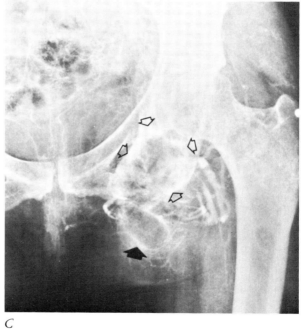

C

Figure 80-5. Chondrosarcoma of the ischium in a 33-year-old woman with a 5-month history of pain and tenderness in the left buttock. (A) There is an osteolytic lesion in the ischium. The cortex is expanded, and a fracture is seen (*arrow*). (B) The arteriogram exhibits a faint blush around the periphery of the lesion in the arterial phase. (C) The venous phase again shows the tumor blush at the margins of the lesion (*open arrows*). The tumor can be seen extending through the fracture site into the soft tissue (*solid arrow*).

contain calcification. This is one bone tumor that may appear completely benign roentgenographically. If the lesion progresses, it will become less well defined and eventually penetrate the cortex.

The angiographic pattern of chondrosarcomas is varied, ranging from normal to hypervascular [84]. Large tumors may be hypovascular, exhibiting only displacement of the normal surrounding arteries (Fig. 80-3). At the other end of the spectrum, the tumor may exhibit florid neovascularity, and large abnormal veins may be seen draining the tumor (Fig. 80-4). The lesion may display a tumor stain (Fig. 80-5), but this is not a prominent feature.

Despite the varied angiographic pattern, angiography contributes valuable information in the evaluation of chondrosarcomas. Lagergren et al.

[40] demonstrated a relationship between the degree of vascularity and the degree of differentiation of the tumor. The highly vascular tumors are poorly differentiated and have a poor prognosis (Fig. 80-6). The most vascular area of the tumor corresponds to the most aggressive portion of the tumor. This is the area that should be subjected to biopsy. The displacement of surrounding normal vessels, the peripheral reactive

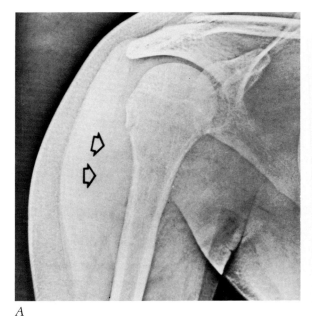

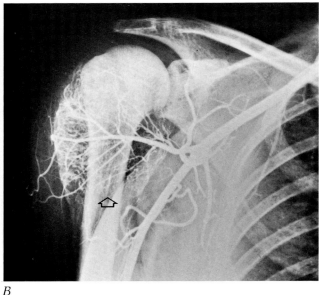

A   B

Figure 80-6. A poorly differentiated chondrosarcoma of the humerus in a 20-year-old woman. The patient presented with a 3-month history of pain and swelling in the shoulder. (A) The xerogram shows displacement of the soft tissue (*arrows*). However, the bone appears normal. (B) The florid neovascularity clearly outlines the extent of the tumor. Vertical streaks of contrast material are seen within the medullary cavity (*arrow*), indicating the origin of the tumor. The patient developed pulmonary metastases 7 months after primary resection of the tumor.

vascularity, and the neovascularity all contribute to defining the extent of the lesion. Therefore, angiography usually accurately delineates the extent of the tumor [31] (Fig. 80-6; see also Fig. 80-4).

It is important to remember that the lack of abnormal vascularity does not completely rule out malignancy in chondroid tumors. Some slow-growing chondrosarcomas will have a deceptively normal vascular pattern.

Bone Tumors of Osteoblastic Origin

BENIGN TUMORS

Osteoid Osteoma
Osteoid osteoma is a small, painful, benign neoplasm of bone. It is a not uncommon entity. Ninety percent of the patients are below the age of 25 years, and it is more prevalent in males than in females with a ratio of 2 to 1.

Osteoid osteoma has been observed in nearly all the bones of the body. Ordinarily, however, it affects the diaphysis of the tibia and femur.

Radiographically, the changes are related to the central nidus and its location. The tumor usually presents as a small radiolucent intracortical nidus less than 1 cm in size surrounded by a dense area of sclerosis. The nidus may contain calcium or be completely radiolucent. In this situation, the diagnosis is obvious; however, the lesion does not always present the classic roentgen picture. The surrounding dense sclerosis may obscure the central nidus, or, if the lesion is located in cancellous bone, relatively little sclerosis may be present. Occasionally, when the osteoid osteoma is located adjacent to a joint, it lacks the classic roentgen findings and instead appears as a synovitis [54, 62].

Angiography can be extremely helpful when the diagnosis is in doubt. The findings at angiography are characteristic [42, 47, 54]. A small vessel with an irregular lumen supplies a circumscribed highly vascular area in bone. An intense circumscribed blush appears early in the arterial phase and persists into the late venous phase (Figs. 80-7, 80-8). This pattern easily allows differentiation from osteomyelitis, Brodie's abscess, and stress fractures, which lack the intense vascular blush seen in osteoid osteoma.

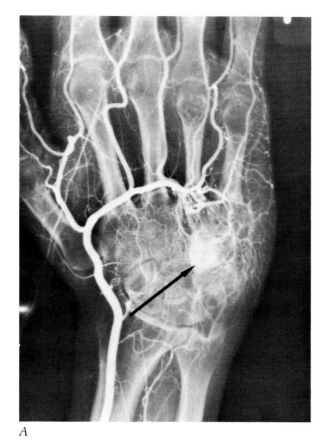

A

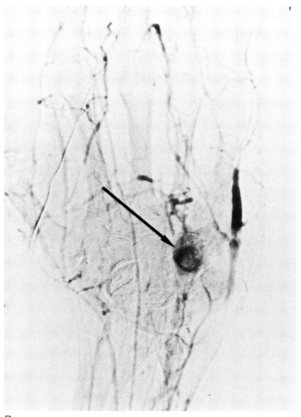

B

Figure 80-7. Osteoid osteoma of the hamate in a 29-year-old man complaining of increasing pain, swelling, and limitation of motion of the left wrist of 18 months' duration. (A) The arterial phase shows an intense circumscribed vascular blush in the hamate (*arrow*). (B) The venous phase of the arteriogram (subtraction film) shows the persistence of the blush (*arrow*). (From O'Hara et al. [54].)

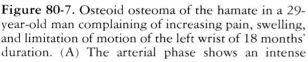

Osteoblastoma

Benign osteoblastoma is a rare neoplasm of bone. The lesion is similar to osteoid osteoma in histologic appearance and in age incidence. It differs, however, in size, location, and roentgen appearance. The tumor principally affects the vertebrae and the bones of the limbs. It has an affinity for the vertebral arch, chiefly in the transverse and spinous processes, although the bodies may also be affected. In the tubular bones, the lesion is eccentrically located in the metaphysis or shaft.

The radiographic features are not distinctive, and lesions vary in size and density, ranging from 2 to 12 cm in size. The lesion is expansile and readily breaks the cortex. The soft tissue component may be surrounded by a thin calcific shell. There is usually no periosteal reaction.

The roentgenograms are often misleading, and angiography may be helpful. The angiographic

pattern of osteoblastomas, however, has not been clearly defined. Yaghmai [81] reported the angiographic features of one lesion, stating that it contained mild hypervascularity. On the other hand, osteoblastomas may be extremely vascular and exhibit an intense tumor stain (Fig. 80-9). This is not surprising because of the lesion's histologic similarity to osteoid osteoma.

MALIGNANT TUMORS

Osteosarcoma

Osteosarcoma is a malignant bone tumor characterized by the predominant production of osteoid matrix by tumor cells. Osteosarcomas have been subdivided, on the basis of histologic pattern, into many types: sclerosing, osteolytic, medullary, and telangiectatic. This classification is, however, of little prognostic significance. Osteosarcoma is the most common primary tumor

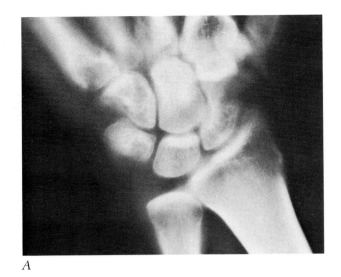

A

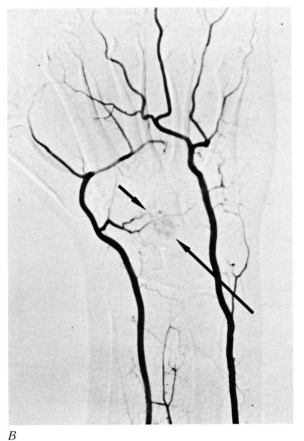

B

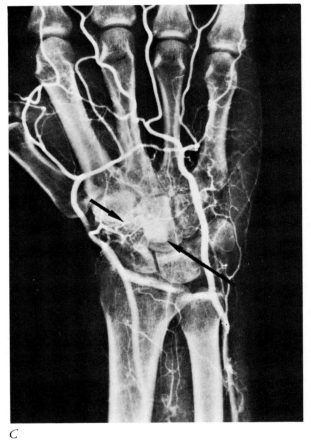

C

Figure 80-8. Osteoid osteoma of the capitate bone in a 28-year-old man suffering from pain in the right wrist for the last 2 years. (A) A magnified tomogram of the wrist demonstrates sclerosis of the distal part of the wrist with a suggestion of a lucent area abutting the area of sclerosis. (B) A subtraction roentgenogram of the early arterial phase demonstrates a small irregular vessel (*short arrow*) supplying a vascular lesion in the capitate (*long arrow*). (C) The angiogram in the later arterial phase again shows the irregular vessel (*short arrow*). The intense persistent blush of the lesion is clearly seen (*long arrow*). (From O'Hara et al. [54].)

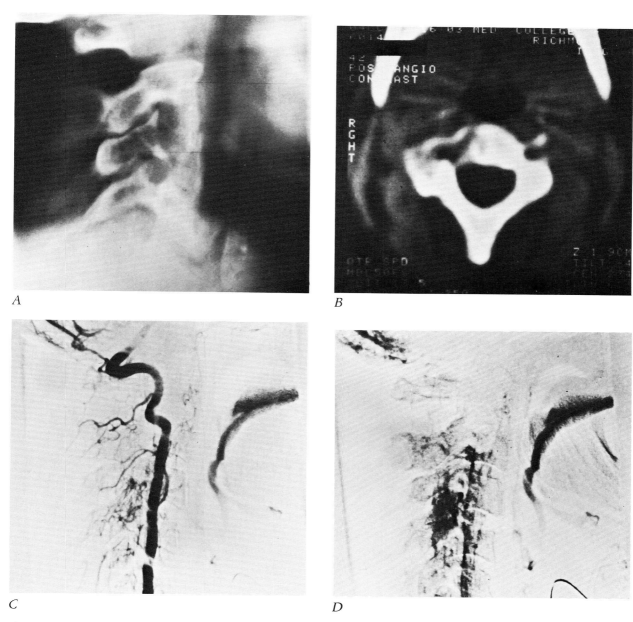

Figure 80-9. Osteoblastoma of the cervical spine in a 42-year-old woman who complained of right arm pain. (A) A tomogram of the cervical spine demonstrates an expansile lytic lesion involving the posterior elements of the third cervical vertebra. (B) A CT scan shows the expansion and thinning of the lateral mass and pedicle of the third cervical vertebra. (C) The vertebral angiogram reveals a highly vascular lesion supplied by tortuous vessels. (D) A persistent intense tumor blush is present. (Courtesy of Frederick S. Vines, M.D.)

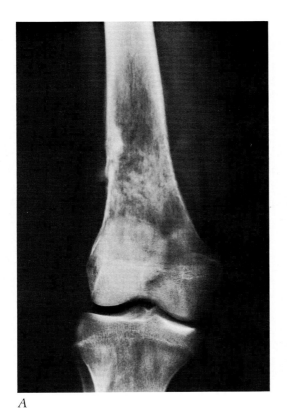

A

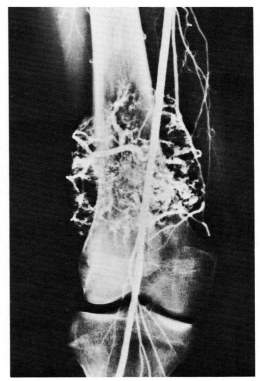

B

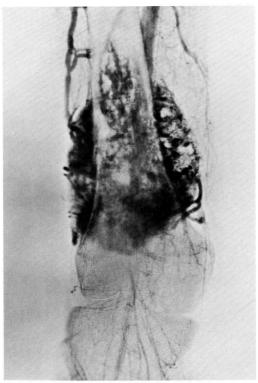

C

Figure 80-10. Osteosarcoma of the distal femur in a 15-year-old girl. (A) A destructive mixed lesion is seen in the distal femur. Soft tissue calcification is present on the lateral side of the femur. (B) The arteriogram exhibits considerable neovascularity, and encasement of some vessels is seen. (C) An intense tumor blush is present, and abnormal veins demonstrate the extension of the tumor into the soft tissue on both the medial and lateral aspects of the bone.

of bone, multiple myeloma excluded. The lesion usually occurs in the second decade of life. It is more often found in males than in females, with a ratio of 2 to 1. Osteosarcomas occurring in older age groups are usually associated with a preexisting bone disorder such as Paget's disease, postirradiated bone, or osteochondromas.

The metaphyseal area of long bones is by far the most common site of origin of osteosarcoma. It occurs most often in the lower end of the femur, upper end of the tibia or femur, and upper humerus.

The radiographic picture of osteosarcoma is usually a combination of bone destruction (lysis), bone formation (increased density), and periosteal reaction (periosteal new bone forma-

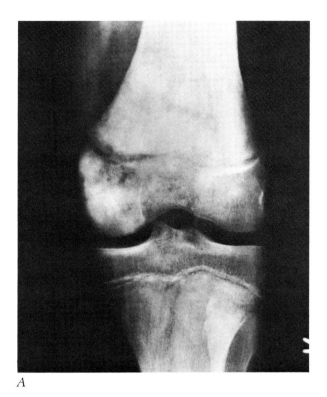

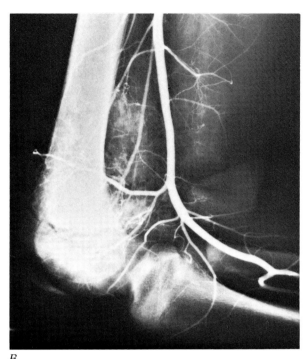

A   *B*

Figure 80-11. Osteosarcoma of the distal femur in a 13-year-old boy with intermittent leg pain of several years' duration. (A) A sclerotic lesion is noted in the metaphysis, and it appears to have crossed the epiphyseal plate—an unusual situation. (B) The arteriogram demonstrates the lesion in the distal femur and surrounding soft tissue. (C) The subtraction film enhances the visualization of the vessels, clearly showing the involvement of the epiphysis and the soft tissue extension.

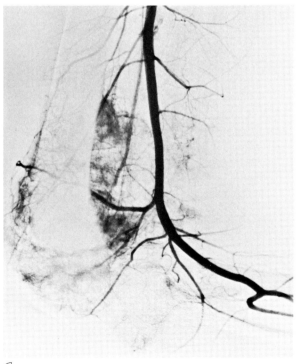

tion). Commonly, osteosarcomas produce a Codman's triangle due to subperiosteal bone formation that is stimulated by the advancing tumor. The tumor may present a roentgen picture ranging from very dense to (rarely) a purely osteolytic lesion.

Although the varied tissue component of osteosarcomas creates a spectrum of vascular architecture, osteosarcomas are usually hypervascular [41]. The vessels supplying the tumor may be enlarged. Neovascularity and hypervascularity are invariably present [81] (Fig. 80-10). Subtraction films are very helpful in evaluating the vascular pattern in sclerotic osteosarcomas (Fig. 80-11). A tumor stain is usually present (Fig. 80-12). Encasement of the vessels is often seen

C

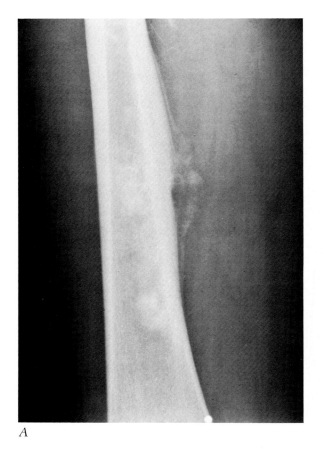

A

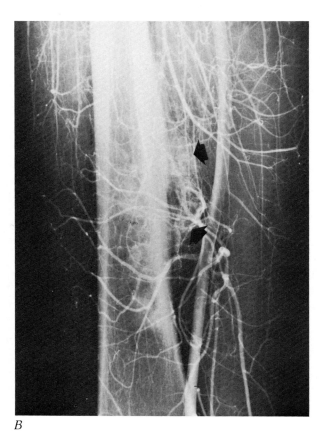

B

Figure 80-12. Osteosarcoma involving the diaphysis of the femur in a 14-year-old girl with a 1-month history of thigh pain. (A) A sclerotic lesion is present in the femur, and a small amount of periosteal new bone formation is seen forming a Codman's triangle. (B) The magnification film shows the tumor blush most marked in the area of the periosteal new bone formation (*arrows*). This is the most active area of the tumor and the best site for biopsy.

(see Fig. 80-10). A vascular sunburst pattern with small vessels running perpendicular to the shaft of the bone may be seen in some cases [59].

Early-draining veins are present in most of the tumors. The veins are usually dilated and often displaced by the tumor (see Fig. 80-10). The tumor may invade the veins, causing obstruction of the venous flow.

Most, if not all, osteosarcomas penetrate the cortex and invade the surrounding soft tissues before they are discovered [64, 86]. This greatly aids the angiographic diagnosis of malignancy because the abnormal vascularity in the surrounding soft tissue is readily visualized even when the plain film findings are subtle or nonexistent (Fig. 80-13).

Angiography is extremely helpful in osteosarcomas. It demonstrates that the tumor is malignant, delineates the best site for biopsy, and accurately depicts the degree of soft tissue extension. However, skip areas within the medullary canal are not always detected [31]. Computed tomography may prove to be helpful in detecting these skip metastases, but experience is limited [7].

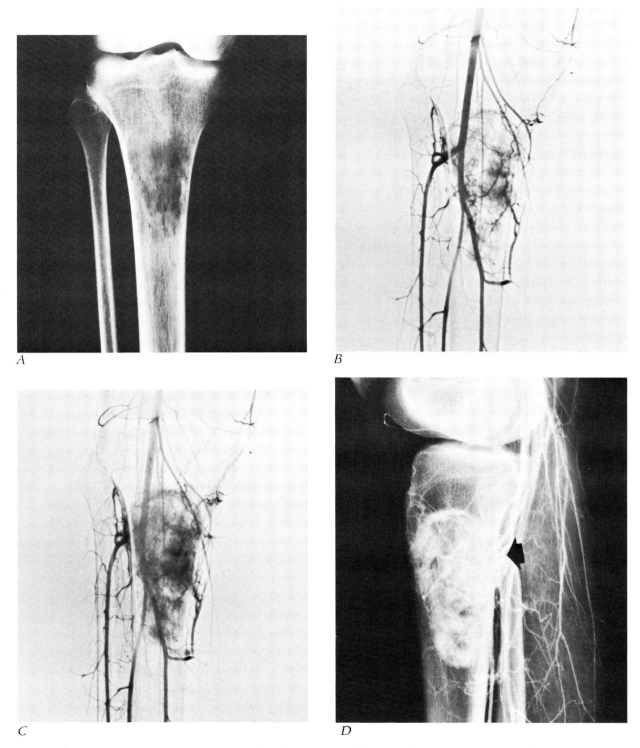

A

B

C

D

Figure 80-13. Osteosarcoma of the proximal tibia in a 27-year-old woman complaining of leg pain of 4 weeks' duration. (A) A radiolucent destructive lesion with a permeative pattern is present in the proximal tibia. (B) The arterial phase reveals some neovascularity. (C) An intense tumor stain is present. (D) The lateral film clearly shows extension of the lesion outside the bone (*arrow*) although this was not apparent on the plain films. The biopsy was interpreted as indicating a giant cell tumor. However, because of the arteriogram, the tissue was reviewed by a consultant, who considered the tumor to be an osteosarcoma.

Bone Tumors of Marrow Origin

PLASMA CELL MYELOMA

Plasma cell myeloma is a primary malignant tumor of bone characterized by a neoplastic proliferation of plasma cells of the bone marrow. It is the most common primary malignant bone tumor. While the age range is from 25 to over 80 years, 75 percent of the patients are between the ages of 50 and 70 years. The most frequently involved bones are vertebra, rib, skull, pelvis, and femur.

Radiographically, multiple myeloma is usually a destructive lesion, although it may uncommonly be partly or dominantly sclerotic. The hallmark of the disease is the sharply circumscribed "punched-out" lesion. The lesions are usually multiple, and in such cases the diagnosis is obvious. However, uncommonly the disease may appear as a solitary focus. It is in this situation that angiography may be helpful.

The angiographic findings in myeloma have been described by Laurin et al. [44]. In their review of 10 cases, 9 were found to be solitary on admission, and all of the lesions exhibited various degress of hypervascularity. The arteries were slightly enlarged in the majority of cases. Neovascularity was present in 9 of the 10; in the other case, the arterial detail was obscured by an intense vascular blush. A diffuse tumor blush was present in all instances, and subtraction films were of help in demonstrating the blush. Early venous filling was observed in 9 cases. Soft-tissue extension of the tumor, which was present in all cases, helped differentiate the lesions from benign hypervascular lesions. In addition to the 10 hypervascular cases just cited, an isolated instance of hypovascular multiple myeloma has been described [86].

EWING'S SARCOMA

Ewing's sarcoma is an uncommon primary malignant tumor of the bone that apparently arises from immature reticulum cells of the bone marrow. It is the fourth most prevalent primary malignant bone tumor. Ewing's sarcoma is mainly a tumor of youth and adolescence, usually occurring between the ages of 5 and 30 years. It is more frequent in males than in females, with a ratio of 2 to 1.

Ewing's sarcoma has occurred in almost all the bones of the body. The tubular bones are most likely to be involved in younger patients, but in patients over the age of 20 the flat bones are the most frequent sites. While the tumor classically involves the diaphyses, it may affect the metaphyses or epiphyses.

The radiographic picture is that of a rapidly growing tumor with destructive and reparative processes going on simultaneously. In the long bones, cortical destruction may be associated with "onionskin" lamination of the periosteum. In the flat bones, mottled destruction is associated with patchy sclerosis.

The degree of vascularity, as depicted by angiography, varies in Ewing's sarcomas, but most of these tumors have a sparse vascular bed [26, 86]. A faint tumor stain is often visualized in the late capillary phase. Circumscribed avascular regions, representing areas of tumor necrosis, are likely to be present in these tumors. Figure 80-14 demonstrates a Ewing's sarcoma with unusually intense vascularity. Ewing's sarcoma tends to penetrate the cortex, and a soft tissue component accompanies the tumor as a rule. The extension of the tumor is usually well delineated by arteriography (Fig. 80-14). Neovascularity is often visible at the periphery of the tumor, and encasement of small vessels may be seen. Displacement of adjacent major vessels is often present.

RETICULUM CELL SARCOMA

Reticulum cell sarcoma of bone is an isolated focus of this disease that apparently arises from the medullary cavity. The tumor has been reported in almost every bone in the body; however, it has a predilection for the long bones. It is a tumor of adults.

Radiographically, reticulum cell sarcoma appears as a destructive lesion, often with little periosteal response. The angiographic findings are similar to those of Ewing's sarcoma [86]. In the early stages of the tumor, angiography may appear deceptively innocent [70].

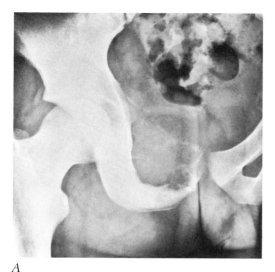

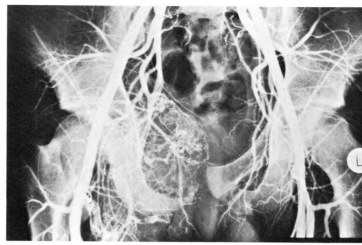

A   B

Figure 80-14. Ewing's sarcoma of the pubic bone in a 16-year-old boy with a 1-month history of a lump in his groin. (A) The plain radiograph of the pelvis reveals a large lytic lesion destroying the right pubic bone. (B) The pelvic arteriogram demonstrates a large hypervascular tumor extending into the soft tissues. (C) Arteriography, with magnification, exhibits florid neovascularity, displacement of the surrounding vessels, and arteriovenous shunting. Extension of the tumor into the veins is seen (*arrow*).

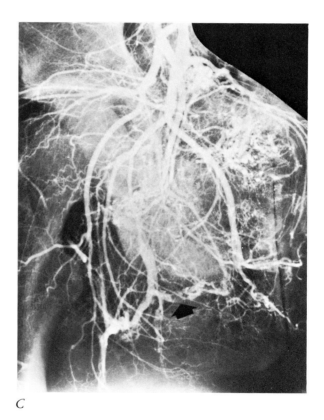

C

Bone Tumors of Uncertain Origin

GIANT CELL TUMOR

Giant cell tumor is an uncommon, aggressive tumor that develops within bone and apparently arises from the mesenchymal cells of the connective tissue framework. Microscopically, the lesion is composed of a moderately vascularized stroma, plump spindle- or ovoid-shaped cells, and regularly interspersed giant cells. Because these multinucleated giant cells are almost ubiquitous in bone lesions, many tumors must be differentiated from giant cell tumors. Giant cell tumors are rare before the age of 20 or after the age of 55. The lesion is more common in females than in males. These tumors have a tendency to recur if they are not completely removed. The incidence of malignancy is estimated at about 20 percent. A review of reported giant cell tumors, however, failed to reveal any known metastases at the time of original diagnosis [64]. Therefore, complete removal is essential.

Roentgenographically, the lesion appears as an osteolytic lesion, with an indistinct margin in the epiphyseal end of a long bone. The tumor begins as an eccentric lesion but may progress to involve the entire diameter of the bone. There is an absence of periosteal new bone formation and reactive bony sclerosis. The tumor invariably arises in the epiphysis and secondarily involves the metaphysis. The classic appearance is that of a

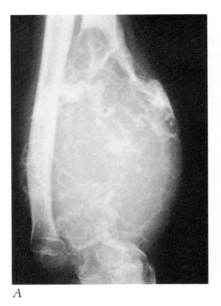
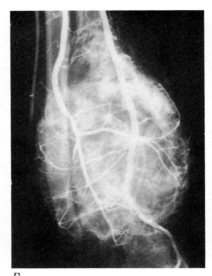
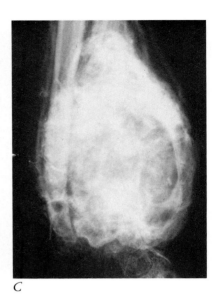

A   *B*   *C*

Figure 80-15. Giant cell tumor in a 29-year-old man complaining of pain and swelling of 5 years' duration. (A) The plain film reveals a large, expansile, multiloculated bone lesion. (B) The arteries supplying the tumor are increased in size and draped around the periphery of the lesion. (C) An intense nonhomogeneous blush is present within the tumor. (From Yaghmai [86].)

radiolucent expansile lesion, and light trabeculation is often present. Giant cell tumors have a propensity for the distal femur, proximal tibia, and distal radius, but the lesion has been reported in almost all the tubular bones and many of the flat bones as well.

The angiographic appearance of giant cell tumors has been described in several series [25, 43, 49, 56, 86]. The tumors are usually hypervascular (Fig. 80-15). The blood supply is derived primarily from the surrounding tissue, and the vessels are dilated. A prominent arterial network is present on the surface of the tumors, and these vessels often have a corkscrew appearance. Abundant neovascularity and an intense blush are present. Early venous filling takes place in about 20 percent of the tumors. Venous pooling may also be seen. Vessel encasement and occlusion may also be present. The synovial tissue in the vicinity of the tumor may look hyperemic at angiography, causing occasional confusion with extraosseous extension of the tumor [9]. Approximately 10 percent of the tumors are avascular or hypovascular [56, 86]. The avascular lesions are often necrotic or hemorrhagic or they have been previously treated.

Angiography has an important role in the preoperative evaluation of giant cell tumors. It accurately depicts the intraosseous extent of the tumor and defines the extraosseous extent in 89 percent of patients [56]. This is of particular importance in view of the high recurrence rate of the tumor and its ability to become malignant after treatment.

ANEURYSMAL BONE CYST

Aneurysmal bone cyst is an uncommon benign lesion of bone consisting of blood-filled spaces and solid areas containing spindled stroma, osteoid, and multinucleated giant cells. The lesions are most frequent in the second and third decades, although 78 percent of the patients are less than 20 years old. The lesion is more prevalent in females than males. It may involve almost any bone but has a predilection for the long bones, particularly the femur, and the spine. The majority of aneurysmal bone cysts in the long bones are located in the metaphysis, but they may extend into the epiphysis.

The classic appearance is that of an osteolytic, eccentric, expansile lesion that causes marked ballooning of a paper-thin cortex. Fine trabeculation is present within the lesion.

The angiographic findings in aneurysmal bone cysts have been described in several reports [8, 21, 48, 49, 86]. These cysts are generally less vascular than giant cell tumors. Although the arteries supplying them may be somewhat increased in size, the arterial network seen on their periphery is not as prominent as in the giant cell tumor. A peripheral blush of contrast material may be present, and often areas of contrast blush are interspersed with areas of no vascularity.

Some aneurysmal bone cysts are highly vascular, and differentiating them from giant cell tumors is impossible [48, 49, 58, 86]. However, a poorly vascularized tumor devoid of arteriovenous fistulas and soft tissue invasion is probably an aneurysmal bone cyst.

Bone and Soft Tissue Tumors of Fibrous Tissue Origin

Tumors of fibrous tissue origin may originate in either soft tissue or bone, and many spread to involve the adjacent structures. For this reason, they are discussed together. Additionally, fibrous histiocytomas are included here because of their microscopic and radiographic similarity to fibrous tissue tumors.

BENIGN TUMORS

Nonossifying Fibroma (Fibroma)

Nonossifying fibroma is a benign bone lesion derived from fibrous tissue. The lesion usually occurs between the ages of 8 and 20. It is commonly located in the shaft of a long bone.

Radiographically, the lesion presents as an ovoid radiolucent defect with scalloped, sclerotic edges. A nonossifying fibroma generally has a typical plain film appearance, and angiography is very seldom indicated. The interosseous forms of fibroma have a benign angiographic appearance [49, 76, 83].

Soft tissue fibromas have a slight hypervascularity, but the vessels look normal [83].

Desmoid Tumor

The desmoid tumor is a benign fibrous tumor that usually arises in the soft tissue. On rare occasions, it may arise as a primary bone tumor. Although the tumor is benign, it is locally invasive.

Angiographically, no abnormal vessels are seen; however, the tumor may displace the adja-

---

Figure 80-16. Desmoid tumor of upper calf in a 51-year-old woman. (A) The plain film demonstrates a soft tissue mass in the upper calf. The bones have a normal appearance. (B) The arteriogram shows displacement of the popliteal artery by the tumor (*arrows*). A faint blush is present, but there are no abnormal vessels.

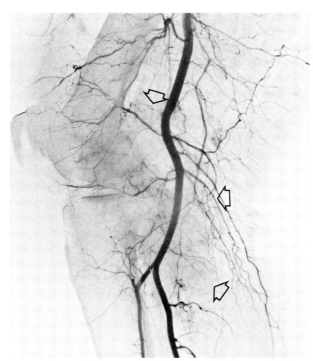

A

B

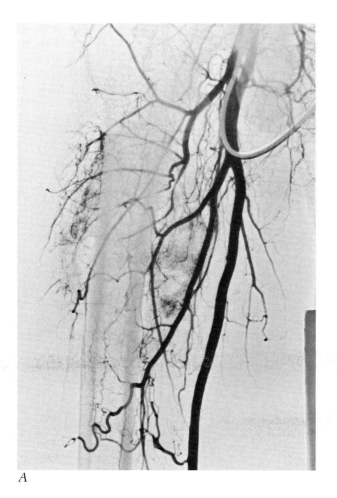

A

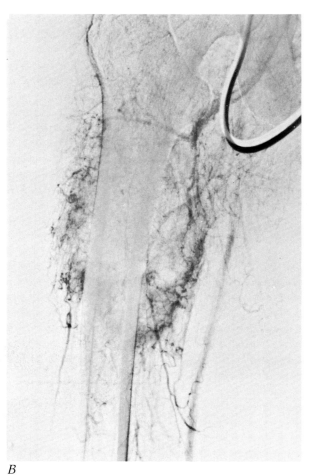

B

Figure 80-17. Fibrosarcoma of the thigh in a 63-year-old man. (A) The early arterial phase reveals a large hypervascular mass in the soft tissue of the right thigh. (B) The late arterial phase exhibits florid neovascularity, early venous drainage, and an avascular center in the lower portion of the tumor.

cent vessels. The vascularity is usually normal [83], but a faint blush may occasionally be present (Fig. 80-16).

MALIGNANT TUMORS

Fibrosarcoma
Fibrosarcomas are malignant tumors arising from the fibrous elements either in the medullary cavity of bone or in the soft tissue. Fibrosarcoma is a relatively rare bone tumor. It has a predilection for the long bones, particularly about the knee. Fibrosarcoma of the bone occurs at any age but is most common in the second, third, and fourth decades. When it arises in preexisting lesions, such as Paget's disease, it occurs in older patients. Soft tissue fibrosarcomas usually occur in children or young adults.

Roentgenographically, the tumor most often originates eccentrically in the metaphysis of a long bone; less commonly it may arise in a periosteal location. It appears as a destructive lesion, and it is not unusual for the tumor to erode through the cortex into the soft tissue. A bone sequestrum may be present. The margin of the lesion is poorly defined, and reactive bone formation is sparse.

Fibrosarcomas of bone and soft tissue origin exhibit varying degrees of vascularity. Some have a highly vascular appearance (Fig. 80-17), and others are poorly supplied with vessels. However, fibrosarcomas usually have increased vascularity when compared to the surrounding tissue [39, 83]. The degree of hypervascularization and the degree of malignancy in fibrosarcomas show good correlation; a highly malignant tumor is

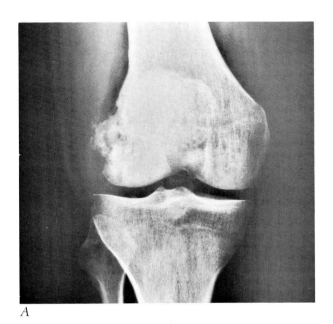

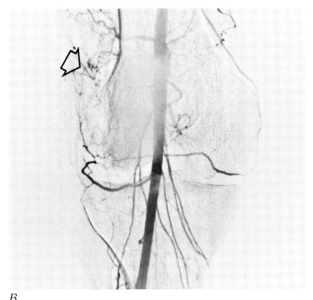

A

B

Figure 80-18. Fibrosarcoma of the distal femur in a 43-year-old man. The patient gave a 2½-year history of knee pain, beginning after minor trauma. He was originally treated for infection by his local physician. (A) An irregular destructive lesion is present in the distal femur, and the cortex is destroyed. (B) The small vessels are displaced (*arrow*), demonstrating the soft tissue extension of the tumor. A faint tumor blush is seen.

usually richly supplied by vessels [11, 39, 83]. Furthermore, in fibrosarcomas of nonhomogeneous vascularity, the areas of the tumor showing the greatest vascularity are the most malignant [39]. Displacement of the major arteries and veins is a frequent finding. Encroachment and invasion of the major vessels are seen more often in fibrosarcomas than in other malignant tumors of bone. Yaghmai [83] studied 35 malignant fibrosarcomas by angiography and demonstrated neovascularity in every instance. Osseous fibrosarcoma often breaches the cortex to invade the soft tissue (Fig. 80-18).

Fibrosarcomas reveal considerable variability in their angiographic appearance, and slow-growing fibrosarcomas may look deceptively innocent, especially in the early stage [70, 77].

Malignant Fibrous Histiocytoma
Malignant fibrous histiocytoma is a malignant tumor of probable histiocytic origin [18, 19]. It may arise either as a primary lesion in the bone or as a lesion in the soft tissue. A host of labels has been applied to the tumors depending on their location and predominance of fibrous, histiocytic, or xanthomatous elements. The tumors may occur at any age, but the typical age is 55 years.

Soft tissue tumors are found most often in the extremities and the chest wall. Radiographically, the soft tissue masses are usually well defined and lack distinguishing features. The roentgen appearance, when the bone is involved, is that of a malignant process. The osseous lesions are frequently purely osteolytic.

Marked destruction is seen in the form of moth-eaten and permeative patterns. An ill-defined margin is often present. Extension into the soft tissue and pathologic fractures are often seen.

Malignant fibrous histiocytomas of the bone are usually hypervascular and exhibit a diffuse capillary blush (Fig. 80-19). Hudson et al. [32] found neovascularity in 6 of the 10 patients with primary bone malignant fibrous histiocytoma whom they studied angiographically. Laking of contrast material and arteriovenous shunts may also be present. Displacement of vessels is often found.

Soft tissue fibrous histiocytomas have a similar angiographic appearance. A circumscribed hypervascular mass is observed (Fig. 80-20). Neovascularity, early-draining veins, and displacement or encasement of vessels may also be present [80].

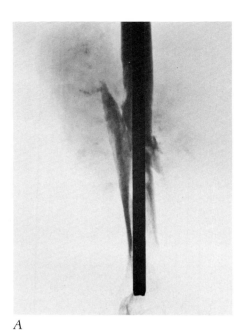 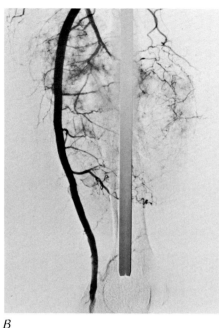 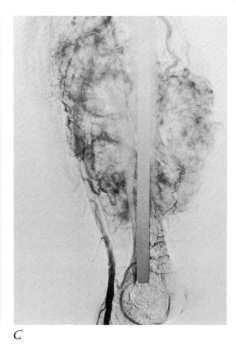

A   *B*   *C*

Figure 80-19. Malignant fibrous histiocytoma of the femur in a 69-year-old man. Tha patient sustained a fracture of his femur when he was kicked by a cow, and an intramedullary rod was inserted. Three weeks later he developed pain in his thigh. Lung metastases were present 6 months later. (A) An intramedullary rod is seen in place through a fracture in the femur. A large soft tissue mass is apparent. (B) The superficial femoral artery is displaced by a hypervascular mass containing fine neovascularity. (C) A diffuse blush is seen, arteriovenous shunts are present, and large veins drain the tumor.

Figure 80-20. Recurrent malignant fibrous histiocytoma of the upper arm in a 60-year-old man. The original tumor was excised 3 years previously. (A) A circumscribed hypervascular mass is demonstrated in the soft tissue of the upper arm. (B) An intense blush, fine neovascular vessels, and early-draining veins are present.

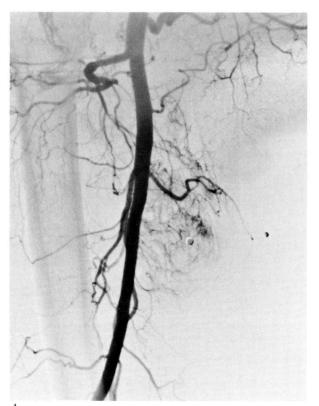 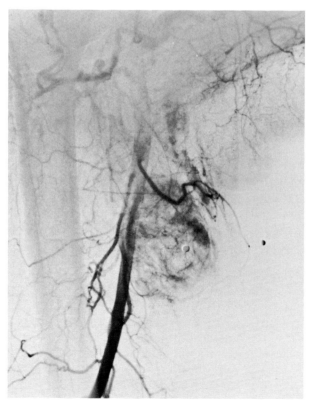

A   *B*

Bone and Soft Tissue Lesions of Vascular Origin

BENIGN LESIONS

Hemangioma

There is confusion in the literature concerning the classification of hemangiomas, partly because of the problem of nomenclature. It is difficult to determine whether hemangiomas are true neoplasms or congenital malformations. They are not considered true neoplasms despite the fact that they infiltrate and have the potential to grow. They may be designated as congenital hamartomas, representing mesodermal rests of basal formative tissue. Hemangiomas may occur primarily in the bone or soft tissue. They all have abnormal arteriovenous communications.

Hemangiomas can be grouped into four categories: (1) capillary hemangiomas, (2) cavernous hemangiomas, (3) venous hemangiomas, and (4) arteriovenous malformations. Capillary hemangiomas are composed of fine capillary loops that tend to spread outward in a "sunburst" pattern. Cavernous hemangiomas are aggregations of larger thin-walled vessels and sinusoidal blood spaces. The shunts in these lesions are probably at the level of the arterioles and small veins. Both these lesions lack smooth muscle cells in the vessel walls. Venous hemangiomas have thickened walls containing muscle cells. The vascular malformation is another subcategory of hemangioma consisting of abnormal arteriovenous communications, resulting from a failure of differentiation of the common embryologic anlage into artery and vein.

Osseous hemangiomas are rather uncommon lesions. They are found in patients of all ages but are more prevalent in the fifth decade of life. Hemangiomas occur most frequently in the vertebrae, skull, and long bones, but they also occur in the jaws.

Radiographically, hemangioma of the spine is usually a single lesion, although two or more vertebral bodies may be involved. There is a slight loss of bone density of the vertebral body. The hallmark is a vertical-striped pattern, the "corduroy cloth" appearance. Compression of the vertebra causes loss of the characteristic picture. Most hemangiomas of the spine are asymptomatic, but occasionally spinal cord compression is present.

Hemangiomas of the skull and flat bones usually exhibit a round area of rarefaction with central reticulations assuming a "honeycomb" appearance. The striations may be exaggerated or extend at right angles from the bone, giving a sunburst pattern. In the extremities hemangiomas may appear as well-circumscribed lytic lesions with scattered trabeculae coursing

---

Figure 80-21. Recurrent hemangioma in the heel of a 26-year-old woman. (A) Early and (B) late arterial phases show numerous enlarged tortuous vessels with early visualization of the veins.

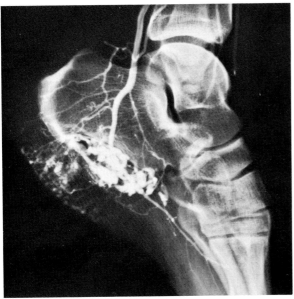
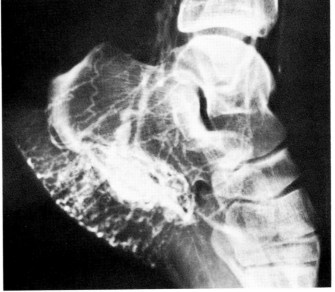

A   B

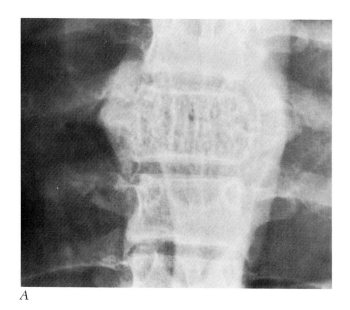

A

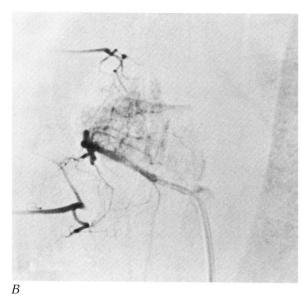

B

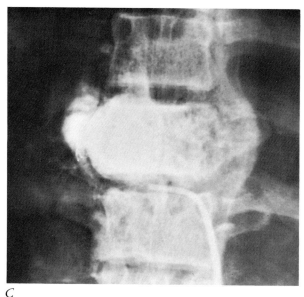

C

Figure 80-22. Hemangioma of a dorsal vertebra in an asymptomatic 14-year-old girl. (A) The typical striated appearance of a vertebral body hemangioma is present. Note the accompanying paravertebral mass. (B) A selective injection of an intercostal artery reveals early opacification of the vertebral body. (C) The late phase shows a diffuse blush of contrast material in the vertebral body and adjacent soft tissue. Injection of the opposite intercostal artery revealed a similar opacification of the other half of the vertebral body and adjacent paravertebral mass.

through them. Sometimes the bony contour is expanded. If the trabecular pattern is not evident, identification of hemangiomas may be difficult and they may simulate malignancy.

Hemangiomas more frequently involve the soft tissues. These lesions are the most common tumors of skeletal muscles and are second only to lipomas as the most common soft tissue tumors of the extremities [4]. They are frequently associated with overlying skin abnormalities. On the plain radiographs, hemangiomas may demonstrate phleboliths, periosteal elevation, cortical thinning, osteoporosis, and bone loss due to lysis or erosion. Enlargement of the adjacent bone may also be present.

The angiographic appearance of hemangiomas has been described in several series [3, 4, 45, 55, 86]. A continuum of angiographic patterns exists. The hemangioma may be very vascular with coarse, irregular, enlarged arteries and pooling of contrast material, and arteriovenous shunting may be found (Fig. 80-21). In the osseous form, dilated vascular spaces may be encountered, or the lesion may exhibit only a heavy, even tumor stain (Fig. 80-22). Many hemangiomas show fine-caliber arteries with smooth walls and orderly distribution with some staining in the area. Pooling of contrast may be seen (Fig. 80-23) but is not necessarily present.

Arteriovenous malformations may be localized [61] (Fig. 80-24) or diffuse (Fig. 80-25). The feeding arteries are enlarged and moderately tortuous. The smaller vessels are numerous and markedly tortuous. There is rapid circulation, with essentially simultaneous visualization of the arteries and veins. In large lesions, the shunts may not be seen in all parts of the limb. A striking feature is the considerable dilatation of the veins.

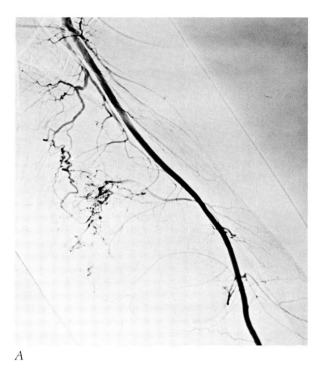

A

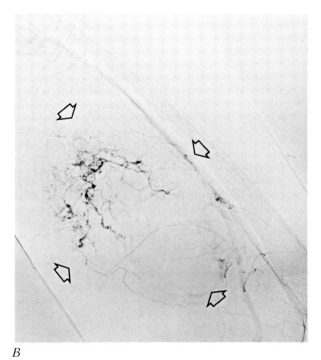

B

Figure 80-31. A malignant neurofibrosarcoma of the thigh in a 17-year-old girl. (A) A large oval mass displaces the superficial femoral artery and surrounding soft tissue vasculature. (B) The extent of the mass becomes more apparent in the later arterial phase (*arrows*). Extensive neovascularity is present in one area of the lesion. The remainder of the lesion is relatively avascular.

new bone formation and bony destruction indicate a malignant process. If the interface of the tumor with the soft tissue is well defined, the lesion is probably benign. An indistinct margin is consistent with malignancy or inflammation. Tumors that may appear radiolucent include lipomas, hamartomas, and teratomas.

The value of angiography in soft tissue tumors has been described in several series [20, 30, 36, 37, 46, 50, 51, 60, 66, 71]. However, it is important to correlate the angiographic findings with the clinical findings and with the plain film appearance.

The angiographic pattern of benign soft tissue tumors is usually one of avascularity and stretching or displacement of vessels around the tumor mass. Exceptions to this rule are lesions of vascular origin. Glomus tumors are highly vascular, are characterized by enlarged feeding vessels, and exhibit an intense blush. Early venous filling is often seen [37]. Hemangiomas have already been discussed.

Tumors of nerve origin are also an exception. While benign nerve tissue tumors may be avascular, they may contain very tortuous vessels or neovascularity [15]. Angiography often cannot distinguish between a benign nerve sheath tumor and a malignant one (Fig. 80-31) with certainty, although the presence of vascular encasement usually indicates a malignant tumor.

Malignant tumors of the soft tissue are in most cases more abundantly vascularized than the adjacent soft tissues (Fig. 80-32). The highly malignant tumors show an intense vascularity. Neovascularity, pooling of contrast material, a tumor blush, encasement, and arteriovenous shunts may also be present. Tumors demonstrating neovascularity are frankly malignant or have a propensity to local recurrence and metastases even though they have the histologic picture of a benign lesion. Sharp delineation of the borders of the mass favors the diagnosis of neoplasm. Hemangiomas and inflammatory lesions do not have sharp margins. Liposarcomas, myxofibrosarcomas, rhabdomyosarcomas, mesenchymal sarcomas, and malignant fibrous histiocytomas are usually highly vascular. Fibrosarcomas are often highly vascular, but a few are poorly supplied with vessels [5]; the highly vascular tumors are the most malignant [39, 83]. Angiography does

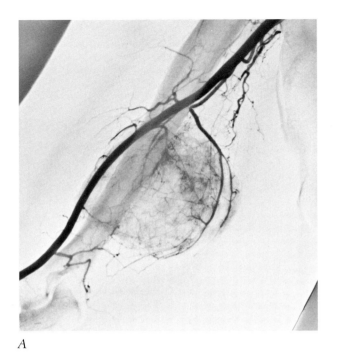

A

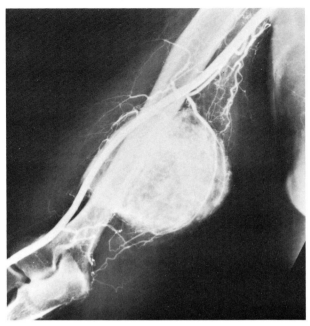

B

Figure 80-32. A pleomorphic high-grade sarcoma in the soft tissues of the upper arm of a 62-year-old woman. The mass had been present for 6 months. (A) A circumscribed hypervascular mass containing neovascularity displaces the brachial artery. (B) The late arterial phase reveals an intense homogeneous blush.

Figure 80-33. An atypical intramuscular lipoma, grade I liposarcoma, in the upper leg of a 58-year-old man. The tumor had been present for many years and was slowly enlarging. The plain film demonstrated a radiolucent mass in the thigh. The vessels are displaced by the mass (*arrows*), but no abnormal vascularity is evident.

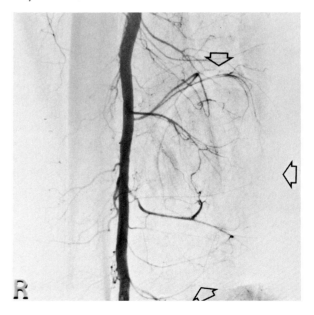

not distinguish one sarcoma from another. This is of little consequence, however, because, despite differences in histogenesis, analysis of the rates of local recurrence and metastasis of these sarcomas reveals that their rates are almost the same [63]. The exceptions are low-grade fibrosarcoma and grade I liposarcoma (Fig. 80-33). These tumors are poorly vascularized and are locally invasive but do not usually metastasize.

The angiogram provides a fairly clear impression of the size of the tumor and its relationship to the surrounding tissues [37]. It can also demonstrate unsuspected satellite lesions [46]. This aids the surgeon in the decision as to what type of surgery should be performed, whether amputation or radical excision [63]. If arteriography shows that a major vessel is displaced or that a nonexpendable bone is involved, amputation is preferable [63].

Angiography can aid in the selection of a biopsy site, delineate the vascular supply of the lesion, and detect local recurrences [46]. Angiography is of most value when the surgeon and the angiographer confer during the procedure and when questions posed by the surgeon are answered during the angiographic procedure.

Myositis Ossificans

Myosistis ossificans circumscripta is a reactive lesion occurring in the soft tissues, at times near bone and periosteum. The lesion is characterized by fibrous, osseous, and cartilaginous proliferation and metaplasia. A history of trauma can be obtained in most cases, but in a certain number of patients no antecedent injury can be elicited. Localized myositis ossificans occurs most often in children and young adults. The lesion has a predilection for areas prone to trauma. It arises in the large muscle groups, in and around the elbow, thigh, buttocks, shoulder, and calf. While there are many unanswered questions concerning its pathogenesis, the microscopic evolution of the lesion has been well documented [1]. It is important to understand the stages of myositis ossificans when interpreting the histology, plain films, and angiograms. Three stages of maturation are recognized. The developing lesion also demonstrates three zones of maturation, and if this is not recognized the lesion is easily mistaken for a malignancy. The maturation proceeds inward from the periphery, the central area being the last to ossify.

The first stage is one of a rapidly developing soft tissue mass. There is usually no evidence of calcification. During this time of tissue necrosis and regeneration, angiography may show a hypervascular mass [24].

The second or active stage begins in the second week and continues for 12 to 14 weeks. In the first 3 to 6 weeks, the microscopic zonal pattern of maturation that is characteristic of the entity develops. The plain films exhibit faint calcification, and periosteal reaction is present if the underlying bone is injured. At 6 to 8 weeks, the lacy pattern of new bone is sharply circumscribed about the periphery and may have an eggshell-like appearance. The angiographic features during the active stage are characterized by hypervascularity and a poorly defined stain in the mass [22, 33, 37, 82]. The criteria for malignancy (neovascularity, pooling of contrast material, and arteriovenous shunting) are usually absent, allowing the diagnosis of a benign process to be established [33, 82]. However, a disturbing hypervascular pattern with markedly irregular vessels may be seen during this stage [51]. It is important to review the clinical history and the plain films before interpreting the angiograms.

Figure 80-34. Posttraumatic exostosis, myositis ossificans, in a 27-year-old man who sustained an injury 8 months before these films were obtained. (A) A calcified mass is seen extending from the pubic bone (arrows). (B) The arteriogram exhibits a normal vascular pattern.

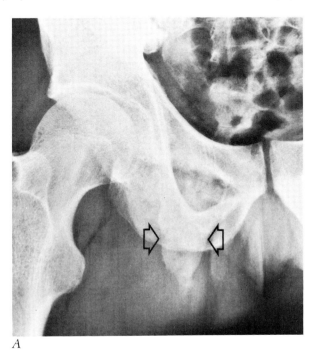

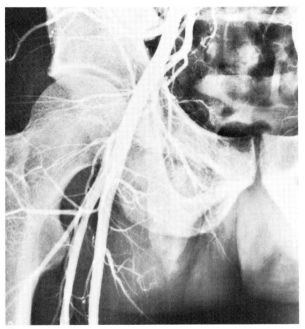

A

B

The third stage is the healing stage, which usually begins at around 16 weeks and lasts 5 to 6 months. The lesion gradually shrinks in size and may persist as a hard mass or undergo almost total regression. Occasionally in this stage myositis ossificans will take on the appearance of an exostosis (Fig. 80-34). Angiographic findings in this stage are variable. The pattern is less vascular than in the active stage and may be normal (Fig. 80-34).

Embolization of Bone and Soft Tissue Tumors

Transcatheter selective arterial embolization of bone and soft tissue tumors has been utilized in several clinical situations. It has served as an adjunct to surgery to control inoperable bleeding [17]. It has been used in hemangiomas either for palliation [67] or to decrease intraoperative blood loss [29, 78] and lessen the chance of recurrence [78]. It has also been employed to relieve chronic pain in patients with pelvic tumors [17, 79].

Feldman et al. [17] first succeeded in alleviating the pain of a patient with metastasis to the right ilium by embolizing the branches of the right internal iliac artery and the fourth lumbar artery in 1975. The relief of pain lasted until the patient's death 2½ months later. These authors also described the successful use of preoperative embolization with Gelfoam to decrease intraoperative blood loss in a man with large giant cell tumors of both fibulas.

Wallace et al. [79] reported the use of therapeutic arterial occlusion of the internal iliac artery for symptomatic relief of pain. They were successful in eight of nine patients.

The embolization of pelvic tumors is performed by first obtaining selective arteriograms to delineate accurately the vascular supply to the lesion (Fig. 80-35). The vascular supply to these neoplasms is frequently through the internal iliac artery; additional blood supply may originate from the lower lumbar, the middle sacral, the circumflex iliac, and the external pudendal arteries. The major vessels of supply are embolized first with 2 × 3 mm Gelfoam particles, followed by Gianturco coils to occlude the vessels permanently (Fig. 80-35).

The patients will experience severe pain requiring narcotics, beginning shortly after embolization and subsiding in 3 to 7 days. Temperature elevation ranging from 38.8 to 39.8° C will occur, subsiding in 72 to 96 hours. If a persistent sacral artery is present on the side to be embolized, the

Figure 80-35. Recurrent chondrosarcoma of the pelvis in a 66-year-old man with persistent pain following irradiation. (A) A large hypervascular lesion is present in the iliac bone. The tumor extends into the soft tissue. (B) The right internal iliac artery is totally occluded following selective embolization with Gelfoam particles and the insertion of Gianturco coils. One week after the procedure the patient experienced a marked decrease in his pain.

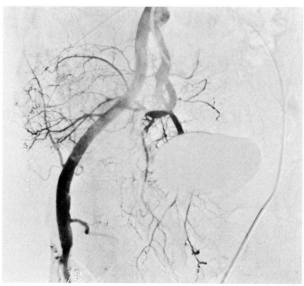

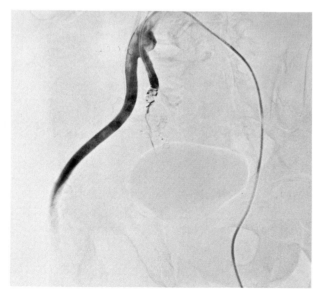

A   B

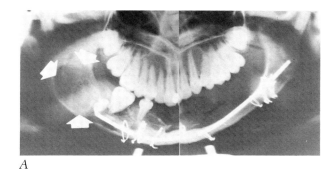

A

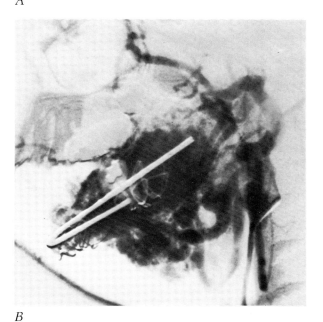

B

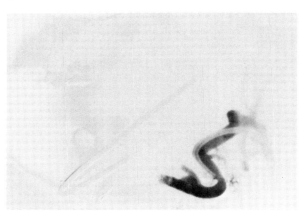

C

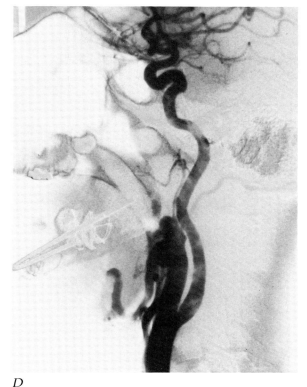

D

Figure 80-36. Recurrent hemangioma in a 12-year-old girl who presented with loosening of the teeth. (A) Panorex shows the sequelae of the previous resection of the left mandible at age 2. A large multilocular radiolucent defect is seen in the right mandible (*arrows*). (B) A selective right external carotid angiogram shows a large hypervascular hemangioma involving the soft tissue and bone of the right jaw. (C) A selective injection of the facial artery demonstrates complete occlusion of the artery following transcatheter embolization with Gelfoam. (D) A common carotid arteriogram shows absence of filling of the hemangioma after selective embolization of the feeding vessels. The patient did well for 6 months and then developed bleeding from the gums. The soft tissue hemangioma appeared well controlled; the hemangioma within the mandible was the source of the hemorrhage. (From C. J. Tegtmeyer and T. E. Keats, The Mouth, Tongue, Jaws and Salivary Glands. In J. G. Teplick and M. E. Haskin [eds.], *Surgical Radiology: A Complement in Radiology Imaging to the Sabiston-Davis-Christopher Textbook of Radiology.* Philadelphia: Saunders, 1981.)

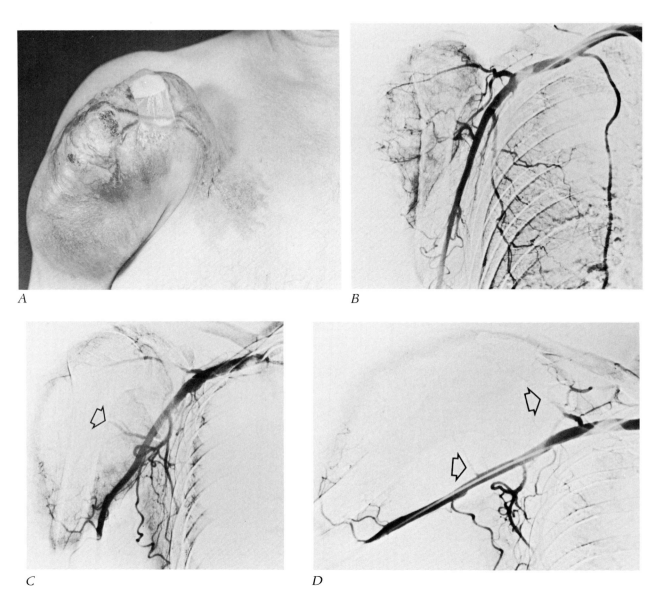

A

B

C

D

Figure 80-37. Recurrent liposarcoma in a 61-year-old man. (A) The huge tumor of the shoulder is seen with large vessels coursing across the surface of the lesion. (B) A hypervascular mass is present, which contains florid neovascularity and a tumor stain. (C) The embolization procedure was performed in stages. The circumflex humeral artery (*arrow*) was occluded with Gelfoam. (D) Two weeks later, the branch of the thoracicoacromial artery supplying the tumor was occluded (*upper arrow*). The occluded circumflex artery is again seen (*lower arrow*). Following this occlusion the patient experienced intense pain. Surgery was subsequently performed with minimal blood loss.

procedure is contraindicated because embolization of this artery may result in sacral nerve injury and footdrop.

Embolization with Gelfoam particles has been successfully employed in the treatment of hemangiomas. It has been utilized to control pain associated with a peripheral hemangioma [52], and to decrease the size of a hemangioma and control a persistent left-to-right shunt [67]. Voigt et al. [78] reported the use of Gelfoam embolization in 10 patients with deforming vascular malformations in the craniofacial area. The procedure allowed reconstructive surgery to be carried out with decreased blood loss, and good cosmetic results were obtained. No recurrences were seen, but the follow-up was short, only 6 to 9 months.

The surgery for deforming hemangiomas of the craniofacial region is difficult, and recurrences are not uncommon. Embolization prior to surgery may be very helpful (Fig. 80-36). Gelfoam embolization usually provides only temporary relief, however, because of the breakdown of the Gelfoam and the formation of new collateral vessels. Therefore, if surgery is contemplated, it should take place shortly after embolization for optimum results.

The embolization of soft tissue tumors may result in severe, prolonged muscle pain if acute muscle ischemia takes place. The pain usually subsides in a week, without permanent sequelae, but its severity can be distressing for the patient and unnerving for the angiographer. Doppman and Di Chiro [13] reported two cases with this complication, and we have encountered it in one patient in whom a recurrent sarcoma of the shoulder was embolized (Fig. 80-37).

Cautious use of embolization seems indicated in certain situations: for palliation of pain in patients with inoperable tumors, preoperatively to decrease blood loss during resection, and in hemangiomas to decrease blood loss and help prevent recurrences. It may also be helpful in hemangiomas to relieve symptoms and decrease the size of the lesion when resection is not contemplated.

ACKNOWLEDGMENT

I want to extend my gratitude to Pat West and Geelee Tegtmeyer for their help in the preparation of this chapter.

References

1. Ackerman, L. V. Extra-osseous localized non-neoplastic bone and cartilage formation (so-called myositis ossificans): Clinical and pathological confusion with malignant neoplasms. *J. Bone Joint Surg.* [Am.] 40:279, 1958.
2. Ayella, R. J. Hemangiopericytoma. *Radiology* 97:611, 1970.
3. Bartley, O., and Wickbom, I. Angiography in soft tissue hemangiomas. *Acta Radiol.* (Stockh.) 51:81, 1959.
4. Bliznak, J., and Staple, T. W. Radiology of angiodysplasias of the limb. *Radiology* 110:35, 1974.
5. Cockshott, W. P., and Evans, K. T. The place of soft tissue arteriography. *Br. J. Radiol.* 37:367, 1964.
6. Dahlin, D. C. *Bone Tumors: General Aspects and Data on 6,221 Cases* (3rd ed). Springfield, Ill.: Thomas, 1978.
7. de Santos, L. A., Bernardino, M. E., and Murray, J. A. Computed tomography in the evaluation of osteosarcoma: Experience with 25 cases. *AJR* 132:535, 1979.
8. de Santos, L. A., and Murray, J. A. The value of arteriography in the management of aneurysmal bone cyst. *Skeletal Radiol.* 2:137, 1978.
9. de Santos, L. A., and Prando, A. Synovial hyperemia in giant cell tumor of bone: Angiographic pitfall. *AJR* 133:281, 1979.
10. De Villiers, D. R., Farman, J., and Campbell, J. A. H. Pelvic haemangiopericytoma: Preoperative arteriographic demonstration. *Clin. Radiol.* 18:318, 1967.
11. Dibbelt, W. Über die Blutgefässe der Tumoren. *Arb. Pathol. Anat. Bakt.* 8:114, 1912.
12. Doan, C. A. The circulation of the bone-marrow. *Contrib. Embryol.* 14:27, 1922.
13. Doppman, J. L., and Di Chiro, G. Paraspinal muscle infarction: A painful complication of lumbar artery embolization associated with pathognomonic radiographic and laboratory findings. *Radiology* 119:609, 1976.
14. Drinker, C. K., Drinker, K. R., and Lund, C. C. The circulation in the mammalian bone-marrow. *Am. J. Physiol.* 62:1, 1922.
15. Dunnick, N. R., and Castellino, R. A. Arteriographic manifestations of ganglioneuromas. *Radiology* 115:323, 1975.
16. Ekelund, L., Laurin, S., and Lunderquist, A. Comparison of a vasoconstrictor and a vasodilator in pharmacoangiography of bone and soft-tissue tumors. *Radiology* 122:95, 1977.
17. Feldman, F., Casarella, W. J., Dick, H. M., and Hollander, B. A. Selective intra-arterial embolization of bone tumors: A useful adjunct in the management of selected lesions. *AJR* 123:130, 1975.
18. Feldman, F., and Lattes, R. Primary malignant fibrous histiocytoma (fibrous xanthoma) of bone. *Skeletal Radiol.* 1:145, 1977.
19. Feldman, F., and Norman, D. Intra- and extraosseous malignant histiocytoma (malignant fibrous xanthoma). *Radiology* 104:497, 1972.
20. Finck, E. J., and Moore, T. M. Angiography for mass lesions of bone, joint, and soft tissue. *Orthop. Clin. North Am.* 8:999, 1977.
21. Fuhs, S. E., and Herndon, J. H. Aneurysmal bone cyst involving the hand: A review and report of two cases. *J. Hand Surg.* 4:152, 1979.
22. Goldman, A. B. Myositis ossificans circumscripta: A benign lesion with a malignant differential diagnosis. *AJR* 126:32, 1976.
23. Gomez-Reino, J. H., Radin, A., and Gorevic, P. D. Pseudoaneurysm of the popliteal artery as a complication of an osteochondroma. *Skeletal Radiol.* 4:26, 1979.

24. Gronner, A. T. Muscle necrosis simulating a malignant tumor angiographically: Case report. *Radiology* 103:309, 1972.

25. Gunterberg, B., Kindblom, L.-G., and Laurin, S. Giant-cell tumor of bone and aneurysmal bone cyst. A correlated histologic and angiographic study. *Skeletal Radiol.* 2:65, 1977.

26. Halpern, M., and Freiberger, R. H. Arteriography as a diagnostic procedure in bone disease. *Radiol. Clin. North Am.* 8:277, 1970.

27. Han, S. K., Henein, M. H. G., Novin, N., and Giargiana, F. A., Jr. An unusual arterial complication seen with a solitary osteochondroma. *Am. Surg.* 43:471, 1977.

28. Hawkins, I. F., Jr., and Hudson, T. Priscoline in bone and soft-tissue angiography. *Radiology* 110:541, 1974.

29. Hemmy, D. C., McGee, D. M., Armbrust, F. H., and Larson, S. J. Resection of a vertebral hemangioma after preoperative embolization: A case report. *J. Neurosurg.* 47:282, 1977.

30. Herzberg, D. L., and Schreiber, M. H. Angiography in mass lesions of the extremities. *AJR* 111:541, 1971.

31. Hudson, T. M., Haas, G., Enneking, W. F., and Hawkins, I. F., Jr. Angiography in the management of musculoskeletal tumors. *Surg. Gynecol. Obstet.* 141:11, 1975.

32. Hudson, T. M., Hawkins, I. F., Jr., Spanier, S. S., and Enneking, W. F. Angiography of malignant fibrous histiocytoma of bone. *Radiology* 131:9, 1979.

33. Hutcheson, J., Klatte, E. C., and Kremp, R. The angiographic appearance of myositis ossificans circumscripta: A case report. *Radiology* 102:57, 1972.

34. Joffe, N. Haemangiopericytoma: Angiographic findings. *Br. J. Radiol.* 33:614, 1960.

35. Kadir, S., Athanasoulis, C. A., and Waltman, A. C. Tolazoline-augmented arteriography in the evaluation of bone and soft-tissue tumors. *Radiology* 133:792, 1979.

36. Kindblom, L.-G., Merck, C., and Svendsen, P. Myxofibrosarcoma: A pathologico-anatomical, microangiographic and angiographic correlative study of eight cases. *Br. J. Radiol.* 50:876, 1977.

37. Lagergren, C., and Lindbom, Å. Angiography of peripheral tumors. *Radiology* 79:371, 1962.

38. Lagergren, C., Lindbom, Å., and Söderberg, G. Hypervascularization in chronic inflammation demonstrated by angiography: Angiographic, histopathologic, and microangiographic studies. *Acta Radiol.* (Stockh.) 49:441, 1958.

39. Lagergren, C., Lindbom, Å., Söderberg, G. Vascularization of fibromatous and fibrosarcomatous tumors: Histopathologic, microangiographic and angiographic studies. *Acta Radiol.* (Stockh.) 53:1, 1960.

40. Lagergren, C., Lindbom, Å., and Söderberg, G. The blood vessels of chondrosarcomas. *Acta Radiol.* (Stockh.) 55:321, 1961.

41. Lagergren, C., Lindbom, Å., and Söderberg, G. The blood vessels of osteogenic sarcomas: Histologic, angiographic and microradiographic studies. *Acta Radiol.* (Stockh.) 55:161, 1961.

42. Lateur, L., and Baert, A. L. Localisation and diagnosis of osteoid osteoma of the carpal area by angiography. *Skeletal Radiol.* 2:75, 1977.

43. Laurin, S. Angiography in giant cell tumors. *Radiologe* 17:118, 1977.

44. Laurin, S., Åkerman, M., Kindblom, L.-G., and Gunterberg, B. Angiography in myeloma (plasmacytoma): A correlated angiographic and histologic study. *Skeletal Radiol.* 4:8, 1979.

45. Levin, D. C., Gordon, D. H., and McSweeney, J. Arteriography of peripheral hemangiomas. *Radiology* 121:625, 1976.

46. Levin, D. C., Watson, R. C., and Baltaxe, H. A. Arteriography in diagnosis and management of acquired peripheral soft-tissue masses. *Radiology* 103:53, 1972.

47. Lindbom, Å., Lindvall, N., Söderberg, G., and Spjut, H. Angiography in osteoid osteoma. *Acta Radiol.* (Stockh.) 54:327, 1960.

48. Lindbom, Å., Söderberg, G., Spjut, H. J., and Sunnqvist, O. Angiography of aneurysmal bone cyst. *Acta Radiol.* (Stockh.) 55:12, 1961.

49. Lundström, B., Lorentzon, R., Larsson, S.-E., and Boquist, L. Angiography in giant-cell tumours of bone. *Acta Radiol.* [*Diagn.*] (Stockh.) 18:541, 1977.

50. Margulis, A. R., and Murphy, T. O. Arteriography in neoplasms of extremities. *AJR* 80:330, 1958.

51. Martel, W. M., and Abell, M. R. Radiologic evaluation of soft tissue tumors. A retrospective study. *Cancer* 32:352, 1973.

52. Mitty, H. A., and Kleiger, B. Partial embolization of large peripheral hemangioma for pain control. *Radiology* 127:671, 1978.

53. Murray, J. A. Synovial sarcoma. *Orthop. Clin. North Am.* 8:963, 1977.

54. O'Hara, J. P., III, Tegtmeyer, C., Sweet, D. E., and McCue, F. C. Angiography in the diagnosis of osteoid-osteoma of the hand. *J. Bone Joint Surg.* [*Am.*] 57:163, 1975.

55. Pochaczevsky, R., Sussman, R., and Stoopack, J. Arteriovenous fistulas of the maxillofacial region. *J. Can. Assoc. Radiol.* 23:201, 1972.

56. Prando, A., de Santos, L. A., Wallace, S., and Murray, J. A. Angiography in giant-cell bone tumors. *Radiology* 130:323, 1979.

57. Probst, F. P. Extra-articular pigmented villonodular synovitis affecting bone. The role of angiography as an aid in its differentiation from similar bone-destroying conditions. *Radiologe* 13:436, 1973.

58. Ring, S. M., Beranbaum, E. R., Madayag, M. A., and Nicolosi, C. R. Angiography of aneurysmal bone cyst. *Bull. Hosp. Joint Dis.* 33:1, 1972.

59. Rittenberg, G. M., Schabel, S. I., Vujic, I., and Meredith, H. C. The vascular "sunburst" appearance of osteosarcoma: A new angiographic finding. *Skeletal Radiol.* 2:243, 1978.

60. Rosenberg, J. C. The value of arteriography in the treatment of soft tissue tumors of the extremities. *J. Int. Coll. Surg.* 41:405, 1964.

61. Scottie, D., Edeiken, J., and Madan, V. Arteriovenous malformation of the hand with involvement with bone. *Skeletal Radiol.* 2:151, 1978.

62. Sherman, M. S. Osteoid osteoma associated with changes in an adjacent joint. Report of two cases. *J. Bone Joint Surg.* 29:483, 1947.

63. Simon, M. A., and Enneking, W. F. The management of soft-tissue sarcomas of the extremities. *J. Bone Joint Surg. [Am.]* 58:317, 1976.

64. Spjut, H. J., Dorfma, H. D., Fechner, R. E., and Ackerman, L. V. *Tumors of Bone and Cartilage. Atlas of Tumor Pathology* (2nd series, fasc. 5). Washington, D.C.: Armed Forces Institute of Pathology, 1971.

65. Srinivasan, C. K., Patel, M. R., Pearlman, H. S., and Silver, J. W. Malignant hemangioendothelioma of bone: Review of the literature and report of two cases. *J. Bone Joint Surg. [Am.]* 60:696, 1978.

66. Stanley, P., and Miller, J. H. Angiography of extremity masses in children. *AJR* 130:1119, 1978.

67. Stanley, R. J., and Cubillo, E. Nonsurgical treatment of arteriovenous malformations of the trunk and limb by transcatheter arterial embolization. *Radiology* 115:609, 1975.

68. Steckel, R. J. Usefulness of extremity arteriography in special situations. *Radiology* 86:293, 1966.

69. Steinbach, H. L. Angiography of Bones and Joints. In H. L. Abrams (ed.), *Angiography* (2nd ed.). Boston: Little, Brown, 1971.

70. Strickland, B. The value of arteriography in the diagnosis of bone tumours. *Br. J. Radiol.* 32:705, 1959.

71. Templeton, A. W., Stevens, E., and Jansen, C. Arteriographic evaluation of soft tissue masses. *South. Med. J.* 59:1255, 1966.

72. Tilling, G. The vascular anatomy of the long bones: A radiological and histological study. *Acta Radiol. [Suppl.]* (Stockh.) 161:1, 1958.

73. Trueta, J. The normal vascular anatomy of the human femoral head during growth. *J. Bone Joint Surg. [Br.]* 39:358, 1957.

74. Unni, K. K., Ivins, J. C., Beabout, J. W., and Dahlin, D. C. Hemangioma, hemangiopericytoma, and hemangioendothelioma (angiosarcoma) of bone. *Cancer* 27:1403, 1971.

75. Viamonte, M., Jr., Roen, S., and LePage, J. Nonspecificity of abnormal vascularity in the angiographic diagnosis of malignant neoplasms. *Radiology* 106:59, 1973.

76. Voegeli, E., and Fuchs, W. A. Arteriography in bone tumours. *Br. J. Radiol.* 49:407, 1976.

77. Voegeli, E., and Uehlinger, E. Arteriography in bone tumors. *Skeletal Radiol.* 1:3, 1976.

78. Voigt, K., Schwenzer, N., and Stoeter, P. Angiographic, operative, and histologic findings after embolization of craniofacial angiomas. *Neuroradiology* 16:424, 1978.

79. Wallace, S., Granmayeh, M., de Santos, L. A., Murray, J. A., Romsdahl, M. M., Bracken, R. B., and Jonsson, K. Arterial occlusion of pelvic bone tumors. *Cancer* 43:322, 1979.

80. Yaghmai, I. Malignant giant cell tumor of the soft tissue: Angiographic manifestations. *Radiology* 120:329, 1976.

81. Yaghmai, I. Angiographic features of osteosarcoma. *AJR* 129:1073, 1977.

82. Yaghmai, I. Myositis ossificans: Diagnostic value of arteriography. *AJR* 128:811, 1977.

83. Yaghmai, I. Angiographic features of fibromas and fibrosarcomas. *Radiology* 124:57, 1977.

84. Yaghmai, I. Angiographic features of chondromas and chondrosarcomas. *Skeletal Radiol.* 3:91, 1978.

85. Yaghmai, I. Angiographic manifestations of soft-tissue and osseous hemangiopericytomas. *Radiology* 126:653, 1978.

86. Yaghmai, I. *Angiography of Bone and Soft Tissue Lesions.* New York: Springer, 1979.

87. Yaghmai, I., Shamza, A. Z., Shariat, S., and Afshari, R. Value of arteriography in the diagnosis of benign and malignant bone lesions. *Cancer* 27:1134, 1971.

2. Lymphangiography

Technique and Complications of Lymphography

WALTER A. FUCHS

Radiologic demonstration of lymph vessels and lymph nodes is mainly achieved only by direct lymphangiography, which is performed by injecting contrast material directly into the lymph vessels, lymph nodes, or occasionally lymph cysts. Indirect lymphangiography is used solely in animal experimentation. The contrast agents in this technique are introduced outside the lymphatic system either orally or by injection into subcutaneous tissue, muscle, joints, serous cavities, or solid organs. No contrast agent for indirect lymphangiography of the human body exists. Therefore, clinical lymphangiography demonstrates only those lymph vessels and nodes connected with the subcutaneous lymphatics of the extremities. Radiologic investigation of the lymphatic systems of the internal organs remains outside the range of diagnostic possibilities for the present.

Clinical Lymphangiography

Clinical lymphangiography is performed essentially according to the direct technique of Kinmonth [20, 21] in which injection of contrast material is preceded by the subcutaneous injection of a vital dye. The dye facilitates visualization of the lymph vessels during the surgical cutdown for their direct puncture [14].

INSTRUMENTS

Several types of needles and catheters are used for puncture of the lymphatic vessel. Automatic injectors have been constructed for the slow and continuous injection of the viscous oily contrast material. The quantity injected is automatically adjusted to the prevailing pressure within the lymph vessels to avoid accidental rupturing of a lymph vessel. Injection by hand, or by a simple injector that utilizes weights, cannot precisely control the injection pressure and is therefore not advisable. The contrast agent is kept at body temperature.

VITAL STAINING

Lymph vessels are stained by the subcutaneous injection of vital dye to make possible their visualization and dissection. Only the lymphatics absorb the dye and become visible through the skin as fine, greenish-blue streaks a few minutes

1979

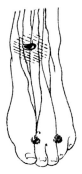

Figure 81-1. Interdigital injection of a vital dye using local anesthesia and a transverse incision of the skin.

after injection. A 1 percent dye solution is prepared by diluting one part of 2 percent patent blue-violet with an equal part of 2 percent procaine without epinephrine. The sites of injection are the interdigital webs, in which a great number of lymphatics find their source. Active or passive movements of the extremity or region injected increase lymph flow and speed up dye absorption.

SURGICAL DISSECTION

The vital dye injection sites are swabbed with skin disinfectant, and the subcutaneous injections are made. When the subcutaneous lymph vessels are sufficiently stained to be recognized as fine, greenish-blue streaks through the skin, the procedure may be started (Fig. 81-1). The area of incision is chosen at a place in which the stained lymphatics are clearly seen. A local anesthetic is injected subcutaneously, and a superficial transverse incision (2–4-cm long) is made. The subcutaneous lymphatics become visible as fine, greenish-blue vessels within the subcutaneous tissue. They are lifted with curved forceps, and the adherent fat and fibrous tissue are stripped away (Fig. 81-2). Complete stripping is essential for a successful puncture; it ensures that the needle tip will lie in the lumen of the vessel and not

Figure 81-2. A lymph vessel is lifted up with curved forceps, and the adherent fat and fibrous tissue are stripped away.

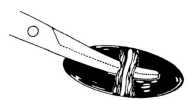

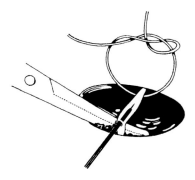

Figure 81-3. A silk loop is placed around the lymphatic and pulled upward to obstruct and dilate the vessel. The lymphatic is stretched by curved forceps and is punctured by the needle on the edge of the forceps. The stylet is withdrawn.

in surrounding tissue. A loop of silk thread is then placed around the vessel near the proximal border of the incision, and the lymphatic is pulled upward slightly by the silk, thereby producing a fold that obstructs the vessel.

The tip of the puncture needle is placed exactly over the upper edge of the curved forceps and introduced into the lumen of the vessel with a gentle rotating movement (Fig. 81-3). The needle is carefully set down, the curved forceps is removed, and a silk knot is tightened over the needle (Fig. 81-4). A soft polyethylene tube that has been filled with contrast agent is then connected to the needle by means of a Luer-Lok and to the syringe that has been placed in position on the automatic injector.

After the injection is completed, the incision is cleaned of any traces of oil by copious irrigation with sterile saline. Antiseptic powder is applied, and the skin is closed with interrupted sutures. The stitches are removed 10 days later. Following the injection of oily contrast material, the patient should remain in the horizontal position for about 1 to 2 hours. The patient should remain in bed until the next day, and ambulatory patients should be driven home.

Figure 81-4. The blunt needle tip is advanced within the vessel, and a silk knot is tightened over the rough part of the needle.

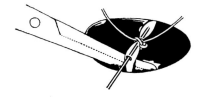

RADIOGRAPHIC TECHNIQUE

The radiographic technique includes routine exposures of the inguinal, iliac, and aortic areas immediately after the contrast injection (filling phase) and 24 hours later (storage phase). A standard chest film is also taken with the second series to demonstrate whether lung changes have been caused by the contrast material. The standard 90-kV exposure is correct when the structure of the lymph nodes is shown in good detail.

Preliminary screening with an image intensifier and television may become necessary in special cases to observe the extent of filling obtained. Laminography is very valuable as a supplementary method to distinguish between fused and superimposed lymph nodes [5]. In obese patients and in the event of the superimposition of bony structures, the lymphangiographic pattern of lymph nodes is demonstrated in detail. Direct roentgenographic magnification with an x-ray tube combining a high x-ray output with a fine focal spot produces very sharp images at two to three times linear magnification [7, 25]. Logetronic detail enhancement by the photographic technique yields additional definition of the structural pattern of lymph nodes because small details are accentuated. The subtraction technique cannot be applied for lymphangiography because it is difficult to obtain roentgenograms of identical position, both prior to the investigation and after the lymph nodes are contrast-filled.

Foot Lymphangiography

VITAL STAINING

Subcutaneous injection of 1 to 2 cc of 1 percent dye solution is made into each of the first and fourth interdigital webs. The anteromedial and anterolateral subcutaneous lymphatics are thus demonstrated.

SURGICAL DISSECTION

The region of the first metatarsal bone is usually the most appropriate site for incision because the anteromedial lymphatics are easily dissected.

CONTRAST INJECTION

For adults, a 5- to 7-cc injection is used on each side in bilateral visualization. The unilateral injection dose is 8 to 10 cc with provision made for some contralateral filling of the aortic lymph nodes. For children, 1 to 4 cc is sufficient to fill the entire retroperitoneal lymph system unilaterally. The injection rate is set at 0.1 to 0.15 cc per minute at a pressure of 1.4 atmospheres.

RADIOGRAPHIC TECHNIQUE

Films of the lower extremities are required only in cases of edema after malignant invasion. The following routine exposures are made twice, immediately after injection and 24 hours later: inguinal and pelvic region, anteroposterior and right and left oblique films; thoracic duct and thoracic region, anteroposterior and lateral films; upper abdominal region, lateral projection (optional); and standard chest roentgenogram (24 hours only).

Cavography combined with *urography* is routinely performed by some investigators simultaneously with the 24-hour roentgenography. A bilateral femoral venous injection of 20 cc each of a water-soluble contrast agent is used. The rationale for doing this combined study is to demonstrate lymph node disease within the upper lumbar (aortic) region compressing the inferior vena cava, and to investigate stasis or dislocation of the ureter by malignant disease.

Arm Lymphangiography

VITAL STAINING

Injection of 0.5 cc of the 1 percent dye solution is made into each of the interdigital webs of the hand.

SURGICAL DISSECTION

The group of lymphatics demonstrated (i.e., either the radial or the ulnar group) corresponds to the side of the carpus chosen as the site for incision and injection.

CONTRAST INJECTION

For demonstration of the lymph vessels and nodes of the upper extremity and axilla, 4 to 5 cc of oily contrast material is required. The speed of injection should not exceed 0.1 cc per minute to prevent rupture of the delicate lymph vessels.

RADIOGRAPHIC TECHNIQUE

The following routine exposures are made twice, immediately after injection and 24 hours later: forearm, anteroposterior and lateral films; upper arm, anteroposterior and lateral films; axillary and supraclavicular regions, anteroposterior and right and left oblique films with an angle of 25 degrees; and standard chest roentgenogram.

Contrast Material and Vital Dyes

VITAL DYES

The standard dye for direct lymphangiography is patent blue-violet, which is injected intradermally or subcutaneously. Patent blue-violet is a triphenylmethane dye with the molecular weight of 1,159.4. Alphazurine 2 G is a blue dye, similar to patent blue-violet, which has been frequently used in the United States. The prepared dye solution should be made sterile by autoclaving in sealed ampules. Other dyes that have been used are Evans blue, brilliant blue, direct sky blue, and Prontosil rubrum. An 11 percent water solution of patent blue-violet is isotonic with body fluids, and 0.2 to 0.5 cc, diluted in 1.5 to 3.0 cc of 1 percent procaine or other local anesthetic, is injected subcutaneously in the web space between toes or fingers. The patent blue-violet is then absorbed and transported from the tissue, mainly by the lymphatics, and is excreted in the urine. The blue coloration progressively clears from the injected area and is essentially gone at 2 weeks.

CONTRAST MATERIAL

Oily contrast material is far superior to the water-soluble media for visualizing the lymph nodes and lymph vessels because it does not diffuse through the wall of the lymphatics. Therefore, detailed opacification of lymph nodes distant from the injection site is achieved. Water-soluble organic iodide contrast agents are now seldom used for lymphangiography because they diffuse rapidly from lymph vessels and nodes and thus obscure details of structure. The standard contrast agent used for lymphangiography is an iodized oil known commercially as Ethiodol in the United States and as Lipiodol Ultra-Fluid in European countries [9, 11].

Ethiodol is synthesized from the natural oil of poppy seeds and consists of the iodized glyceryl esters of oleic, linolenic, palmitic, and stearic acids [17]. It is yellow and has a specific gravity of 1.280 at 15° C. The viscosity is 53.6 centipoises at 20° C and 30.2 centipoises at 37° C. The iodine content is 37 percent. Stored in closed ampules and protected from light, Ethiodol is stable. Progressive liberation of iodine takes place when it is heated or in contact with air. Decomposition is indicated by discoloration. Solutions of contrast agent with a darker color should never be used.

Ethiodol injected directly into a peripheral lymphatic fills the lymph vessels and nodes. The opaque material remains in the nodes for several months. The oily contrast material is phagocytized by polynuclear giant cells and metabolized by esterases to sodium iodine. After the oily substance is eliminated from the nodes, the foreign body reaction subsides. Sodium iodine is excreted mainly by the kidneys, but the pancreas, liver, and salivary glands also take part in its elimination [23]. Contrast medium in excess of that retained in the nodes enters the systemic veins via the thoracic duct or lymphaticovenous communications. From the great veins it passes into the lung capillaries. Some of the contrast material is removed via the pulmonary circulation. The macrophages in the alveolar spaces phagocytize parts of the agent, which is later removed by the sputum. With increase of the administered dose, the lung becomes a less efficient filter for the oily particles, and the amounts reaching other organs such as the liver, spleen, kidneys, and bone marrow are greater.

Complications of Lymphangiography

WOUND INFECTION

Wound infection is rare after lymphangiography when adequate cleansing of the skin, strict aseptic technique, and careful dressing of the wound are carried out. Lymphangitis is uncommon but may occasionally be observed in preexisting lymphedema. Slight swelling of the extremity rarely occurs. Delayed wound healing is seen as a result of excessive skin tension because of movement. Extravasation of the oily contrast material from the lymph vessels is related to excessive injection pressure and is common in lymphatic obstruction [10].

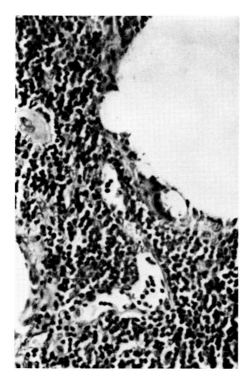

Figure 81-5. Foreign body reaction. Granulation tissue with inflammatory cell infiltration and giant cells surround oil droplets.

FOREIGN BODY REACTION

Foreign body reaction and considerable dilatation of the marginal and intermediary sinuses occur within a few hours after lymphangiography [27, 29]. The number of giant cells increases until the fourteenth day after administration of the contrast material. Granulation tissue and inflammatory cell infiltration surround oil droplets of various sizes (Fig. 81-5). The increased size of lymph nodes observed on the lymphangiogram in the first days after contrast injection can be attributed to the dilatation of the sinuses filled with contrast material and to the foreign body reaction. A significant decrease in phagocytic reaction is observed after 3 to 6 weeks, and the foreign body reaction subsides almost completely within 12 to 15 months. Small, circumscribed areas of fibrosis and scar reaction in the marginal sinuses and fibrous encapsulation of oil droplets may be observed as irreversible changes. These structural alterations of the lymph nodes are too minute to be demonstrated by lymphangiography. When the nodes have been examined by a second lymphangiography several months later, no change in the structural pattern of normal lymph nodes and no impairment of lymph circulation have been encountered.

SPREAD OR EXTENSION OF A NEOPLASM

The question of whether lymphangiography causes a neoplasm to spread has not been conclusively answered. A few clinical and experimental observations indicate the possibility of propagation of tumor cells by lymphangiography, but very extensive clinical experience with this method gives strong evidence that lymphangiography with oily contrast material does not increase the number of metastases.

SENSITIVITY REACTIONS TO CONTRAST MEDIA AND TO IODINE

Sensitivity reactions are very rare, occurring with an incidence of approximately 0.1 percent [10, 22]. Dermatitis and erythematous skin reactions have been observed [30]. Sialadenitis is occasionally encountered and is considered to be a hypersensitivity of the salivary gland to iodine. Corticoids and antihistamines are utilized to treat these reactions. Adverse reactions to the blue dye are infrequent; the incidence is 1 in 700 examinations [10, 22]. A few cases of nonfatal anaphylactic reactions to patent blue-violet have been reported [24].

LUNG COMPLICATIONS

Lung complications of lymphangiography are caused by embolism of the iodized oil into the pulmonary capillaries [2, 4, 6, 8, 10, 12, 13, 16, 22, 31]. After each lymphangiogram oily contrast material not retained in the lymph nodes enters the venous circulation. Miliary or reticular deposits of oily substance in the lungs are visible on the roentgenograms within 24 hours after injection in about 10 percent of the patients (Figs. 81-6, 81-7). Most of these patients have neither clinical symptoms nor respiratory impairment, but scintiscanning of the lungs after the injection of a radioactive tracer material shows that lung embolization has occurred in every case.

No significant impairment of ventilation is observed as a result of lymphangiography. Wedging of the small lipid particles temporarily decreases the capillary bed available for diffusion of gases [12, 16]. The maximum decrease in diffusing capacity ranges between 12 and 60 percent and is

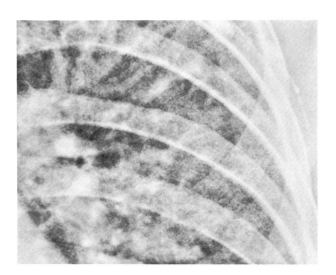

Figure 81-6. Pulmonary oil embolism. Reticular deposits of oily substance are visible.

noted between 3 and 72 hours. Recovery time may vary from 21 to 256 hours. The decreased diffusing capacity is due to the decrease in capillary blood volume, which is between 28 and 60 percent of normal.

Twenty-four hours after lymphangiography the oily contrast material is not found exclusively in the capillary bed of the lung but is scattered in the interstitial tissue of the lung. The oily substance leaves the lung partially via the vascular system. Lipid material also traverses the capillary endothelium into the interstitial tissue and later into the alveolar spaces, in which it is phagocytized by macrophages that are later expectorated. Reactive granulation tissue within the alveolar walls and areas of focal atelectases due to small infarctions are frequently encountered. These histologic inflammatory reactions subside within a few months after lymphangiography. The mechanical vascular occlusive phase, which sometimes causes acute symptoms, is followed in some patients by a chemical phase. In the chemical phase a lung response may develop that consists of edematous and inflammatory changes as a reaction to the fatty acids released by hydrolysis. The fatty acids damage the vessel endothelium and alveolar membranes, causing hemorrhage and exudation [10]. The chemical phase is marked by fever, hemoptysis, and varying degrees of respiratory distress.

Radiographic investigations demonstrate the change of the finely stippled pattern of uncomplicated oil embolism to massive bronchopneumonic infiltration in the perihilar and basal

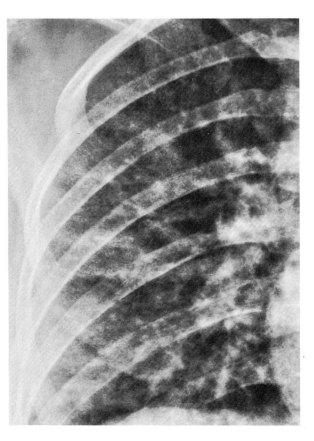

Figure 81-7. Chemical pneumonia. Miliary deposits of oily contrast substance and bronchopneumonic infiltration 5 days after lymphangiography.

areas (Fig. 81-7). Clinical and radiologic symptoms usually disappear within 10 to 14 days, and the patient returns to normal without residual effects.

In a survey of 32,000 lymphangiograms, in approximately 0.5 percent of cases serious pulmonary complications were reported [22]. They included hemoptysis, infarction, edema, and pneumonia. Because lung complications are clearly related to oily contrast–material embolism, the amount of oil reaching the lungs must be kept to a minimum. The dosage of oily material injected in the adult patient has been reduced from 10 to 15 cc for each leg to 5 to 6 cc. Low dosage is appropriate in cases of irradiation fibrosis of lymph nodes because only small amounts of contrast material are retained in these nodes. The same dosage applies to lymphatic obstruction because oily material enters the lung by way of lymphaticovenous anastomoses.

Pulmonary function tests are necessary in every patient with a history of pulmonary disease, prior radiation therapy to the chest, or metastatic neoplasm or lymphoma in the lung [12, 16]. In poor-risk patients unilateral left lymphangiography completed by vena cavography is the safest procedure. General anesthesia should not be administered in the immediate postlymphangiography period because lung diffusion is diminished. The aims of treatment of lung complications due to acute vascular obstruction are to improve oxygenation of blood and to maintain blood circulation [10]. Dyspnea, tachypnea, tachycardia, and cyanosis require immediate administration of oxygen. Digitalis should be given parenterally in case of heart failure. Hypotension and shock must be treated. Intermittent positive pressure respiration may be needed. Intravenous administration of ethyl alcohol is advised to block the activity of lipase. Low-molecular-weight dextran is recommended to combat the sludging phenomenon of the blood.

HEPATIC OIL EMBOLISM

Hepatic oil embolism is rarely a cause of complications of lymphangiography (the incidence is approximately 0.2 percent) [1, 3, 10]. Severe lymphatic obstruction in the common iliac and lower aortic region and occlusion of the pelvic veins must be present to shunt the oily contrast material through lymphaticovenous anastomoses and then via a venous collateral circulation into the portal venous system. The complication does not produce symptoms. Finely stippled deposits of oily material are seen radiographically (Fig. 81-8). Hepatic oil embolism occurs in all lymphangiography, but impairment of hepatic function has not been observed [15].

CEREBRAL OIL EMBOLISM

Cerebral oil embolism has been reported in a few cases as a complication of lymphangiography [10, 18, 19, 26, 28]. When excessive doses of oily material reach the venous circulation, the lung does not retain all of it and embolisms of oily material reach the brain.

Fever and pain in the back and groin, weakness, headache, unpleasant taste sensations, and nausea are transitory symptoms requiring no medication. Iodine sialitis and thyroiditis have been reported. Hemolytic crisis and thrombocytopenic purpura may be attributed to the oily material used in lymphangiography.

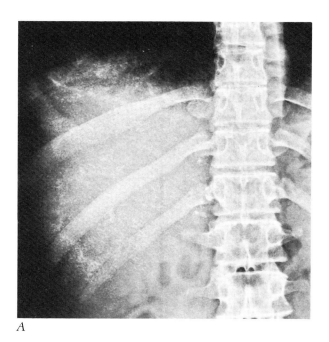

A

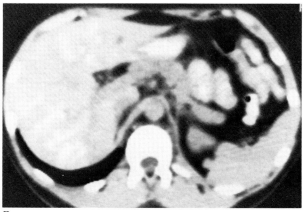

B

Figure 81-8. Hepatic oil embolism. (A) Reticular deposits of oily material visible in the portal venous system. (B) High-density deposits of oily contrast substance demonstrated at CT.

CARDIOVASCULAR REACTIONS

Such complications as hypertensive crisis and hypotensive reaction have been observed in a few cases [10, 13].

The incidence of fatal cases is generally extremely low. However, most patients examined by lymphangiography are frequently critically ill, and caution has, therefore, to be applied to prevent major complications.

References

1. Bodie, J. F., and Linton, D. S., Jr. Hepatic oil embolization as a complication of lymphangiography. *Radiology* 99:317, 1971.
2. Bron, K. M., Baum, S., and Abrams, H. L. Oil embolism in lymphangiography. Incidence, manifestations and mechanism. *Radiology* 80:194, 1963.
3. Chavez, G. M., Picard, J., and Davis, D. Liver opacification following lymphangiography; pathogenesis and clinical significance. *Surgery* 63:564, 1968.
4. Clouse, M. E., Hallgrimsson, J., and Wenlund, D. E. Complications following lymphography with particular reference to pulmonary oil embolization. *AJR* 96:972, 1966.
5. De Roo, T., Thomas, P., and Kropholler, R. W. The importance of tomography for the interpretation of the lymphographic picture of lymph node metastases. *AJR* 94:924, 1965.
6. Desprez-Curely, J. P., Bismuth, V., Langier, A., and Descamps, J. Accidents et incidents de la lymphographie. *Ann. Radiol.* (Paris) 5:577, 1962.
7. Ditchek, T., and Scanlon, G. T. Direct magnification lymphography. *J.A.M.A.* 199:654, 1967.
8. Dolan, P. A. Lymphography: Complications encountered in 522 examinations. *Radiology* 86:876, 1966.
9. Fischer, H. W. Experiences in seeking an Ethiodol emulsion for lymphography. *Invest. Radiol.* 1:29, 1966.
10. Fischer, H. W. Complications. In W. A. Fuchs, J. W. Davidson, and H. W. Fischer (eds.), *Lymphography in Cancer*. New York: Springer, 1969.
11. Fischer, H. W. Contrast Media. In W. A. Fuchs, J. W. Davidson, and H. W. Fischer (eds.), *Lymphography in Cancer*. New York: Springer, 1969.
12. Fraimow, W., Wallace, S., Lewis, P., Greening, R. R., and Cathcart, R. T. Changes in pulmonary function due to lymphangiography. *Radiology* 85:231, 1965.
13. Fuchs, W. A. Complications in lymphography with oily contrast media. *Acta Radiol.* (Stockh.) 57:427, 1962.
14. Fuchs, W. A. Investigation Techniques. In W. A. Fuchs, J. W. Davidson, and H. W. Fischer (eds.), *Lymphography in Cancer*. New York: Springer, 1969.
15. Fuchs, W. A., Preisig, R., and Bucher, H. Liver Function After Lymphography. In M. Viamonte, P. R. Koehler, M. Witte, and C. Witte (eds), *Progress in Lymphology*. Stuttgart: Thieme, 1970. Vol. II.
16. Gold, W. M., Youker, J., Anderson, S., and Nadel, J. A. Pulmonary function abnormalities after lymphangiography. *N. Engl. J. Med.* 273:519, 1965.
17. Guerbet, M. Étude expérimentale de la toxicité du Lipiodol ultrafluide par voie intraveineuse ou lymphatique. *J. Radiol. Electrol. Med. Nucl.* 45:887, 1964.
18. Jay, J. C., and Ludington, J. C. Neurologic complications following lymphangiography. Possible mechanisms and a case of blindness. *Arch. Surg.* 106:863, 1973.
19. Jochem, W., and Buchelt, L. A case of cerebral embolism after lymphography. *Radiology* 93:711, 1969.
20. Kinmonth, J. B. Lymphography in man: A method of outlining lymphatic trunks at operation. *Clin. Sci. Mol. Med.* 11:13, 1952.
21. Kinmonth, J. B., Taylor, G. W., and Kemp Harper, R. Lymphangiography: A technique for its clinical use in the lower limb. *Br. Med. J.* 1:940, 1955.
22. Koehler, P. R. Complications of Lymphography. In M. Viamonte, P. R. Koehler, M. Witte, and C. Witte (eds.), *Progress in Lymphology*. Stuttgart: Thieme, 1970. Vol. II.
23. Koehler, P. R., Meyers, W. A., Skelly, J. F., and Schaffer, B. Body distribution of Ethiodol following lymphangiography. *Radiology* 82:866, 1964.
24. Kopp, W. L. Anaphylaxis from alphazurine 2G during lymphography. *J.A.M.A.* 198:200, 1966.
25. Love, R. W., and Takaro, T. Lymphangiography with direct roentgenographic magnification. New application for an old technique. *Radiology* 87:123, 1966.
26. Nelson, B., Rush, E. A., Takasugi, M., and Wittenberg, J. Lipid embolism to the brain after lymphography. *N. Engl. J. Med.* 273:1132, 1965.
27. Oehlert, W., Weissleber, H., and Gollasch, D. Lymphogramm und histologisches Bild normaler und pathologisch veränderter Lymphknoten. *ROEFO* 104:751, 1966.
28. Rasmussen, K. E. Retinal and cerebral fat emboli following lymphography with oily contrast media. *Acta Radiol.* [*Diagn.*] (Stockh.) 10:199, 1970.
29. Ravel, R. Histopathology of lymph nodes after lymphangiography. *Am. J. Clin. Pathol.* 46:335, 1966.
30. Redman, H. C. Dermatitis as a complication of lymphangiography. *Radiology* 86:323, 1966.
31. Sokol, G. H., Clouse, M. E., Kotner, L. M., and Sewell, J. B. Complications of lymphangiography in patients of advanced age. *AJR* 128:43, 1977.

Normal Radiologic Anatomy of the Lymphatics and Lymph Nodes

WALTER A. FUCHS

Normal Structural Roentgen Anatomy

The basic topographic anatomy of lymph vessels and lymph nodes in the inguinal, pelvic, lumbar, and axillary regions is constant, but considerable variation is encountered in size, shape, number, and structure of the lymph nodes. Normal lymph nodes vary between 1 and 30 mm in diameter, depending on the functional load, constitutional elements, and age. They may be round, oval, elongated, or bean-shaped with a slight indentation at the hilar region. Lymph nodes consist of lymphatic tissue, which is connected with the lymphatic circulation by afferent and efferent lymphatics (Figs. 82-1, 82-2) [2, 4, 20, 21]. The sinus system of the lymph nodes includes the marginal sinus, situated close to the lymph node capsule of fibrous tissue, and extensions of the marginal sinus, the intermediate sinuses, which converge toward the hilus where they unite to form the terminal sinuses. The lymphatic tissue is formed by a netlike stroma of reticular fibers and both free and fixed reticulohistiocytic, lymphatic, and plasmatic cells. Myeloid and mast cells are also present. Loose lymphatic tissue, consisting of a meshwork of reticular fibers and reticulohistiocytic cells, fills the sinuses, which are the main channels for lymph circulation [26, 32].

The diffuse lymphatic tissue of the nodes is formed by a dense network of reticular fibers and uniformly distributed cells of the lymphatic group. The nodular lymphatic tissue of the lymph nodes includes follicles, which are rounded, and dense accumulations of predominantly lymphatic cells embedded in a very loose reticular stroma. The diffuse lymphatic tissue is arranged into a rather compact cortex, and a medulla, which consists of a coarse network of medullary cords. The cortex is divided into lymphatic lobules by trabeculae of dense connective tissue arising from the capsule. The lymph follicles, which are not permanent structures, are localized predominantly in the cortex but may also be found in the medullary cords. The functions of the nodules are lymph filtration and cell production, chiefly of lymphatic and plasma cells. Depending on the functional state of the lymph node, primary and secondary nodules may be present. These differ in that the primary follicle has a more uniform structure whereas the secondary follicle contains a so-called germinal center.

In lymphangiography the filling phase immediately after injection of a contrast medium

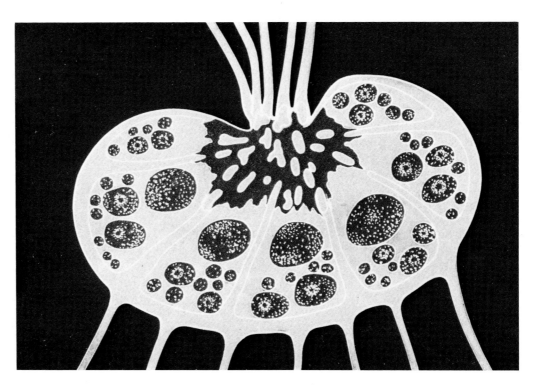

Figure 82-1. Schematic representation of structural lymph node anatomy.

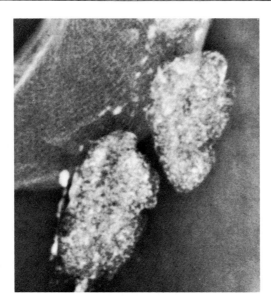

Figure 82-2. Lymphographic storage pattern of normal lymph nodes.

demonstrates both lymph vessels and lymph nodes (Fig. 82-3A) [6–9]. Contrast medium enters a node through the numerous afferent lymphatics joining its marginal lymph sinus, passes through the medullary sinuses in streaks, and leaves the lymph node by way of efferent lymphatics from the hilus. Generally, there are more afferent than efferent lymphatics. Often the contrast medium first passes directly from the afferent to the efferent lymph vessels of a lymph node without demonstrating the entire sinus system. Then gradually, as more contrast material enters the node, the entire sinus system is visualized. Direct connections between efferent lymphatics of a lymph node and afferent lymphatics of other nodes are observed frequently.

During the storage phase, which is 2 to 24 hours after injection, the contrast material leaves the lymph vessels and accumulates in the lymph nodes (Fig. 82-3B). Contrast filling of the lymph vessels for more than 24 hours must generally be regarded as a sign of impaired lymphatic circulation. The oily contrast agent is retained as drops in the lymph nodes by the network of fibrous and reticulohistiocytic cells [4]. Intracellular deposits of contrast medium are rare because reabsorption of the fluid takes place very slowly. The major portion of the contrast material remains embedded in the meshwork of the reticulum cells, which phagocytize it for about 5 to 9 months. The marginal sinus of the nodes and the peripheral parts of the intermediary sinuses are most densely filled with contrast fluid. Small structural changes in the lymph nodes may be

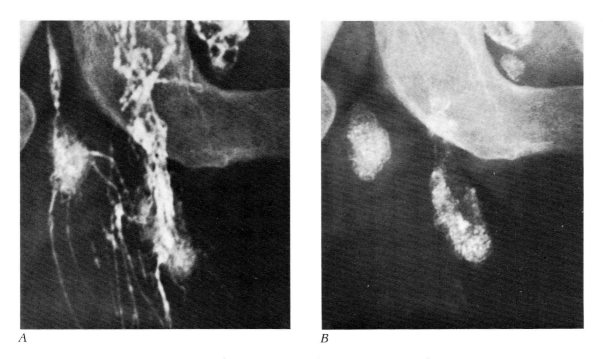

A   B

Figure 82-3. Normal inguinal lymph nodes. (A) Filling phase. (B) Storage phase.

Figure 82-4. Fibrolipomatosis of inguinal lymph nodes. (A) Filling phase. (B) Storage phase.

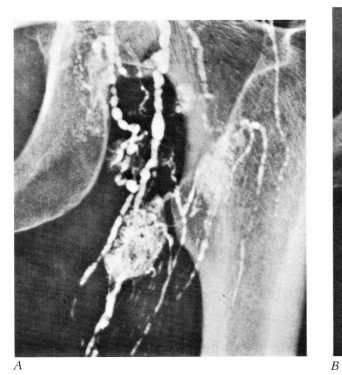
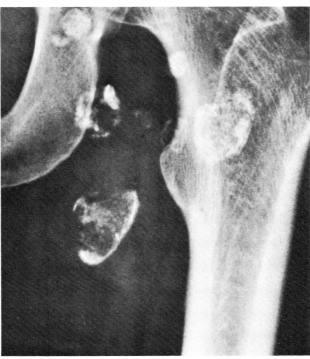

A   B

obscured by an excessive amount of contrast medium within the sinuses. The follicular lymphatic tissue of the nodes is not penetrated by oily contrast agent. Small, round filling defects of varied sizes corresponding to the different lymph follicles lead to a fine homogeneous, reticular appearance [27]. In the medullary parts without nodules, however, the distribution may appear to be irregular.

The size of lymph nodes and vessels as determined by lymphangiography tends to decrease in old age, but size is more dependent upon the functional state than upon age [11]. With the same qualification in mind, it is generally found that children and young women have fine, delicate lymphatics.

Fibrolipomatosis is considered a manifestation of the normal physiologic involution of the lymph nodes. It is characterized by the replacement of the central parts of the lymph nodes by connective and fatty tissue [6, 7, 9, 17]. Lymphatic structures are left only in the periphery of the nodes. The intermediary sinuses traversing the fibrolipomatous tissue stay intact (Fig. 82-4A). Lymphography results in a large central filling defect permeated by the intermediary sinuses, because only the reticular meshwork of the lymphatic tissue is able to retain the contrast substance (Fig. 82-4B). Consequently, careful analysis of the radiographic pattern of the intermediary sinuses during the lymphographic filling phase is of paramount importance in the diagnostic evaluation of filling defects.

Involutive changes are very common in inguinal and axillary lymph nodes, because they are the primary regional lymph node groups of the extremities, and therefore are most often affected by inflammatory lesions. The external iliac and the aortic node groups at the level of L1–L2 manifest similar, but less extensive, involutive changes. Fibrolipomatosis is more pronounced in patients of the middle and older age groups.

Topographic Anatomy

LOWER EXTREMITY

The lymphatics of the lower extremities [3, 8, 14, 16, 25] consist of a subcutaneous prefascial and a deep subfascial lymph system. The lymph from the capillary network of the skin and the subcutis drains through delicate lymphatics into groups of larger, longitudinal lymph vessels situated above the fascia. They are closely connected with the largest subcutaneous veins. The deep subfascial lymph vessels collect the lymph from the muscles, fascia, and joints. The valves in lymphatics direct the flow, contrary to veins, from the deep to the superficial lymphatic system. At present, lymphangiography as a routine procedure can outline only the prefascial lymphatics.

According to their relationship to the veins, the lymph vessels of the leg are divided into an anterior vena saphena magna group and a posterior vena saphena parva group. The anterior group is composed of a medial and a lateral bundle of lymphatics. The anteromedial group follows a straight and almost parallel course on the medial side of the leg and comprises 5 to 6 vessels in the lower leg and 10 to 20 vessels in the thigh (Fig. 82-5).

The vessels of the anterolateral group of lymphatics, five to six in number, course distally on the peroneal side of the leg and cross in a wide curve toward the medial side at the level of the knee, where they become of large diameter and tortuous (Fig. 82-6). Above the knee these lymphatic trunks are always situated medially in close connection with the great saphenous vein until they join the superficial inguinal lymph nodes.

The posterior prefascial lymphatic group, which accompanies the lesser saphenous vein, consists of only one to three prefascial collecting trunks that reach one to three subfascial lymph nodes in the popliteal region (Fig. 82-7). The latter nodes are connected to the deep inguinal or iliac nodes by subfascial lymphatics, which follow the deep blood vessels on the medial aspect of the thigh (Fig. 82-8). The collecting subcutaneous prefascial lymph vessels branch dichotomously as they course proximally. Despite this division, they retain equal diameters of about 0.75 to 1.0 mm. Normally, there are no anastomoses among the various superficial groups of vessels.

INGUINAL REGION

The lymph nodes of the inguinal region [3, 5, 8, 11, 12, 17, 25, 29, 31] are subdivided into a superficial and a deep group (Figs. 82-9, 82-10). The superficial inguinal lymph nodes are separated into a superior and an inferior group. On the lymphangiogram the perineal and genital groups of superior superficial inguinal lymph nodes are rarely demonstrated because these nodes are very seldom connected with afferent lymphatics from the lower extremity. The crural

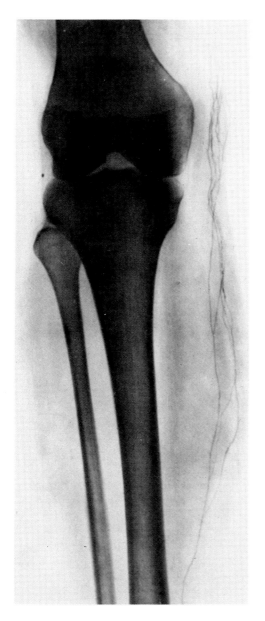

Figure 82-5. Anteromedial group of subcutaneous lymphatics.

group of superior superficial inguinal lymph nodes is situated cranially in the inguinal region and cannot be differentiated on the lymphangiogram from the deep inguinal lymph nodes. The configuration of both groups is similar—round and small. Afferent and efferent lymphatics do not provide a distinction between two groups. For this reason the superior superficial inguinal lymph nodes receiving afferent lymphatics from the right and the deep inguinal nodes have been grouped together.

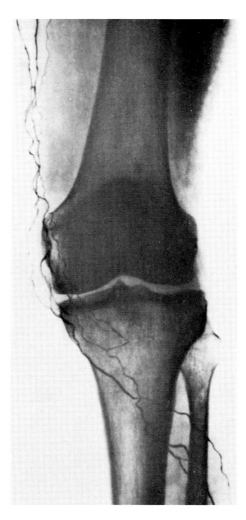

Figure 82-6. Anterolateral group of subcutaneous lymphatics.

The most cranial of the deep inguinal nodes is the largest and most constant. It is situated in the inguinal fossa close to the lacunar ligament and medial to the femoral vein in intimate relationship with the medial external iliac lymph nodes. The inferior superficial inguinal lymph nodes (subinguinal lymph nodes) localized around the hiatus saphenus are regularly filled with contrast material because their afferent lymphatics drain the lymph from the lower extremity.

PELVIC REGION

According to their relationship to the iliac blood vessels, the lymph nodes of the pelvic region [3, 5, 8, 11, 12, 17, 18, 23, 25, 29, 31] are divided into the external, internal, and common iliac node groups (Fig. 82-11).

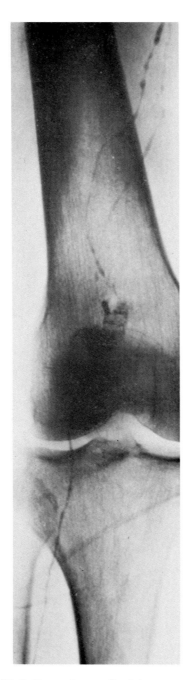

Figure 82-7. Posterior prefascial group of lymphatics connected with two popliteal lymph nodes.

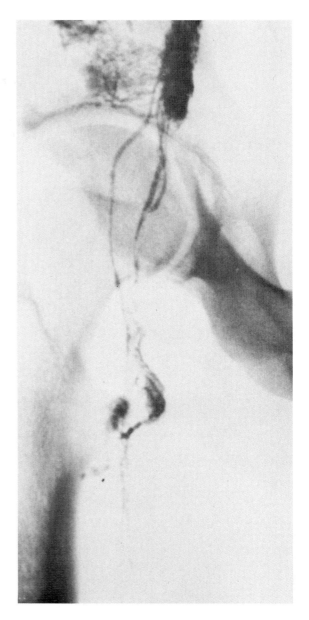

Figure 82-8. Lymphatics of the posterior prefascial group connected with deep inguinal lymph nodes and intermediate and lateral external iliac lymph nodes.

The external iliac lymph nodes are situated along the external iliac artery and vein and are continuous with the inguinal lymph nodes (Figs. 82-12, 82-13). They are subdivided into the lateral, intermediate, and medial external iliac node groups, which are connected by numerous lymphatics. The lateral external iliac lymph node chain is localized along the lateral aspect of the external iliac artery within a cleft formed by the artery with the psoas muscle. The medial external iliac lymph node group is positioned medial and dorsal to the external iliac vein near the pelvic wall and between the external iliac artery and the obturator nerve.

The common iliac lymph nodes are arranged along the common iliac vessels and are a direct continuation of the lateral, intermediate, and medial node groups of the external iliac area (Figs. 82-12, 82-13). The lateral iliac lymph

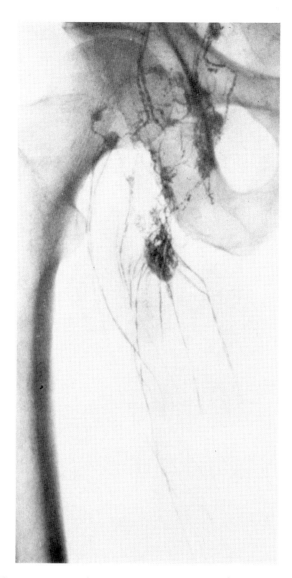

Figure 82-9. Subcutaneous lymphatics of the anterior medial group enter inferior superficial inguinal (subinguinal) lymph nodes and deep inguinal lymph nodes.

nodes are situated at the lateral aspect of the common iliac artery and on the inner margin of the psoas muscle. Their afferent lymphatics arise from the lateral external iliac lymph nodes. The efferent lymphatics reach the lateral aortic lymph nodes on the corresponding side. The intermediate common iliac lymph nodes are found on the posterior aspect of the common iliac artery and vein and are continuous with the intermediate external iliac lymph node group. The medial common iliac lymph nodes are localized on the medial aspect of the common iliac artery and vein. The lymphatics and nodes of both sides form a triangular arrangement.

All lymph nodes situated within the region of supply of the internal iliac artery and its branches make up the internal iliac lymph nodes, also called hypogastric lymph nodes (Fig. 82-13) [15, 18, 31]. According to their relation to parietal and visceral arterial branches, they are divided into parietal and visceral lymph node groups. The parietal lymph node group is composed of the superior and inferior gluteal lymph nodes and the lateral, sacral, and obturator lymph nodes, which are occasionally contrast-filled by foot lymphangiography. The visceral lymph nodes are only partially connected with the visceral arterial branches and are situated close to the related organs. They comprise the vesical, rectal, and parauterine lymph node groups. The internal iliac lymph nodes, which are not contrast-filled by foot lymphangiography, receive lymph from the joints and muscles of the pelvis and from the organs in the pelvic region, the upper third of the vagina, uterus, ovaries, prostate, vesicular gland and urinary bladder, and areas of the penis and the rectum. They are connected to the common iliac and aortic node group by efferent lymphatics.

LUMBAR (AORTIC) REGION

The lumbar lymph nodes [3, 8, 11, 12, 17, 18, 29, 31] are situated on the anterior aspect of the lumbar vertebrae and around the abdominal aorta and inferior vena cava. Anatomically they are divided into the right intermediate and left lumbar node groups (Fig. 82-14). In the lymphangiogram only one intermediate and two lateral lymph node chains are discernible (Fig. 82-15): the exact position of the preaortic and retroaortic node groups in relation to the abdominal aorta cannot be determined on roentgenograms. Unilateral injection of contrast material leads to retrograde contrast filling of the common iliac lymph nodes of the contralateral side in about half the cases, which therefore may not be interpreted as a pathologic finding. Visualization of contralateral lymph nodes at the level of the fourth to fifth lumbar vertebrae by anastomosing lymphatics is also observed in about 50 percent of normal lymphangiograms.

The right lumbar lymph nodes, situated on the right side of the abdominal aorta, are grouped according to their relation to the inferior vena cava into the precaval, interaorticocaval, retrocaval, and laterocaval nodes. In the lymphangiogram they are projected upon the right aspect of the

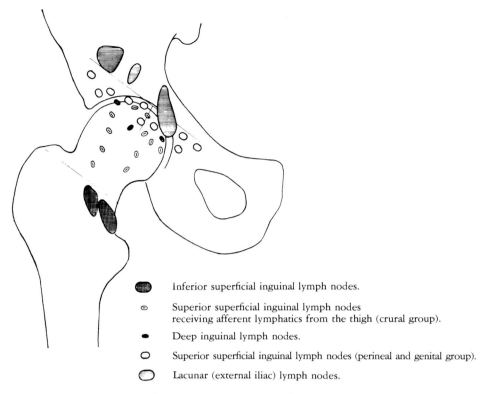

Inferior superficial inguinal lymph nodes.

Superior superficial inguinal lymph nodes receiving afferent lymphatics from the thigh (crural group).

Deep inguinal lymph nodes.

Superior superficial inguinal lymph nodes (perineal and genital group).

Lacunar (external iliac) lymph nodes.

Figure 82-10. Topographic anatomy of the inguinal lymph nodes. (From Fuchs [8].)

vertebral bodies and up to 2 cm further laterally. The number of right lumbar lymph nodes that are contrast-filled by lymphangiography is considerably smaller than that of the other two lumbar node chains (Fig. 82-16). This is in contrast to anatomic findings, which show the right lumbar lymph node group comprising the greatest number of nodes. In 70 percent of cases the upper border of the right lymph nodes filled with contrast material reaches the level of the third lumbar vertebra or below, in about 20 percent it reaches the second lumbar vertebra, and in only 10 percent does it reach the first lumbar vertebra.

The intermediate lumbar lymph nodes (preaortic and retroaortic lymph nodes) are projected onto the vertebral bodies of the lumbar spine in lymphangiography. Contrast filling of the intermediate lymph nodes is considerably more frequent than is found with the right lumbar lymph node group. It reaches the level of the first lumbar vertebra in 50 percent of cases and the second lumbar vertebra in 40 percent. In only 10 percent is the upper border of this chain situated at or below the third lumbar vertebra.

The left lumbar lymph nodes are situated between the psoas muscle and the abdominal aorta and form a chain of 5 to 10 nodes. On the lymphangiogram they are projected onto the left lateral aspect of the lumbar spine and up to 2 cm further laterally. They receive afferent lymphatics from the lateral common iliac lymph nodes and are connected to the other aortic lymph node chains. Radiologically the left lumbar lymph node group is the most constant of all lumbar node groups and comprises the largest number of contrast-filled nodes. Clustering of lymph nodes is seen below the left renal artery and vein. It reaches the level of the first and second lumbar vertebrae in about 90 percent of cases and the level of the third lumbar vertebra in 10 percent.

Contrast filling of lumbar lymphatics and lumbar lymph nodes on the dorsal aspect of the lumbar fossa is a rare variation.

UPPER EXTREMITY

In the forearm and arm [8, 15, 25] the subcutaneous lymphatics are divided into a medial ulnar (basilic) group and a lateral radial (cephalic) group.

The ulnar group of lymphatics drains primarily the third, fourth, and fifth finger and the ulnar

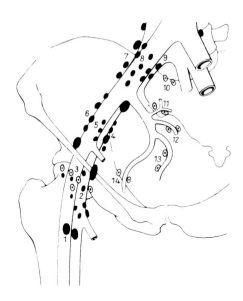

Inguinal lymph nodes:

1 Inferior superficial inguinal (subinguinal) lymph nodes
2 Superior superficial and deep inguinal lymph node group
3 Superior superficial inguinal lymph nodes (perineal and genital group)

Pelvic lymph nodes:

4 Medial external iliac lymph nodes
5 Intermediate external iliac lymph nodes

6 Lateral external iliac lymph nodes
7 Lateral common iliac lymph nodes
8 Intermediate common iliac lymph nodes
9 Medial common iliac lymph nodes
10 Promontorial (subaortic) lymph nodes
11 Lateral sacral lymph nodes
12 Superior gluteal lymph nodes
13 Inferior gluteal lymph nodes
14 Obturator lymph nodes

● Routinely demonstrated by lymphography; ⊖ Inconstantly demonstrated by lymphography

Figure 82-11. Topographic roentgen anatomy of the inguinal and iliac lymph nodes (oblique projection). (From Fuchs [8].)

side of the hand and forearm (Fig. 82-17). The majority of these lymph channels run along with the basilic vein to the cubital region. Above this point they follow the medial border of the biceps muscle to reach the prefascial axillary lymph nodes. One to two lymphatics may accompany the basilic vein through the deep fascia and join the deep subfascial lymph vessels of the upper arm.

The radial group of lymphatics drains the first and second digits and the radial side of the hand and forearm. These lymphatics are situated on the lateral side of the wrist and join the cephalic vein in the forearm. They follow the vein to the level of the olecranon, at which point most of them curve medially to enter the lateral group of axillary lymph nodes. A few lymphatics continue with the cephalic vein to reach the infraclavicular lymph nodes. The collecting lymphatics from the deltoid region pass over the anterior and poste-

rior axillary folds to end in axillary lymph nodes. The skin of the scapular region is drained by lymph vessels that end in the subcapsular groups of axillary nodes or follow the transverse cervical vessels to the interior deep cervical lymph nodes. The deep lymph channels of the arm follow the muscles, vessels, and nerves and end at the lateral axillary lymph nodes. They are less numerous than the superficial vessels, with which they communicate at intervals. A few deep lymph nodes are connected with the deep lymphatic system.

AXILLARY REGION

The axillary lymph nodes [8, 15, 25] are the first regional nodes of the whole upper limb and are divided into five groups (Fig. 82-18).

The lateral axillary group is situated medial and posterior to the axillary vein. The afferent lymphatics of this group drain the lymph of the entire

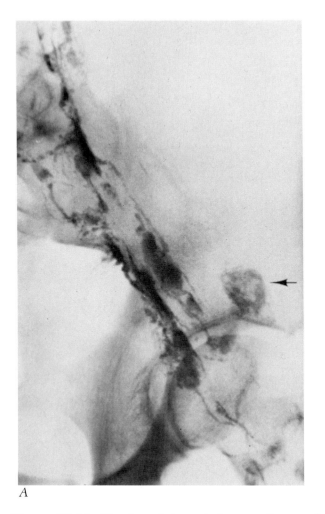 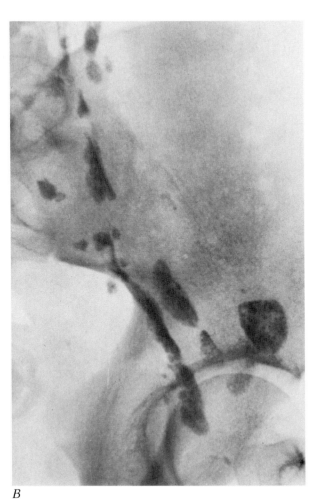

A

B

Figure 82-12. The lateral (*arrow*), intermediate, and medial external iliac lymph node chains connected by numerous lymphatics. (A) Filling phase. (B) Storage phase.

upper extremity, except for the regions drained by radial subcutaneous vessels following the cephalic vein. The efferent vessels join the central and apical axillary lymph nodes or the inferior deep cervical lymph nodes.

The anterior or pectoral group of axillary lymph nodes is located along the inferior border of the lesser pectoral muscle near the lateral thoracic vessels. The afferent lymphatics of this group drain the skin and muscles of the anterior and lateral walls of the thorax, the abdominal wall above the umbilicus, and the central and lateral areas of the mammary gland. The efferent lymph vessels enter the central and apical axillary node group.

The posterior or subcapsular axillary lymph nodes are placed along the lower margin of the posterior wall of the axilla close to the axillary

vessels. The afferent lymphatics of this group drain the skin and muscles of the lower part of the neck and of the dorsal aspect of the body as far inferiorly as the iliac crests. The efferent lymphatics enter the apical and central groups of axillary nodes.

The central axillary lymph node group is situated near the base of the axilla. The group has no drainage area of its own but receives efferent lymphatics from most of the other axillary lymph node groups. The efferent lymphatics of the group enter the apical axillary lymph nodes.

The apical axillary lymph nodes are situated within the apex of the axilla medial to the axillary vein, dorsal to the superior portion of the lesser pectoral muscle, and cranial to the superior margins of the pectoral muscles. The only direct territorial afferents of this group are those that ac-

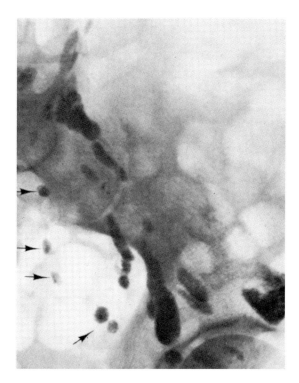

Figure 82-13. Contrast filling of multiple parietal internal iliac lymph nodes: superior and inferior gluteal nodes, lateral sacral nodes, and fusion of the medial external iliac nodes.

company the cephalic vein. The nodes receive efferent lymphatics from all the other axillary lymph node groups. The efferent vessels of the apical axillary group unite to form the subclavian trunk, which opens either directly into the junction of the internal jugular and subclavian veins or into the jugular lymphatic trunk. On the left side the subclavian trunk may enter the thoracic duct directly. A few efferents of the apical axillary lymph nodes are usually connected with inferior deep cervical nodes.

Lymphangiography by injection of contrast material into a lymph vessel of the radial or ulnar group of lymphatics in the forearm demonstrates only a few lymph nodes of the lateral axillary group (Fig. 82-19). Complete contrast filling of all lateral axillary lymph nodes is not achieved because each lymphatic of the forearm may enter a different node. The efferent lymphatics of the contrast-filled lateral axillary lymph nodes drain into a few nodes of the central and apical groups of axillary nodes. From the apical axillary node group, efferent lymphatics are demonstrated, uniting to form the subclavian trunk. Occasion-

ally, some supraclavicular and deep cervical lymph nodes are filled with contrast material.

THORACIC DUCT

The frequency of lymphographic demonstration of the thoracic duct varies [1, 8, 10, 13, 19, 22, 24, 28, 30]. It depends on the amount of contrast material, the timing of the films, and the positioning of the patient.

On the basis of its embryologic development, the thoracic duct is subdivided into abdominal, thoracic, and cervical sections.

The *abdominal section of the thoracic duct* is formed by the union of the two lumbar trunks, originating from the efferent lymphatics of the upper lumbar lymph nodes and the intestinal trunk, which collect the lymph from the gastrointestinal tract. The intestinal trunk is not a constant finding, because the efferent lymphatics of the abdominal organs usually unite to form a few larger lymph vessels, which enter the thoracic duct or one of the lumbar trunks directly. Extensive variations of the abdominal section of the thoracic duct are encountered. The entry of trunks into the thoracic duct is most frequently localized between T12 and L2, but it may be situated between T11 and L3–4. The cisterna chyli, an ampullaceous enlargement of the thoracic duct at its origin, was found mainly when the origin of the thoracic duct was low. Large reticular lymph trunks, but no cisterna chyli, are frequently observed (40–50%), particularly when the origin of the thoracic duct is close to T11. Rare configurations are ampullaceous dilatation of the lumbar trunks and numerous anastomosing small lymphatics. A beadlike appearance of the lower thoracic duct may be found, especially in cases of low origin. The configuration of the cisterna chyli may be conical, ampullaceous, fusiform, or moniliform.

Lumbar trunk *visualization by lymphography* occurs in about 25 percent of cases. In the lymphogram, lumbar trunks are demonstrated as large, oblique lymph vessels, with medially directed courses originating from several small efferent lymphatics. Topographic localization and configuration of the *lumbar trunks* are variable because of partial contrast filling. A single lumbar trunk (Fig. 82-20) or two lumbar trunks (Figs. 82-21, 82-22) as well as three lumbar trunks (Fig. 82-23) are commonly found; a reticular configuration of the lumbar trunks is demonstrated occasionally (5% of cases). In 30 percent the lumbar

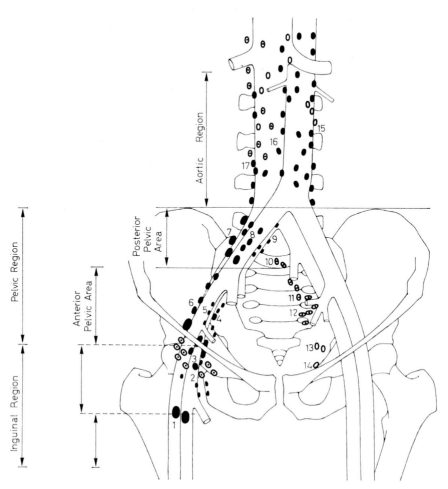

Figure 82-14. Topographic roentgen anatomy of the inguinal, iliac, and aortic lymph nodes (anteroposterior projection). *1* = inferior superficial inguinal (subinguinal) lymph nodes, *2* = superior superficial (crural group) and deep inguinal lymph node group, *3* = superior superficial inguinal lymph nodes (perineal and genital group), *4* = medial external iliac lymph nodes, *5* = intermediate external iliac lymph nodes, *6* = lateral external iliac lymph nodes, *7* = lateral common iliac lymph nodes, *8* = intermediate common iliac lymph nodes, *9* = medial common iliac lymph nodes, *10* = promontorial (subaortic) lymph nodes, *11* = lateral sacral lymph nodes, *12* = superior gluteal lymph nodes, *13* = inferior gluteal lymph nodes, *14* = obturator lymph nodes, *15* = left aortic lymph nodes, *16* = preretroaortic lymph nodes, *17* = right aortic lymph nodes. ● Routinely demonstrated by lymphangiography; ⊙ facultatively demonstrated by lymphangiography. (From Fuchs [8].)

trunks are situated at L1, in 39 percent at L2, and in 15 percent at L3. In a few cases, the beginning of the thoracic duct is found to be above T12 or below L4. The diameter of the lumbar trunks varies between 1 and 6 mm, with an average of 2 mm.

On the lymphogram, the cisterna chyli is recognized as a large lymph trunk situated between T12 and L3 and formed by the union of the lumbar trunks from which the thoracic duct originates. Its size is definitely larger than that of all the surrounding vessels. In 30 to 80 percent of cases the cisterna chyli is visualized by lymphography. It is mainly situated at the level of T12 (10%), L1 (40–50%), and L2 (30–40%). The cisterna chyli is usually projected over the vertebral bodies. Its configuration may be reticular, ampullaceous (Fig. 82-23), conical (see Fig. 82-22), or fusiform (see Fig. 82-20) with about equal frequency. Its diameter ranges between 2 and 16 mm, with an average of 4 to 6 mm.

Contrast filling of retrocrural lymph nodes situated dorsal to the diaphragmatic crura is observed in about half the cases. These lymph

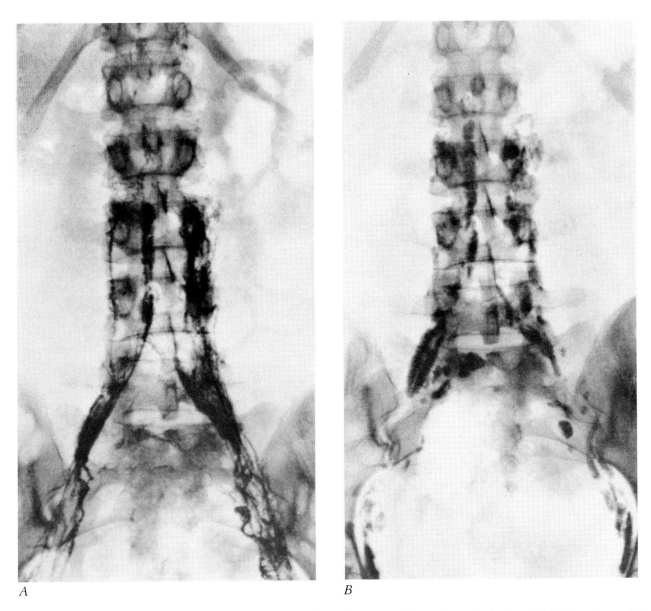

A   *B*

Figure 82-15. Lumbar lymph nodes, development of the three aortic lymph node chains. (A) Filling phase. (B) Storage phase.

nodes are situated at the level of T12 and L1 (Fig. 82-24).

The topographic anatomy of the *thoracic section of the thoracic duct* shows considerable variation. After passage through the diaphragm at the aortic opening, the first part of the thoracic section of the thoracic duct is situated, in 60 percent of cases, in the posterior mediastinum, on the right side of the aorta. Continuing at about the level of T5–6, the thoracic duct crosses obliquely to the left dorsal to the thoracic aorta. It leaves the thoracic cavity between the left subclavian artery

and the esophagus. In the older age group, four types of anatomic variations are observed: left-sided duct in 36 percent of cases, midline position in 20 percent, oblique course in 17 percent and right-sided duct in 6 percent. Because of the close connection of the two structures, the topographic-anatomic position of the thoracic duct depends largely on that of the thoracic aorta. With increasing age the elongation of the aorta, due to arteriosclerosis, causes a displacement of the thoracic duct from the right side toward the midline and the left. In addition, the elongation

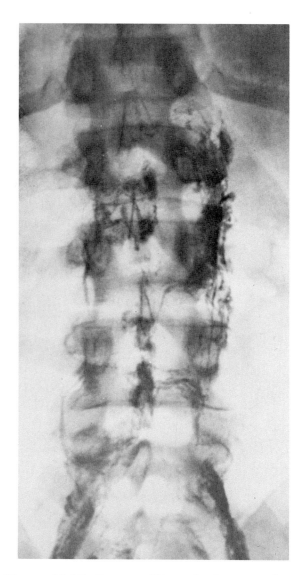

Figure 82-16. Contrast filling of a large number of lumbar nodes situated at the level of the left renal blood vessels. There is sparse filling of the right lumbar nodes above the fourth lumbar vertebra.

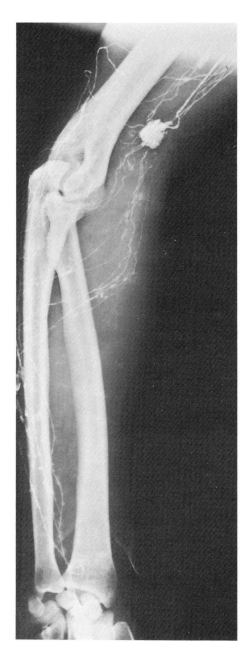

Figure 82-17. Ulnar group of lymphatics. Lymph channels follow the basilic vein and the medial border of the biceps muscle. Contrast filling of cubital lymph node.

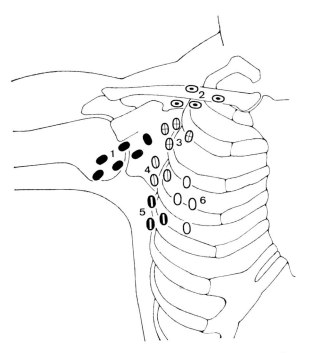

Figure 82-18. Topographic roentgen anatomy of the axillary lymph nodes. *1* = lateral axillary lymph nodes, *2* = supraclavicular lymph nodes, *3* = apical axillary lymph nodes, *4* = central axillary lymph nodes, *5* = posterior or subscapular axillary lymph nodes, *6* = anterior or pectoral axillary nodes. (From Fuchs [8].)

of the aortic arch leads to elongation or angulation of the thoracic duct. The presence of a hemithoracic duct, situated on the left side of the main trunk of the thoracic duct, is rather frequent. Numerous narrow lymphatic channels that course away from the main trunk for short distances, often to nodes alongside, and then return to the thoracic duct are occasionally observed. Duplication of the thoracic duct, with one duct situated on each side of the thoracic aorta, is another rare anatomic variation. Cranially, both trunks may join together.

The thoracic section of the thoracic duct is frequently connected with posterior mediastinal lymph nodes. Efferent lymph vessels of the thoracic wall, the heart, and the mediastinum enter the thoracic section of the thoracic duct. On *lymphograms,* the thoracic section of the thoracic duct is filled with contrast material in about 75 percent of cases. The upper part of the thoracic duct is visualized most frequently, and the entire thoracic duct is demonstrated in only about 10 percent of cases.

The thoracic section of the thoracic duct may divide into a caudal subsection, situated between the diaphragm and T3, and a cranial subsection reaching the supraclavicular region (Fig. 82-25). This subdivision is important, because the

Figure 82-19. Axillary lymphangiogram. Contrast filling of lateral, central, and apical axillary lymph nodes.

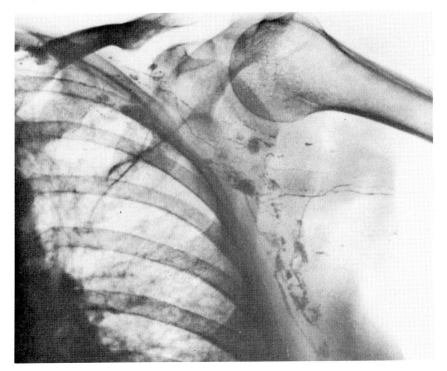

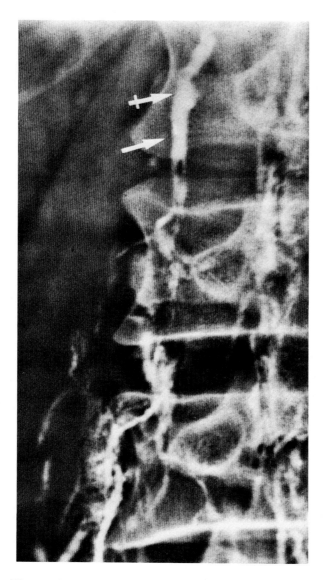

Figure 82-20. Solitary lumbar trunk (*arrow*) in continuous connection with the fusiform cisterna chyli (*barred arrow*).

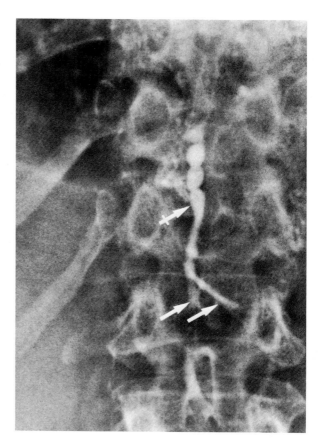

Figure 82-21. Two lumbar trunks (*arrows*) entering the beadlike cisterna chyli (*barred arrow*).

thoracic duct is projected onto the vertebral bodies up to the region of T3. In about two-thirds of the cases, the lower subsection of the thoracic duct is situated to the left of the midline (see Fig. 82-27). In one-third its position is median, and only in rare cases is it projected to the right of the midline. The upper subsection of the thoracic duct, above T3, is mainly localized on the left side. Duplication of the thoracic duct is present in one case out of ten (see Fig. 82-29). Very seldom, both lymph trunks are situated to the left of the midline, or separate trunks on each side of the midline are recognized. When present, partial duplication of the thoracic duct is observed predominantly in the lower thoracic section of the thoracic duct. A reticular configuration of the thoracic duct is seen in about 20 percent of cases (Fig. 82-26), but only rarely is the entire thoracic section reticular. The largest diameter of the thoracic section of the thoracic duct is usually measured at the level of T2. In most instances, the maximum diameter ranges between 4 and 6 mm. Posterior mediastinal lymph nodes connected with the thoracic duct are demonstrated in 15 percent of cases at the level of T4–T8 (see Fig. 82-30). In 4 percent of cases retrosternal lymph nodes situated in the anterior mediastinum, arising from the thoracic duct with netlike lymphatics, are contrast-filled by lymphography. In 4 percent of cases lymph nodes of the hilar region of the lungs are demonstrated, and in 6 percent paratracheal lymph nodes are demonstrated.

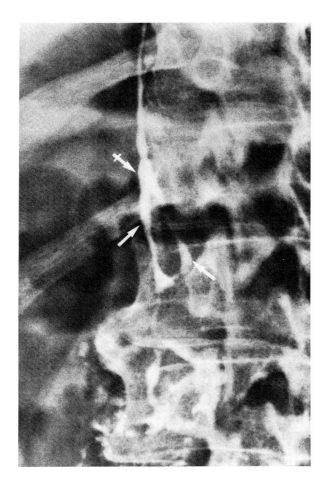

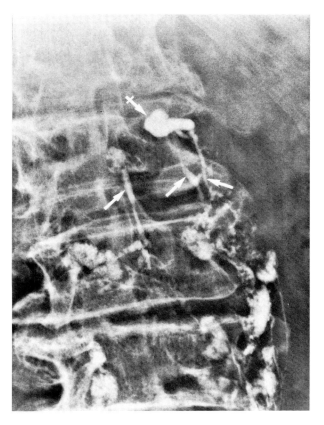

Figure 82-23. Three lumbar trunks (*arrows*) entering the ampullaceous cisterna chyli (*barred arrow*).

Figure 82-22. Two lumbar trunks (*arrows*) in connection with the conical cisterna chyli (*barred arrow*).

The *cervical section of the thoracic duct* runs through the left upper thoracic aperture toward the subclavian triangle to enter the veins. In only one-fourth of the cases is a single channel present. In half the cases a double channel is observed. Multiple branching, accompanied by multiple entry points, may also be seen. The thoracic duct may enter the internal jugular vein, the venous angle, and either the subclavian or the innominate vein. An ampullaceous dilatation of the terminal part of the thoracic duct containing one or two valves is observed in 50 percent of cases.

The cervical part of the thoracic duct is frequently connected with cervical and supraclavicular lymph nodes by numerous lymphatics with a bidirectional flow. The left subclavian and left mediastinal trunks—collecting the lymph from the left thorax, the left arm, and the cervical region—enter the cervical section of the thoracic

duct. On the right side, identical lymphatic trunks are in direct connection with the venous system, or in rare cases with a right lymphatic duct. On *lymphograms* the cervical section of the thoracic duct is demonstrated in 65 to 90 percent of patients. In 90 percent of cases it enters the venous system on the left side (Fig. 82-27); in about 3 percent on the right side (Fig. 82-28); and in 5 percent bilaterally (Fig. 82-29). In about 50 percent of cases only one lymph trunk is present; in 25 percent two branches of the cervical section of the thoracic duct are encountered; and in 25 percent three or more lymphatic vessels. An ampullaceous configuration at the terminus of the thoracic duct is observed in half the patients. Usually, there is only a single ampullaceous trunk, while rarely two or three ampullaceous trunks are present. Supraclavicular lymph nodes are visualized in about half of all lymphograms. They are generally situated on the left side (40%) and in only about 5 percent of cases on the right side. Occasionally (2%), lymph nodes are dem-

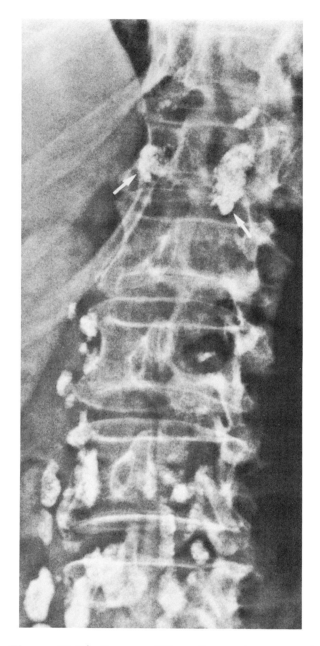

Figure 82-24. Contrast filling of several retrocrural lymph nodes at the level T10–11 (*arrows*).

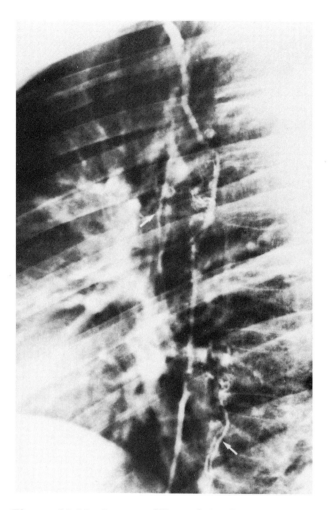

Figure 82-25. Contrast filling of the thoracic section of the thoracic duct and several small concomitant lymph trunks (*arrows*) and posterior mediastinal lymph nodes.

onstrated within both the left and right supraclavicular regions (Fig. 82-30).

In about 2 percent of cases left axillary lymph nodes are filled with contrast material (Fig. 82-31). Left cervical lymph nodes are visualized on 3 percent of lymphograms. Rarely is a single right cervical lymph node demonstrated by lymphography. Contrast filling of the supraclavicular, cervical, axillary, paravertebral, mediastinal, and pulmonary hilar lymph nodes is of clinical significance. Visualization of these lymph nodes is not a definitive sign of collateral circulation and is, therefore, not a sign of a pathologic condition. All these nodes, which are closely connected with the thoracic duct, are necessarily demonstrated

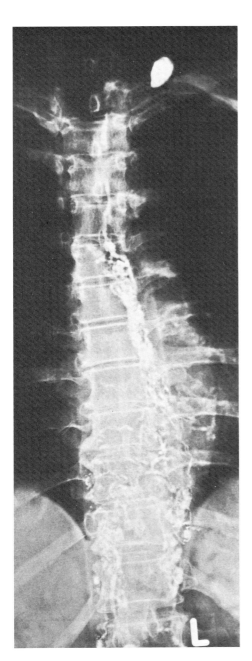

Figure 82-26. Netlike configuration of the thoracic duct.

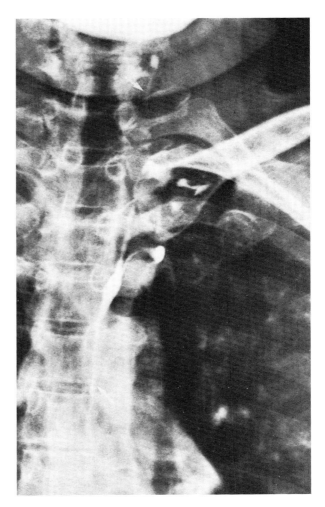

Figure 82-27. Left lateral position of the thoracic duct. Triple entering of the cervical section into the external jugular (*arrow*) and subclavian vein.

by lymphography when they are the last regional lymph nodes of the system, draining the abdominal retroperitoneal organs and the lower extremities. In cases of malignant tumors in these areas, metastatic spread into these node groups must be considered. Cancer cells within the thoracic duct are relatively frequent. Malignant cells are likely to migrate into these lymph node groups connected with the thoracic duct. Cancer metastases in the supraclavicular lymph nodes are frequently demonstrated by lymphography. Cancer metastases in paravertebral, tracheobronchial, and anterior mediastinal lymph nodes occur occasionally in later stages of the disease.

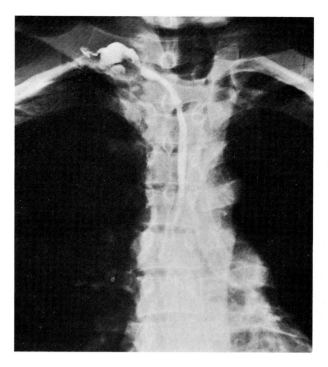

Figure 82-28. Right-sided ampullaceous entering of the thoracic duct.

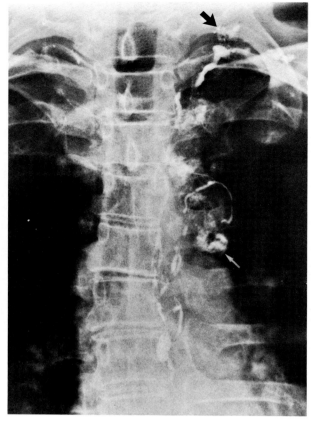

Figure 82-30. Contrast filling of posterior mediastinal (*white arrow*), retrosternal (*black arrow*), and bilateral supraclavicular lymph nodes.

Figure 82-29. Bilateral entering of the netlike cervical section of the thoracic duct.

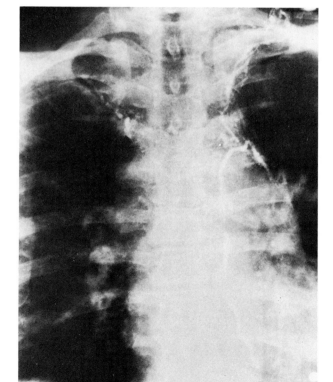

Figure 82-31. Contrast filling of supraclavicular and axillary lymph nodes from thoracic duct (pulmonary oil embolism).

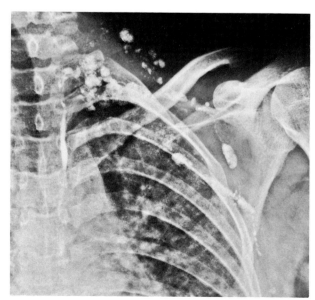

References

1. Baltaxe, H. A., and Constable, W. C. Mediastinal lymph node visualization in the absence of intrathoracic disease. *Radiology* 90:94, 1968.
2. Bargmann, W. *Histologie und mikroskopische Anatomie des Menschen* (7th ed.). Stuttgart: Thieme, 1977.
3. Barthels, P. Das Lymphgefässystem. In K. von Bardeleben (ed.), *Handbuch der Anatomie des Menschen*. Jena: Fischer, 1909.
4. Bourquin, J. Histologische Grundlagen des Lymphadenogramms. *Radiologe* 8:150, 1968.
5. Cunéo, B., and Marcille, M. Topographie des ganglions iliopelviens. *Bull. Soc. Anat.* 76:653, 1901.
6. Ditchek, T., Blahut, R. J., and Kittleson, A. C. Lymphadenography in normal subjects. *Radiology* 80:175, 1963.
7. Fischer, H. W., Lawrence, M. S., and Thornbury, J. R. Lymphography of the normal adult male. *Radiology* 78:399, 1962.
8. Fuchs, W. A. Normal Anatomy. In W. A. Fuchs, J. W. Davidson, and H. W. Fischer (eds.), *Lymphography in Cancer*. New York: Springer, 1969.
9. Fuchs, W. A., and Böök-Hederström, G. Inguinal and pelvic lymphography. *Acta Radiol.* (Stockh.) 56:340, 1961.
10. Fuchs, W. A., and Galeazzi, R. Die Röntgenanatomie des Ductus thoracicus. *Radiologe* 10:180, 1970.
11. Fuchs, W. A., and Pfammatter, Th. Die topographische Röntgenanatomie der inguinalen und retroperitonealen Lymphknoten. *Radiologe* 10:262, 1970.
12. Herman, P. G., Benninghoff, D. L., Nelson, J. H., and Mellins, H. Z. Roentgen anatomy of the ilio-pelvic-aortic lymphatic system. *Radiology* 80:182, 1963.
13. Idanov, D. A. Anatomie du canal thoracique et des principaux collecteurs lymphatiques du tronc chez l'homme. *Acta Anat.* (Basel) 37:35, 1959.
14. Jacobsson, S., and Johansson, S. Normal roentgen anatomy of the lymph vessels of upper and lower extremities. *Acta Radiol.* (Stockh.) 51:321, 1959.
15. Jossifow, G. M. *Das Lymphgefässsystem des Menschen*. Jena: Fischer, 1930.
16. Kaindl, F. K., Mannheimer, E., Pfleger-Schwarz, L., and Thurnher, B. *Lymphangiographie und Lymphadenographie der Extremitäten*. Stuttgart: Thieme, 1960.
17. Kolbenstvedt, A. Normal lymphographic variation of lumbar, iliac and inguinal lymph vessels. *Acta Radiol. [Diagn.]* (Stockh.) 15:662, 1974.
18. Kubik, S. Die normale Anatomie des Lymphsystems unter besonderer Berücksichtigung der Sammelgebiete der Lymphknoten der unteren Körperhälfte. *Strahlentherapie [Sonderb.]* 69:8, 1969.
19. Kubik, S. Lagevarianten, Lage- und Formveränderungen der Pars thoracalis des Ductus thoracicus. *ROEFO* 122:1, 1975.
20. Leiber, B. *Der menschliche Lymphknoten: Anatomie, Physiologie und Pathologie nach Ergebnissen der Vergleichenden Klinischen und histologischen Zytodiagnostic.* Munich-Berlin: Urban & Schwarzenberg, 1961.
21. Lennert, K. *Handbuch der speziellen pathologischen Anatomie und Histologie.* Berlin: Springer, 1960.
22. Poirier, P. *Traité d'Anatomie Humaine.* Paris: Masson, 1898.
23. Rosenberger, A., and Abrams, H. L. Radiology of the thoracic duct. *AJR* 111:807, 1971.
24. Rouvière, H. *Anatomie des Lymphatiques de l'Homme.* Paris: Masson, 1932.
25. Rusznyak, I., Földi, M., and Szabo, G. *Physiologie und Pathologie des Lymphkreislaufs.* Jena: Fischer, 1957.
26. Tjernberg, B. Lymphography. An animal study on the diagnosis of V × 2 carcinoma and inflammation. *Acta Radiol. [Suppl.]* (Stockh.) 214, 1962.
27. Van Pernis, P. A. Variations of the thoracic duct. *Surgery* 28:806, 1949.
28. Weissleder, H. Das pathologische Lymphangiogramm des Ductus thoracicus. *ROEFO* 101:573, 1964.
29. Wirth, W. Zur Röntgenanatomie des Lymphsystems der inguinalen pelvinen und aortalen Region: 1. *ROEFO* 105:441, 1966; 2. *ROEFO* 105:636, 1966.
30. Wirth, W., and Frommhold, H. Der Ductus thoracicus und seine Variationen. Lymphographische Studie. *ROEFO* 112:450, 1970.
31. Wirth, W., and Kubik, S. Lymphographic Roentgen Anatomy. In M. Viamonte and A. Rüttimann (eds.), *Atlas of Lymphography*. Stuttgart: Thieme, 1980.
32. Yoffey, J. M., and Courtice, F. C. *Lymphatics, Lymph and Lymphoid Tissue* (2nd ed.). Cambridge, Mass.: Harvard University Press, 1956.

The Thoracic Duct

ALEXANDER ROSENBERGER

The growing recognition of the importance of the lymphatic system and thoracic duct in circulatory physiology, metastatic changes, and immunologic processes has led to an increased interest in the study of their anatomy, physiology, and pathology. The thoracic duct is the central collecting trunk of all the lymph vessels of the body with the exception of those of the right side of the head and neck, the right upper limb, the right hemithorax, the right side of the heart, and the convex surface of the liver [1]. The first description of the thoracic duct in man is attributed to Pecquet in 1651; by the end of the eighteenth century the gross anatomy of the thoracic duct had been thoroughly explored.

In order to have a better understanding of the anatomy and anatomic variations of the thoracic duct, a succinct review of the development of the lymph system is necessary. In the human embryo six lymph sacs can be found, from which lymph vessels are derived: two paired jugular and posterior lymphatic sacs and two unpaired ones, namely, the retroperitoneal sac and the cisterna chyli. There are two opinions as to the origin of these lymph sacs. According to the first, lymphatic spaces develop from the mesenchyma forming capillary plexuses from which the lymph sacs are derived. The second theory connects the lymph vessels to the venous system, considering the lymphatics as offshoots from the endothelium of the veins, forming plexuses. These plexuses lose their connection with the veins and are transformed into lymph sacs. The lymph vessels originate from the lymph sacs. With the exception of the cisterna chyli, the lymph sacs are transformed in a later stage into lymph nodes [1].

In the embryo the thoracic duct is a paired structure formed by an anastomotic outgrowth of the jugular sac and the cisterna chyli; there are numerous transverse connections between the two sides. The jugular sac lies at the junction of the subclavian vein with the anterior cardinal vein. The cisterna chyli lies anterior to lumbar vertebrae L3–4. In embryonic life numerous valves can be present in the thoracic duct. They appear about the fifth month but may disappear prior to birth.

Anatomy of the Thoracic Duct

The thoracic duct begins at the upper end of the cisterna chyli, usually at the height of the twelfth thoracic vertebra. It originates from the union of

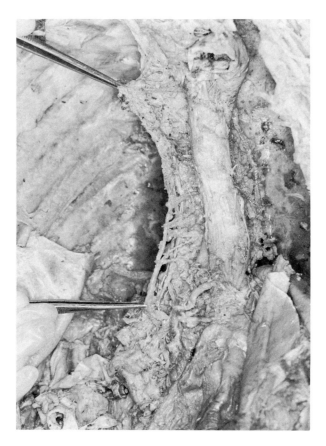

Figure 83-1. Anatomic preparation of the entire thoracic duct. Because of removal of the mediastinal organs, the duct lies lateral to the spine in its course. In the middle part a network of small channels is present, giving the duct a plexuslike appearance.

three roots, the right and left lumbar trunk and the intestinal trunk; these trunks can meet at an identical site or successively.

With the aorta on its left and the azygos vein on its right, the thoracic duct enters the thoracic cavity through the aortic hiatus of the diaphragm (Fig. 83-1). It courses anterior and to the right of the dorsal spine in the posterior mediastinum. At about the fifth thoracic vertebra level it turns to the left side of the spine. At about the height of the third thoracic vertebra it leaves the aortic arch and lies between the mediastinal pleura and the left side of the esophagus. In its course upward it arches forward above the dome of the pleura between the left common carotid artery and the left subclavian artery to reach about the level of the seventh cervical vertebra, the anteriorly situated left internal jugular vein, or the junction of the latter with the left subclavian vein. Before entering the veins it usually re-

ceives the lymph coming from the jugular, mammary, and subclavian trunks draining the lymph from their respective regions, whereas the left bronchomediastinal trunk can open separately into the great veins. In the neck the arch of the thoracic duct lies 3 to 4 cm above the clavicle, anterior to the vertebral vessels, sympathetic trunk, and thyrocervical vessels. In its course the thoracic duct collects lymph vessels from lumbar, posterior intercostal, and posterior mediastinal lymph nodes.

The slightly right-to-left sweep of the thoracic duct in the thorax is easily explained by its phylogenesis. Originally a paired structure with numerous transverse anastomoses, in its ultimate form it is an unpaired structure, its caudal part belonging to the embryonic right vessel and its cranial portion to the left vessel, whereas the middle part originates from the transverse anastomoses.

Radiologic Studies of the Thoracic Duct

In vivo the thoracic duct can be studied by cannulation of the duct in the neck and retrograde injection of contrast material under operative conditions [2, 3]. Lymphangiography with oily contrast material based on the principles of Kinmonth [4] represents a physiologic way to study the thoracic duct. Briefly this technique consists of identification and cannulation of a superficially situated lymph vessel on the dorsum of the foot and slow injection of the oily contrast material into the vessel. When satisfactory opacification of the thoracic duct is achieved, controlled by television-monitored fluoroscopy or radiographs, the morphology of the thoracic duct is studied by anteroposterior, lateral, and oblique radiographs of the chest. Lately the cross-sectional anatomy of the contrast-filled thoracic duct as seen on computed tomography (CT) has been studied [5] (Fig. 83-2A, B).

The functional aspects of the flow of opacified lymph in the thoracic duct may be visualized by cine or 70-mm camera technique [6]. Studies are done during quiet and deep respiration, apnea, and the Valsalva maneuver. Posture changes from the recumbent to the upright position and their influence on lymph flow can be studied in this way too.

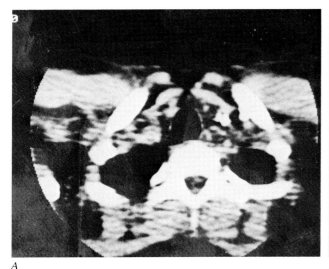
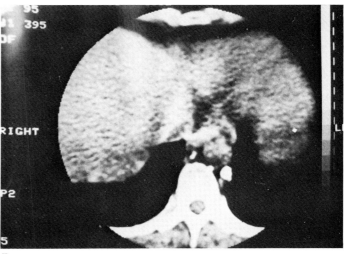

A   *B*

Figure 83-2. Computed tomography study of the contrast-filled duct. (A) Cervical portion of the duct. The point of emptying into the great veins is well seen. (B) Visualization of the abdominal portion of the duct at the level of the diaphragmatic crura. Some lymph nodes opacified by contrast material are also delineated.

Radiologic Anatomy of the Thoracic Duct

In studying the thoracic duct one can divide it into three portions: abdominal, thoracic, and cervical segments. It has to be anticipated that the landmarks used in the radiologic description are sometimes different from those mentioned in the anatomic study.

ABDOMINAL PART OF THE THORACIC DUCT

The abdominal part of the thoracic duct consists of the cisterna chyli and a short segment of the duct below the diaphragm.

The cisterna chyli is formed by the confluence of the two lumbar trunks draining the lymph of the lower extremities, pelvis, and abdominal organs and the intestinal trunk carrying the lymph from the gastrointestinal tract [7, 8]. In the lymphangiogram only the lumbar trunks can be visualized, usually as 2-mm-wide vessels originating from the confluence of small lymph vessels and coursing in an oblique fashion upward to reach the cisterna chyli or the opposite vessel (Fig. 83-3). The union of the lumbar trunks usually lies at the level of T12–L2 [7]. The intestinal trunk is demonstrated only in experimental lymphangiog-raphy or (seldom) in the presence of lymphatic obstruction, in which case it serves as a collateral pathway.

The cisterna chyli is the initial saclike dilated portion of the thoracic duct. Its shape may show various forms [9]: round, oval, commalike, linear, beaded, inverted V, or inverted Y (Fig. 83-4A–D). The size of the cisterna shows a wide range of variations too: 2 to 16 mm in width in lymphangiography [7] and 5 to 7 cm in length [10]. These measurements were made on radiographs, which reproduce static aspects of the cisterna chyli, whereas cine studies [6] have demonstrated different calibers in the same individual depending on the state of relaxation or contraction of the cisterna.

The location of the cisterna may be anywhere between T12 and L3 [7, 10, 11, 12]; in 77 percent of cases, it lies in the midline anterior to the vertebral column. In our series [13] it was situated at the height of T12 in 36 percent of cases and at L2 in the rest.

THORACIC PART OF THE THORACIC DUCT

The thoracic part of the thoracic duct is the segment from the entrance of the duct into the

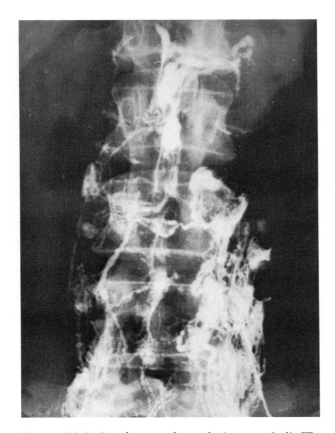

Figure 83-3. Lumbar trunks and cisterna chyli. The lumbar trunks are converging toward the cisterna chyli, which overlies the midline of the spine at L2. The caliber of the latter is larger than that of the thoracic duct above it and the lumbar trunks below it.

thoracic cavity through the aortic hiatus to an arbitrary point where the duct lies between the esophagus and the aortic arch.

The thoracic duct as visualized in lymphangiographic studies [7, 8, 10, 14] courses at the midline of the spine or slightly to the right of it. At the height of T5–6 it changes its course progressively to the left of the spine (Fig. 83-5A). At the level of the carina the duct crosses the main left bronchus as viewed in the anteroposterior radiograph and ascends parallel but dorsal to the left lateral wall of the trachea (Fig. 83-5A). Over the dorsal aspect of the aortic arch it turns ventrally as seen in the lateral chest radiograph to course toward the thoracic inlet (Fig. 83-5B).

The duct can be visualized in its entire length during the lymphangiographic studies in the minority of the cases (about 7%) [7]. Usually only certain parts of it can be illustrated, the lower segments being demonstrated less often than the cranial portions.

The width of the duct varies on average between 2 and 6 mm, but diameters between 0.5 and 12.0 mm [15] have been described. This great range in visualization of different parts of the thoracic duct as well as the variations in the caliber is related to many factors: quantity of contrast material injected, tonus of the duct, positioning of the patient, timing of the radiographs, and individual differences.

CERVICAL PORTION OF THE THORACIC DUCT

The cervical portion of the thoracic duct is the terminal part of the duct between the thoracic inlet and the point of its emptying into the large veins of the neck. In the anteroposterior radiograph the duct turns cranially and slightly to the left, resembling an inverted J (Fig. 83-6A); it either courses parallel to the clavicle or arches 2 to 3 cm above it. Sometimes this terminal part has a more vertical course (Fig. 83-6B).

The highest portion of the duct in the neck lies at C6–T2 [14], but during coughing it may move upward [15]. The cervical segment is visualized in 65 to 90 percent of lymphangiograms [7, 8]. The duct terminates in various fashions; there may be a single duct (25%) or it can divide into two to four channels, which open separately or reunite before entering the veins. Three channels have been found in 15 percent of cases, four channels in 6 percent of cases. These figures are in striking contrast to reports in anatomic dissections, in which one terminal was found in 90 percent of cases [16]. Sometimes an ampullalike dilatation of the cervical portion of the duct can be observed (Fig. 83-7). The cervical portion of the duct empties into the left great veins of the neck in 92 to 95 percent, on the right side in 2 to 3 percent, and bilaterally in 1.0 to 1.5 percent [7, 8, 10] (see Fig. 83-6A).

In 60 percent of the patients the duct empties into the internal jugular vein. In the remaining cases the site of emptying may be the subclavian vein (15%), between the external and internal jugular veins (7%), in the angle between the external jugular and subclavian veins (2.5%), and in the innominate vein (1.5%).

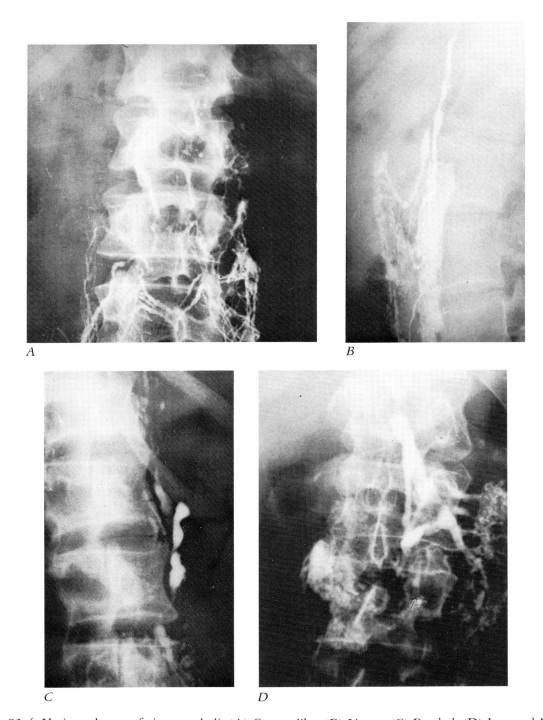

Figure 83-4. Various shapes of cisterna chyli. (A) Commalike. (B) Linear. (C) Beaded. (D) Inverted Y.

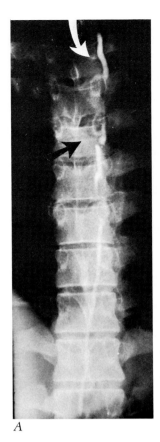
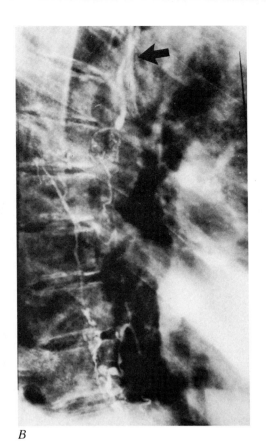

A   B

Figure 83-5. Thoracic part of the thoracic duct opacified by contrast material in the whole length. (A) Anteroposterior view, showing progressive course of the duct from right to left. At the level of the left main bronchus (*black arrow*) it reaches the left side of the spine and ascends parallel to the left wall of the trachea (*white arrow*). The distance between the duct and the tracheal wall should not exceed 1 cm. (B) Lateral view of a double thoracic duct. The anterior channel (*arrow*) is the main carrier of the lymph.

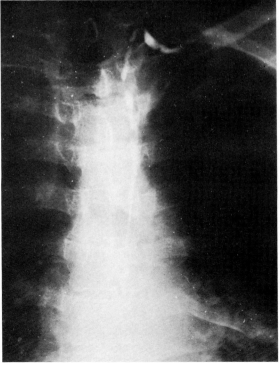
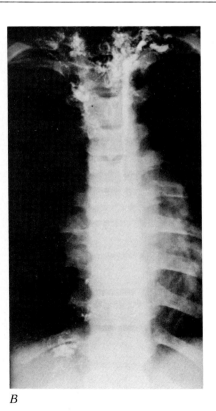

A   B

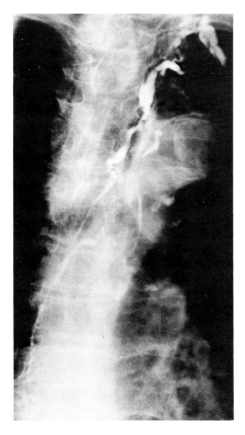

Figure 83-7. Ampullalike dilatation of the terminal portion of the thoracic duct. Below this level doubling of the thoracic duct is visible.

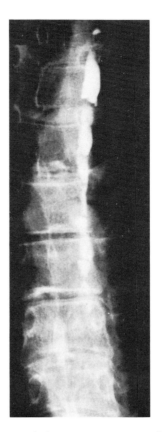

Figure 83-8. Beaded appearance given by numerous valves in the upper half of the duct. The valves of the thoracic duct are bicuspid. They may vary in number (see Fig. 83-5A), and their visualized size depends on whether they are opening or closing.

VALVES

Bicuspid valves can be seen in the course of the thoracic duct, their function being to ensure unidirectional flow of the lymph. In the lymphangiogram the open valve resembles a fish mouth; the closed valve produces a localized bulging of the lateral contour of the duct, giving it a beaded appearance (Fig. 83-8). The function of the valve can be studied in cine or rapid-filming studies [6]. As to the number of valves present in the duct, findings differ widely, but all agree that they are more numerous in the upper portion. One valve at least is always present in the high upper cervical segment.

Lymph Nodes Along the Thoracic Duct

Filling of lymph nodes in the supraclavicular area around the terminal portion of the duct (one of them is the Virchow-Troisier node [17]) can be seen in the large majority of lymphangiograms and is a normal finding. Filling of lymph nodes in the posterior mediastinum (Fig. 83-9A) and along the posterior intercostal vessels (Fig. 83-9B) emptying into the duct can be seen in 20 percent of studies. In exceptional cases filling of middle mediastinal, carinal (Fig. 83-10A), hilar (Fig. 83-10B), and anterior mediastinal lymph nodes (Fig. 83-11) can occur.

Filling and visualization of these nodes probably represent a normal finding and are due to bidirectional flow in the lymph channels connecting these nodes with the thoracic duct. Pathologic architecture of mediastinal lymph

◀ Figure 83-6. Cervical portion of the thoracic duct. (A) The cervical portion is formed by one channel arching above the clavicle. (B) Numerous glands surrounding the terminal portion of the duct. Note also the opacification of the right duct.

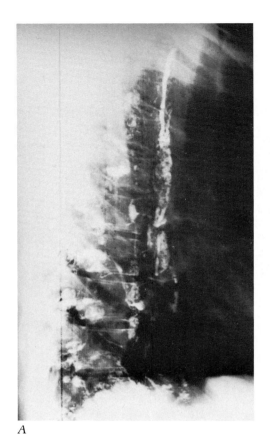

A

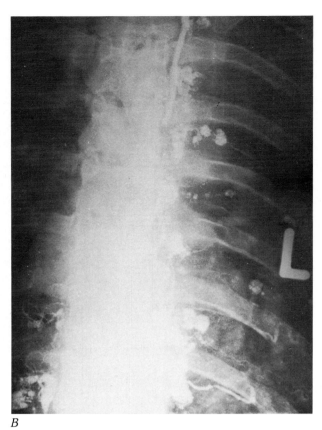

B

Figure 83-9. Filling of posterior mediastinal nodes and intercostal vessels. These structures can be seen in 20 percent of the studies. (A) Lateral view of a thoracic duct with filling of numerous posterior mediastinal glands. (B) Filling of intercostal lymph vessels mainly in the left lower half of the thorax.

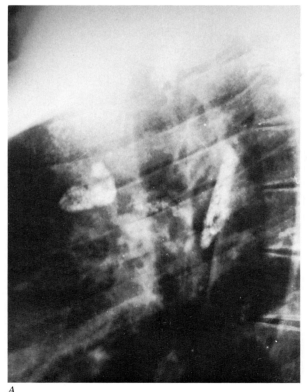

A

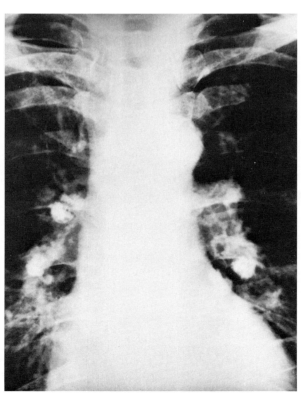

B

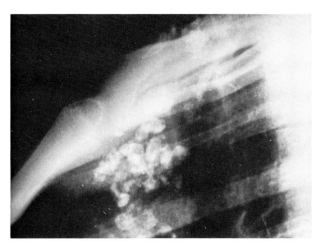

Figure 83-11. Filling of a group of anterior superior mediastinal lymph nodes.

nodes as visualized by lymphangiography has the same implications as anywhere else in the body.

Variations in the Thoracic Duct

The thoracic duct is subject to many variations, and Rouvière [9] remarks that articles dealing with duct variations are more numerous than those devoted to its normal anatomy.

The variations in the appearance of the thoracic duct can be explained by its embryologic development. In the absence of lumbar trunks the lymph vessels form a netlike structure, thereafter uniting to form the duct [7]. In the absence of the cisterna chyli the lumbar trunks may ascend to a higher level before uniting (Fig. 83-12). Most variations in the aspect of the thoracic duct occur in its thoracic portion (40%) [2]. The crossing of the duct from right to left at the height of T5–6 may be abrupt instead of progressive. In some cases the entire course of the duct may be left-sided or right-sided. There are different opinions about the multiplicity of the channels in the duct in the thoracic segment. Whereas anatomists state [18] that doubling occurs only above the level of T5–6, lymphangiographic

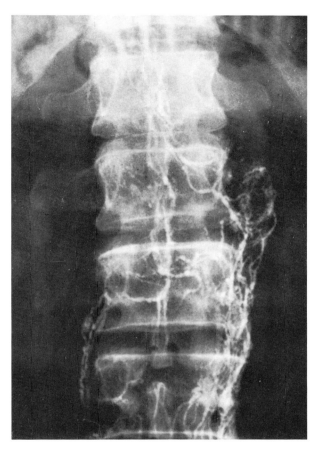

Figure 83-12. In the absence of the cisterna chyli the lumbar trunks form a netlike structure and reach up to the level of the body of L1.

studies [7, 14, 19] have shown two or three channels at every level in about 10 percent of cases. Double thoracic ducts can terminate in a single duct at the level of the third to eighth thoracic vertebra (Fig. 83-13). Bilateral superior mediastinal thoracic ducts (Fig. 83-14; see also Fig. 83-5B) are not necessarily related to double ducts at lower levels. In 3 percent of cases, many small lymph vessels arise from the lower portion of the duct and reach the duct again higher up. The large number of anastomoses between them can give the duct a plexuslike appearance. Wide variations in the number and site of emptying of the thoracic duct in its cervical portion are well known from anatomic and lymphangiographic studies. The knowledge of these variations is most important to clinicians, for the cervical portion of the duct is easily subject to trauma and to surgical manipulation.

◀ Figure 83-10. Filling of middle mediastinal nodes and hilar nodes. (A) Lateral view illustrating filling of middle mediastinal lymph nodes. (B) Filling of hilar nodes. In this case the hilar nodes are bilateral, a finding that is more the exception than the rule.

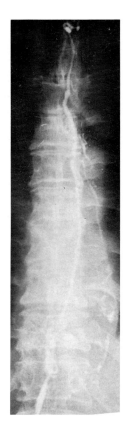

Figure 83-13. Doubling of the thoracic duct up to the level of T4.

Figure 83-14. Doubling of cervical portion of the thoracic duct with filling of lymph nodes around the two channels.

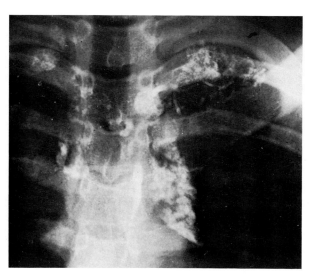

Functional and Experimental Aspects of the Thoracic Duct

The role of lymph circulation is to return tissue-fluid proteins and large molecules from the interstitial space to the bloodstream. Fat from the intestine enters the lymph too, giving it a milky appearance. The constituents of lymph are similar to those of plasma, but the protein content of lymph is lower, reflecting the permeability of functionally different blood-lymph barriers [20, 21]. The main sources of the proteins in the lymph are the liver and the intestine. The coagulation properties of lymph are lower than the coagulation properties of blood [20, 22]. The flow rate of thoracic duct lymph is about 1 cc per minute and the pressure of lymph is about 11 cm H_2O.

Flow of lymph [23] depends on formation of tissue fluid, movement of tissue fluid into the lymphatics, and factors that move the lymph along the lymphatic vessels. The flow of lymph in the thoracic duct is a passive phenomenon, depending on lymph formation and distensibility of the duct. Factors influencing lymph flow in the thoracic duct are residual pressure from the pumping action of the heart, active and passive movement of the muscular system [9], suction effect of the negative intrathoracic pressure, movements of the diaphragm, and, possibly, transmitted pulsations from the great intrathoracic vessels [19]. The flow in the duct, as shown in animal observation and in man, is rhythmic, the valves ensuring a unidirectional stream. Cine and 70-mm camera radiologic studies are very useful in the observation of these phenomena [6, 9, 19, 24]. The thoracic duct possesses an autonomic innervation, the influence of which causes relaxation and contraction of the duct, thus influencing lymph propulsion [25].

The thoracic duct functions as the major pathway of immunologically active lymphocytes and proteins to blood; pathogenic microorganisms may also be transported by the duct. Many experimental studies concerned with the immunologic aspects of the thoracic duct have been carried out [26, 27].

Radiologic Aspects of the Abnormal Thoracic Duct

The pathology of the thoracic duct as demonstrated by lymphangiography is mentioned in the radiologic literature only in the form of case reports. No systematic studies dealing with the abnormal duct have been made. Pathology of the thoracic duct is rarely mentioned as an entity in the textbooks of medicine, surgery, or pathology.

CONGENITAL MALFORMATIONS

Malformations and variations of congenital origin have already been mentioned. It is presumed that in some cases of Noonan's syndrome [28], a congenital disease, the pulmonary lymphangiectasis may be caused by interruption of the thoracic duct [29]. Congenital defects, stenosis, or atresia of the thoracic duct is presumed to cause bilateral hydrochylothorax, thus leading to bilateral pulmonary hypoplasia in neonates [30].

INJURY

Injury of the thoracic duct can be divided into spontaneous rupture, blunt trauma, penetrating wounds, and iatrogenic complications, like incidental puncturing of the duct [31], or surgery in the posterior mediastinum. The main consequence of duct injury is chylothorax [32]. Leakage of lymph into the mediastinum can lead to its spill into the pleura if the pleura is lacerated by an initial trauma or by the weight of the mediastinal collection. Lymphangiography can demonstrate the site of the lesion and the individual pattern of the duct [33].

INFLAMMATION

Tuberculosis and syphilis can cause changes in the lymphatic vessels. Theoretically similar changes should occur in the thoracic duct, too. Nevertheless, there is no radiologic documentation of inflammatory lesions of the thoracic duct.

TUMORS

Tumors of the thoracic duct are unusual; references to primary malignancy occurring in the duct could not be found in the literature. Lymphangioma is a benign tumor composed of lymphatic vessels and supporting connective tissue and lymph nodules. It is described in pathology textbooks as rarely occurring in the thoracic cavity [34], but reference in the radiologic literature could not be found. The thoracic duct is the main pathway of lymph drainage for the organs below the diaphragm to the lesser circulation. It is a known fact that the incidence of lung metastases from primary tumors below the diaphragm is higher than from suprathoracic tumors [35].

Secondary involvement of the thoracic duct can occur by embolization of malignant cells arrested in the thoracic duct or by invasion from contiguous structures.

MEDIASTINAL MASSES

Mediastinal masses can cause displacement, kinking, tortuosity, and obstruction of the

Figure 83-15. Partial obstruction of the thoracic duct at the venous angle.

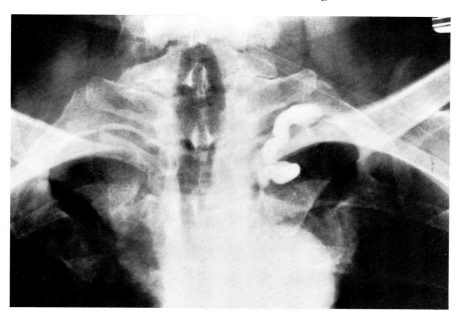

thoracic duct, according to the site and the size of the mass. A useful radiologic measurement for evaluating the presence of a mediastinal mass is the distance between the thoracic duct and the left wall of the trachea in the anteroposterior radiograph. This distance should not exceed 10 mm [10] (see Fig. 83-5A); a wider separation points toward a mediastinal mass. Computed tomography of the thoracic duct is an additional method for evaluating mediastinal masses [5].

OBSTRUCTION

Intrinsic or extrinsic pathology may lead to obstruction of the thoracic duct (Fig. 83-15). Extrinsic obstruction can be caused by mediastinal masses [36] or mediastinal fibrosis. Pathology inside the duct may be due to filariasis [19] or metastasis [35].

The suspicion of thoracic duct obstruction should arise if lymphangiography reveals a sharp cutoff of the contrast medium in the course of the duct associated with dilatation distal to it, visualization of lymphatic collaterals such as an intestinal trunk, lymphaticovenous communications [10, 37, 38], and delayed emptying. Because of the known variety in the radiologic appearance of the normal thoracic duct, the size of the duct, visualization of intercostal lymphatics, or filling of mediastinal lymph nodes as a single criterion for thoracic duct obstruction is inadequate.

References

1. *Gray's Anatomy* (35th ed.). Philadelphia: Saunders, 1973. Pp. 168, 727.
2. Dumont, A. E., and Witte, M. H. Clinical usefulness of thoracic duct cannulation. *Adv. Intern. Med.* 15:51, 1969.
3. Ellis, F. G. Technique for intermittent collection of thoracic duct lymph. *Surgery* 60:1251, 1966.
4. Kinmonth, J. B. Lymphangiography by radiological methods. *Clin. Radiol.* 6:217, 1955.
5. Adler, B. O., and Rosenberger, A. Computerized tomography of the thoracic duct: An anatomic study. *Cardiovasc. Intervent. Radiol.* 4:224, 1981.
6. Adler, B. O., and Rosenberger, A. Observations on physiological aspects of the thoracic duct with 70 mm camera. Unpublished data.
7. Fuchs, W. A., and Galeazzi, R. L. Die Röntgenanatomie des Ductus thoracicus. *Radiologe* 10:180, 1970.
8. Wirth, W., and Fromhold, H. Der Ductus thoracicus und seine Variationen. Lymphographische Studie. *ROEFO* 112:450, 1970.
9. Rouvière, H. *Anatomie des Lymphatiques de l'Homme.* Paris: Masson, 1932.
10. Rosenberger, A., and Abrams, H. L. The Thoracic Duct. In H. L. Abrams (ed.), *Angiography* (2nd ed.). Boston: Little, Brown, 1971.
11. Kausel, H. W., Reeve, T. S., Stein, A. A., Alley, R. D., and Stranahan, A. Anatomic and pathologic study of the thoracic duct. *J. Thorac. Cardiovasc. Surg.* 34:631, 1957.
12. Zhdanov, D. A. Anatomie du canal thoracique et des principaux collecteurs lymphatiques du tronc chez l'homme. *Acta Anat.* (Basel) 37:20, 1959.
13. Rosenberger, A., Adler, O., and Abrams, H. The thoracic duct: Structural, functional and radiologic aspects. *CRC Crit. Rev. Radiol. Sci.* 3:523, 1972.
14. Hidden, G., and Florent, J. Étude radioanatomique du canal thoracique opacifié par lymphographie pédieuse. *J. Chir.* (Paris) 91:373, 1966.
15. Pomerantz, M. J., Herdt, J. R., Rockoff, S. D., and Ketcham, A. S. Evaluation of the functional anatomy of the thoracic duct by lymphangiography. *J. Thorac. Cardiovasc. Surg.* 46:568, 1963.
16. Greenfield, J., and Gottlieb, M. I. Variation in the terminal portion of the human thoracic duct. *Arch. Surg.* 73:955, 1956.
17. Negus, D., Edwards, J. M., and Kinmonth, J. B. Filling of cervical and mediastinal nodes from the thoracic duct and the physiology of Virchow's node; studies by lymphography. *Br. J. Surg.* 57:267, 1970.
18. Van Permis, P. A. Variations of the thoracic duct. *Surgery* 26:806, 1949.
19. Rocca-Rosetti, S., Marrocu, F., Cossu, F., and Sulis, E. La lymphographie dans l'étude de la morphophysiologie systeme du canal thoracic. *J. Belge Radiol.* 48:306, 1965.
20. Rusznyak, I., Foldi, M., and Szabo, G. *Lymphatics and Lymphatic Circulation* (2nd English ed.). New York: Pergamon, 1967.
21. Bergström, K., and Werner, B. Proteins in human thoracic lymph. Studies on distribution of some proteins between lymph and blood. *Acta Chir. Scand.* 131:413, 1966.
22. Chrobák, L., Bartós, V., Brzek, V., and Hnízdová, D. Coagulation properties of human thoracic duct lymph. *Am. J. Med. Sci.* 253:69, 1967.
23. Hall, J. G. Flow of lymph. *N. Engl. J. Med.* 281:720, 1969.
24. Weissleder, H. Das pathologische Lymphangiogramm der Ductus thoracicus. *ROEFO* 101:573, 1964.
25. Vajda, J. Innervation of lymph vessels. *Acta Morphol. Acad. Sci. Hung.* 14:197, 1966.

26. Fitts, C. T., Williams, A. V., Graber, C. D., Artz, C. P., and Hargerst, T. S.   Thoracic duct lymph: Its significance in dialysis and immunology. *Surg. Clin. North Am.* 49:533, 1969.
27. Graber, C. D., Fitts, C. T., Williams, A. V., Artz, C. P., and Othersen, H. B.   Recovery of immune responsiveness after cessation of thoracic duct drainage in calves and men. *Ann. Surg.* 171:241, 1970.
28. Noonan, J. A., Walters, L. R., and Reeves, J. T.   Congenital pulmonary lymphangectasia. *Am. J. Dis. Child.* 120:314, 1970.
29. Baltaxe, J. A., Lee, J. G., Ehlers, K. H., and Engle, M. A.   Pulmonary lymphangectasia demonstrated by lymphangiography in 2 patients with Noonan's syndrome. *Radiology* 115:149, 1975.
30. Swischuk, L. E., Richardson, C. J., Nichols, M. M., and Ingman, M. J.   Bilateral pulmonary hypoplasia in the neonate. *AJR* 133:1057, 1979.
31. Schwartz, E.   Puncture of the thoracic lymph duct with chylothorax: A rare complication of aortography. *Radiology* 75:248, 1960.
32. Hyde, P. V. B., Jersky, J., and Gishen, P.   Traumatic chylothorax. *S. Afr. J. Surg.* 12:57, 1974.
33. Heilman, R. D., and Collins, V. P.   Identification of laceration of the thoracic duct by lymphangiography. *Radiology* 81:470, 1963.
34. Robbins, S. L. *Pathologic Basis of Disease.* Philadelphia: Saunders, 1974, P. 630.
35. Celis, A., Kuthy, J., and del Castillo, E.   The importance of the thoracic duct in the spread of malignant disease. *Acta Radiol.* (Stockh.) 45:169, 1956.
36. Wallace, S., Jackson, L., Dodd, G. D., and Greening, R. R.   Lymphatic dynamics in certain abnormal states. *AJR* 91:1187, 1964.
37. Edwards, J. M., and Kinmonth, J. B.   Lymphovenous shunts in man. *Br. Med. J.* 4:579, 1969.
38. Escobar-Prieto, A., Gonzalez, G., Templeton, A. W., Cooper, B. R., and Palacios, E.   Lymphatic channel obstruction: Patterns of altered flow dynamics. *AJR* 113:366, 1971.

Lymphangiopathies

WALTER A. FUCHS

Lymphedema

Lymphedema is caused by an abnormal increase in the interstitial fluid associated with lymphatic insufficiency. A distinction is made between lymphedema secondary to a well-defined cause and primary lymphedema.

PRIMARY LYMPHEDEMA

In primary lymphedema a number of different etiologies may be described from the standpoints of radiologic and clinical features, sex incidence, familial tendencies, age of onset, and associated deformities [23].

Congenital lymphedema includes Milroy's disease [31], a rare hereditary abnormality of the lymph system. Lymphedema may be present at birth or may develop during puberty or adolescence. The disease is believed to be predominantly inherited and female sex–linked. The form known as Meige's disease occurs chiefly in females with onset in adolescence and is considered to be female sex–linked [30]. In Turner's syndrome primary lymphedema is associated with dysgenesis of the ovaries and other deformities. The testicular feminization syndrome is a subvariety of this group associated with primary amenorrhea and lymphedema.

Nonhereditary congenital lymphedema is much more frequent. Lymphedema praecox is the most common form of primary lymphedema and is found mainly in females [26, 43]. It is caused by congenitally anomalous lymphatics, but lymphedema does not develop until between the ages of 9 and 25 years. Injury, surgery, or other forms of trauma or stress lead to insufficiency of the lymph circulation, primarily within the malformed lymph trunks. In lymphedema tarda symptoms appear after the age of 35 years.

Lymphangiopathia obliterans is another cause of primary lymphedema [21]. It is characterized by a pronounced proliferation and hyaline degeneration of the intima of the lymph vessels. This process causes progressive narrowing of the lumen with ultimate occlusion. The disorder occurs chiefly in young women. Its etiology is not known, but it is assumed to be a degenerative vascular process. At first it is limited to one extremity, but the contralateral limb becomes involved some years later. Differentiation between congenital hypoplasia of the lymphatics and obliterative lymphangiopathy can be established only by histologic examination.

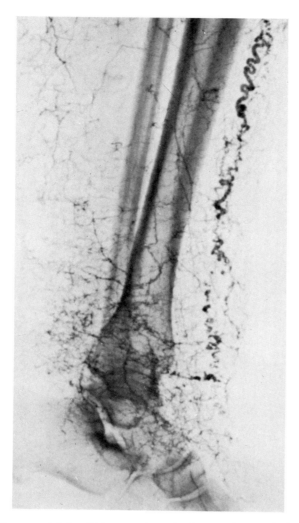

Figure 84-1. Primary lymphedema—hyperplasia. There are numerous dilated and tortuous lymphatics and dermal backflow.

The radiologic signs in primary lymphedema are hyperplasia and hypoplasia [17, 20, 24, 39]. In hyperplasia the lymph vessels are dilated and tortuous (Fig. 84-1; see Figs. 84-4A, B, 84-11A). The varicosity may be confined to a section of a lymph trunk, or it may involve larger regions of the lymph system. Dermal backflow is often associated with hyperplasia and is due to contrast filling of dermal lymphatics caused by valvular insufficiency. Retrograde filling of interstitial lymphatics is also frequently observed. In hypoplasia the lymph vessels are fewer and smaller than normal. Sometimes subcutaneous lymph trunks cannot be found, and the term *aplasia* is then used (Fig. 84-2). If blue dye is injected subcutaneously, it will spread rapidly in the dermal plexus of the dorsum of the foot and ankle. In some cases a solitary lymph trunk is observed, which is usually dilated and tortuous (Fig. 84-3).

Chylous reflux designates the condition in which the direction of chyle flow from the intestines is abnormal because of congenital abnormalities or disease of the lymphatic system [7, 23, 25]. Dysplasia of the lymphatic system, congenital insufficiency of lymphatic valves, atresia of lymph vessels, traumatic laceration of lymphatic structures, and obstruction due to inflammatory or malignant lesions are the major causes of chylous reflux. Proximal to the obstruction of lymph flow, the lymphatics are severely dilated. Their valves become incompetent, with consequent lymph flow. The intralymphatic pressure is considerably increased, and lymph vessels may rupture, with subsequent fistula formation.

Chylous edema is the result of retrograde flow of the intestinal lymph to the pelvis, genitals, and

Figure 84-2. Primary lymphedema—aplasia. There is dermal backflow of the vital dye after subcutaneous injection. No subcutaneous lymphatics were found at dissection.

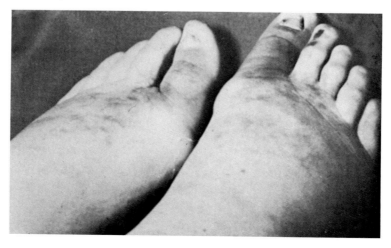

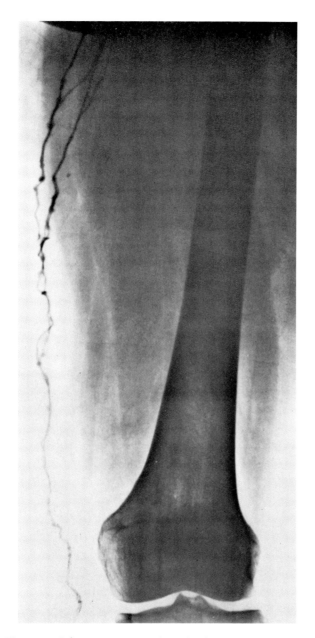

Figure 84-3. Primary lymphedema—hypoplasia. There is a solitary dilated and tortuous lymph trunk.

lower limbs (Fig. 84-4C). It leads to vessel dilatation and tortuosity in both the superficial and deep lymphatics. Progressive dilatation of the dermal lymphatics causes formation of chyloderma. Rupture of the vesicles results in chylorrhea. In rare cases of long-standing lymphedema, sarcomatous degeneration occurs (Stewart-Treves syndrome) [42]. Lymphangiomatosis of the bone may be due to incompetent lymphatic valves [33, 48]. Retrograde lymph flow from the pelvic region gradually leads to cystlike areas of bone destruction, which vary in size and contain oily contrast material after lymphangiography (Fig. 84-5).

SECONDARY LYMPHEDEMA

Secondary lymphedema is due to inflammatory lesions of the lymphatic and venous systems as well as to trauma, parasite invasion, tumor infiltration, surgical excision, or radiotherapy [11, 16, 18, 23].

Inflammatory Lesions
In lymphangitis, lymphangiography reveals multiple occlusions of otherwise normal lymph channels (Fig. 84-6). Peripheral to the occlusions the lymph vessels are distended and tortuous and often show backflow into dermal and intestinal lymphatics. Generally, many more lymphatics are contrast-filled than normal lymphangiograms show. Frequently a diffuse or localized extravasation of contrast agent is seen. Histologic examination shows inflammation, with a dense, perivascular cellular infiltration.

In the venous postthrombotic syndrome the prefascial lymphatics may exhibit certain changes after obliterative inflammations of the deep venous system. The contrast material flows in a retrograde direction into very fine lymphatics that join the major lymphatic channels. In chronic venous ulceration, the opaque material enters into the dermal lymph plexus and is seen at the periphery of the ulcers as minute deposits of contrast medium.

Filariasis
Filariasis, due to infection with *Wuchereria bancrofti,* is the most frequent cause of secondary lymphedema and one of the commonest diseases in the world [2, 23, 38]. Stenosis and complete obstruction of the lymphatics by inflammatory and sclerotic processes or by the parasite itself, as well as extensive collateral circulations and dermal backflow, are observed. Inflammatory reaction occurs in the regional lymph nodes but does not block lymph flow.

Noninflammatory Lesions
Malignant infiltration of lymph vessels and lymph nodes is a major cause of obstruction of lymph flow and secondary lymphedema. Details of pathogenesis and radiologic appearance are discussed in Chapter 86.

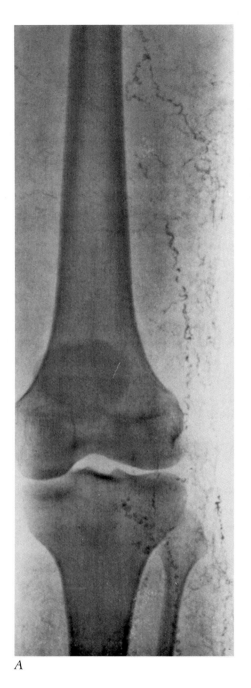

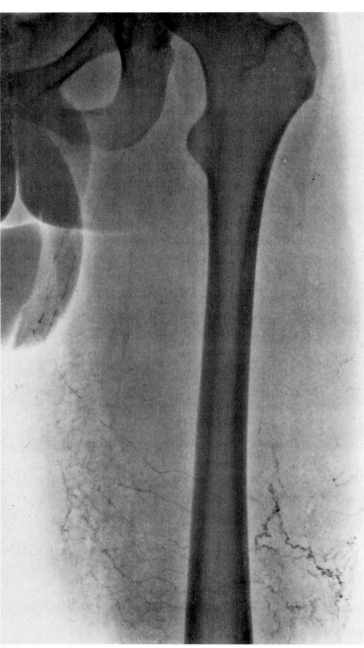

A

B

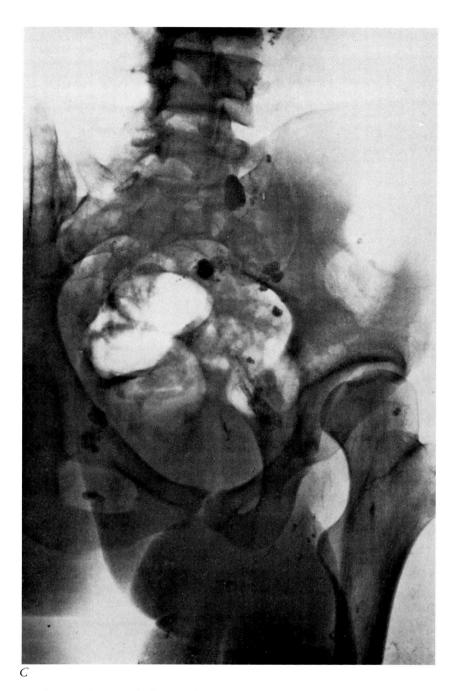

C

Figure 84-4. Primary lymphedema—chylous reflux. (A and B) Hyperplasia of the dilated, tortuous lymphatics in the left lower leg and thigh. (C) Chylous reflux. Contrast material fills the contralateral lymph nodes and lymphatics of the scrotum. There is dysplasia of the retroperitoneal lymphatic system.

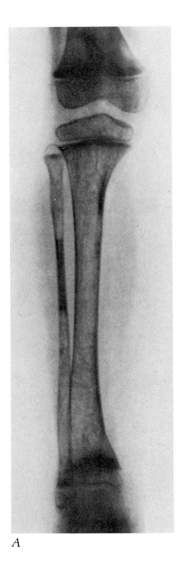

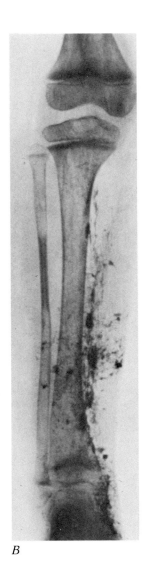

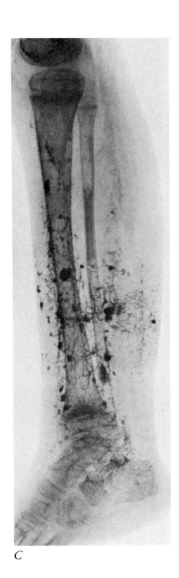

A
B
C

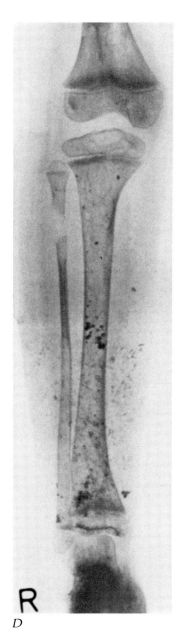

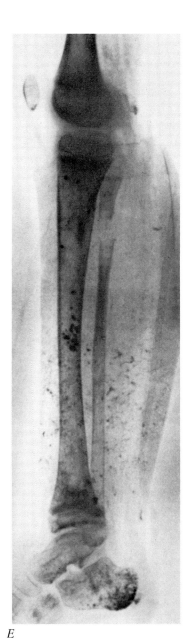

D

E

Figure 84-5. Lymphangiomatosis of the bone. (A) Cystlike areas of bone destruction. The areas are irregular in shape and vary in size within the tibia and fibula. (B and C) Lymphangiography. Primary lymphedema with hyperplasia of the lymphatics and extravasation of contrast material. (D and E) Accumulation of oily substance within the cystlike areas in the calcaneus. The diagnosis was confirmed by biopsy of the fibula 10 days after lymphangiography.

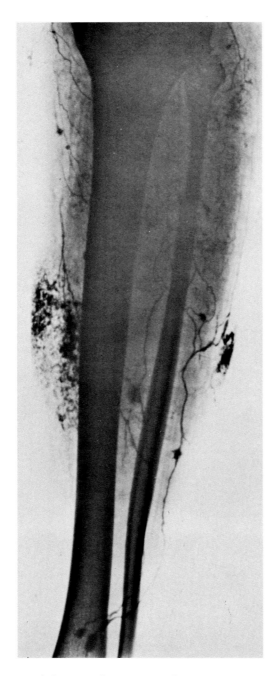

Figure 84-6. Secondary lymphedema—lymphangitis. There is obstruction of numerous subcutaneous lymphatics, extensive collateral circulation, and dermal and interstitial backflow.

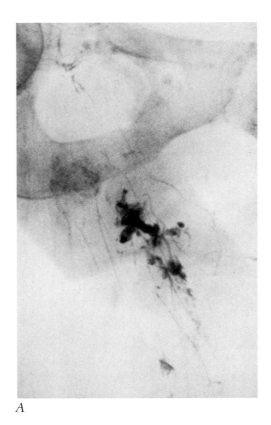

A

Figure 84-7. Postoperative lymphedema. (A) Extravasation of contrast material into the operation area, new formation of efferent lymphatics, and collateral circulation 3 months after inguinal lymphadenectomy. (B) Scar formation in the axilla after surgery and radiotherapy of breast cancer. Newly formed lymphatics traverse the area of operation. Collateral circulation is via the cephalic lymphatic chain.

Postoperative Lymphedema

Experimental animal studies indicate that regeneration of lymph vessels occurs approximately 20 days after surgical incision. In lymphangiography, extravasation of contrast material into the operation site is observed (Fig. 84-7; see Figs. 84-12, 84-13) [1, 23, 44]. Regeneration of lymphatics progresses from afferent lymph vessels. In cases of large incisions, repair proceeds via direct regeneration from the major lymph trunks. Collaterals bypassing the operation area are encountered when not all anatomic connections have been interrupted (Fig. 84-7B). Lymphaticovenous anastomoses develop to restore the balance of lymph flow. Complete repair of lymphatic circulation is achieved usually between 2 and 11 months postoperatively but will be retarded by infection, venous alterations, and irradiation.

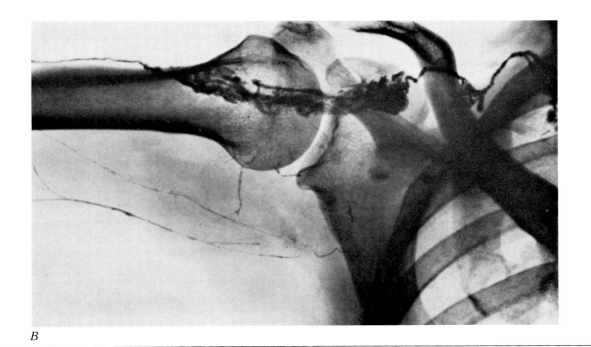

B

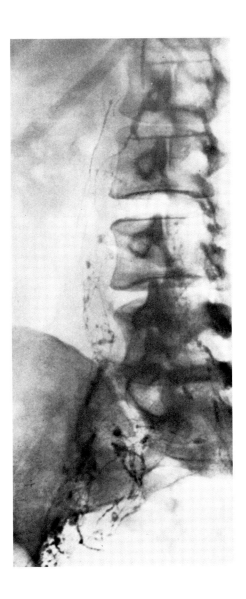

Figure 84-8. Irradiation fibrosis. Multiple fine lymphatics and lymph nodes after radiotherapy of Hodgkin's disease with 7,500 rads.

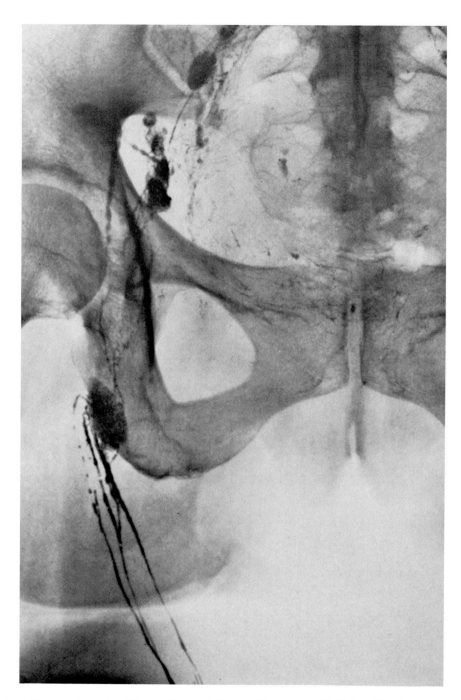

Figure 84-9. Irradiation fibrosis. There is partial obstruction of the lymphatic circulation leading to collaterals within the pelvic area 3 years after radiotherapy (6,000 rads) of a carcinoma of the uterine corpus.

Irradiation Fibrosis

The sensitivity of the lymphatics to irradiation is low. Slight changes in the lymph vessel wall occur when doses of 4,000 rads are applied. A high dosage of 15,000 rads is necessary to alter the lymphatic circulation significantly [14]. The impairment of lymphatic circulation due to irradia- tion mainly is consequent to scar formation in adjacent, highly radiosensitive connective tissue. No alterations of the lymphatic circulation occur in the normal or slightly altered lymphatic system when a therapeutic radiation dose is applied (Fig. 84-8). Small, delicate lymph vessels and small lymph nodes with structural patterns still intact are encountered. The small irradiated lymph nodes are not able to retain large amounts of contrast material. Irradiation of lymph nodes and lymph vessels extensively infiltrated by malignant disease frequently causes partial or complete obstruction of the lymph vessel, due to necrosis and secondary scar formation within the connective tissue (Fig. 84-9). Formation of a collateral circulation follows. Complete fibrosis and replacement of the lymphatic tissue make visualization of the lymph nodes impossible by lymphangiography. Secondary inflammations seem to play an important role in producing these obstructive fibrotic changes.

Retroperitoneal Fibrosis

Idiopathic retroperitoneal fibrosis is a relatively uncommon clinical entity. The etiology of this disease is still unknown, but it is considered to be a hypersensitivity or autoimmune phenomenon [22, 46]. Lymphangiography reveals complete or partial obstruction of the lymphatic circulation (Fig. 84-10B) [5, 10, 19, 45]. Collateral lymphatics within the pelvic and inferior aortic region are contrast filled. Fibrotic induration of the retroperitoneal connective tissue leads to external compression of the lymphatics. The lymph vessels superior to the fourth lumbar vertebra are

Figure 84-10. Retroperitoneal fibrosis. (A) Low lumbar obstruction of the right ureter. (B) Partial obstruction of the lymphatic and venous circulation. (C) Pre- vertebral mass lesion surrounding the abdominal aorta and inferior vena cava (*arrows*). *MP* = psoas muscle.

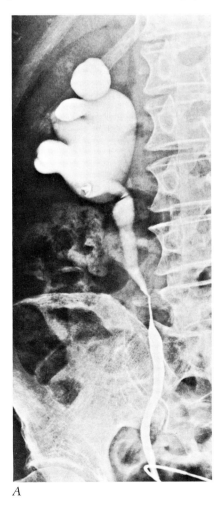

A

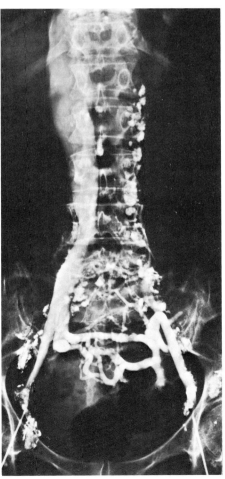

B

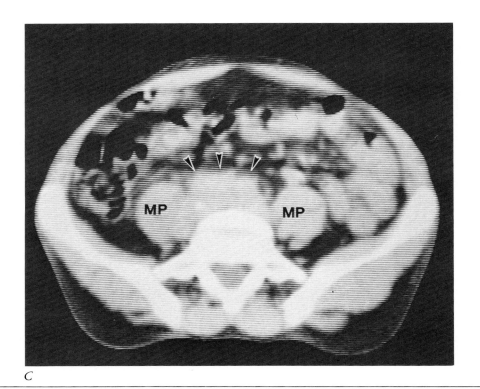

C

usually not visualized, and irregular filling defects within the iliac and aortic lymph nodes may be observed. Cavography demonstrates dislocation, compression, and complete obstruction of the inferior vena cava and pelvic veins, and the end result is an extensive collateral circulation. Urography shows urinary stasis with dilatation of the ureters and hydronephrosis (Fig. 84-10A). Computed tomography demonstrates a retroperitoneal mass lesion obliterating the vascular contours and extending toward the ureters (Fig. 84-10C). In structure and density it cannot be differentiated from malignant disease.

Lymph Fistula

CHYLOPERITONEUM

The presence of chyle in the peritoneal cavity is due to congenital atresia in the newborn or to obstruction of the lymphatic circulation in the adult [7, 8, 23, 32]. Malignant tumors are the most frequent cause of chyloperitoneum. The compression or obliteration of lymph channels may occur at any point between the abdominal wall and the entry of the thoracic duct into the venous system. Dilatation of the lymph trunks and valve insufficiency lead to reversal of lymph flow. Extravasation of contrast material into the peritoneal cavity and the retroperitoneal area may be demonstrated by lymphangiography (Fig. 84-11B). Traumatic rupture, inflammatory adenopathies, pancreatic lesions, and thrombosis of the subclavian vein are occasionally responsible for chylous effusion.

LYMPHOINTESTINAL FISTULA

Exudative enteropathy may be related to congenital abnormalities of the intestinal lymph channels. Diffuse dilatation of the lymphatics of the intestinal mucosa, called intestinal lymphangiectasis, then occurs [4, 12, 29, 34, 37, 40]. Blockage of the lymph circulation by tumor, pancreatitis, or constrictive pericarditis has been reported as a direct cause of exudative enteropathy. When the site of obstruction is situated in the thoracic duct or retroperitoneal area, lymphangiography demonstrates interruption, stasis, and even reversal of lymph flow. Fistulas into the intestines may occasionally be visualized. If the obstacle is confined to the visceral lymph channels, the lymphangiogram appears normal. The cause of chylous effusion is valve insufficiency, due to either malformation, mainly malignant, or inflammatory obstruction. Occasionally, the fistula is acquired after injury. Chylous disease occurs

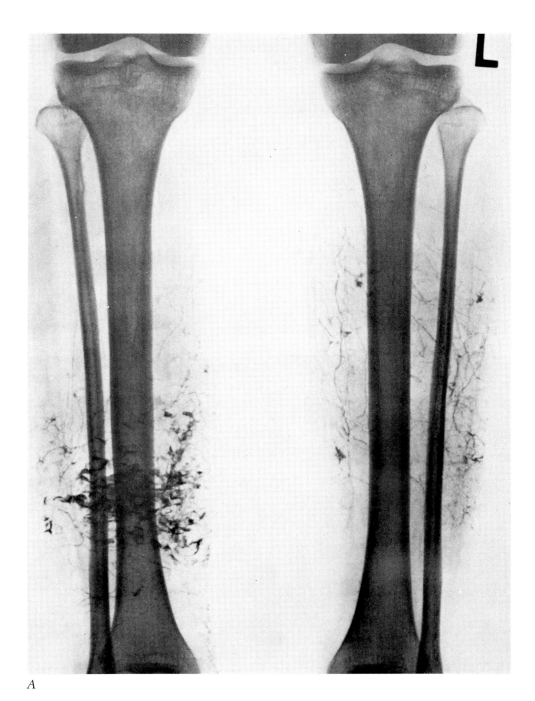

A

Figure 84-11. Primary lymphedema, chyloretroperitoneum, and chylothorax due to congenital abnormalities and secondary obstruction of lymph flow. This 28-year-old woman was operated on for valvular pulmonary stenosis and atrial septal defects. (A) Primary lymphedema of both legs. There are numerous fine interstitial and dermal lymphatics. (B) Bilateral extravasation of contrast material into the retroperitoneal space and dilatation of the thoracic duct. There is no chyluria. (C) Effusion of contrast medium along the peribronchial sheaths into the right pleural cavity and into the mediastinum. Fine intrapulmonary, mediastinal, and supraclavicular lymphatics act as collaterals. The severe dilatation of the thoracic duct was due to obstruction caused by an inflammatory reaction after insertion of a catheter into the subclavian vein during extracorporeal circulation.

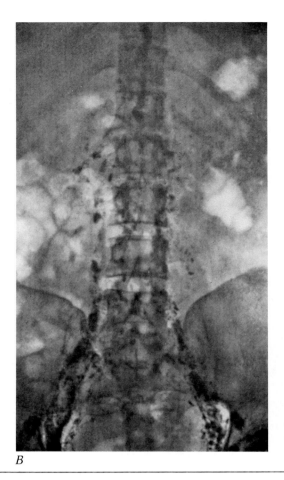

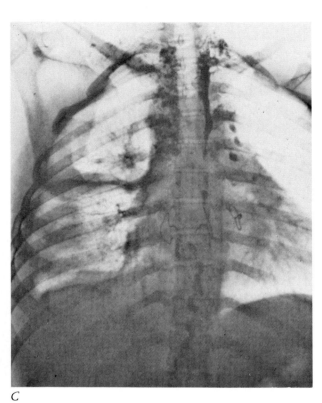

B   *C*

when the lymphatic circulation is decompensated and all collateral channels are exhausted.

CHYLURIA

The common etiology of chyluria is filariasis. Lymphangiography demonstrates unilateral or bilateral renal lymphatic reflux and multiple lymphocalyceal fistulas related to obstruction of lymph flow at the origin of the thoracic duct [2, 6, 27, 36, 38, 41]. Lymphedema of the legs and genital organs is found invariably as a manifestation of general invasion of the lymphatic system by the parasite.

CHYLOTHORAX

Trauma is the most frequent cause of effusion of lymph in the pleural cavities. It results from penetrating trauma and injury to the thoracic duct by operative or diagnostic procedures [3, 32]. Spontaneous chylothorax is related to blockage of the thoracic duct by malignant tumor and

inflammatory and parasitic disease, as well as to congenital malformations [15]. Lymphangiography makes it possible to determine the anatomic site and the type of laceration. It permits differentiation between congenital malformations and acquired conditions. In the presence of an obstruction, lymphangiography shows dilatation of the thoracic duct and effusion of contrast material along the peribronchial sheaths into the pleural cavity and mediastinum (see Fig. 84-11C).

Lymphocele

Lymphocyst formation is a complication of lymphadenectomy [13, 35, 47]. The lymphatics which have been cut continue to pour lymph into the space left at the site of operation. If the lymph drainage from the operation area is not readily reestablished by the proliferation of new lymphatics, cyst formation occurs (Figs. 84-12,

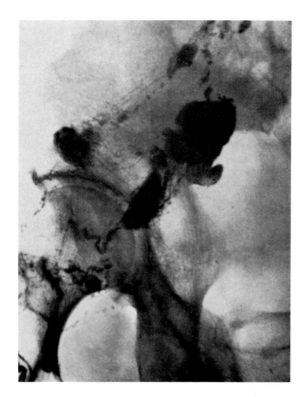

Figure 84-12. Postoperative lymphocyst 4 months after lymphadenectomy in carcinoma of the uterine cervix. Drainage of the operation area is by efferent lymphatics.

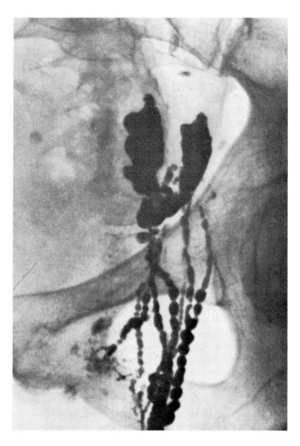

Figure 84-13. Postoperative lymphocyst 10 days after lymphadenectomy in carcinoma of the uterine cervix. Interruption of the lymph circulation and dilatation of the afferent lymphatics are seen.

84-13). The cyst may be demarcated, or it may continue to fill, extending beyond the operation site. It can persist for months or years. Preoperative irradiation probably contributes to lymphocyst formation, and irradiation delays its absorption. Lymphangiography provides a direct method of diagnosing lymphocysts because they are more densely filled with contrast material than the structured lymph nodes. Lymphocysts remain densely opaque when only traces of residual contrast medium are left in the lymph nodes. By enlarging and compressing adjacent structures, lymphocysts can cause pelvic pain, urinary symptoms, alterations in bowel habits, and edema of the external genitalia and extremities. It is important that lymphocysts be recognized as such and not confused with recurrent malignancies, so that the patient can be appropriately treated. Traumatic lymphocysts occur rarely and only are localized to the area traumatized.

Lymphogenic Neoplasm

Cavernous lymphangioma and cystic hygroma originate from a peripheral sequestration of primary lymphatic cavities [9]. In children they constitute 6 percent of all benign tumors. *Cavernous lymphangioma* consists of multiple cavities lined with endothelium and surrounded by fibrous tissue. *Cystic hygroma* contains larger cavities lined with endothelium and filled with clear or hemorrhagic fluid. These lymphatic cavities are localized in the face, neck, mediastinum, and axillae. Because they are sequestered from lymph flow, lymphangioma and hygroma are only rarely demonstrable by intravascular lymphangiography but may be visualized by direct puncture (Fig. 84-14). Mesenteric and retroperitoneal cysts induce symptoms by compression of the digestive and urinary tracts. Sudden rupture results in an acute abdomen.

Lymphangiomyomas are congenital and usually

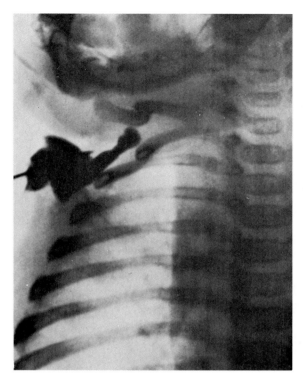

Figure 84-14. Cavernous lymphangioma in the right axillary region. There is partial contrast filling by direct puncture; no efferent lymphatics are seen.

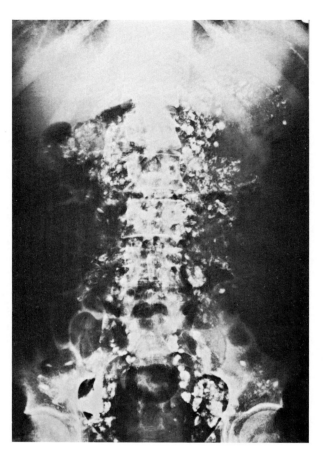

Figure 84-15. Lymphangiomyomatosis with numerous multicystic lesions within the retroperitoneum.

occur in females in the retroperitoneum or mediastinum (Fig. 84-15) [28]. Lymphography demonstrates multicystic lesions, chylothorax, and chylous ascites.

Lymphangiosarcoma (Stewart-Treves syndrome) represents a malignant degeneration in primary or secondary lymphedema, usually following radical mastectomy [42].

References

1. Abbes, M.   Les altérations de la circulation lymphatique après amputation du sein. *Ann. Chir.* 20:660, 1966.
2. Akisada, M., and Tani, S.   Filarial chyluria in Japan: Lymphography, etiology, and treatment in 30 cases. *Radiology* 90:311, 1968.
3. Althaus, U., and Fuchs, W. A.   Chylothorax nach kardiovaskulären Eingriffen. *Schweiz. Med. Wochenschr.* 102:44, 1972.
4. Amos, J. A. S.   Multiple lymphatic cysts of the mesentery. *Br. J. Surg.* 46:588, 1969.
5. Beltz, L., and Lymberopoulos, S.   Die retroperitoneale Fibrose. *Urologe* [A] 5:276, 1966.
6. Bernageau, J., Bismuth, V., Desprez-Curely, J. P., and Bourdon, R.   La lymphographie dans les chyluries. *J. Radiol. Electrol. Med. Nucl.* 45:529, 1964.
7. Bismuth, V., and Bourdon, R.   Les ascites chyleuses de l'adulte: Apport de la lymphographie (5 cas). *J. Radiol. Electrol. Med. Nucl.* 45:413, 1964.
8. Camiel, M. R., Benninghoff, D. L., and Herman, R. G.   Chylous ascites with lymphographic demonstration of lymph leakage into the peritoneal cavity. *Gastroenterology* 47:188, 1964.
9. Castellino, R. A., and Finkelstein, S.   Lymphographic demonstration of a retroperitoneal lymphangioma. *Radiology* 115:355, 1975.
10. Clouse, M. E., Fraley, E. F., and Litwin, S. B.   Lymphangiographic criteria for diagnosis of retroperitoneal fibrosis. *Radiology* 83:1, 1964.
11. Collette, J. M.   La lymphographie dans les lymphostases acquises. *Ann. Radiol.* (Paris) 1:211, 1958.
12. Desprez-Curely, J. P., Bismuth, V., and Bourdon,

R. Hypoprotéinémie idiopathique et stéatorrhé: Démonstration radiographique d'une fistule intestinale. *Ann. Radiol.* (Paris) 1:744, 1958.

13. Dodd, G. D., Rutledge, F., and Wallace, S. Postoperative pelvic lymphocysts. *AJR* 108:312, 1970.

14. Engeset, A. Irradiation of lymph nodes and vessels: Experiments in rats, with reference to cancer therapy. *Acta Radiol. [Suppl.]* (Stockh.) 229:1, 1964.

15. Freundlich, I. M. The role of lymphangiography in chylothorax. A report of six nontraumatic cases. *AJR* 125:617, 1975.

16. Fuchs, W. A., Rüttimann, A., and del Buono, M. S. Zur Lymphographie bei chronisch-sekundären Lymphödemen. *ROEFO* 92:608, 1960.

17. Gough, M. H. Primary lymphoedema: Clinical and lymphangiographic studies. *Br. J. Surg.* 53:917, 1966.

18. Gregl, A., and Kienle, J. Lymphangiographie beim peripheren Lymphödem. *ROEFO* 105:622, 1966.

19. Haertel, M., Bollmann, J., Vock, P., and Zingg, E. Computertomographie und retroperitoneale Fibrose (Morbus Ormond). *ROEFO* 131:504, 1979.

20. Jacobsson, S., and Johansson, S. Lymphangiography in lymphedema. *Acta Radiol.* (Stockh.) 57:81, 1962.

21. Kaindl, F., Mannheimer, E., Pfleger-Schwarz, L., and Thurnher, E. *Lymphangiographie und Lymphadenographie der Extremitäten.* Stuttgart: Thieme, 1960.

22. Kerr, W. S., Suby, H. I., Vickert, A., and Praley, P. Idiopathic retroperitoneal fibrosis: Clinical experiences with 15 cases, 1956–1967. *J. Urol.* 99:575, 1968.

23. Kinmonth, J. B. *The Lymphatics: Diseases, Lymphography and Surgery.* London: Arnold, 1972.

24. Kinmonth, J. B., and Taylor, G. W. Lymphatic circulation in lymphedema. *Ann. Surg.* 139:129, 1954.

25. Kinmonth, J. B., and Taylor, G. W. Chylous reflux. *Br. Med. J.* 1:529, 1964.

26. Kinmonth, J. B., Taylor, G. W., Tracy, G. D., and Marsh, J. D. Primary lymphoedema. *Br. J. Surg.* 45:1, 1957.

27. Koehler, R., Chiang, T. C., Lin, C. T., Chen, K. C., and Chen, K. Y. Lymphography in chyluria. *AJR* 102:455, 1968.

28. Kruglik, G. D., Reed, J. C., and Daroca, P. J. RPC from the AFIP. *Radiology* 120:583, 1976.

29. Leonidas, J. C., Kopel, F. B., and Danese, C. A. Mesenteric cyst associated with protein loss in the gastrointestinal tract: Study with lymphangiography. *AJR* 112:150, 1971.

30. Meige, H. Dystrophie oedémateuse héréditaire. *Presse Med.* 6:341, 1898.

31. Milroy, W. F. An undescribed variety of hereditary oedema. *N.Y. Med. J.* 56:505, 1892.

32. Nix, J. T., Albert, M., Dugas, J. E., and Wendt, D. L. Chylothorax and chylous ascites: A study of 302 selected cases. *Am. J. Gastroenterol.* 28:40, 1957.

33. Nixon, G. W. Lymphangiomatosis of bone demonstrated by lymphangiography. *AJR* 110:582, 1970.

34. Oh, C., Danese, C. A., Dreiling, D. A., and Elmhurst, M. D. Chylous cysts of mesentery. *Arch. Surg.* 94:790, 1967.

35. Parker, J. J., and Schmutzler, K. J. Chylous lymphocyst. *Radiology* 98:569, 1971.

36. Picard, J. D. La lymphographie au cours de chyluries (à propos de 30 observations). *J. Urol. Nephrol.* (Paris) 73:671, 1967.

37. Pomerantz, M., and Waldmann, T. A. Systemic lymphatic abnormalities associated with gastrointestinal protein loss secondary to intestinal lymphangiectasia. *Gastroenterology* 45:703, 1963.

38. Rajaram, P. C. Lymphatic dynamics in filarial chyluria and prechyluric state: Lymphographic analysis of 52 cases. *Lymphology* 3:114, 1970.

39. de Roo, T. The value of lymphography in lymphedema. *Surg. Gynecol. Obstet.* 124:755, 1967.

40. Servelle, M., Rouffilange, F., Andrieux, J., Soulie, J., Sequin, P., and de Leersnider, D. Lymphographie des chylifères intestinaux. *Sem. Hop. Paris* 44:881, 1968.

41. Servelle, M., Turiaf, J., Rouffilange, F., Scherer, G., Perrot, H., Frentz, F., and Turpyn, H. Chyluria in abnormalities of the thoracic duct. *Surgery* 54:536, 1963.

42. Stewart, F. W., and Treves, N. Lymphangiosarcoma in postmastectomy lymphedema: A report of six cases in elephantiasis chirurgica. *Cancer* 1:64, 1948.

43. Taylor, G. W. Chronic lymphoedema. *Br. J. Surg.* 54:898, 1967.

44. Tsangaris, N. T., and Yutzy, C. V. Lymphangiographic study of postmastectomy lymphedema. *Surg. Gynecol. Obstet.* 123:1228, 1966.

45. Virtama, P., and Helfia, T. Lymphography and cavography in retroperitoneal fibrosis. *Br. J. Radiol.* 40:231, 1967.

46. Wagenknecht, L. V. *Retroperitoneale Fibrosen.* Stuttgart: Thieme, 1978.

47. Weingold, A. B., Olivo, E., and Marino, J. Pelvic lymphocyst: Diagnosis and management. *Arch. Surg.* 95:304, 1967.

48. Winterberger, A. R. Radiographic diagnosis of lymphangiomatosis of bone. *Radiology* 102:321, 1972.

Benign Lymph Node Disease

WALTER A. FUCHS

Involutive Changes

Fibrolipomatosis, a manifestation of the normal physiologic involution of the lymphatic system [6], is characterized by the complete replacement of the central parts of the lymph nodes by connective and fatty tissue (Fig. 85-1). Lymphatic structures are left only in the periphery of the nodes, as incomplete cortical margins, and consequently the lymphangiographic appearance of those nodes is characterized by large central filling defects. The intermediary sinuses are preserved and are therefore contrast filled during the filling phase of lymphography (Fig. 85-2). Fibrolipomatosis is most common in the inguinal and axillary lymph nodes because they are the primary regional node groups of the extremities and are the nodes most often affected by inflammatory lesions. The external iliac lymph nodes and the lymph node groups at the level of the first to second lumbar vertebrae manifest similar but less extensive involutive changes. Fibrolipomatosis is more pronounced in patients of the middle and older age groups.

Reactive Hyperplasia

Reactive hyperplasia is characterized histologically by a proliferative process in which histioreticular and lymphocytic cells may take part. Hyperplasia may involve the medulla and cortex separately, but medullary and follicular hyperplasia may also be present simultaneously. The lymphangiographic node pattern of reactive hyperplasia is similar to that of a nonspecific hyperplasia inflammatory reaction. The large follicles and the wide sinuses give rise to larger, evenly distributed, filling defects (Fig. 85-3). No impairment of the lymph circulation is present [14].

Reactive hyperplasia is encountered in regional lymph nodes of primary tumors or of operation sites and should be regarded as a reactive change induced by inflammatory toxic products and metabolic agents of tumor cells. The presence of reactive hyperplasia in regional lymph nodes of a primary tumor implies the presence of a defense mechanism within these nodes.

2041

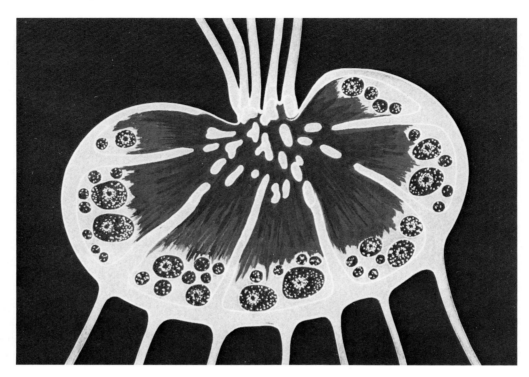

Figure 85-1. Fibrolipomatosis (schematic drawing). Extensive fibrolipomatous replacement of centrally lo-cated lymphatic tissue leading to central filling defects. Contrast-filled marginal lymphatic tissue.

Figure 85-2. Fibrolipomatosis of the inguinal lymph nodes. (A) Filling phase with an intact intermediary sinusoidal system. (B) Storage phase. Contrast-filled marginal sinus system.

Figure 85-3. Reactive hyperplasia. Enlarged inguinal and external iliac lymph nodes with a homogeneous storage pattern.

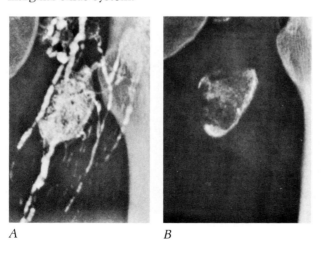

A   B

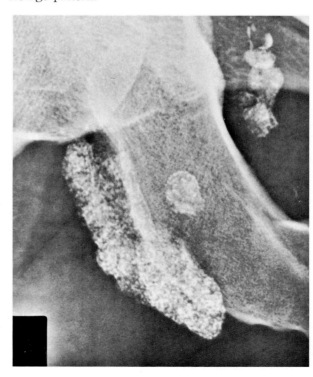

Inflammatory Disease

Classification of inflammatory reactions of lymph nodes is best made on the basis of morphologic change and not on the basis of etiology. The cellular reactions are not specific, even though they may be characteristic of a certain group of agents. In lymphangiography, the observed patterns are necessarily less specific. The morphologic alterations distinguished are hyperplastic inflammatory changes, granulomatous epithelial cell changes, and abscess-forming and necrotizing changes.

HYPERPLASTIC INFLAMMATORY CHANGES

The characteristic histologic changes of inflammatory reactions in lymph nodes are generalized hyperplasia of the lymphatic tissue with consequent node enlargement and new follicle formation [14]. The newly formed follicles cause filling defects that alter the structural pattern seen in the lymphadenogram. The number and size of the follicles vary from node to node, depending on the degree of the inflammatory reaction. Therefore, marked variations in the structural lymphangiographic architecture of the nodes arise.

The lymphangiographic pattern of an inflamed node resembles that of an enlarged node [15]. A great variety of structural patterns in hyperplastic inflammatory disease are encountered, however. Large follicles and wide sinuses produce large filling defects within coarse, opaque strands. An increase in follicle size will loosen up the storage pattern, which always presents a regular, harmonious structure. In some cases, extensive filling defects by very large follicles may dominate the lymphadenogram (Fig. 85-4).

The storage phase of the lymphadenogram is most often characterized by a reticular pattern in which contrast droplets are localized within small sinuses. When sinuses are wide, coarse droplets within them may dominate the lymphadenogram. Hyperplastic inflammatory changes of lymph nodes occur as nonspecific reactive phenomena in general infectious disease, infectious mononucleosis, measles and other viral infections, and syphilis [2], as well as in rheumatic arthritis, ankylosing spondylitis [5], and psoriatic arthropathy.

Figure 85-5. Tuberculosis. Enlargement of the common left iliac and aortic lymph nodes with large central filling defects and loosening of the storage pattern.

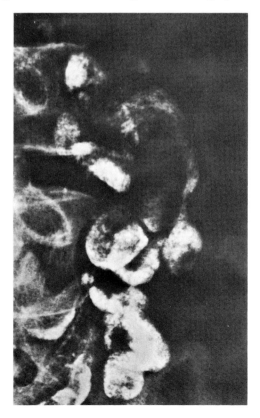

Figure 85-4. Chronic hyperplastic inflammatory reaction. Enlarged inguinal lymph nodes with large follicular filling defects.

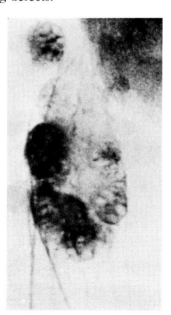

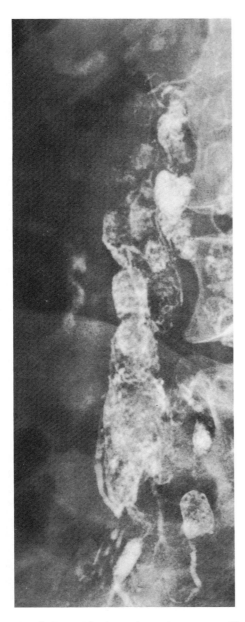

Figure 85-6. Sarcoidosis. Enlarged common iliac and lumbar lymph nodes with structural loosening because of lacunar filling defects.

GRANULOMATOUS EPITHELIOID CELL INFLAMMATORY CHANGES

Granulomatous epithelioid cell reactions are encountered in chronic inflammatory diseases of widely varying etiology [10]: tuberculosis, sarcoidosis, toxoplasmosis, brucellosis, syphilis, histoplasmosis, coccidioidomycosis, tularemia, leprosy, blastomycosis, Crohn's disease, and parasitic diseases.

In *tuberculosis,* filling defects of various sizes in enlarged lymph nodes are the structural alterations of the lymphangiographic pattern that are most often encountered [1, 3, 4, 10]. The multiple well-demarcated central and marginal filling defects are due to the tuberculous granuloma (Fig. 85-5). The pathologic lymph nodes are slightly enlarged and are situated predominantly within the lumbar area. These changes are nonspecific and may resemble malignancy [9]. Calcifications within lymph nodes may occasionally be recognized. Impairment of the lymphatic circulation may be present.

The lymphangiographic pattern of *sarcoidosis* has been described as similar to that of malignant lymphoma [1, 10, 12, 13]. The pattern of enlarged lumbar lymph nodes manifests structural loosening because of lacunar filling defects and droplike deposits of contrast material (Fig. 85-6). Lymphatic obstruction is extremely rare. Brucellosis, syphilis, and leprosy have been seen to produce the same type of lymphangiographic pattern as has nonspecific inflammation.

Histoplasmosis is reported to produce lymph node involvement that is also similar in appearance to that of malignant lymphoma [16]. The lymphangiographic pattern of toxoplasmosis is also that of a nonspecific hyperplastic reaction.

In *Bancroft's filariasis,* signs of reactive inflammatory reaction are observed in the early stages of the disease. Poor opacification of the lymph nodes is observed in the later stages of filariasis, when permanent chyluria and stasis of the lymph circulation caused by extensive fibrosis are present.

The lymphangiographic findings in *Whipple's disease* are general enlargement of the iliac and aortic lymph nodes, filling defects, and loosening of the structural pattern [15].

ABSCESS-FORMING AND NECROTIZING CHANGES

Abscess-forming and necrotizing changes develop in inguinal lymphogranuloma (Nicolas-Favre disease), lymphogranuloma venereum, cat-scratch disease, and abscess-forming lymphadenitis.

Radiation Fibrosis

Irradiation of the lymph nodes causes the alteration and destruction of lymphocytes, even when small doses are used. However, repopulation

86

Malignant Metastatic Disease

WALTER A. FUCHS

Formation of Cancerous Metastases

Lymph node metastases are formed by emboli of small groups of cancer cells that reach the marginal sinuses via afferent lymphatics. Tumor cells are deposited in close proximity to the entry points of the afferent lymph vessels and in the intermediary sinuses. Because malignant cells from a primary tumor reach a regional lymph node by way of numerous afferent lymphatics, multiple foci of malignant growth may implant in the periphery of the node (Fig. 86-1A). With increasing growth of the malignant cell formation, irregular destruction of the marginal area of the affected lymph node occurs. Further malignant infiltration of the node leads to compression of the lymphatic tissue, destruction of the capsule, and obliteration of the intermediary sinus. In advanced stages, the entire lymph node is infiltrated, and the afferent lymphatics are obstructed (Fig. 86-1B). Lymph flow is blocked, and a collateral circulation develops [26].

Metastases from a cancerous organ do not necessarily implant in the primary regional lymph nodes of the organ. Malignant infiltration may occur in only secondary and tertiary regional node groups. Primary regional lymph nodes may be bypassed via direct anastomoses between afferent and efferent lymphatics. Some of the major lymphatic channels may not be linked directly with the primary regional nodes, and some of the intermediate sinuses in lymph nodes may be so large that they do not act as filters. Malignant metastases to nonregional lymph node groups may also occur when lymphatic vessels are obstructed. Consequent dilatation of the afferent lymphatics renders their valves defective and leads to retrograde flow, collateral lymph circulation, and atypical metastatic spread.

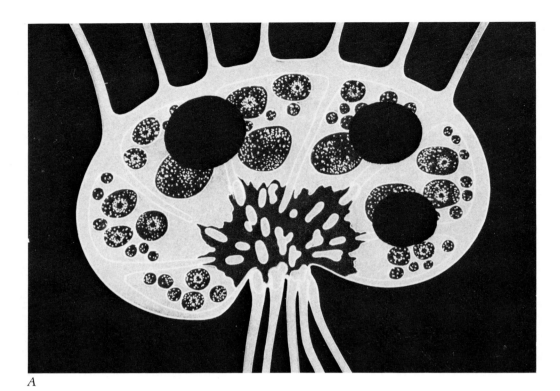

A

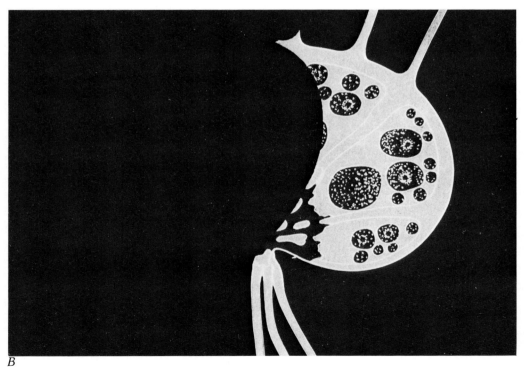

B

Figure 86-1. Formation of cancer metastases. (A) Multiple foci of malignant growth implanted in the periphery of the nodes destroying the sinus system. (B) Advanced malignant metastatic invasion with destruction of lymphatic tissue and blockage of afferent lymphatics.

Principles of Lymphographic Diagnosis

The lymphographic symptoms of malignant metastatic spread comprise as *direct diagnostic signs* nodal filling defects and lymph node enlargement, whereas obstruction of the lymphatic circulation and displacement of adjacent lymph nodes and lymphatics are considered *secondary indirect symptoms*. This triple combination of (1) large marginal filling defects, (2) enlargement of the lymph node, and (3) lymph stasis may be called the metastatic triad [9, 10, 28, 29].

NODAL FILLING DEFECTS

Tumor metastases will appear as filling defects, since malignant tissue is impervious to oily contrast material. Malignant metastatic foci may, however, be recognized as such only if they produce filling defects that differ in size and shape from those of the follicles. Areas of neoplastic growth must, therefore, be larger than the largest follicle in a particular node before lymphographic recognition becomes possible. The minimum size of malignant cellular deposits recognizable by lymphography is considered to be within the range of 2 to 10 mm, with an average of 5 mm (Fig. 86-2; see Figs. 86-14, 86-15). Lymph follicles become enlarged by *inflammation* and *reactive hyperplasia*, conditions that in the case of carcinoma occur concomitantly within the regional lymph nodes. The defects due to nonspecific inflammation reaction appear larger, but they retain their form and regular distribution throughout the node [26]. With increasing size of the tumor foci, compression and then obstruction of the marginal and the intermediate sinus take place. The filling defects become irregular in shape but are well demarcated in the case of direct infiltration; they are more regular if invasion is less prominent. The destruction of the sinus system, leading to permanent filling defects in the filling and retention phase of the lymphogram, is a diagnostic feature (see Figs. 86-2, 86-5, 86-14) of particular importance for differentiation from

Figure 86-2. Carcinoma of uterine cervix stage 2. Small marginal and central filling defects within normal-sized lumbar lymph nodes. (A) Filling phase showing the destruction of sinus system. (B) Storage phase. (C) Follow-up study after 3 months showing increase in node size and large filling defects due to malignant metastatic deposits.

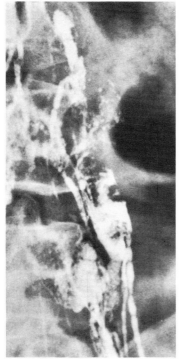
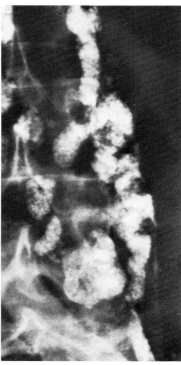
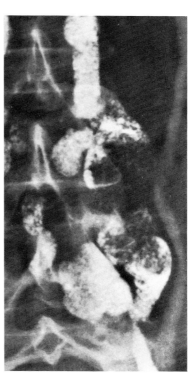

A   *B*   *C*

filling defects due to *fibrolipomatosis,* in which the marginal and intermediary sinus system stays intact. *Granulomatous inflammatory alterations* within a lymph node may produce identical changes, since destruction of the lymphatic structure by granulation tissue takes place. Well-demarcated marginal and central filling defects and obliteration of the sinus system are then observed on the lymphogram, identical with the findings produced by malignant deposits [26].

The genesis of cancer metastases leads to their peripheral deposition in a node, whereas filling defects of fibrolipomatosis are predominantly situated in the hilar region. Malignant growth tends to infiltrate the entire lymph node, obstructing the lymphatic circulation and displacing the remaining lymphatic tissue toward the periphery of the node (see Figs. 86-4–86-6, 86-8, 86-12).

The *demarcation* of regular and irregular filling defects due to malignant deposits is well defined, whereas those of fibrolipomatosis are somewhat unevenly delineated. On the combined evidence of localization, contour appearance, and, particularly, presence or absence of obstruction of the intermediate and marginal sinuses, the distinction between fibrolipomatosis and neoplastic disease is made reliably in most cases. However, interpretation of inguinal lymph nodes and the most caudally situated external iliac and axillary lymph nodes may be difficult because involutive changes in these node groups are common findings. Tangential projections, tomography, and follow-up studies will help to confirm doubtful lymphographic diagnoses.

Follow-up studies at short regular intervals are of great diagnostic importance in doubtful cases since the lymphographic diagnosis will become significantly more accurate by comparing size and structure of suspicious lymph nodes (see Figs. 86-2, 86-15). Lymph nodes that were previously normal, or did not show conclusive pathologic findings, may enlarge and develop central and marginal filling defects due to metastatic foci. Alteration of form, increase in size of lymph nodes, and displacement or separation of contrast-filled lymphatic tissue indicate the presence of malignant disease. A slight but definite increase in size, with a subsequent gradual decrease, is observed in normal lymph nodes; it is due to reactive inflammatory changes induced by the oily contrast material. Comparative analysis of follow-up roentgenograms taken at intervals of 2 weeks, for periods as long as 6 months, is necessary for careful evaluation.

Second-look lymphography by reinjection of contrast material becomes necessary if an inadequate amount of contrast material is present within the lymph nodes at the time of follow-up.

Differentiation between certain histologic types of carcinoma on the basis of the topographic arrangement of filling defects caused by metastatic foci within lymph nodes is not possible because the process of malignant metastatic spread into regional lymph nodes is independent of the histologic type of a malignant tumor. But the growth rate of the malignant tissue depends on its histologic structure, and a degree of differentiation on the basis of the growth rate should be possible. Measurement of the time it takes for the node size to double yields additional information on the biologic behavior of certain types of carcinoma (see Figs. 86-2, 86-14). The number of malignant cell deposits within a lymph node may be another important factor influencing the lymph node architecture and facilitating diagnosis. In malignant melanoma, central filling defects within enlarged lymph nodes are frequent findings, not commonly seen in other histologic types of lymph node metastases (see Fig. 86-16) [8, 22]. The central position of the defects may be explained by the fact that the number of tumor cells invading the lymphatic system is quite large. The numerous malignant cell groups not only are deposited within the marginal sinuses of a lymph node but may invade the entire node, leading to large central filling defects seen in the lymphogram. Malignant metastatic spread of testicular tumors in aortic lymph nodes often causes a particular lymphographic finding: diffuse multifocal infiltration of the lymphatic tissue due to neoplastic disease (see Figs. 86-7–86-9). In the early stages of the metastatic process, the malignant tissue produces marked loosening of the lymphatic structure within the lymph nodes, which have still preserved their basic structural appearance. The lymphographic findings then closely resemble those of primary malignant lymphoma. With increasing tumor growth the entire lymph node is invaded by malignant tissue, and only displaced remainders of the lymphatic tissue are visualized by lymphography.

SIZE AND SHAPE OF LYMPH NODES

The size of lymph nodes affected by cancer spread is generally increased, particularly in fast-growing tumors. However, the affected nodes may remain normal in size (see Figs. 86-2, 86-13). The degree of malignant involvement must be considerable before the size and shape of a lymph node are altered. The size of lymph nodes shows a good deal of variation. Normal-sized inguinal and iliac lymph nodes may measure up to 3 cm in diameter, and aortic lymph nodes may have a maximum length of 4 cm but with a width never exceeding 1.5 cm. Parietal internal iliac lymph nodes are normally small and may, when enlarged, still be smaller than nodes in other regions. It is important to compare the size of the questionable lymph node with the size of the corresponding contralateral lymph node group. The evaluation of enlargement thus requires substantial experience.

DISLOCATION AND ABSENCE OF LYMPH VESSELS AND LYMPH NODES

Dislocation of lymph vessels and lymph nodes is of limited value in the diagnosis of malignant metastatic disease. It may be regarded as a reliable indirect diagnostic sign only if malignant invasion of lymph nodes is simultaneously observed (see Figs. 86-6, 86-7A, 86-8). The reason is that great anatomic variations of the lymph system and the dislocation of lymph vessels and lymph nodes are associated with tortuous arteriosclerotic arteries in the elderly patient. Topographic boundary lines to localize certain groups of lymphatics and lymph nodes are of equally limited significance.

The absence of a node or a node group that is usually filled with contrast material is without diagnostic significance since the lymphatic system is subject to innumerable variations. Additional signs of lymph flow obstruction must be present before such "empty regions" may be considered pathologic findings. This is particularly the case for the aortic area, where numerous connections between the various node groups are present.

OBSTRUCTION OF THE LYMPHATIC CIRCULATION

Lymph stasis is visualized on the lymphogram as dilated afferent lymphatics, which remain contrast-filled after injection. Node groups distal to the site of obstruction are not demonstrated when blockage is complete (Fig. 86-3; see Fig. 86-11). A stenosis of the vessel just before the occlusion is also a common finding. Impeded flow results in increased intralymphatic pressure, and extravasation of contrast medium may occur during injection. In addition, a collateral circulation bypassing the obstruction develops, so that

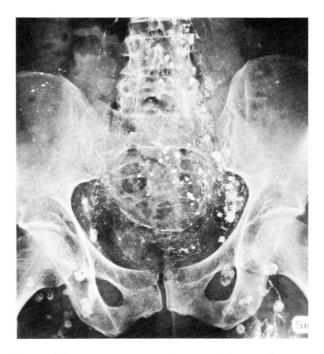

Figure 86-3. Recurrent carcinoma of the uterine cervix. Extensive obstruction of the lymphatic circulation within the iliac and lower aortic area due to recurrent malignancy following surgery and radiotherapy. Retroperitoneal and perivesical collaterals are demonstrated. Metastatic lower left aortic lymph nodes are shown.

lymph vessels appear that are not normally visible (Fig. 86-3). The collaterals are contrast-filled by a reversed flow, consequent on the process of lymph stasis, with vessel dilatation and the resulting valve insufficiencies. Collateral lymph flow in perivascular fibrous sheaths and perineural sheaths is occasionally observed. However, differentiation of these conditions from simple extravasation may be difficult. A persistent contrast filling of a few solitary lymph vessels up to 24 hours after contrast injection may not be attributable to lymph stasis (see Fig. 86-11). The only conclusive symptom of lymphatic obstruction is abrupt nonfilling of lymphatics immediately following contrast injection, together with contrast filling of collateral lymphatics. Dilatation of the lymphatics, change of vessel caliber with incomplete filling of lymph vessels, and extravasation of contrast material may be due to technical shortcomings and are therefore not diagnostic. Obstruction of lymph vessels and development of collaterals occur in more advanced cases of malignant metastatic spread and are therefore less frequently observed.

The *topographic anatomy of collateral lymphatic circulation* is determined by the topographic-anatomic localization of lymphatic obstruction. The extent of collateral flow depends mainly on the degree of lymphatic obstruction. Blockage of a subcutaneous lymph vessel group in the *lower extremity* leads to the formation of collaterals in unaffected areas. Obstruction of the lymph vessels of the saphena magna region introduces lymphatic collaterals in the saphena parva region and vice versa. Additional cutaneous, subcutaneous, interstitial, and deep collateral lymphatics are commonly filled with contrast material. Obstruction of the lymph flow in the *inguinal region* will cause collaterals via subcutaneous lymphatics in the thigh, in the outer genital organs (scrotum, vulva), across the perineum to the opposite side, and in lymphatics of the lateral and medial aspects of the anterior abdominal wall. Interruption of the lymphatic circulation in one of the *external iliac lymph node chains* leads to collateral circulation via the remaining nonobstructed external iliac lymphatics (Fig. 86-3). Lymph vessels situated medially in the pelvic region serve as collaterals to the contralateral side. Lymph vessels of the urinary bladder, uterus, and rectum may also act as collaterals. Laterally situated collateral lymphatics of the lower lumbar region are frequently observed. Extravasation of contrast agent into the abdominal cavity and the lumen of pelvic organs may occasionally be demonstrated by lymphography. In rare cases direct collaterals to the axillary region are found. In subtotal and total blockage of the lymphatic circulation in the common iliac lymph node group, retroperitoneal lymph vessels and nodes in the parietal lumbar region act as collaterals. Aortic lymph nodes distal to the obstruction site may then be contrast-filled via these particular groups of lymphatics (Fig. 86-3).

Obstruction of the *aortic lymph vessels and nodes* produces collateral circulation to lymph vessels of the contralateral side (see Fig. 86-6). The unaffected lymph nodes situated distal to the malignant infiltration are usually filled with contrast medium. Because of the numerous physiologic connections between the aortic lymph node chains, the lymph nodes invaded by malignant growth are easily bypassed. Lymphography may then not demonstrate blocked infiltrated lymphatics, and collateral circulation will not be demonstrated as such. The numerous anatomic variations of contrast-filled aortic lymph nodes lead to further difficulties of interpretation.

False-negative lymphographic findings due to unrecognized tumor-induced nonfilling of lymph nodes must, therefore, be taken into account.

Obstruction of the *thoracic duct* leads to dilatation of the cisterna chyli and the lumbar trunks (see Fig. 86-9A). Valvular insufficiency develops, and reflux of lymph may occur to the intestinal, pleural, peritoneal, renal, and hepatic lymphatics, with consequent chylothorax, chylous ascites, and chyluria [25]. Lymphography demonstrates extravasation of contrast material into the pleural and peritoneal cavities and to the renal pelvis. Contrast filling of collateral intercostal lymph channels and axillary lymphatics is occasionally observed. Lymphaticovenous anastomoses to the inferior and superior vena cava and the portal venous system frequently occur. The mechanism of collateral circulation in obstruction of the thoracic duct has been studied experimentally by ligation of the thoracic duct in dogs. The results of the investigations reproduce exactly the pathophysiologic data observed in malignant obstruction of the thoracic duct and resemble those seen in congenital lymphatic malformation.

Clinical Indications for Lymphangiography

The clinical indication for lymphography in epithelial malignancies is the detection of malignant metastatic spread to regional lymph nodes—that is, N staging [7]. The proved presence of malignant lymph node metastases dramatically affects both the therapeutic approach and the prognostic outlook in every type of malignant neoplasm. Therefore, radiologic and cytohistologic diagnosis of malignant metastatic deposits within lymph nodes is of paramount importance.

GYNECOLOGIC TUMORS

The treatment of *carcinoma of the uterine cervix* depends not only on the continuous extension of the primary tumor but also on the discontinuous fashion of metastatic spread to regional lymph nodes (see Fig. 86-2). Consequently, lymphography gives important information concerning planning of both the surgical and the radiotherapeutic approach [2, 10, 12, 13, 15, 21]. Since therapeutic measures rely mainly on the degree of lymphatic metastatic spread to the regional lymph nodes, it is evident that lymphography must be done prior to all therapeutic interventions.

In about 15 to 25 percent of all cases in clinical stages 1 and 2, lymphatic metastatic spread can be demonstrated by lymphography, which may show that tumor infiltration is more advanced than could be judged by clinical investigations. In clinical stage 3 disease, malignant lymph node metastases are demonstrated by lymphography in about 30 to 50 percent of patients.

Two-thirds of all pathologic lymphograms show tumor spread in the external iliac lymph nodes only. In 15 percent, metastatic spread is exclusively localized in the aortic lymph nodes at the level of L4–5, a group of lymph nodes that is normally not excised at retroperitoneal lymphadenectomy. In 10 percent of all cases, lymphatic metastatic spread is demonstrated in both the iliac and the aortic lymph nodes.

Carcinoma of the corpus uteri shows, contrary to general opinion, a relatively high percentage of lymph node metastases as demonstrated by lymphography—10 to 20 percent in clinical stages 1 and 2 and 20 to 40 percent in clinical stage 3 disease. Malignant metastatic spread most commonly occurs to the aortic (lumbar) and common iliac lymph nodes (Fig. 86-4) [10, 28].

In *carcinoma of the vulva and vagina,* false-negative lymphographic findings are relatively frequent. The first regional lymph node group in the inguinal region, the medial superior superficial inguinal lymph nodes, is not demonstrated by lymphography. Furthermore, fibrolipomatosis and chronic inflammation make the diagnostic evaluation of the inguinal lymph nodes rather difficult. The indication for lymphography is the necessity to evaluate the external iliac lymph nodes prior to surgery and radiotherapy, in which case pathologic lymphographic findings may be expected in about one-third of the patients (Fig. 86-5) [10, 20, 28].

In *malignant tumors of the ovaries,* lymphatic metastatic spread is more common than is generally thought (Fig. 86-6). Because of the high frequency of positive lymphographic findings, clinical stages 1, 2, and 3 are changed into clinical stage 4 in 40 to 50 percent of the cases. These data demonstrate clearly the need for lymphography for accurate staging in this type of tumor [1, 10, 18, 20, 28]. Negative lymphographic findings are, however, sometimes in sharp contrast to the large-sized primary tumors, which

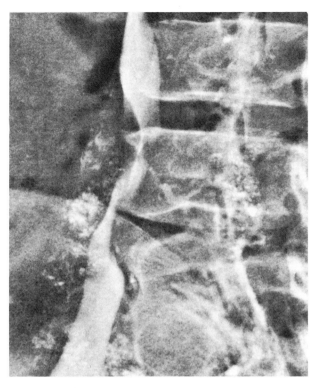

Figure 86-4. Carcinoma of corpus uteri stage 2. Filling defects by metastatic deposits within right common iliac lymph nodes. Compression and indentation of the right common iliac vein are due to enlarged metastatic lymph nodes.

Figure 86-5. Carcinoma of the vagina. Marginal and central filling defects obstructing the sinus system within enlarged medial external iliac lymph nodes due to malignant metastases. Partial obstruction of afferent lymphatics is seen.

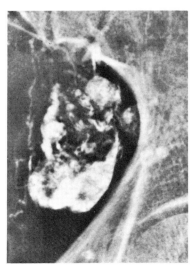

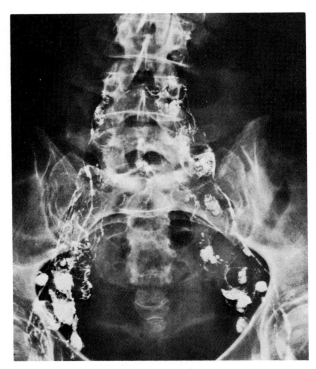

Figure 86-6. Ovarian carcinoma. Extensive metastatic deposits within enlarged bilateral aortic lymph nodes leading to obstruction of the afferent lymphatic circulation.

themselves lead to a dislocation of the lymph vessels and lymph nodes.

TUMORS OF THE GENITOURINARY TRACT

In *malignant testicular tumors,* the clinical indications for lymphography are well established [4, 10, 11, 14, 17, 28]. The first regional lymph nodes of the testicles are the aortic (lumbar) lymph nodes at the level of L2–3 (Figs. 86-7, 86-8). Thus they cannot be investigated by clinical methods. Consequently, lymphography should be performed in all cases for the classification of the tumor stage. Cavography is routinely undertaken as an additional method because lymphography does not show all aortic lymph nodes, particularly those that are not situated in the vicinity of the inferior vena cava. False-negative lymphographic findings occur in about one-third of cases. The frequency of lymphographic metastatic spread increases with increased malignancy of the neoplastic disease (Fig. 86-9). Positive lymphographic findings are observed in about 30 percent of cases of seminoma,

40 percent of teratocarcinoma, 60 percent of embryonal carcinoma, and 80 percent of choriocarcinoma [11].

The indications for lymphography in *carcinoma of the penis* are acceptable only if a diagnostic evaluation of the external iliac lymph nodes is necessary prior to lymphadenectomy or radiotherapy (Fig. 86-10) [10]. This limitation must be attributed to the fact that the first regional lymph node groups, the medial superior superficial inguinal lymph nodes, are not demonstrated by lymphography, and that fibrolipomatosis and chronic inflammation often render the lymphographic interpretation very difficult.

With *carcinoma of the prostate* the lymphographic findings have shown that lymphatic metastatic spread is much more common than was previously thought (Fig. 86-11). Metastases are demonstrated lymphographically in more than 50 percent of cases [3, 4, 10, 16, 23, 24, 30]. In clinical stage 1, pathologic lymphograms are relatively rare, whereas the frequency of positive lymphographic findings in stage 2 is about 40 percent and in stage 3 up to 75 percent. Skeletal metastases are as frequent in patients with as without lymph node metastases.

In *malignant tumors of the urinary bladder* lymphography is not indicated in the presence of superficial tumors limited to the mucosa and submucosa, because malignant spread to regional lymph nodes then seldom occurs. In cases in which malignant invasion of the muscular structures has been demonstrated, or even perivesical infiltration clinically diagnosed, malignant metastases in regional lymph nodes are common [4, 10, 28]. Lymphography will then demonstrate metastatic foci within the external iliac lymph nodes in more than one-third of cases (Fig. 86-12). If lymphatic metastatic spread is demonstrated by lymphography, no radical surgery, including cystectomy and lymphadenectomy, or aggressive radiotherapy need be performed because the survival rate is not altered by these invasive measures.

In *malignant renal tumors* the surgical approach, and particularly the prognosis of the disease, may be altered by the presence and extent of lymphatic metastatic spread. In the advanced stages of the malignancy, positive lymphographic findings within the regional aortic lymph nodes may be expected in 30 to 40 percent of cases (Fig. 86-13). Sympathicoblastoma of the *adrenal gland* has a high frequency of lymph node metastases [19, 22]. The great extent of lymphatic involve-

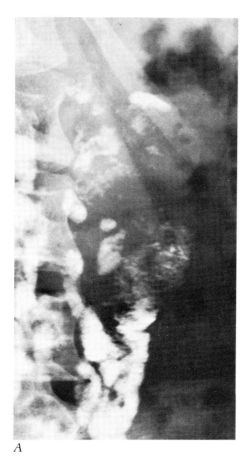
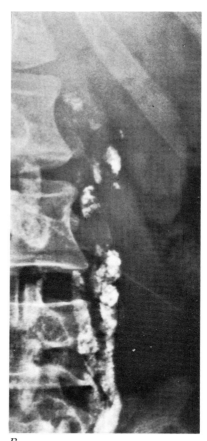

A

B

Figure 86-7. Seminoma of left testicle. (A) Metastatic spread to enlarged left aortic lymph nodes containing extensive filling defects. (B) Follow-up study after adequate radiotherapy showing marked reduction of lymph node size.

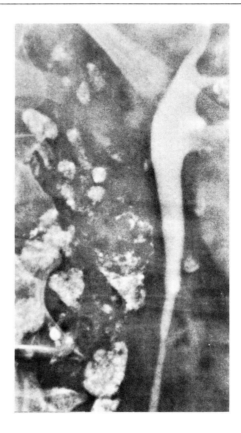

Figure 86-8. Embryonal carcinoma of left testicle. Multiple confluent filling defects within enlarged left aortic lymph nodes are due to metastatic deposits.

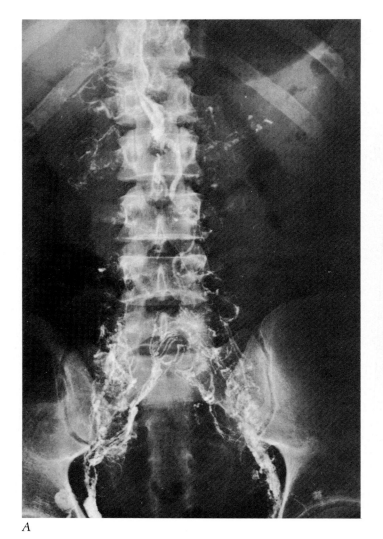

A

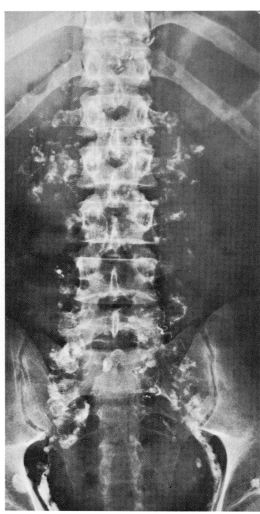

B

Figure 86-9. Choriocarcinoma of right testicle. Extensive metastatic spread within aortic and common iliac lymph nodes. Moderate obstruction of other lymphatic circulation. Partial blockage of the cisterna chyli is evident. (A) Filling phase. (B) Storage phase.

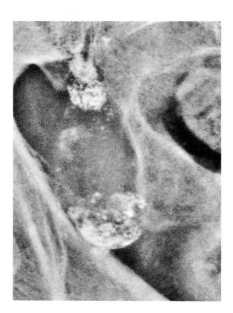

Figure 86-10. Carcinoma of the penis. Malignant metastases within enlarged medial external iliac lymph nodes containing extensive confluent filling defects.

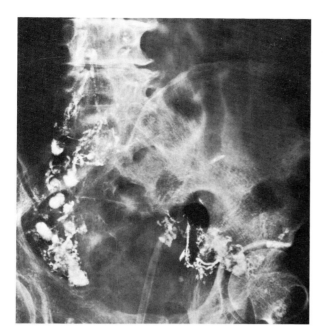

Figure 86-11. Carcinoma of the prostate. Obstruction of the lymphatic circulation due to extensive metastatic spread to the left and right iliac lymph nodes. Stasis of afferent lymphatic circulation is demonstrated.

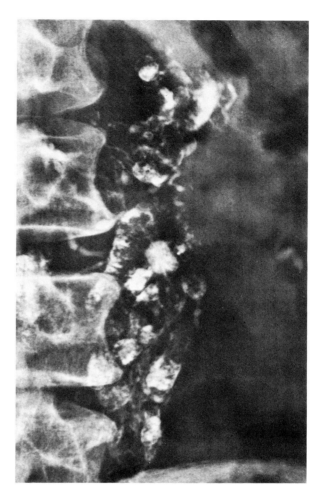

Figure 86-13. Carcinoma of the left kidney. Extensive metastatic spread within multiple enlarged left aortic lymph nodes containing numerous filling defects. Partial obstruction of lymphatic circulation is seen.

Figure 86-12. Carcinoma of the urinary bladder. Confluent filling defects due to metastatic deposits within enlarged external iliac lymph nodes.

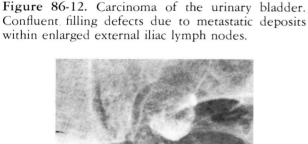

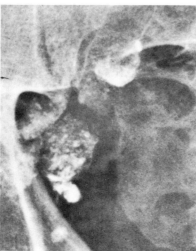

ment explains the relatively poor prognosis of most of the cases.

MALIGNANT TUMORS OF THE GASTROINTESTINAL TRACT

There is no clinical indication for lymphography in malignant tumors of the gastrointestinal tract with the possible exception of carcinoma of the rectum. In all other anatomic localizations of malignant tumors of the gastrointestinal tract lymphography does not demonstrate the regional lymph node groups [10].

In rectal carcinoma, metastatic spread to the regional lymph nodes demonstrated by lymphography is mainly observed in cases with clinically advanced tumor infiltration (Fig. 86-14). Con-

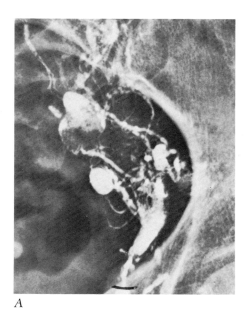

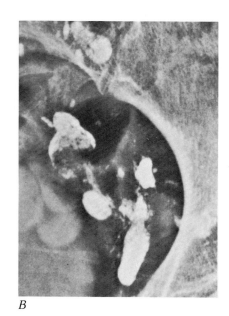

A

B

Figure 86-14. Carcinoma of the rectum. Metastatic deposits within a slightly enlarged medial external iliac lymph node. Large confluent marginal filling defects are destroying the sinus system. (A) Filling phase. (B) Storage phase.

Figure 86-15. Melanoma of the right thigh. (A) Inguinal lymph node with fibrolipomatosis and small marginal filling defect destroying the sinus system. (B) Follow-up study 4 months later shows massively enlarged lymph nodes due to progressive growth of malignant tissue.

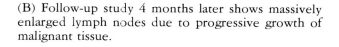

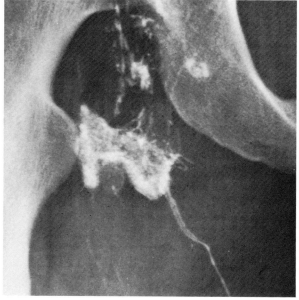

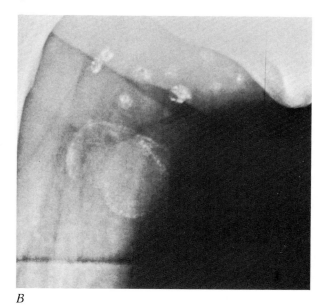

A

B

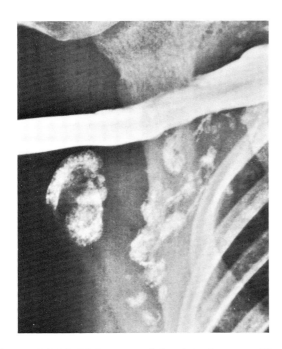

Figure 86-16. Melanoma of the right forearm. Sharply demarcated large central filling defect within an enlarged axillary lymph node is due to tumor metastases.

sequently, since lymphography seems to give no additional diagnostic information that would influence the therapeutic approach in a given patient, its clinical indications are questionable.

CARCINOMA OF THE BREAST

In carcinoma of the breast there is no indication for lymphographic investigations. Lymphography of the upper extremity demonstrates only a few lymph nodes within the axillary region. In the case of lymphedema of the upper extremity, differentiation between postsurgical and postirradiation changes and recurrence of malignant tumor is not possible.

NEOPLASMS OF THE SKIN

In *malignant melanoma* a clinical indication for lymphography is present only if the primary tumor is situated within an area where lymphography may demonstrate the regional lymph nodes (Figs. 86-15, 86-16) [5, 8, 22, 28]. Accurate knowledge of the topographic anatomy is, therefore, of particular importance. Filling defects caused by chronic inflammation and involution may lead to inconclusive diagnosis. The lymphographic findings may, however, facilitate the

evaluation of prognosis in a particular patient, since a threefold difference in the survival rate is observed in cases of negative or positive findings [8, 27].

Lymph node metastases of *skin carcinoma* are again demonstrated by lymphography only when the regional lymph nodes are within the drainage area of the dissected lymph vessel. Because the regional lymph nodes of the skin are often affected by inflammatory and involutive changes, lymphographic diagnosis is likely to be inconclusive.

References

1. Athey, P. A., Wallace, S., Jing, B.-S., Gallagher, H. S., and Smith, J. D. Lymphography in ovarian cancer. *AJR* 123:106, 1975.
2. Benninghoff, D. L., Herman, P. G., and Nelson, J. H. Clinicopathologic correlation of lymphography and lymph node metastases in gynecological neoplasms. *Cancer* 19:885, 1966.
3. Castellino, R. A., Ray, G., Blank, N., Govan, D., and Bagshaw, M. Lymphography in prostatic carcinoma: Preliminary observation. *J.A.M.A.* 223:877, 1973.
4. Cosgrove, M. D., and Metzger, C. K. Lymphangiography in genitourinary cancer. *J. Urol.* 113:93, 1975.
5. Cox, K. R., Hare, W., and Bruce, T. Lymphography in melanoma: Correlation of radiology with pathology. *Cancer* 19:637, 1966.
6. de Roo, T. Lymphangiographic studies in a series of 55 patients with malignant melanoma. *Lymphology* 6:6, 1973.
7. Dunnick, N. R., and Castellino, R. A. Lymphography in patients with suspected malignancy or fever of unexplained origin. *Radiology* 125:107, 1977.
8. Fischer, B., Göthlin, J., and Fuchs, W. A. Die Lymphographie beim malignen Melanom. *ROEFO* 121:224, 1974.
9. Fuchs, W. A. *Lymphographie und Tumordiagnostik.* Berlin: Springer, 1965.
10. Fuchs, W. A. Diagnosis of Cancer Metastases. In W. A. Fuchs, J. W. Davidson, and H. W. Fischer (eds.), *Lymphography in Cancer.* Berlin, Heidelberg, New York: Springer, 1969.
11. Fuchs, W. A., and Girod, M. Lymphography as a guide to prognosis in malignant testicular tumours. *Acta Radiol.* (Stockh.) 16:305, 1975.
12. Fuchs, W. A., and Seiler-Rosenberg, G. Lymphography in carcinoma of the uterine cervix. *Acta Radiol. [Diagn.]* (Stockh.) 16:353, 1975.
13. Ginaldi, S., Wallace, S., Jing, B. S., and Bernardino, M. E. Carcinoma of the cervix: Lymphangiography and computed tomography. *AJR* 136: 1087, 1981.

14. Jonsson, K., Ingemansson, S., and Ling, L. Lymphography in patients with testicular tumours. *Br. J. Urol.* 45:548, 1973.

15. Kolbenstvedt, A. Lymphography in the diagnosis of metastases from carcinoma of the uterine cervix stages I and II. *Acta Radiol. [Diagn.]* (Stockh.) 16:81, 1975.

16. Loening, S. A., Schmidt, J. D., Brown, R. C., Hawtrey, C. E., Fallon, B., and Culp, D. A. A comparison between lymphangiography and pelvic node dissection in the staging of prostatic cancer. *J. Urol.* 117:752, 1977.

17. Maier, J. G., and Schamber, D. T. The role of lymphangiography in the diagnosis and treatment of malignant testicular tumors. *AJR* 114:482, 1972.

18. Markovits, P., Bergiron, C., Chauvel, C. H., and Castellino, R. A. Lymphography in the staging, treatment planning, and surveillance of ovarian dysgerminomas. *AJR* 128:835, 1977.

19. Musumeci, R. E., Fossati-Bellani, F., Damascelli, B., Uslengh, C., and Bonadonna, G. Usefulness of lymphography in childhood neoplasia. *Cancer* 29:51, 1972.

20. Parker, B. R., Castellino, R. A., Fuks, Z. Y., and Bagshaw, M. A. The role of lymphography in patients with ovarian cancer. *Cancer* 34:100, 1974.

21. Piver, M. S., Wallace, S., and Gastro, J. R. The accuracy of lymphangiography in carcinoma of the uterine cervix. *AJR* 111:278, 1971.

22. Rauste, J., Tallroth, K., and Wiljasalo, M. Lymphographic changes caused by lymph node metastases in carcinoma of the suprarenal glands. *Lymphology* 9:19, 1976.

23. Sherwood, T., and O'Donoghue, E. P. N. Lymphograms in prostatic carcinoma: False-positive and false-negative assessments in radiology. *Br. J. Radiol.* 54:15, 1981.

24. Spellmann, M. C., Castellino, R. A., Ray, G. R., Pistenna, D. A., and Bagshaw, M. A. An evaluation of lymphography in localized carcinoma of the prostate. *Radiology* 125:637, 1977.

25. Takashima, T., and Benninghoff, D. L. Lymphatic venous communications and lymph reflux after thoracic duct obstruction: An experimental study in the dog. *Invest. Radiol.* 1:188, 1966.

26. Tjernberg, B. Lymphography. An animal study on the diagnosis of V × 2 carcinoma and inflammation. *Acta Radiol. [Suppl.]* (Stockh.) 214:1962.

27. Veronesi, U., Cascinelli, N., and Preda, F. Prognosis of malignant melanoma according to regional metastases. *AJR* 111:301, 1971.

28. Viamonte, M., Rüttimann, A., Gerteis, W., Bismuth, V., and Desprez-Curely, J. P. Metastatic Disease. In M. Viamonte and A. Rüttimann (eds.), *Atlas of Lymphography*. Stuttgart: Thieme, 1980.

29. Wiljasalo, M. Lymphographic differential diagnosis of neoplastic diseases. *Acta Radiol. [Suppl.]* (Stockh.) 247:1965.

30. Zingg, E. J., Fuchs, W. A., Héritier, P., and Göthlin, J. Lymphography in carcinoma of the prostate. *Br. J. Urol.* 46:549, 1974.

Malignant Lymphoma

WALTER A. FUCHS

The term *malignant lymphoma* covers all primary neoplasms of lymphoreticular tissues. Several classifications of subtypes, based on analysis of the cellular composition and pattern of a lymph node, have been proposed. The cellular composition of malignant lymphoma embraces primitive reticular cells or their histiocytic derivatives, including the stem-cell type, and derivatives from lymphocytes or their precursors. In each of these cellular subtypes a nodular or diffuse pattern may occur (Fig. 87-1) [20, 25]. For the diagnosis of *Hodgkin's lymphoma,* characteristic Reed-Sternberg cells must be identified. All other cellular compositions of malignant lymphoma have been named *non-Hodgkin's lymphoma.*

In Hodgkin's disease several subtypes of node pattern have been proposed [21] based on the type and arrangement of cellularity: lymphocytic predominance, nodular sclerosis, mixed cellularity, and lymphocytic depletion. These various histologic features may be manifestations of differences in the host response and may be related to clinical stages and survival.

Malignant lymphoma often initially affects only one lymph node group or extranodal site.

It is evident, as diagnosis of malignant lymphoma is based on cellular characteristics identified on the microscopic level, that specific lymphographic patterns corresponding to each subtype of the malignant lymphomas cannot be identified (Fig. 87-2). In spite of attempts at correlation there is no pathognomonic lymphographic pattern in malignant lymphoma that can replace the histologic examination [4, 9, 16, 18, 23, 24].

Principles of Lymphographic Diagnosis

SIZE OF LYMPH NODES

Increase in size of numerous lymph nodes or lymph node groups is an important diagnostic feature. The size of the nodes may range from slight (more than 1.5 cm diameter) to enormous enlargement. The lumbar (aortic) nodes and (aortic) lymph channels, which are normally in close connection to the spine, then extend more than 2 cm off the lateral border of the spine and 3 cm off the anterior border.

2061

Lymphosarcoma, lymphocytic ——————————— Lymphocytic, well differentiated, diffuse
                                                                    — Lymphoblastic
Lymphosarcoma, lymphoblastic ————————— Lymphocytic, poorly differentiated, diffuse
                                                                    — Mixed lymphocytic-histiocytic, diffuse
Reticulum cell sarcoma ——————————————— Histiocytic, diffuse
                                                                    — Undifferentiated (pleomorphic), diffuse
                                                                    Undifferentiated (Burkitt type), diffuse
Giant follicular lymphoma ———————————————— All of the above in nodular form

Figure 87-1. Classification of non-Hodgkin's lymphoma according to Rappaport [25].

Figure 87-2. Lymphographic pattern in malignant lymphoma. (A) Lacunar filling defects due to multiple rounded foci of lymphomatous growth. (B) Lacunar filling defects due to multiple irregularly shaped lymphomatous areas. (C) Solitary filling defects due to lymphomatous tissue confined to a section of a lymph node. (D) Large confluent filling defects due to lymphomatous tissue leading to a complete distortion of the lymph node pattern.

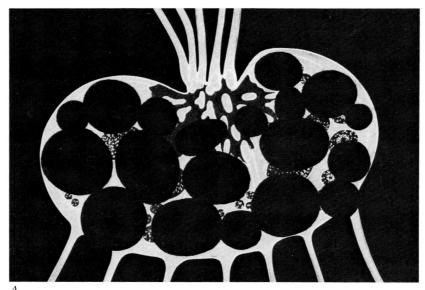

A

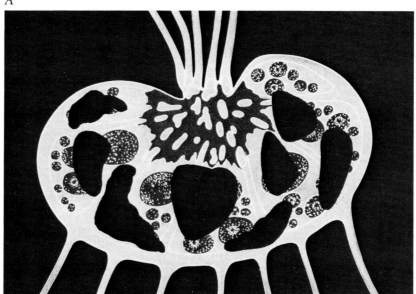

B

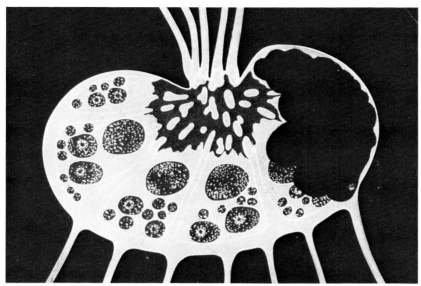

C

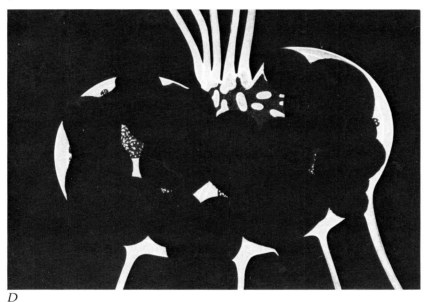

D

PATTERN OF NODES

Slightly enlarged lymph nodes usually show filling defects due to lymph follicles or nodular agglomerations of pathologic cell groups. These are homogeneously distributed within the entire node, so that the normal structural pattern of the lymph node does not seem to be altered (Fig. 87-3; see also Figs. 87-15, 87-22). Such nodular changes of *reactive hyperplasia* are nonspecific, since this lymphographic pattern may occur concomitantly in many other forms of neoplastic or inflammatory disease, as well as in immunologic disorders [6].

With increasing malignant cellular alterations within the lymph node, its size becomes moderately larger and the lymphogram demonstrates multiple contiguous *lacunar filling defects* within the entire node [9, 10]. The filling defects may be well demarcated or confluent. The marginal sinuses—that is, the contours of the nodes—may be well demonstrated and therefore intact or infiltrated by neoplastic tissue and thus appear irregular (Figs. 87-4, 87-5; see also Figs. 87-14, 87-15). In rare cases the filling defects are confined to a section of a lymph node, producing a lymphographic pattern similar to that of metastatic disease in epithelial carcinoma (Fig. 87-6).

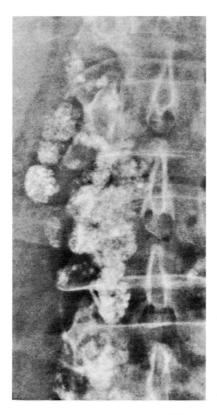

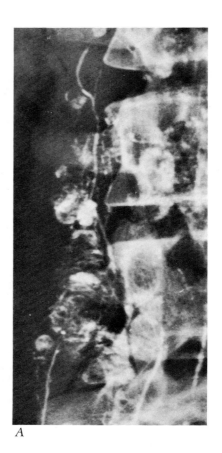

A

Figure 87-3. Hodgkin's lymphoma. Slightly enlarged aortic lymph nodes in reactive hyperplasia with homogeneously distributed filling defects due to pathologic tissue (proved by staging laparotomy).

If the malignant cellular infiltration of the lymph nodes is more advanced and the nodes have become substantially enlarged, the filling defects are confluent, the marginal sinuses are often obliterated, and the remaining lymphatic tissue is replaced and displaced by the neoplastic cellular formations (see Figs. 87-13, 87-16, 87-17, 87-19) [10, 11, 18, 27]. In this stage of the disease the lymphographic storage pattern of the nodes is completely distorted and has a *cystic, foamy* (see Figs. 87-9, 87-12, 87-16, 87-18), *irregular,* and *spotty coarse* (see Figs. 87-17–87-19), or *granular* or *reticular* structure (Fig. 87-7; see also Figs. 87-10, 87-11, 87-19). At times only

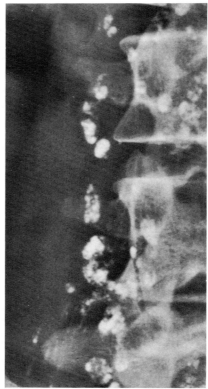

B

Figure 87-4. Hodgkin's lymphoma. (A) Moderately enlarged iliac lymph nodes with multiple lacunar filling defects. (B) Reduction of lymph node size following radiotherapy.

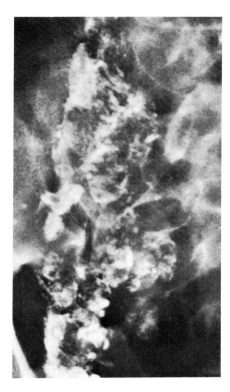

Figure 87-5. Hodgkin's lymphoma. Enlarged common iliac lymph nodes with multiple large-sized contiguous filling defects.

Figure 87-6. Hodgkin's lymphoma. Solitary filling defect confined to a section of an aortic lymph node (verified by staging laparotomy).

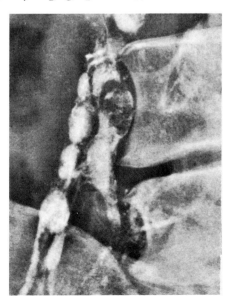

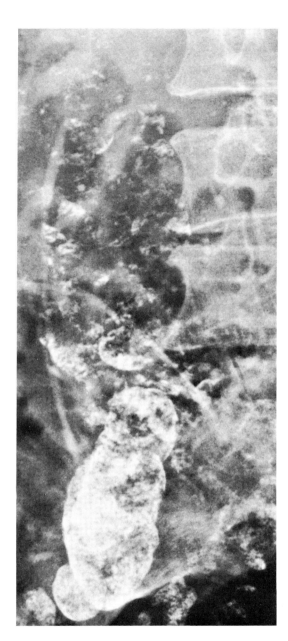

Figure 87-7. Hodgkin's lymphoma. Markedly enlarged aortic and iliac lymph nodes with completely distorted cystic storage pattern.

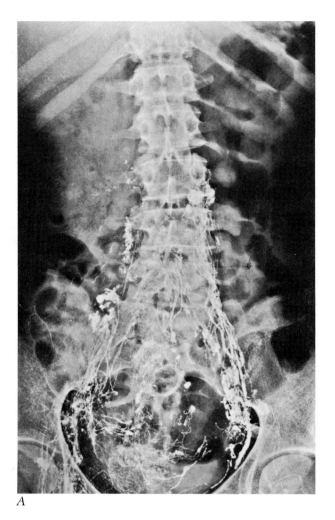

A

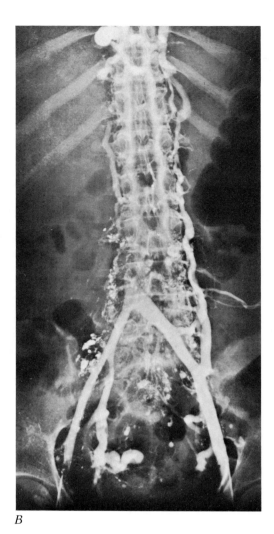

B

Figure 87-8. Hodgkin's lymphoma. (A) Extensive fibrosis of lymph nodes and lymphatic obstruction with collateral circulation in recurrent disease within aortic lymph nodes following radiotherapy. (B) Obstruction of inferior vena cava and extensive collateral venous flow. Hepatic oil embolism is shown.

the marginal sinuses are capable of storing contrast material, giving the nodes a bubblelike appearance. With extracapsular infiltration of malignant disease the outline of the lymph nodes becomes indistinct (see Figs. 87-11, 87-16, 87-17, 87-19).

In the most advanced stages of malignant cellular invasion within the lymph nodes—that is, when the entire lymphatic tissue is replaced by malignant cells—no oily contrast material is captured and stored. Identification and evaluation of the diseased lymph nodes may then become difficult. The extent of this type of advanced malignant disease can be best appreciated by evaluating the altered pathways of the distorted lymph flow.

OBSTRUCTION OF THE LYMPHATIC CIRCULATION

Stasis and obstruction of lymph vessels are substantial only in advanced lymphomatous disease (see Figs. 87-9, 87-13, 87-17) and quite rare compared to the statsis and obstruction found in malignant metastatic spread of epithelial tumors.

Secondary fibrosis leading to obstruction of the lymphatic circulation is, however, relatively frequent in cases of recurrence following radiotherapy and chemotherapy (Fig. 87-8). Numerous small tortuous lymphatics are contrast-filled as collateral channels. The lymph nodes may then be completely obliterated or replaced by neoplastic tissue.

Prolonged retention of contrast material in pathologic lymph nodes is occasionally observed for up to 2 or 3 years, whereas the normal non-involved lymph nodes have completely metabolized the contrast substance within a few months.

Diagnostic Accuracy

In malignant lymphoma, the lymphogram, which gives a gross radiologic display of the lymph node architecture, is highly accurate in detecting gross structural changes regardless of their specific etiology (Figs. 87-9–87-19). Particular lymphographic patterns are, however, not pathognomonic for any specific disease process [11, 18, 23, 27, 28]. In a careful study of consecutive previously untreated patients, Castellino et al. [6, 22] have demonstrated by a meticulous lymphographic-histologic correlation that lymphography in both Hodgkin's disease and non-Hodgkin's lymphoma has an overall diagnostic accuracy of over 90 percent in the evaluation of

Figure 87-9. Lymphosarcoma. Markedly enlarged iliac lymph nodes with cystic foamy storage pattern. Slight stasis of the lymphatic circulation is demonstrated.

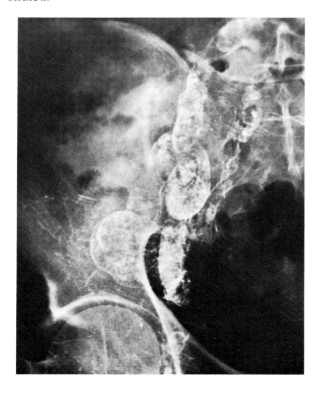

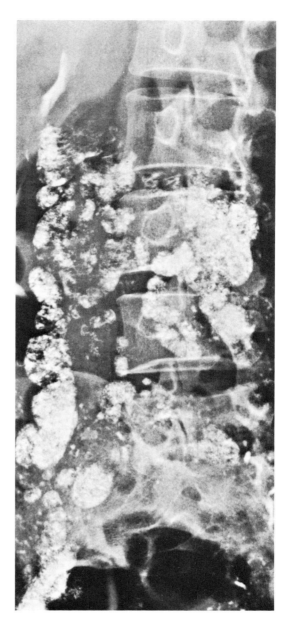

Figure 87-10. Lymphosarcoma. Enlarged iliac and aortic lymph nodes with granular and irregular coarse storage patterns.

lymph nodes demonstrated on the lymphogram (Figs. 87-20, 87-21). In *Hodgkin's disease* the overall accuracy for lymphographically visualized nodes was 92 percent with a specificity of 100 percent and a sensitivity of 75 percent. In *non-Hodgkin's lymphoma,* the overall accuracy was 91 percent with a specificity of 92 percent and a sensitivity of 89 percent. A later study of 632 patients by Marglin and Castellino [22] demonstrated an overall accuracy for lymphographically visualized nodes in Hodgkin's disease of 92 per-

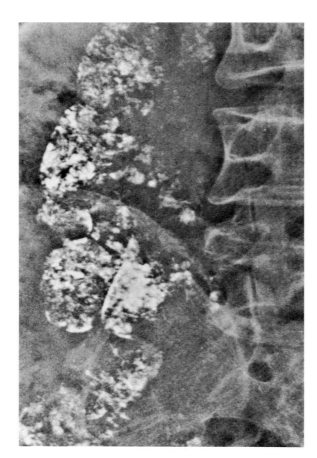

Figure 87-11. Lymphosarcoma. Markedly enlarged iliac and aortic lymph nodes with spotty coarse irregular storage pattern. Destruction of lymph node outline is due to extracapsular infiltration.

cent, with a specificity of 92 percent and a sensitivity of 93 percent. The overall accuracy for lymphographically visualized nodes in non-Hodgkin's disease was 88 percent, with a specificity of 86 percent and a sensitivity of 89 percent.

False-negative lymphograms are caused by microscopic lymph node involvement without significant distortion of nodal structure. False-positive lymphographic results are due to the demonstration of filling defects produced by obliteration of the sinus system, whether by fibrosis, proliferation of histiocytes, expansion of adjacent lymph follicles, hyaline deposition, or vascular abnormality (Figs. 87-22–87-25).

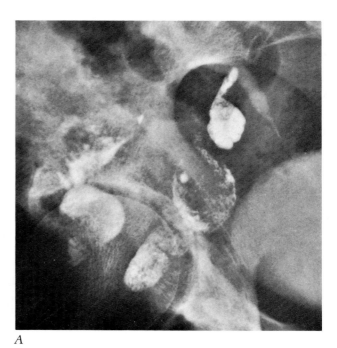

A

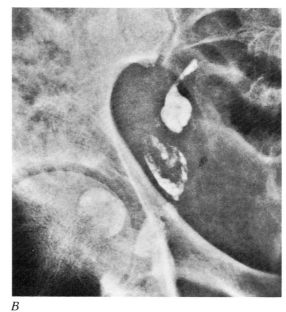

B

Figure 87-12. Lymphosarcoma. Enlarged medial external iliac lymph node with cystic bubblelike appearance. (A) Reactive hyperplasia of the neighboring nodes. (B) Marked decrease of lymph node size following radiotherapy.

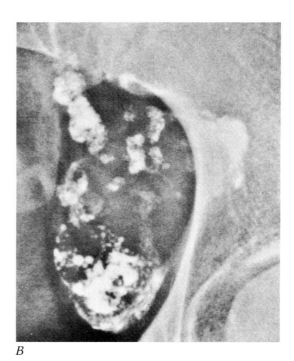

A

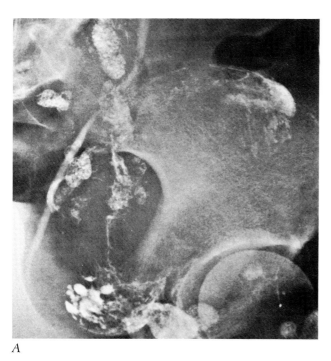

B

Figure 87-13. Reticulosarcoma. Extensive enlargement of external iliac lymph nodes with only marginal netlike storage pattern. (A) Displacement of left ureter and urinary bladder; slight stasis of lymphatic circulation. (B) Marked reduction of tumor mass following radiotherapy.

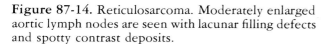

Figure 87-14. Reticulosarcoma. Moderately enlarged aortic lymph nodes are seen with lacunar filling defects and spotty contrast deposits.

Figure 87-15. Giant follicular lymphoma. Enlarged aortic and common iliac lymph nodes with lacunar filling defects and partially obliterated lymphoid tissue. Reactive hyperplasia of iliac lymph nodes. Displacement of right ureter is demonstrated.

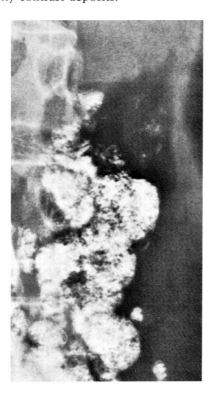

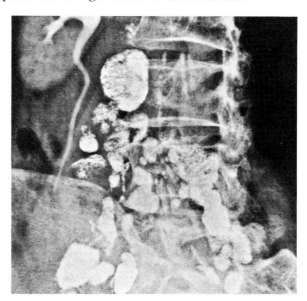

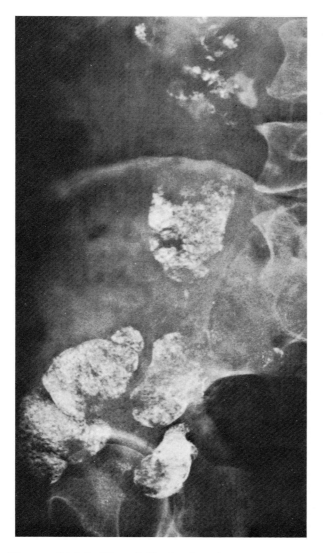

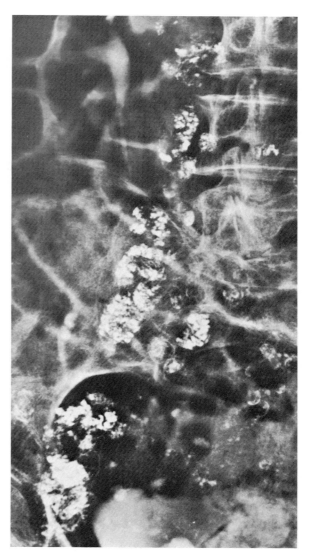

Figure 87-16. Giant follicular lymphoma. Massively enlarged iliac and aortic lymph nodes with cystic foamy pattern and partial obliteration of lymphatic tissue in upper aortic nodes.

Figure 87-17. Giant follicular lymphoma. Generally enlarged iliac and aortic lymph nodes with spotty coarse storage pattern. Slight obstruction of the lymphatic circulation. No stasis of right ureter.

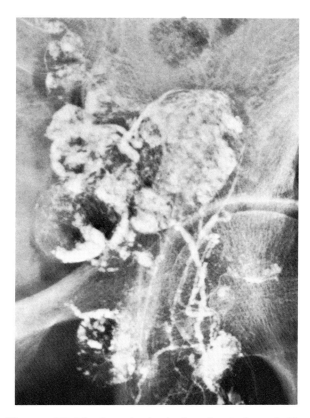

Figure 87-18. Lymphatic leukemia. Enlarged iliac lymph nodes with cystic foamy and partially spotty storage pattern.

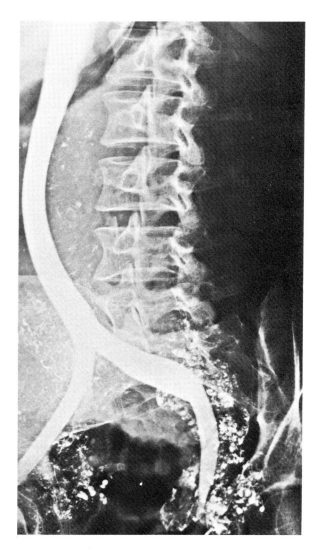

Figure 87-19. Lymphatic leukemia. Extensive malignant involvement of the massively enlarged aortic and iliac lymph nodes. Spotty and reticular storage pattern. Displacement of inferior vena cava is shown.

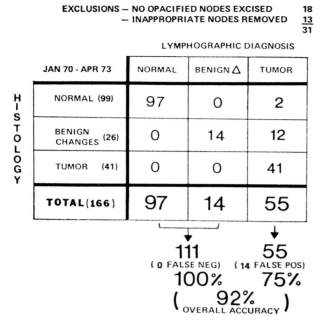

EXCLUSIONS — NO OPACIFIED NODES EXCISED   18
— INAPPROPRIATE NODES REMOVED   13
31

LYMPHOGRAPHIC DIAGNOSIS

JAN 70 - APR 73	NORMAL	BENIGN △	TUMOR
H NORMAL (99)	97	0	2
I **S** BENIGN CHANGES (26)	0	14	12
T **O** **L** TUMOR (41)	0	0	41
O **G** **Y** **TOTAL** (166)	97	14	55

111
(0 FALSE NEG)
100%
55
(14 FALSE POS)
75%

(92% OVERALL ACCURACY)

Figure 87-20. Lymphographic-histologic correlation in Hodgkin's disease. (From Castellino et al. [6].)

Figure 87-21. Lymphographic-histologic correlation in non-Hodgkin's lymphoma. (From Castellino et al. [6].)

EXCLUSIONS — NO OPACIFIED NODES EXCISED   32
— INAPPROPRIATE NODES REMOVED   8
40

LYMPHOGRAPHIC DIAGNOSIS

JULY 71 - APR 73	NORMAL	BENIGN △	TUMOR
H NORMAL (32)	32	0	0
I **S** BENIGN CHANGES (8)	0	4	4
T **O** **L** TUMOR (34)	2	1	31
O **G** **Y** **TOTAL** (74)	34	5	35

39
(3 FALSE NEG)
92%
35
(4 FALSE POS)
89%

(91% OVERALL ACCURACY)

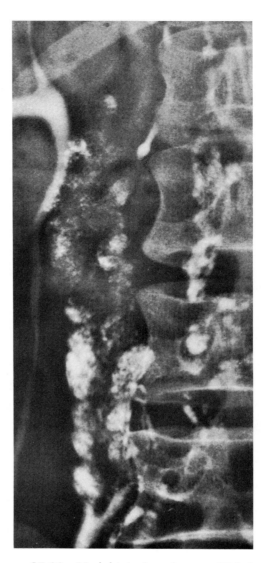

Figure 87-22. Hodgkin's lymphoma. Slightly enlarged aortic lymph nodes with partially confluent follicular filling defects due to malignant tissue (verified by staging laparotomy).

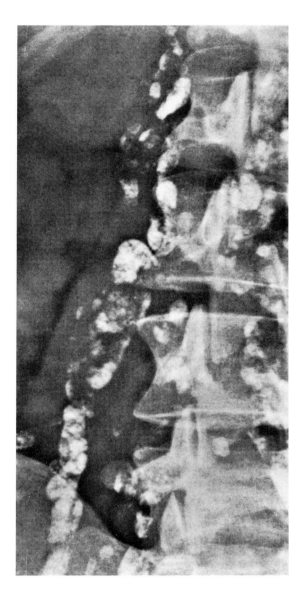

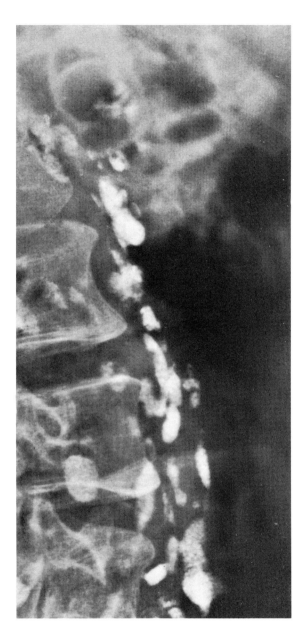

Figure 87-23. Reactive hyperplasia and fibrolipomatosis in slightly enlarged aortic lymph nodes in a patient with supradiaphragmatic Hodgkin's lymphoma (verified by staging laparotomy).

Figure 87-24. Hodgkin's lymphoma in normal-sized aortic lymph nodes, some of them showing follicular filling defects, in a patient with supradiaphragmatic Hodgkin's lymphoma (verified by staging laparotomy).

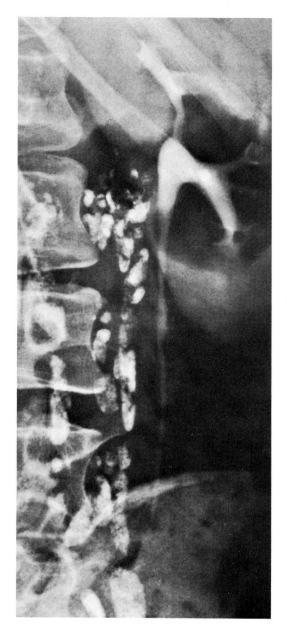

Figure 87-25. Fibrosis of normal-sized aortic lymph nodes showing filling defects due to hyaline deposition in a patient with supradiaphragmatic Hodgkin's lymphoma (verified by staging laparotomy).

Staging

In Hodgkin's disease, the stage or extent of disease at the time of diagnosis is the most important single guide to prognosis and treatment [3, 8, 12]. Lymphography and staging laparotomy with splenectomy both play a critical part in the staging process [2]. Positive lymphograms transfer about one-third of the early cases of Hodgkin's disease, i.e., stages 1 and 2, into stage 3 [1, 8, 19]. However, staging laparotomy revealed that abdominal lymphoma is present in about 25 percent of lymphographically negative asymptomatic patients in the early clinical stages 1A and 2A [17]. This substantial reduction of the accuracy rate of lymphography is due to the anatomic fact that many of the lumbar (aortic) lymph nodes, and particularly the celiac and splenic lymph node groups, are not visualized by lymphography.

In general, patients with unequivocally positive lymphograms do not require additional operative confirmation of the abdominal lymph node involvement. However, in patients with negative lymphograms, abdominal spread of malignant disease is established only by staging laparotomy.

In advanced stage 3 of Hodgkin's disease, the topographic anatomic extent of the abdominal lymph node involvement may provide a more detailed *prognostic evaluation* [5, 15]. The survival rate for patients with disease present in the aortic lymph nodes only is considerably better than for those with additional involvement of unilateral or bilateral iliac and inguinal nodes.

Therapy Planning and Control

Planning external irradiation of malignant lymphoma involves the exact topographic-anatomic localization of the portal fields [1, 5, 12]. This is accurately done on the basis of the lymphographic findings. During staging, laparotomy, and lymphadenectomy, intraoperative radiographic controls are facilitated when based on lymphographic findings.

Control roentgenograms at 4 to 6 months, following contrast injection and repeat studies, directly demonstrate the results of radiotherapy and chemotherapy [7, 13, 14, 26] (see Figs. 87-4, 87-12, 87-13). Follow-up studies with plain roentgenograms at regular time intervals permit evaluation of changes in size and storage pattern, indicating stability, recurrence, or progression of the disease.

References

1. Abrams, H. L., Takahashi, M., and Adams, D. F. Usefulness and accuracy of lymphangiography in lymphoma. *Cancer Chemother. Rep.* 52:157, 1968.

2. Aisenberg, A. C. The staging and treatment of Hodgkin's disease. *N. Engl. J. Med.* 22:1228, 1978.

3. Aisenberg, A. C., and Qazi, R. Abdominal involvement at the onset of Hodgkin's disease. *Am. J. Med.* 57:870, 1974.

4. Bottomley, J. P., Bradley, J., and Whitehouse, G. H. Waldenström's macroglobulinaemia and amyloidosis with subcutaneous calcification and lymphographic appearances. *Br. J. Radiol.* 47:232, 1974.

5. Castellino, R. A., Bagshaw, M. A., and Zboralske, F. F. Oncologic diagnostic radiology. *Radiology* 101:453, 1971.

6. Castellino, R. A., Billingham, M., and Dorfman, R. F. Lymphographic accuracy in Hodgkin's disease and malignant lymphoma with a note on the "reactive" lymph node as a cause of most false-positive lymphograms. *Invest. Radiol.* 9:155, 1974.

7. Castellino, R. A., Fuks, Z., Blank, N., and Kaplan, H. S. Roentgenologic aspects of Hodgkin's disease: Repeat lymphangiography. *Radiology* 109:53, 1973.

8. Castellino, R. A., Goffinet, D. R., Blank, N., Parker, B. R., and Kaplan, H. S. The role of radiography in the staging of non-Hodgkin's lymphoma with laparotomy correlation. *Radiology* 110:329, 1974.

9. Davidson, J. W. Hodgkin's Disease. In W. A. Fuchs, J. W. Davidson, and H. W. Fischer (eds.), *Lymphography in Cancer.* Berlin, Heidelberg, New York: Springer, 1969.

10. Davidson, J. W., and Clarke, E. A. Radiographic features of Hodgkin's disease. *Lymphology* 5:95, 1972.

11. de Roo, T. *Atlas of Lymphography.* Philadelphia: Lippincott, 1975.

12. Desforges, J. F., Rutherford, C. J., and Piro, A. Hodgkin's disease. *N. Engl. J. Med.* 301:1212, 1979.

13. Dunnick, N. R., Fuks, Z., and Castellino, R. A. Repeat lymphography in non-Hodgkin's lymphoma. *Radiology* 115:349, 1975.

14. Fabian, C. E., Nudelman, E. J., and Abrams, H. L. Postlymphangiogram film as an indicator of tumor activity in lymphoma. *Invest. Radiol.* 1:386, 1966.

15. Fuchs, W. A., Triller, J., and Haertel, M. Lymphography in Clinical Stage III Hodgkin's Disease. In K. Musshoff (ed.), *Recent Results in Cancer Research.* Berlin: Springer, 1974. Vol. 46.

16. Fuks, Z., Castellino, R. A., Carmal, J. A., et al. Lymphography in mycosis fungoides. *Cancer* 34:106, 1974.

17. Glees, J. P., Gazet, J. C., MacDonald, J. S., and Peckham, M. J. The accuracy of lymphography in Hodgkin's disease. *Clin. Radiol.* 25:5, 1974.

18. Koehler, P. R., and Salmon, R. B. Lymphographic patterns in lymphoma with emphasis on the atypical forms. *Radiology* 87:623, 1966.

19. Lee, B. J., Nelson, J. H., and Schwartz, G. Evaluation of lymphangiography, inferior venacavography, and intravenous pyelography in the clinical staging and management of Hodgkin's disease and lymphosarcoma. *N. Engl. J. Med.* 271:327, 1964.

20. Lennert, K. Pathologisch–histologische Klassifizierung der malignen Lymphome. In A. Stacher, *Leukämien und maligne Lymphome.* Internationale Arbeitstagung über Chemo-und Immunotherapie der Leukosen und Malignen Lymphome, Vienna, 1972. Munich: Urban & Schwarzenberg, 1973.

21. Lukes, R. J., and Butler, J. J. The pathology and nomenclature of Hodgkin's disease. *Cancer Res.* 26:1063, 1966.

22. Marglin, S., and Castellino, R. Lymphographic accuracy in 632 consecutive, previously untreated cases of Hodgkin disease and non-Hodgkin lymphoma. *Radiology* 140:351, 1981.

23. Parker, B. R., Blank, N., and Castellino, R. A. Lymphographic appearances of benign affectations simulating lymphoma. *Radiology* 111:267, 1974.

24. Picard, J. D., Naccache, G., Bilski-Pasquier, G., Debray, J., and Debonnière, C. Contributions à l'étude clinique et lympographique de la maladie de Brill-Symmers. À propos de trente observations. *Ann. Radiol.* (Paris) 9:685, 1966.

25. Rappaport, H. *Atlas of Tumor Pathology*, Section III, Fascicle 8. *Tumors of the Hematopoietic System.* Washington, D.C.: Armed Forces Institute of Pathology, 1966.

26. Steiner, R. M., Harell, G. S., Glatstein, E., and Wexler, L. Repeat lymphangiography in Hodgkin's disease. *Radiology* 97:613, 1970.

27. Weissleder, H. Malignant Lymphoma. In M. Viamonte and A. Rüttimann (eds.), *Atlas of Lymphography.* Stuttgart: Thieme, 1980.

28. Wiljasalo, S. Lymphographic polymorphism in Hodgkin's disease. Correlation of lymphography to histology and duration. *Acta Radiol. [Suppl.]* (Stockh.) 289, 1969.

The Diagnostic Impact of Sonography and Computed Tomography on Lymphography

WALTER A. FUCHS

Lymphography, frequently used in combination with cavography and urography, was hitherto the classic radiologic method of evaluating malignant lymphatic spread within the pelvic and lumbar areas. Considerable clinical experience and knowledge have accumulated during the last 25 years, since the introduction of the method by Kinmonth in 1954. Newer imaging techniques, such as ultrasonography and, particularly, computed tomography (CT), have recently challenged the value of lymphography for the diagnosis of lymph node metastases in epithelial neoplasms and malignant lymphoma.

Ultrasonography

Enlarged aortic and paracaval lymph nodes of more than 3 cm in diameter may be imaged by sonography (Figs. 88-1B, 88-2B, 88-3B) [5, 6, 11, 23, 28, 29]. In such cases the contours of both the abdominal aorta and the inferior vena cava may be obliterated. The enlarged nodes of uniform, very low-amplitude echogenicity will be clearly defined [26]. Anterior displacement of the abdominal aorta may also occur. The sonographic visualization of the iliac lymph nodes is possible only when they are more extensively enlarged [26]. Enlarged mesenteric lymph nodes are demonstrated ventrally adjacent to both the abdominal aorta and the inferior vena cava (Fig. 88-4). Splenic and hepatic hilar lymph nodes may also be visualized when they are substantially increased in size (Fig. 88-5).

Since sonography is capable of evaluating numerous retroperitoneal and intraperitoneal lymph node groups that are not contrast filled at lymphography, the combined application of both techniques gives better results (see Figs. 88-1–88-3). Additional diagnostic information about the topographic extent of pathologic lymph node involvement in malignant lymphoma and malignant testicular tumors may be expected in about 20 percent of cases [23].

Ultrasound-guided biopsy of a lymphomatous mass lesion is readily achieved using a specially designed biopsy transducer, by either compound or real-time technique. Conclusive diagnostic results may be expected in 60 to 80 percent of biopsies [23, 26].

Considerable difficulties in the performance of sonographic investigations may occur when loops of bowel and folds of mesentery cover the lumbar

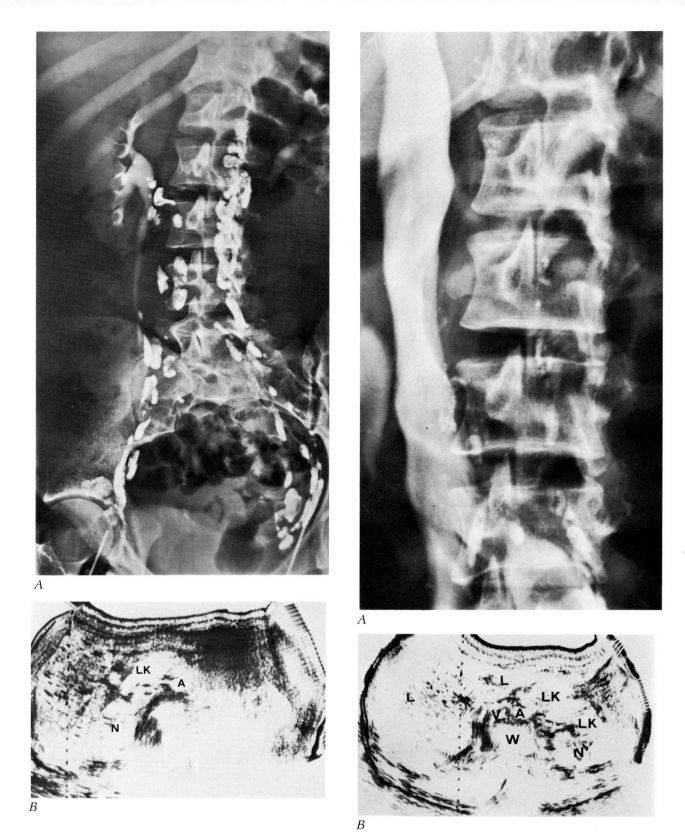

Figure 88-1. Malignant right testicular tumor (embryonal carcinoma). (A) Lymphogram. Incomplete demonstration of slightly enlarged right aortic lymph nodes; slight displacement of right ureter by enlarged nonvisualized lymph nodes. (B) Sonogram. Massively enlarged paracaval lymph nodes (*LK*) are due to metastases. *A* = aorta; *N* = right kidney.

Figure 88-2. Hodgkin's disease. (A) Lymphocavogram. Incomplete contrast filling of enlarged paracaval lymph nodes leads to compression of the inferior vena cava. (B) Sonogram. Massively enlarged left lumbar lymph nodes (*LK*). *L* = liver; *V* = inferior vena cava; *A* = abdominal aorta; *N* = left kidney; *W* = spine.

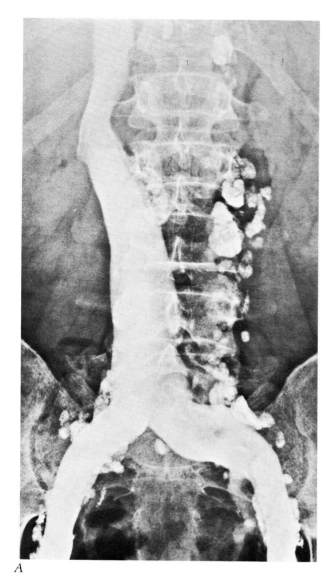

A

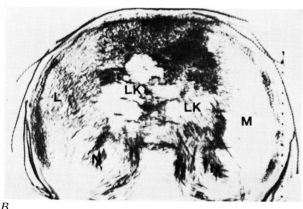

B

Figure 88-3. Non-Hodgkin's lymphoma. (A) Lymphocavogram. Moderately enlarged aortic lymph nodes with abnormal structural pattern. Indentation of inferior vena cava by nonvisualized enlarged lymph nodes. (B) Sonogram. Massively enlarged lumbar, splenic, and hepatic hilar lymph nodes (*LK*). Marked enlargement of liver (*L*) and spleen (*M*) is evident.

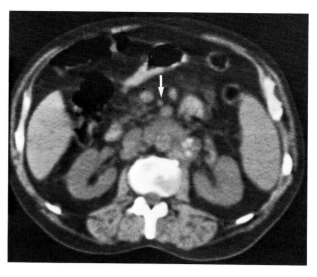

Figure 88-4. Hodgkin's disease. Enlarged aortic lymph nodes only partially contrast filled at lymphography. Enlarged mesenteric lymph nodes (*arrow*) can be seen.

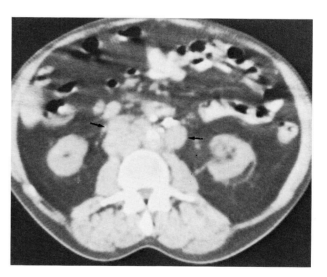

Figure 88-5. Non-Hodgkin's lymphoma (lymphocystic lymphoma). Note pathologic enlargement of paraaortic and paracaval lymph nodes (*arrows*), which are only partially contrast filled at lymphography.

2079

region, particularly in obese patients. Thus diagnostic limitations are imposed on sonography in about one-third of cases.

Computed Tomography

Lymph nodes demonstrated by CT as measuring more than 1.5 to 2.0 cm in the transverse diameter are generally regarded as abnormal. Asymmetric size and configuration of corresponding lymph nodes within the regional lymph node groups are additional signs of abnormality [8, 12, 16, 21, 27, 28]. An increase in the size of lymph nodes is nonspecific and may be due not only to malignant disease but also to inflammatory, involutive, and reactive changes. CT-guided percutaneous needle biopsy may be needed to define the cellular composition of a particular pathologic process (Figs. 88-6, 88-7). The 80 to 90 percent accuracy rate of CT mainly depends on the size and location of the pathologic nodes.

In *epithelial tumors,* CT can demonstrate enlarged regional lymph node groups, indicating the presence of malignant metastatic spread of a primary neoplasm in any anatomic site and thus achieving the *N staging* of a given malignancy [6, 14, 18, 22]. In addition, CT provides extremely valuable information about the full extent of malignant disease because it facilitates the *T staging* of a given malignancy by demonstrating both the location and size of the primary tumor, as well as its extension into the adjacent structures and organs (Fig. 88-8) [13, 16]. Distant

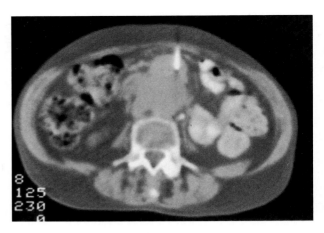

Figure 88-7. Endometrial carcinoma of the uterine corpus. Computed tomography–guided percutaneous biopsy of paraaortic lymph node metastases.

metastatic spread—to the liver, lung, and bone—is readily demonstrated by CT, and thus *M staging* of a given malignancy is achieved.

In *malignant lymphoma,* CT compares favorably with lymphography in the assessment of pelvic and abdominal lymph node involvement, demonstrating the full extent of the disease (see Figs. 88-4, 88-5) [1–4, 8–10, 12, 15, 19, 20, 24, 25, 30]. The overall distribution of lymph node involvement, both above and below the diaphragm, may be assessed by CT more accurately prior to treatment. Extranodal spread to the bone and lungs can be identified, and malignant involvement of either spleen or liver may be suggested.

In the *pelvic area,* CT can demonstrate pathologic enlargement of the external and common iliac lymph nodes, when malignant lymphatic obstruction is not demonstrated in the more centrally located pathologically involved node groups. Enlarged internal iliac lymph nodes that are not contrast filled at lymphography indicate malignant metastatic spread in gynecologic cancer (Fig. 88-8), malignant bladder tumors, carcinoma of the prostate (Fig. 88-9), and carcinoma of the rectosigmoid colon. Contralateral asymmetry of the enlarged nodes is a particularly important diagnostic sign of malignant metastatic spread to the regional lymph nodes [16, 27].

In the *aortic (lumbar) area,* it is extremely uncommon for lymphography to demonstrate the full extent of lymphadenopathies. This particularly applies to lymphoma (see Fig. 88-5) but is also true of malignant testicular (Fig. 88-10) and renal tumors. Compared to CT, in lymphography

Figure 88-6. Embryonal carcinoma of the left testicle. Computed tomography–guided percutaneous biopsy of left paravertebral lymph node metastases.

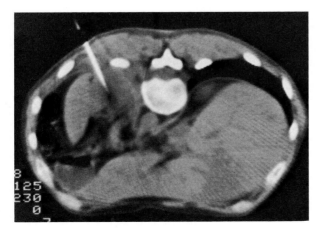

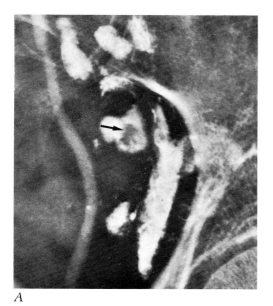

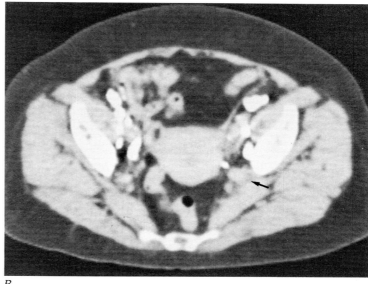

A   B

Figure 88-8. Carcinoma of the uterine cervix. (A) Lymphogram. Centrally situated round filling defect within a slightly enlarged medial external iliac lymph node, a result of malignant metastases (*arrow*). (B) Computed tomogram. Tumorous enlargement of uterus; neoplastic invasion of parauterine tissue. Enlarged metastatic left internal iliac lymph nodes (*arrow*) and enlarged metastatic left external iliac lymph nodes are evident.

Figure 88-9. Carcinoma of the prostate. (A) Lymphogram. Enlarged left external iliac lymph nodes with filling defects suggest the presence of metastases. (B) Computed tomogram. Enlarged metastatic left internal iliac lymph nodes (*arrow*). Enlarged metastatic external iliac lymph nodes are partially contrast filled.

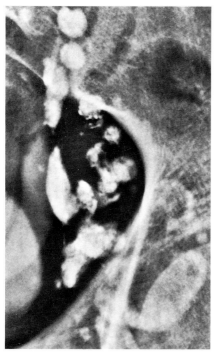

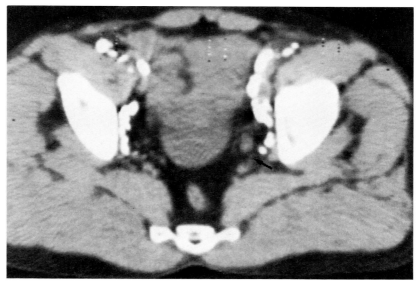

A   B

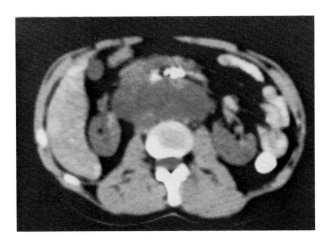

Figure 88-10. Malignant testicular tumor (embryonal carcinoma). Note extensive enlargement of the aortic lymph nodes, which are only partially visualized at lymphography. Hepatic oil embolism is due to tumorous obstruction of the inferior vena cava.

only small parts of the node mass take up the contrast substance [7, 30].

Mesenteric lymph nodes (see Fig. 88-4) and lymph nodes in the porta hepatis and splenic hilus are all outside the scope of lymphography. Owing to the large amount of surrounding fatty tissue, these nodes are easily demonstrated by CT, either as solitary manifestations of lymph node disease or in association with lumbar (aortic) lymph node enlargement [2, 17].

References

1. Alcorn, F. S., Mategrano, V. C., Petasnick, J. P., and Clark, J. W. Contributions of computed tomography in the staging and management of malignant lymphoma. *Radiology* 125:717, 1977.
2. Bernardino, M. E., Jing, B. S., and Wallace, S. Computed tomography diagnosis of mesenteric masses. *AJR* 132:33, 1979.
3. Best, J. J. K., Blackledge, G., Forbes, W. S., Todd, I. D., Eddleston, B., Crowther, D., and Isherwood, I. Computed tomography of abdomen in staging and clinical management of lymphoma. *Br. J. Med.* 2:1675, 1978.
4. Blackledge, G., Best, J. J. K., Crowther, D., and Isherwood, I. Computed tomography (CT) in the staging of patients with Hodgkin's disease: A report on 136 patients. *Clin. Radiol.* 31:143, 1980.
5. Brascho, D. J., Durant, J. R., and Green, L. E. The accuracy of retroperitoneal ultrasonography in Hodgkin's disease and non-Hodgkin's lymphoma. *Radiology* 125:485, 1977.
6. Burney, B. T., and Klatte, E. C. Ultrasound and computed tomography of the abdomen in the staging and management of testicular carcinoma. *Radiology* 132:415, 1979.
7. Dunnick, N. R., and Javadpour, N. Value of CT and lymphography: Distinguishing retroperitoneal metastases from nonseminomatous testicular tumors. *AJR* 136:1093, 1981.
8. Earl, H. M., Sutcliffe, S. B. J., Fry, I. K., Tucker, A. K., Young, J., Husband, J., Wrigley, P. F. M., and Malpas, J. S. Computerised tomographic (CT) abdominal scanning in Hodgkin's disease. *Clin. Radiol.* 31:149, 1980.
9. Ehrlichman, R. J., Kaufman, S. L., Siegelman, S. S., Trump, D. L., and Walsh, P. C. Computerized tomography and lymphangiography in staging testis tumors. *J. Urol.* 126:179, 1981.
10. Ellert, J., and Kreel, L. The role of computed tomography in the initial staging and subsequent management of the lymphomas. *J. Comput. Assist. Tomogr.* 4:368, 1980.
11. Filly, R. A., Marglin, S., and Castellino, R. A. The ultrasonographic spectrum of abdominal and pelvic Hodgkin's disease and non-Hodgkin's lymphoma. *Cancer* 38:2143, 1976.
12. Harell, G. S., Breiman, R. S., Glatstein, E. J., Marshall, W. H. Jr., and Castellino, R. A. Computed tomography of the abdomen in the malignant lymphomas. *Radiol. Clin. North Am.* 15:391, 1977.
13. Hodson, N. J., Husband, J. E., and MacDonald, J. S. The role of computed tomography in the staging of bladder cancer. *Clin. Radiol.* 30:389, 1979.
14. Husband, J. E., Barrett, A., and Peckham, M. J. Evaluation of computed tomography in the management of testicular teratoma. *Br. J. Urol.* 53:179, 1981.
15. Jones, S. E., Tobias, D. A., and Waldman, R. S. Computed tomographic scanning in patients with lymphoma. *Cancer* 41:480, 1978.
16. Kilcheski, T. S., Arger, P. H., Mulhern, C. B., Jr., Coleman, B. G., Kressel, H. Y., and Mikuta, J. I. Role of computed tomography in the presurgical evaluation of carcinoma of the cervix. *J. Comput. Assist. Tomogr.* 5:378, 1981.
17. Kreel, L. The EMI whole body scanner in the demonstration of lymph node enlargement. *Clin. Radiol.* 27:421, 1976.
18. Lackner, K., Weissbach, L., Boldt, I., Scherholz, K., and Brecht, G. Computertomographischer Nachweis von Lymphknotenmetastasen bei malignen Hodentumoren. Ein Vergleich der Ergebnisse von Lymphographie und Computertomographie. *ROEFO* 130:636, 1979.
19. Lee, J. K., Stanley, R. J., Sagel, S. S., Melson, G. L., and Koehler, R. E. Limitations of the postlymphangiogram plain abdominal radiograph as an indicator of recurrent lymphoma: Comparison

to computed tomography. *Radiology* 134:155, 1980.

20. Lee, K. T., McClennan, B. L., Stanley, R. J., and Sagel, S. S.   Computed tomography in the staging of testicular neoplasms. *Radiology* 130:387, 1979.

21. Levine, M. S., Arger, P. H., Coleman, B. G., Mulhern, C. B., Jr., Pollack, H. M., and Wein, A. J.   Detecting lymphatic metastases from prostatic carcinoma: Superiority of CT. *AJR* 137:207, 1981.

22. Marchal, G., Coenen, Y., Wilms, G., and Baert, A. L.   The accuracy of TC-scan in the diagnosis of retroperitoneal metastases of malignant testicular tumours. *ROEFO* 128:746, 1978.

23. Rochester, D., Bowie, H. D., Kunzmann, A., and Lester, E.   Ultrasound in the staging of lymphoma. *Radiology* 124:483, 1977.

24. Schaner, E. G., Head, G. L., Doppman, J. L., and Young, R. C.   Computed tomography in the diagnosis, staging, and management of abdominal lymphoma. *J. Comput. Assist. Tomogr.* 1:176, 1977.

25. Stephens, D. H., Williamson, B. Jr., Sheedy, P.

F., Hattery, R. R., and Miller, W. E.   Computed tomography of the retroperitoneal space. *Radiol. Clin. North Am.* 15:377, 1977.

26. Triller, J., and Fuchs, W. A.   *Abdominelle Sonographie, Lymphknoten.* Stuttgart: Thieme, 1980.

27. Vock, P., Haertel, M., Fuchs, W. A., Karrer, P., Bishop, M. C., and Zingg, E.   Computed tomography in staging of carcinoma of the urinary bladder. *Br. J. Urol.* 54:158, 1982.

28. Walsh, J. W., Amendola, M. A., Konerding, K. F., Tisnado, J., and Hazra, T. A.   Computed tomographic detection of pelvic and inguinal lymph-node metastases from primary and recurrent pelvic malignant disease. *Radiology* 137:157, 1980.

29. Weil, F., Eisenscher, A., Aucant, D., and Bourgoin, A.   Apport de l'échotomographie dans le diagnostic des masses retropéritonéales. *Ann. Radiol.* 18:763, 1976.

30. Zelch, M. G., and Haaga, J. R.   Clinical comparison of computed tomography and lymphangiography for detection of retroperitoneal lymphadenopathy. *Radiol. Clin. North Am.* 17:157, 1979.

VI

Interventional
Techniques

1. Angioplasty

Percutaneous Transluminal Coronary Angioplasty

ANDREAS R. GRÜNTZIG

In 1929, in Germany, Forssmann, in an attempt to devise a method for intracardiac drug injection, introduced a catheter into his own right atrium [1]. With the advent of such experimentation, the era of invasive cardiology had begun.

In the following decades the catheter was used primarily as a diagnostic tool, until in 1964, in the United States, Dotter and Judkins described catheter application to recanalize atherosclerotic obstructions of peripheral arteries [2]. These authors used a coaxial double catheter that could be passed through an obstructed area of the femoral artery in a stepwise fashion, thereby enlarging the stenosed lumen.

Despite the skepticism of the medical community, the method was kept alive and developed further by the German radiologists Porstmann [3] and Zeitler [4].

In 1971, this treatment modality was incorporated into use in Zurich. Several disadvantages of Dotter's coaxial catheter for femoral popliteal obstructions and Porstmann's caged balloon catheter for iliac stenoses led to the modification of the technique in 1974 using a catheter with a distensible (balloon) tip [5]. The relative simplicity of the procedure, as well as the encouraging long-term results, were some of the advantages of the new method [6, 7].

In 1976, the balloon catheter was further modified for coronary angioplasty that was performed first in dogs and later in human cadaver studies [8, 9]. Then in San Francisco, in cooperation with Myler, intraoperative coronary angioplasty was performed to evaluate the use of the technique in dilatation of atherosclerotic plaques in living human beings [10].

Following a period of probing human coronary arteries, I performed the first percutaneous transluminal coronary angioplasty (PTCA) on September 16, 1977, at our center in Zurich. Shortly thereafter, we introduced the technique in cooperation with Kaltenbach in Frankfurt. In March, 1978, Myler, in San Francisco, and Stertzer, in New York, performed the first cases in the United States.

Rationale of the Technique

The dilatation of a chronic atherosclerotic stenosis by means of mechanical forces is made possible because the atheroma obstructing the arterial lumen consists of a variety of components including low-density fatty material and liquid-containing vacuoles that can be compressed, as well as calcified hardened material that is split on dilatation. The two mechanisms, compression and splitting, are involved to a greater or lesser degree depending on the character of the lesion—whether it is hard or soft [11].

In the presence of a good blood flow, organization and fibrosis of this material then takes place, with smoothing of the wall of the recanalized vessel [12]. The healing of this controlled injury has been demonstrated in the follow-up period by hemodynamic, angiographic, and histologic studies after dilatation of peripheral and coronary artery stenosis [6, 13, 14].

Method

The catheter assembly for PTCA consists of two catheters: a guiding catheter and a dilatation catheter. The guiding catheter is introduced at either the groin or the brachial artery, and it is preshaped in such a way that it can be positioned at the orifice of the left or the right coronary artery (Fig. 89-1A). Probing of the bypass graft is made possible by modification of the guiding catheter. The guiding catheter is not tapered at the tip, and thus allows the passage of the dilatation catheter through its inner lumen. To allow the introduction of the dilatation catheter by the Seldinger (femoral) technique, a 9.5 French introducer sheath is advanced over a standard 0.95-mm femoral guidewire. The sheath is intro-

duced under local anesthesia at the groin. The appropriate right or left femoral guiding catheter is then passed through the introducer sheath and advanced into the abdominal aorta. A 1.6-mm guidewire is preloaded into the guiding catheter to facilitate passage through the sheath. The guiding catheter is advanced retrogradely into the ascending aorta and manipulated into the orifice of the coronary artery to be dilated. This catheter remains at the coronary orifice and is positioned in such a way that no obstruction of the orifice occurs. Through this catheter, the dilatation catheter is advanced into the stenotic arterial branch (Fig. 89-1B). The dilatation catheter has an outer diameter of 4.5 French, which is tapered to 0.5 mm (2 French) at the tip. The tip of the dilatation catheter is connected to a short, soft wire that directs the catheter into the artery, avoiding injury to the arterial wall. Although it is fixed in the Grüntzig catheter, other systems are available in which this wire can be removed during manipulation. Just proximal to the guidewire is a side hole connected to the main lumen of the dilatation catheter. The main lumen of the dilatation catheter is connected to a manifold and is used for pressure recording and radiographic contrast medium injections distal to the balloon. To provide a comparison, the aortic pressure at the orifice of the coronary ostium is recorded through the guiding catheter. The simultaneous recording of pressure through the guiding catheter while the dilatation catheter is in place is made possible by use of a Y connector at the end

Figure 89-1. (A) Variety of shapes of available guiding catheters. (B) Guiding catheter and dilatation catheter (inflated balloon) are shown.

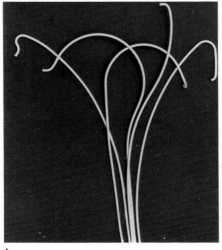

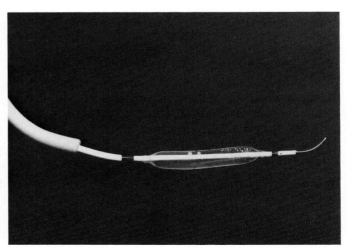

A

B

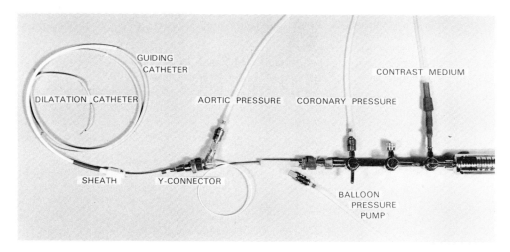

Figure 89-2. Manifold arrangement facilitates simultaneous proximal and distal pressure recording as well as contrast medium injection and balloon inflation.

of the guiding catheter (Fig. 89-2). The balloon is filled with dilute contrast material, which consists of a 50:50 mixture by volume of the contrast agent, such as Renografin-76, and sterile normal saline. This mixture is injected using the second lumen of the dilatation catheter via the respective Luer-Lok connection. Before introduction of the dilatation catheter into the artery, the balloon should be tested using the mixture described above and a pressure equal to that expected during the procedure. The amount of time required for complete inflation and deflation should also be evaluated prior to the use. A vacuum is then established in the balloon inflation lumen of the dilatation catheter and the deflated balloon is folded like an umbrella just prior to the insertion into the Y connector. Balloon withdrawal should be accomplished under the same vacuum conditions. The expandable segment manifests only minimal change over the predetermined outer diameter over a wide range of inflation pressures. The balloon segment is manufactured in a variety of maximal outer diameters, ranging between 3 and 4 mm, designed to adapt to the left anterior descending, circumflex, and right coronary arteries. The pressure distribution throughout the expanded segment is uniform, and thus the inflated balloon will not expand the vessel into an hourglass shape. In addition, expansion of the vessel lumen beyond its natural diameter has to be avoided. It is therefore recommended that the maximal outer diameter of the balloon be smaller than the diameter of the undiseased artery proximal or distal to the stenosis. Should the distensible segment be dam-

aged during the dilatation, the balloon will tear longitudinally—the internal pressure will drop to zero immediately—and only fluid will escape into the artery. The inflation and deflation of the balloon are controlled by a calibrated pressure pump (Fig. 89-3). The use of such an automatic inflation device is recommended highly. The balloon is prepared for insertion by carefully filling it with the contrast mixture and inflating and deflating it several times, first by hand, then using the pressure pump to obtain an air-free system. The balloon is also manipulated in its inflated state to ensure symmetric expansion to detect leaks and air bubbles. Thorough evaluation

Figure 89-3. Automatic pressure pump for inflation of balloon and electronic pressure gauge for measuring balloon pressure are shown.

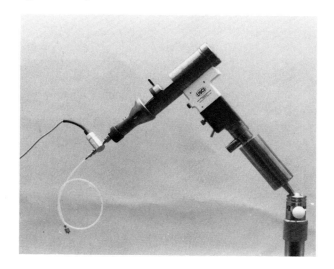

of all equipment is imperative prior to the use of any catheter component.

Brachial artery transluminal angioplasty is performed in standard fashion using the Sones cutdown technique. A flexible guidewire is passed through the Sones catheter to the root of the aorta. Over this guidewire, a brachial guiding catheter is introduced into the aortic root with the assistance of a 3 French Teflon lead catheter. Unlike the femoral guiding catheter, the brachial guiding catheter is not made preformed and tapered, and has side holes. These side holes should prevent wedging of the coronary ostium during engagement of the right and left arteries by Sones-type manipulation. The brachial guiding catheters are approximately 8.5 French in diameter, and one catheter can be used for a stenosis located in either the right or left coronary system.

Procedure

The procedure is carried out with the patient in the fasting state, premedicated with a tranquilizer such as Valium. After local anesthesia of the groin or the brachial cutdown site, a pacing catheter with an additional lumen is inserted into the corresponding vein through an introducer sheath or directly in the case of a cutdown and is advanced into the pulmonary artery. The pacing catheter has several purposes. First, the electrodes are positioned in the right ventricle for capture on demand. Second, the markers on the catheter help in identifying the position of the coronary lesion in space. Third, its lumen may be used for drug injections or pressure measurements.

The guiding catheter is then positioned at the orifice of the appropriate coronary artery or the orifice of the bypass graft without obstructing it. Heparin in a dose of 10,000 units is then administered to avoid clot formation, and sufficient doses of nitrates and calcium antagonists are given sublingually to avoid coronary spasm during the procedure. A single coronary angiogram is obtained in the projection that best displays the lesion as determined from previous arteriography. The use of biplane fluoroscopy aids in orientation and positioning of the dilatation catheter. The stenosis may be repetitively visualized on the monitor using the videotape playback.

If the previous catheterization was performed in another hospital or a considerable period prior to this procedure, the complete set of standard projections, including the left anterior or the right anterior oblique hemiaxial views, is repeated. With these views, lesions of the proximal third of the left anterior descending artery are best displayed because the full extent of the lesion is revealed, overlap of branches is avoided, and the degree of an eccentric stenosis is then accentuated [15, 16].

Once the guiding catheter is positioned at the orifice, the dilatation catheter is very slowly advanced into the coronary artery with the balloon deflated while the coronary pressure is monitored through its tip. Simultaneously, the aortic pressure is recorded through the tip of the guiding catheter. Correct pressure measurements are very important, because the improvement of the distal coronary pressure aids in the decision to terminate the procedure.

Abrupt maneuvers done with force must be avoided. If the lesion is too hard and its lumen too small, passage through the stenosis may not be possible. In this situation, further attempts to advance the dilatation catheter will result in backward displacement of the guiding catheter into the aortic root, indicating the problem. However, if the lesion is soft, a lumen that is smaller than the catheter will allow passage of the dilatation catheter. An example of such a dilatation is shown in Figure 89-4.

Small injections of contrast material through the manifold and the main lumen of the dilatation catheter and coordination with the vertical presence of the electrodes of the preplaced pacing catheter in the outflow tract of the right ventricle aid in the recognition of the coronary anatomy through biplane projection during the maneuver. When the catheter tip traverses the stenosis, the pressure tracing demonstrates a drop in distal pressure as compared with that proximal to the stenosis, with both represented as a phasic waveform (Fig. 89-5).

Once the dilatation catheter is properly positioned, the balloon is immediately inflated to a pressure of 4 to 5 atmospheres (60–75 psi). Inflation of the balloon into a sausage shape is monitored by fluoroscopy. Expansion of the balloon compresses the atheroma, thereby enlarging the lumen. The balloon is then deflated by the pump, and the postdilatation pressures are recorded. A marked rise in distal pressure indicates the successful recanalization of the artery. The

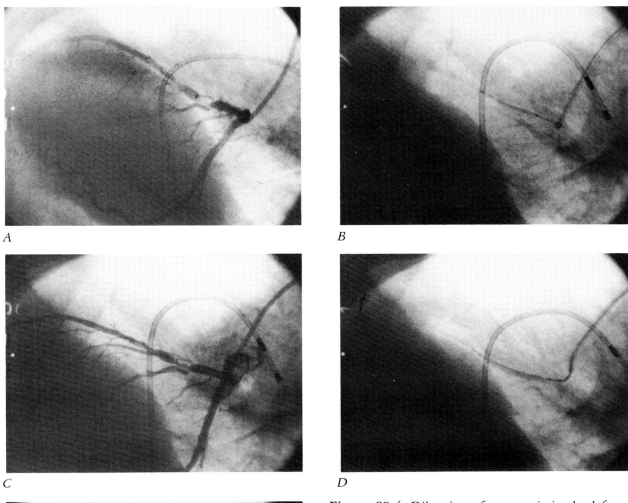

A

B

C

D

E

Figure 89-4. Dilatation of a stenosis in the left anterior descending coronary artery that was initially too small for standard 20-30 catheters (A). Use of a smaller (20-20) catheter (B) results in some increase in luminal size (C), allowing for passage of the larger catheter (D) and marked improvement in vessel lumen (E).

procedure is then terminated, and the pullback pressures are recorded. In the case shown in Figure 89-5, the pullback pressure indicates an excellent hemodynamic result.

Usually the inflation of the balloon with compression of the atheroma is repeated two to four times. The time necessary for passage of the catheter through the stenosis, the inflation and deflations, and the pullback is about 2 to 5 minutes. The time necessary for the whole procedure, including preinterventional and postinterventional angiograms, can be as short as 1 hour or

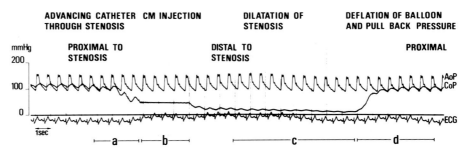

Figure 89-5. Simultaneous coronary pressure tracings proximal and distal to the stenosis are seen: (*a*) crossing the stenosis, (*b*) checking balloon position, (*c*) at inflation of balloon, and (*d*) at deflation of the balloon and pullback. This tracing illustrates a good hemodynamic result with almost no residual pressure gradient.

less. If the coronary anatomy is difficult, as in the case of a sharply angled takeoff of the left anterior descending artery, the selective catheterization becomes laborious. Various techniques may be used to overcome such a situation. Preshaping of the dilatation catheter by using a special type of catheter with a built-in wire (type DG or DJ) and changing the position of the guiding catheter aid in reaching the target. In such cases, the procedure may take 2 hours, with a fluoroscopic time of up to 30 to 40 minutes. It is hoped that future developments in dilatation catheters will reduce these difficulties. Because experience has been accumulated in several centers using our technique for more than 4 years, it is strongly suggested that no operator should apply PTCA without undergoing adequate training in such a center.

The dilatation catheter is finally withdrawn and at least four coronary arteriograms in various orientations, including oblique and hemiaxial views, are performed through the guiding catheter to assess the result of dilatation. The percent stenosis is calculated using the mean value of percent stenosis calculated from three angiographic views of the vessel [17]. The hemodynamic result is estimated by calculating the mean pressure gradient across the stenosis before and after dilatation. It should be noted, however, that the pressure gradient across the stenosis provides only an index of the severity of the lesion because of the influence of the presence of the dilatation catheter on the pressure recording. However, if there is no change in the cardiac output as predicted from heart rate and blood pressure, a decline in the mean pressure gradient after dilatation must represent reduction in stenosis, since the size of the catheter remains the same.

Additional Considerations

The procedure is done when the operative facilities are available for backup. In case of complications, such as total occlusion of an artery at the site of dilatation with impending infarction, coronary bypass must be done immediately in order to avoid a definite infarction. In hospitals with smaller operative programs, the procedure may be scheduled in the afternoon, when the routine work of cardiac surgery is done.

Additional therapy includes the use of acetylsalicylic acid before dilatation, for platelet inhibition. Promptly after the dilatation, long-term adjunctive therapy with aspirin is begun (unless contraindicated), and is maintained for at least 6 months, at which time a control angiography is done. The value of such therapy is currently being evaluated by randomized studies to determine whether this therapy improves vessel patency in the follow-up period.

After dilatation, 12-lead electrocardiogram tracings and testing of cardiac enzymes are repeated every 8 hours for the first 24 hours. The patient should be monitored for at least 6 hours after the procedure. The patient is discharged 2 days after angioplasty, maintained on such medical treatment as the use of nitrate, beta-blocking agents, or calcium antagonists, as is deemed necessary.

Patient Selection

Patients with an accessible stenosis less than 15 mm in length (as judged from coronary arteriograms) and a short history of pain (less than 1 year)

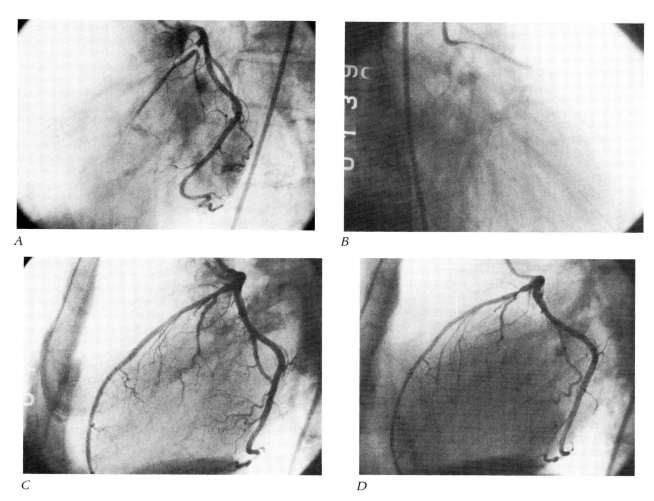

A

B

C

D

Figure 89-6. High-grade proximal left anterior descending coronary artery stenosis (A). Dilated with balloon catheter (B), the excellent result is shown in (C). The 6-month follow-up angiogram (D) showed a partial recurrence, but the patient remained symptom free.

are most suitable for the procedure. The patients should also be suitable candidates for surgery according to symptoms and clinical status.

Results of previous catheterization studies and coronary angiograms of potential candidates for the procedure are reviewed and then discussed with the cardiac surgeons. The possible benefits and risks of the procedure and the alternative treatments are explained to the patient, as is the possibility that he may have to undergo cardiac surgery in case of emergency. After informed consent is obtained, the procedure is performed when the surgeon, anesthesiologist, and operating room with cardiopulmonary bypass equipment are available.

In regard to indications for PTCA, the patient should meet the following criteria: (1) the patient should have disabling angina pectoris; (2) his history of angina pectoris should be short, indicating a more easily compressed atheroma; (3) the disease ideally should be limited to a high-grade stenosis (more than 70%) in one dominant artery; and (4) the left ventricular function at rest should be well preserved. Patients with recurrent arterial stenoses after angioplasty can have vessels dilated a second time. Additional indications such as multivessel disease, recurrence of stenosis after coronary artery bypass surgery, and prophylactic dilatation of moderate stenosis in the presence of mild symptoms are under investigation. Typical examples of successful PTCA procedures are shown in Figures 89-6 to 89-8. Dilatation may also be used in the case of saphenous vein graft closure.

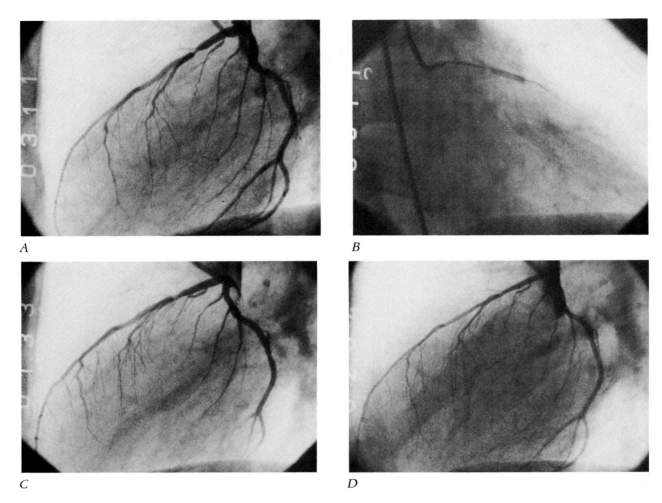

A

B

C

D

Figure 89-7. This is an example of further improvement of vessel patency in the follow-up period (A and B). Stenosis of the proximal left anterior descending coronary artery is shown in (C), illustrating the shady appearance and residual stenosis noted immediately after the procedure. Six months later, however, the artery is markedly improved as shown in (D).

The main reason for limiting PTCA to patients with single-vessel disease is that should a complication of PTCA occur with abrupt reclosure of the dilated segment, the patient will be at considerably decreased risk if only the treated vessel is diseased (allowing vessels to supply and increase collateral flow).

With these restrictive indications, at present only a small percentage of patients undergoing diagnostic coronary arteriography are deemed suitable for the procedure. This figure ranges from 3 to 15 percent depending on the center. The published figure that 7 of 100 consecutively catheterized patients were candidates for dilatation seems reasonable [19].

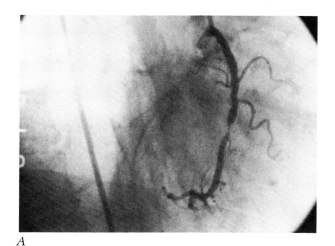

A

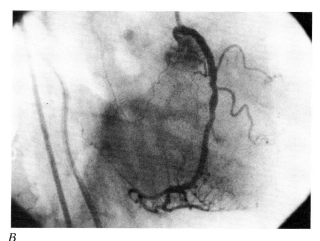

B

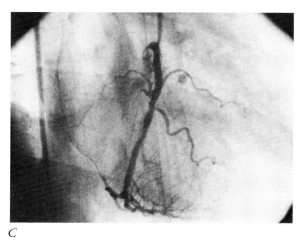

C

Figure 89-8. Stenosis of the right coronary artery in its midportion (A). After dilatation the pressure gradient was eliminated, but the angiographic appearance seemed to be poor, with a small dissection line along the former stenosis (B), and remarkable cleaning noted at 6 months (C).

Results

Since September, 1977, 191 patients with various lesions have undergone PTCA in Zurich. The age range was 26 to 68 years. In all, 130 patients had single-vessel disease with only one major artery having more than a 50 percent obstruction, 18 patients' status was postaortocoronary bypass graft operation with recurrent stenosis and symptoms, and the remainder had double- or triple-vessel involvement. Patients were evaluated on the basis of their clinical status, exercise test, and coronary angiography before and after PTCA, including follow-ups every 3 months for the first year and reangiography every 6 to 9 months after the procedure.

In 87 percent of the patients, we were able to pass the lesion with the dilatation catheter. In this group, the mean duration of angina pectoris since the onset of chest pain had been 9 months with a range of 1 day to 108 months. In 80 percent of patients, anatomic success involving more than

20 percent improvement in the lumen diameter and hemodynamic success as measured by pressure gradients could be noted. Reduction of coronary narrowing of the transluminal diameter from 82 ± 11 to 34 ± 16 percent ($p < 0.001$) was recorded, having been calculated as a mean out of at least three oblique projections. Mean pressure gradient across the lesion was reduced from 56 ± 15 to 19 ± 12 mm Hg ($p < 0.001$) as a result of the dilatation.

Improvement in the anatomy and in the distal coronary pressure led to an increase in the submaximal working capacity consistent with the steady state on bicycle ergometry, from 77 ± 46 to 120 ± 39 watts, and normalization of perfusion scintigram in patients with single-vessel disease.

In 13 percent of patients, the stenosis could not be reached or passed. In these patients, the mean duration of angina pectoris had been 20 months (range 1–192 months). The failures were mainly due to anatomic factors, such as tortuosity of the vessel, sharp angles, troublesome side branches, and tightness and eccentricity of the stenoses.

The mean follow-up time of the primary successes is now 12 months, with a range of 1 to 36 months. Two patients have died [13]. One death was unrelated to PTCA; the second was a sudden death, which occurred unexpectedly in a 45-year-old man with extensive hypertrophy of the medial smooth cells of the left main stem. Based on this latter case, main stem stenoses are not a current indication for me to perform PTCA.

The follow-up angiograms 6 to 9 months after PTCA were available in nearly all patients called in for control. In 50 percent of patients, there was sustained improvement in vessel patency; 25 percent remained unchanged or showed partial recurrence in comparison to the angiogram immediately after PTCA (see Fig. 89-6); in 25 percent, complete recurrences have been observed. Most of these patients with recurrences had a repeated dilatation with primary success. The overall success rate, including the second dilatation, has been calculated according to the life table method at 85 percent.

Similar observations have been made in centers with similar patient volume, such as San Francisco, New York, and Frankfurt. In addition, similar results have been reported in the PTCA registry of the National Heart, Lung, and Blood Institute (NHLBI), which includes data collected from 26 centers in the United States and Europe on 504 patients [20].

Complications

In the 191 attempts, there were no hospital deaths, no evidence of embolization, no central nervous system deficits, two femoral hematomas requiring evacuation, and one femoral occlusion requiring thromboendarterectomy. Thirteen patients underwent aortocoronary bypass graft within 24 hours, and significant elevation of creatine phosphokinase–MB isoenzyme levels (more than 10 units/liter) could be observed in 10 patients, of whom 6 had electrocardiographic evidence of transmural infarction.

The NHLBI registry reported similar experiences. In addition, the reported hospital mortality following PTCA was 1 percent. Two of the deaths occurred in single-vessel disease and four in cases with multiple-vessel involvement.

In most cases, the cause of emergency aortocoronary bypass graft was an intimal dissection or sudden closure of the vessel with clinical and electrocardiographic evidence of impending infarction. Usually it is the forceful manipulation of the catheter that causes intimal dissection, but abrupt vessel closure may also occur after uneventful passage of the stenosis.

The definite risk of infarction and the potential complications resulting from emergency bypass procedures, such as wound infection and sepsis [20], have had repercussions on indications for PTCA. Since coronary arterial dissection also may occur after uneventful dilatation and is therefore intrinsic to the method itself, caution is advised in treating patients with compromised collateral flow and patients without clear-cut indications for bypass surgery. The precise mechanism of the sudden occlusion after uneventful PTCA is not clear. It may be postulated that the fibrous cap of the atheroma ruptures with bleeding and partial dissection, creating a flap that occludes the stenotic area. We believe that early surgical intervention prevented major infarction in those cases. Since the potential complications are both serious and sudden, it is mandatory that a competent surgeon be available for emergency operation should one become necessary. The procedure should not be performed in hospitals lacking this resource.

In conclusion, although PTCA is a relatively simple procedure, it requires special experience and training.

The ideal patient should have a proximal discrete stenosis that is not more than 15 mm in length and is located in the left anterior descending, left circumflex, or right coronary arteries. From the clinical viewpoint, the patient's symptoms should compromise his quality of life and the disease should be controlled unsatisfactorily with beta-blocking agents and nitrates. Failure of the medical therapy and the presence of disabling angina pectoris necessitate consideration of a blood flow augmentation procedure. If these anatomic and clinical conditions are met, the patient may be considered a candidate for coronary bypass surgery. We employ these criteria because, in light of the possibility of complications, there is no justification for risking an unnecessary operation.

In applying these indications, rules, and precautions, the results accumulated in the main centers, as well as in the NHLBI registry, confirm the effectiveness and relative safety of the procedure in patients with single-vessel disease. Work is underway to determine the role of this technique in patients with more extensive coronary artery disease.

References

1. Forssmann, W. Die Sondierung des rechten Herzens. *Klin. Wochenschr.* 8:2085, 1929.
2. Dotter, C. T., and Judkins, M. P. Transluminal treatment of arteriosclerotic obstruction. Description of a technic and a preliminary report of its application. *Circulation* 30:654, 1964.

3. Porstmann, W. Ein neuer Korsett-Ballonkatheter zur transluminalen Rekanalisation nach Dotter unter besonderer Berücksichtigung von Obliterationen an den Beckenarterien. *Radiol. Diagn.* (Berl.) 14:239, 1973.
4. Zeitler, E., Schmidtke, J., and Schoop, W. Die perkutane Behandlung von arteriellen Durchblutungsstörungen der Extremitäten mit Katheter. *Vasa* 2:401, 1973.
5. Grüntzig, A. Die perkutane Rekanalisation chronischer arterieller Verschlüsse (Dotter-Prinzip) mit einem doppellumigen Dilatationskatheter. *ROEFO* 124:80, 1976.
6. Grüntzig, A. *Die perkutane transluminale Rekanalisation chronischer Arterienverschlüsse mit einer neuen Dilatationstechnik.* Baden-Baden: Witzstrock, 1977.
7. Grüntzig, A., and Kumpe, D. Technique of percutaneous transluminal angioplasty with the Grüntzig balloon catheter. *AJR* 132:547, 1979.
8. Grüntzig, A. R., Turina, M. I., and Schneider, J. A. Experimental percutaneous dilatation of coronary artery stenosis (abstract 0319). *Circulation* [Suppl.] 54:II-81, 1976.
9. Grüntzig, A., and Schneider, H. J. Die perkutane Dilatation chronischer Koronarstenosen —Experiment und Morphologie. *Schweiz. Med. Wochenschr.* 107:1588, 1977.
10. Grüntzig, A. R., Myler, R. K., Hanna, E. S., and Turina, M. I. Coronary transluminal angioplasty (abstract 319). *Circulation* [Suppl.] 55, 56:III-84, 1977.
11. Jester, H. G., Sinapius, D., Alexander, K., and Leitz, K. H. Morphologische Veränderungen nach transluminaler Rekanalisation chronischer arterieller Verschlüsse. In E. Zeitler (ed.), *Hypertonie—Risikofaktor in der Angiologie.* Jahrestagung der Deutschen Gesellschaft für Angiologie, Köln, October 2–4, 1975. Baden-Baden: Witzstrock, 1976. P. 76.
12. Leu, H. J., and Grüntzig, A. R. Histopathological Aspect of Transluminal Recanalization. In E. Zeitler, A. Grüntzig, and W. Schoop (eds.), *Percutaneous Vascular Recanalization.* Heidelberg: Springer, 1978. P. 39.
13. Grüntzig, A. R., Senning, A., and Siegenthaler, W. E. Nonoperative dilatation of coronary-artery stenosis. *N. Engl. J. Med.* 301:61, 1979.
14. Engel, H. J., Kaltenbach, M., Kober, G., Scherer, D., and Lichtlen, P. R. Spontaneous regression of coronary obstructions after transluminal dilatation (abstract 605). *Circulation* [Suppl.] 62:III-159, 1980.
15. Aldridge, H. E., McLoughlin, M. J., and Taylor, K. W. Improved diagnosis in coronary cinearteriography with routine use of 110° oblique views and cranial and caudal angulations: Comparison with standard transverse oblique views in 100 patients. *Am. J. Cardiol.* 36:468, 1975.
16. King, S. B., Douglas, J. S., and Morris, D. C. New Angiographic Views for Coronary Arteriography. In W. Hurst (ed.), *The Heart* (4th ed.). New York: McGraw-Hill, 1980. P. 193.
17. Grüntzig, A. Expérience Clinique de Dilatation Intra-arterielle Coronarienne par Catheter. Resultats. *Ann. Cardiol. Angeiol.* (Paris) 28:487, 1979.
18. Turina, M., Grüntzig, A., Krayenbühl, C., and Senning, A. Percutaneous transluminal dilatation of coronary artery stenosis. *Thorac. Cardiovasc. Surg.* 27:199, 1979.
19. Engel, T. R., and Meister, S. G. Coronary percutaneous transluminal angioplasty (ed. note). *Ann. Intern. Med.* 90:268, 1979.
20. Kent, K. (and participants of NHLBI Registry). Percutaneous transluminal coronary angioplasty (PTCA): Update from NHLBI Registry (abstract 609). *Circulation* [Suppl.] 62:III-160, 1980.

Percutaneous Transluminal Dilatation of Renal Artery Stenosis

ANDREAS R. GRÜNTZIG
ULRICH KUHLMANN

Atherosclerotic and nonatherosclerotic renal artery stenoses are the general causes of renal vascular hypertension. Antihypertensive medical therapy may be difficult or may even fail to control the blood pressure. In addition, renal failure can be aggravated in the presence of deteriorated blood flow to the kidney caused by severe arterial stenosis.

In patients with this kind of disease, invasive treatment such as renal vascular surgery has to be considered. Extended experience with surgery has been accumulated over the years. Since the results have been reported to be remarkably good, surgical therapy has been accepted as standard in selected cases. But older patients often fail to respond to surgery [1–3], and the mortality ranges from 5 to 9 percent [1–6]. The mortality is even higher in the presence of concomitant impaired renal function or coronary artery disease [2, 3].

As in peripheral and coronary artery disease, angioplasty seems to be an alternative procedure for treating patients with atherosclerotic stenosis as well as fibromuscular hyperplasia or transplant renal artery stenosis.

Single observations of inadvertent renal artery dilatation in 1963 [7] and intentional dilatation with a Teflon catheter in 1971 [6] have been made previously, but only the introduction of the dilatation catheter technique rendered this method amenable to clinical application. Since its first description [8], the technique has aroused growing interest, and the number of procedures done has increased rapidly [9].

A number of reports of promising results have since appeared that encourage the application of the technique [6, 9–20] and it just might be that "the technique is the most important advance in the management of renal vascular hypertension since the advent of renin measurements" [9]. However, the proper role of the method still has to be defined, and carefully designed prospective studies are needed to compare this procedure to renal artery surgery [9, 11].

Technique

The procedure is basically the same as that for dilatation of the peripheral [21, 22] or the coronary arteries [23]. But the passage of the double-lumen dilatation catheter can be achieved in two different ways. The first system involves the use of a catheter assembly that consists of a

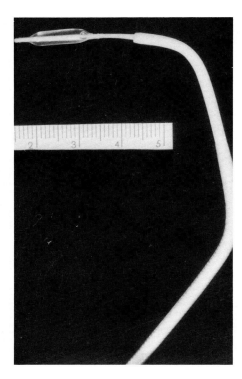

Figure 90-1. Catheter assembly for renal artery dilatation. Note preshaped guiding catheter that directs the dilating catheter into the renal artery.

guiding catheter and a dilatation catheter, while the second method employs a catheter-guidance system.

Using the first method, the ipsilateral femoral artery is punctured, facilitating the selective catheterization of the corresponding renal artery. The guiding catheter is then introduced through an 8 French arterial sheath in the groin. The guiding catheter is not tapered at the tip, and it is preshaped, as shown in Figure 90-1. For passage through the sheath and introduction into the aorta, the guiding catheter is advanced into the aorta and directed into the orifice of the renal artery to be dilated. The catheter remains at the orifice and guides the renal dilatation catheter into the artery. The dilatation catheter has an outer diameter of 4.5 French and is tapered to approximately 3 French at the tip. The main lumen of the dilatation catheter is used for contrast material injection and pressure measurements during the procedure. For purposes of comparison, the aortic pressure at the orifice of the renal ostium is recorded through the guiding catheter using a Y connector at the end of the guiding catheter. Using the second lumen of the dilatation catheter and automatic pressure de-

vices, the balloon is filled with a 50–50 mixture by volume of the contrast agent and sterile normal saline. The balloon segment has a maximal outer diameter of 5 mm obtained by using 3 to 5 atmospheres of pressure (72.5 psi). If smaller diameters are needed, the 3.7-mm coronary dilatation catheter can be used. It is advisable to use a maximal outer diameter of the balloon that is smaller than the diameter of the undiseased part of the renal artery proximal to the stenosis. Judging the size of the artery from the segment distal to the stenosis is useless because of the common presence of poststenotic dilatation.

The second method involves the use of a catheter-guidance system, which consists of a double-lumen dilatation catheter similar to that used for femoral artery dilatation [21]. After the placing of an angiographic catheter (e.g., a Simmons-type "sidewinder" [24]) into the orifice of the artery, a standard guidewire is passed through the stenosis and is followed by the angiographic catheter. During this manipulation, no pressure recording or contrast medium injections are available. After the passage of the catheter through the stenosis, the guidewire is removed and the catheter is available for pressure measurements and contrast medium injections. The guidewire then is placed gently into a side branch of the renal artery. While the guidewire is held carefully in place, the angiographic catheter is removed and exchanged for the dilatation catheter, which then is passed through the stenosis, following the route of the guidewire.

Several different types of dilatation catheters are available for the catheter-guidewire technique. We recommend using balloon sizes not larger than 6-mm maximal outer diameter, and we prefer to use even smaller sizes—to avoid overinflation of the undiseased part of the renal artery and thus the danger of vessel damage. The coaxial guiding-catheter system has the advantage of pressure recording and contrast medium injections while passing the stenosis; in addition, it does not have to be advanced into the peripheral renal branches, a step that could cause irritation of the intima. The disadvantage of the coaxial system is that the guiding catheter limits the balloon size of the dilatation catheter. The maximal size of balloon that can be passed in its deflated and umbrellalike shape through the catheter is 5 mm. In rare instances, a larger balloon might be of use. In these cases, the catheter-guidewire system has to be employed. The disadvantages of the catheter-guidewire system are the relative blindness while crossing the stenosis and the risk of traumatizing peripheral renal branches through guidewire manipulations. Having weighed the advantages and disadvantages of both systems, we prefer the coaxial guiding-catheter system, but we recommend that both systems be available in case one of them fails.

Procedure

The procedure is carried out with the patient in the fasting state and after administration of tranquilizer premedication. After administering local anesthesia to the groin, inserting the arterial sheath, and positioning the guiding catheter, heparin in a dose of 10,000 units is given to avoid clot formation. In young patients, the intrarenal application of nitroglycerin prevents spasm. A selective renal angiogram is obtained in the anteroposterior projection and in angled views if needed. The stenosis is recognized by using the videotape playback. (The procedure should not be done without the playback capacity.) Once the guiding catheter is positioned at the orifice, the dilatation catheter is very slowly advanced into the artery and manipulated through the stenosis while the renal pressure is monitored through its tip. Simultaneously, the aortic pressure is recorded through the tip of the guiding catheter. Correct pressure measurements are very important because the degree of improvement of distal arterial pressure is one measure of the success of the procedure. When the catheter tip traverses the stenosis, a drop in pressure is observed. Once the dilatation catheter is properly positioned, the balloon is immediately inflated at 4 to 5 atmospheres of pressure (60–75 psi).

The balloon is inflated for approximately 5 to 10 seconds by the automatic pressure pump. A marked rise in the distal pressure after deflation of the balloon indicates a successful dilatation and aids in the decision to terminate the procedure. If the distal pressure fails to respond adequately, the inflation of the balloon must be repeated.

Other Aspects of Management

Adjunctive medical therapy originally recommended in coronary dilatation [21, 23] has not been shown to be advantageous. Acetylsalicylic acid (aspirin) (300–600 mg) should be administered daily starting before the procedure, and one tablet per day should be continued after the procedure until the time of restudy, usually 6 to 9 months later.

Despite the tendency to encourage patients to engage in physical activity the day after a peripheral or coronary dilatation, caution is still advised in the case of renal dilatation. After a successful intervention, the blood pressure normalizes within a few hours. Orthostatic hypotension may then develop in some patients. Mobilization of the patient should therefore be done cautiously. If the blood pressure does not normalize, Coumadin therapy is not initiated, but aspirin therapy is continued.

Selection of Patients

As pioneers in the use of this new procedure, we had to employ rather rigid criteria for patient selection, similar to the criteria for reconstructive surgery. The basic criterion was either (1) the presence of hypertension (blood pressure > 160/95 mm Hg) despite adequate medical therapy or (2) intolerable drug side effects. The presence of a lateralizing renal vein renin ratio exceeding 1.5 (affected to unaffected side) aided in the decision. However, according to our previous experience with patients undergoing surgery [26], the elevated renin ratio was not a prerequisite for the case selection.

In regard to the anatomic criteria, the stenosis should be severe (> 75%). If any uncertainty exists about the significance of the stenosis, a pressure gradient of more than 20 mm Hg across the stenosis should be present. The pressure measurements are done with a soft 3 French catheter passed through the diagnostic catheter prior to the procedure.

From the morphologic viewpoint, the technique can be applied to atherosclerotic stenosis as well as to medial or intimal fibromuscular dysplasia. The stenosis should not be too proximal, thus involving the aortic wall, nor too distal, including the side branches.

In case of bilateral stenosis, a two-stage procedure is recommended. In the first stage, the more severely affected side is treated; the other side is treated some days or weeks later. We use the two-stage approach not only because the operation time is shorter for each side but also because the use of less contrast medium is an important consideration in the event of impaired renal function. Also, we do not want to endanger a good result on one side with a complication on the other side. The second procedure can be done if the first procedure resulted in a favorable response of the artery to the dilatation.

Results

From 1977 to 1980, 33 patients underwent renal angioplasty in Zurich. In 31 (94%) of patients, we were able to pass the stenosis, inflate the balloon, and achieve an improvement in the luminal diameter. Of these 31 patients, 23 had atherosclerotic stenosis, as judged from the radiologic criteria [27, 28], and 6 patients had stenosis with typical signs of fibromuscular dysplasia. In the atherosclerotic stenosis group, the mean age was 54 years (the range was 39 to 67 years). All the patients had severe hypertension despite adequate medical therapy. The average blood pressure was 203/113 mm Hg. After dilatation, the blood pressure decreased to 141/91 mm Hg and remained at 141/91 mm Hg in the follow-up period. The follow-up period of this series is on average 12 months (the range is 4 to 24 months).

After dilatation, the pressure gradient across the stenosis measured with the dilatation catheter was reduced as shown in Figure 90-2. Two atherosclerotic patients (9%) had complete recurrence of the stenosis in the follow-up period, and 5 patients (22%) showed partial restenosis at

the time of an elective control study (angiography 6 months later). Four of the cases of partial restenosis were treated with a second percutaneous transluminal angioplasty, again with primary success, and the fifth was normotensive with medical therapy, so that a second dilatation has so far not been necessary. Two patients died from cardiovascular disease in the meantime, and one patient was operated on for an aortic aneurysm.

The mean age in the fibromuscular dysplasia group was 38 years (range was 20 to 48 years), and the average blood pressure was 182/110 mm Hg. The arm blood pressure normalized after dilatation at an average of 137/87 mm Hg. It remained at 136/84 mm Hg in the follow-up period, with a mean of 8 months (the range was 6 to 9 months). The pressure changes before and after dilatation and in the follow-up period are shown in Figure 90-3. There were no recurrences.

In two patients, dilatation of the stenosis of a transplanted kidney artery was done with primary success. But one patient had a complete recurrence after 4 weeks and required surgery; the other patient remained improved.

These clinical results are summarized in Figure 90-4. Using the criteria of the well-known American Cooperative Study [29], the patients were classified as (1) cured, (2) improved, or (3) unimproved, on the basis of their blood pressure response and whether they were taking medication. The cured patients were those not taking medication whose blood pressure was normal in

Figure 90-2. Results of renal artery dilatation in patients with atherosclerotic stenosis (ASS) illustrating the immediate postdilatation drop in pressure gradient and results at the time of restudy.

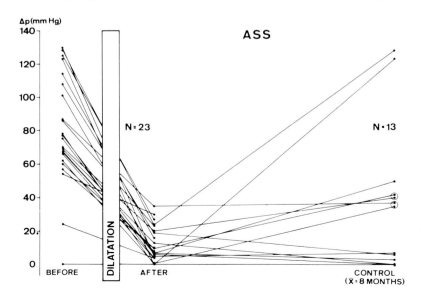

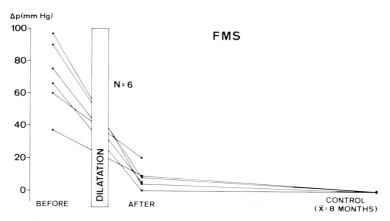

Figure 90-3. Pressure gradient across stenosis pre- and postdilatation in patients with fibromuscular dysplasia (FMS).

the follow-up period. The improved patients were those with improved diastolic blood pressure (< 110 mm Hg without therapy) or those with normalization of diastolic blood pressure (< 95 mm Hg) but still taking antihypertensive drugs. The unimproved patients were those whose diastolic pressure remained above 110 mm Hg despite therapy.

Of the patients with atherosclerotic stenosis, the majority were improved or even cured. Of the fibromuscular disease group, 4 of 6 patients were cured and the remainder improved. Two typical examples of dilatation of atherosclerotic and nonatherosclerotic stenosis are given in Figures 90-5 and 90-6. Our results are comparable to those in published literature. The largest series (153 patients) has been compiled in the European Cooperative Study [25], which reports a primary success rate of 90 percent.

Until now, however, follow-up data from only a few cases and from only a short control period have been available [11, 19, 20]. These reports have used definitions similar to ours to analyze

Figure 90-4. Summary of clinical results in renal artery dilatation in atherosclerotic stenosis (ASS) and fibromuscular dysplasia (FMS) patient groups.

the follow-up data, and the results also are similar to ours and to the results given in Figure 90-4. Surgical results in the case of atherosclerotic stenosis revealed a "cure" rate of 28 percent and improvement of 55 percent, while fibromuscular dysplasia results were 47 percent for each [26]. Considering the limited number of cases, the limited follow-up time of the percutaneous transluminal angioplasty, and the different patient population, it is too early to draw definite conclusions. However, we and others [19] believe that in appropriate, selected cases, the results of angioplasty are comparable to those of surgery.

As is to be expected, dilatation is not without complications. In our atherosclerotic stenosis group, 2 patients experienced acute deterioration of their already impaired renal function as a result of the contrast medium injection. Both patients needed dialysis, and 1 of them remained on chronic dialysis. In 1 patient, orthostatic hypotension caused an episode of transient cerebral ischemia, and in 1 patient Coumadin-related bleeding occurred in the follow-up period. No complications were noted in the fibromuscular dyplasia group or in the transplanted group.

Other complications have been reported, among them intimal dissection with sudden reclosure [18], renal artery rupture [25], perforation of the renal artery [19, 20], and hematoma in the inguinal region. Some of these complications reported might be avoided by modifying the coaxial technique and by using smaller balloon sizes. And, finally, experience has been accumulating in several centers throughout the world, so there is no need to do this procedure in a self-taught fashion. Training can be easily acquired at these centers.

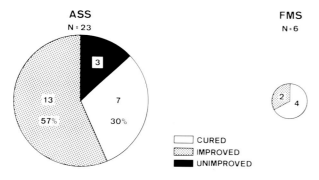

ASS
N = 23

FMS
N = 6

CURED
IMPROVED
UNIMPROVED

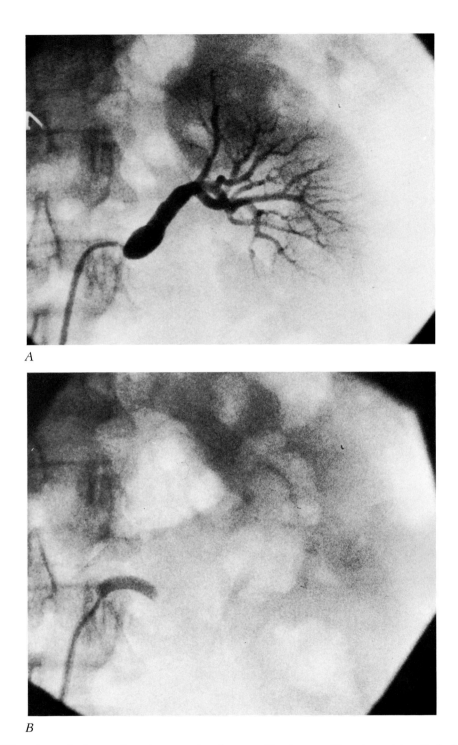

A

B

Figure 90-5. Dilatation of atherosclerotic stenosis of renal artery. Demonstration of predilatation stenosis (A), balloon in place and inflated (B), result im- mediately postdilatation with relief of stenosis (C), and control angiogram 8 months postprocedure with a rea- sonable result (D).

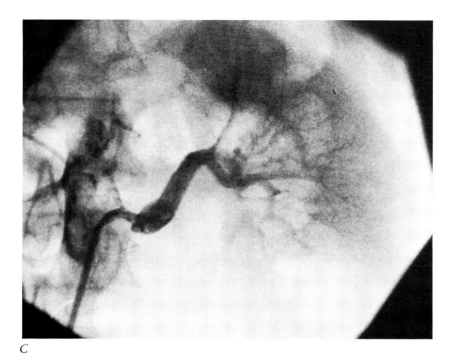

C

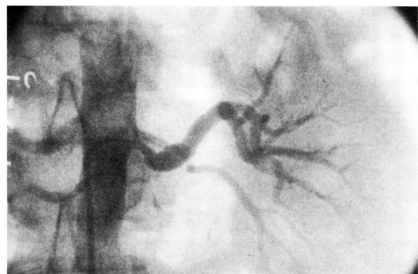

D

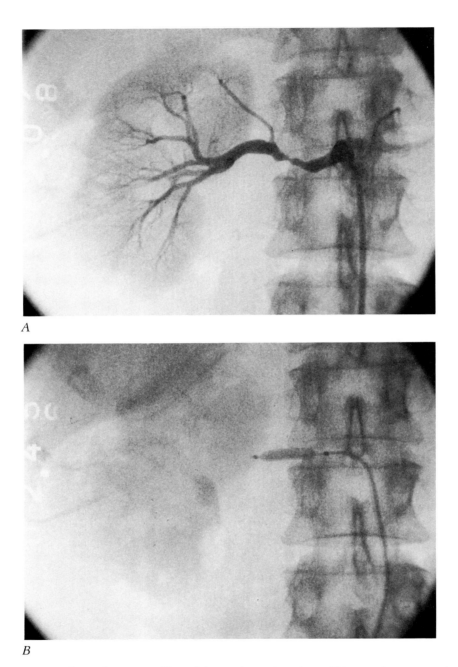

A

B

Figure 90-6. Dilatation of renal artery affected by fibromuscular dysplasia. Predilatation angiogram demonstrating typical lesion of FMS (A), inflated balloon in place (B), results postangioplasty (C), and control angiogram with almost normal appearance of the renal artery (D).

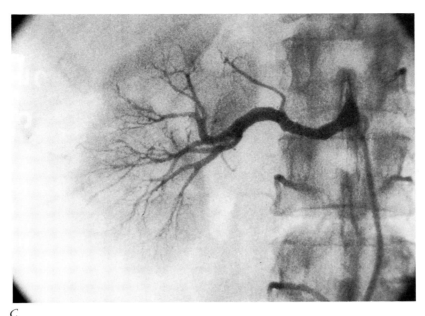

C

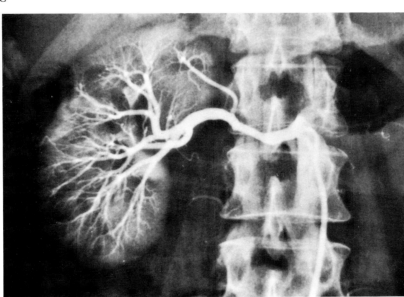

D

Summary

The results indicate that percutaneous transluminal dilatation of renal artery stenosis is effective in the treatment of renal vascular hypertension in properly selected cases. However, since the long-term patency and the complication rate, especially in the light of widespread use of the technique, have not yet been established, caution is advised. Therefore, the following rules for patient selection should be applied: (1) the patient should remain hypertensive (blood pressure > 160/95 mm Hg) despite adequate medical therapy or experience intolerable drug side effects; (2) the patient should agree to have an emergency operation in case of a complication; and (3) the hemodynamic significance of the stenosis should be established before percutaneous transluminal angioplasty by the degree of the stenosis itself, the kidney size, lateralizing renin ratio, the ^{131}I sodium iodohippurate clearance study, or the pressure gradient across the stenosis. Under these circumstances, the technique can be applied, and both reasonable success and patency rates can be expected.

References

1. Foster, J. H., Maxwell, M. H., Franklin, S. S., Bleifer, K. H., Trippel, H., Julian, O. C., De-Camp, P. T., and Varady, P. D. Renovascular occlusive disease. Results of operative treatment. *J.A.M.A.* 231:1043, 1975.
2. Franklin, S. S., Young, J. D., Jr., Maxwell, M. H., Foster, J. H., Palmer, J. M., Cerny, J. and Varady, P. D. Operative morbidity and mortality in renovascular disease. *J.A.M.A.* 231:1148, 1975.
3. Maxwell, M. H. Cooperative study of renovascular hypertension. *Kidney Int.* (Suppl.) 8:V-153, 1975.
4. Shapiro, A. P., McDonald, R. H., Jr., and Scheib, E. Renal arterial stenosis and hypertension: II. Current criteria for surgery. *Am. J. Cardiol.* 37:1065, 1976.
5. Stanley, J. C., and Fry, W. J. Surgical treatment of renovascular hypertension. *Arch. Surg.* 112:1291, 1977.
6. Zeitler, E. Angiographische Probleme zur Diagnostik und Therapie der renovaskularen Hypertonie. In H. Denck, G. Flora, G. Hilbe, and F. Piza (eds.), *Renovaskulare Hypertonie*. Vienna: Verlag der Medizinischen Akademie, 1971. P. 113.
7. Colapinto, R. F. Inadvertent percutaneous transluminal dilatation of a renal artery with a four-year follow-up. *Radiology* 135:605, 1980.
8. Grüntzig, A., Kuhlmann, U., Vetter, W., Lütolf, U., Meier, B., and Siegenthaler, W. Treatment of renovascular hypertension with percutaneous transluminal dilatation of a renal-artery stenosis. *Lancet* 1:801, 1978.
9. Grim, C. E., Yune, H. Y., Weinberger, M. H., Klatte, E. C., and Ryan, M. P. Balloon dilatation for renal artery stenosis causing hypertension: Criteria, concerns, and caution (editorial). *Ann. Intern. Med.* 92:117, 1980.
10. Mahler, F., Krneta, A., and Haertel, M. Treatment of renovascular hypertension by transluminal renal artery dilatation. *Ann. Intern. Med.* 90:56, 1979.
11. Kuhlmann, U., Vetter, W., Furrer, J., Lütolf, U., Siegenthaler, W., and Grüntzig, A. Renovascular hypertension: Treatment by percutaneous transluminal dilatation. *Ann. Intern. Med.* 92:1, 1980.
12. Millan, V. G., and Madias, N. E. Percutaneous transluminal angioplasty for severe renovascular hypertension. *Lancet* 1:993, 1979.
13. Katzen, B. T., Chang, J., Lukowsky, G. H., Edward, G., and Abramson, E. G. Percutaneous transluminal angioplasty for treatment of renovascular hypertension. *Radiology* 131:53, 1979.
14. Weinberger, M. H., Yune, H. Y., Grim, C. E., Luft, F. C., Klatte, E. C., and Donohue, J. P. Percutaneous transluminal angioplasty for renal artery stenosis in a solitary functioning kidney. An alternative to surgery in the high-risk patient. *Ann. Intern. Med.* 91:684, 1979.
15. Martin, E. C., Diamond, N. G., and Casarella, W. J. Percutaneous transluminal angioplasty in non-atherosclerotic disease. *Radiology* 135:27, 1980.
16. Diamond, N. G., Casarella, W. J., Hardy, M. A., and Appel, G. B. Dilatation of critical transplant renal artery stenosis by percutaneous transluminal angioplasty. *AJR* 133:1167, 1979.
17. Sniderman, K. W., Sos, T. A., Sprayregen, S., Sadekkni, S., Cheigh, J. S., Tapia, L., Tellis, V., and Veith, F. J. Percutaneous transluminal angioplasty in renal transplant arterial stenosis for relief of hypertension. *Radiology* 135:23, 1980.
18. Mathias, K. Rau, W., and Kauffman, G. Katheterdilatation einer Arterienstenose nach Nierentransplantation. *Dtsch. Med. Wochenschr.* 104:437, 1979.
19. Schwarten, D. E., Yune, H. Y., Klatte, E. C., Grim, C. E., and Weinberger, M. H. Clinical experience with percutaneous transluminal angioplasty (PTA) of stenotic renal arteries. *Radiology* 135:601, 1980.
20. Tegtmeyer, C. J., Dyer, R., Teates, C. D., Ayers, C. R., Carey, R. M., Wellons, A., Jr., and Stanton, L. W. Percutaneous transluminal dilatation of the renal arteries: Techniques and results. *Radiology* 135:589, 1980.
21. Grüntzig, A. Die perkutane transluminale rekanalisation chronischer arterienverschlusse mit einer neuen dilatationstechnik. Baden-Baden: G. Witzstrock-Verlag, 1977.
22. Grüntzig, A., and Kumpe, D. A. Technique of percutaneous transluminal angioplasty with the Grüntzig balloon catheter. *AJR* 132:547, 1979.
23. Grüntzig, A., Senning, A., and Siegenthaler, W. E. Nonoperative dilatation of coronary-artery stenosis. Percutaneous transluminal coronary angioplasty. *N. Engl. J. Med.* 301:61, 1979.
24. Grable, G. S., and Smith, D. C. The use of the Simmons "sidewinder" catheter in percutaneous transluminal angioplasty of the renal arteries. *Radiology* 137:541, 1980.
25. Richter, E. I., Grüntzig, A., Ingrisch, H., Mahler, F., Mathias, K., Roth, F. J., Sövensen, A., and Zeitler, E. Percutaneous dilatation of renal stenosis. *Ann. Radiol.* (Paris) 23:275, 1980.
26. Vetter, W., Vetter, H., Tenschert, W., Kuhlmann, U., Studer, A., Glänzer, K., Pouliadis, G., Largiadèr, F., Furrer, J., and Siegenthaler, W. Renovaskuläre Hypertonie. Prognostischer

Wert der Seitengen Trennten Reninbestimmung im Wierenvehenblut. *Klin. Wochenschr.* 57:863, 1979.

27. Abrams, H. L. (ed.). *Angiography* (2nd ed.). Boston: Little, Brown, 1971. Pp. 860–863.

28. Bookstein, J. J., Abrams, H. L., Buenger, R. E., Lecky, J., Franklin, S. S., Reiss, M. P., Bleifer, K. H., Klatte, E. C., and Maxwell, M. H. Radiologic aspects of renovascular hypertension. *J.A.M.A.* 220:1218, 1972.

29. Maxwell, M. H., Bleifer, K. H., Franklin, S. S., Varady, P. D., and Deegan, C. Cooperative study of renovascular hypertension. Demographic analysis of the study. *J.A.M.A.* 220:1195, 1972.

Transluminal Angioplasty

CHARLES T. DOTTER

Probably half the readers of this book will one day undergo some form of diagnostic angiography, and some will be candidates for transluminal angioplasty. This method for the percutaneous treatment of vascular obstructions got off to a slow start following its introduction in 1964 [1]. During the ensuing decade, it gained little credence in the United States, and instrumental limitations confined its application to atheromatous lesions of the leg and the pelvic arteries. Technical progress, the demonstration of long-term success, and expanded areas of applicability have led to increasing acceptance in recent years.

Definition

Transluminal angioplasty is a general term for the direct, mechanical treatment of vascular obstructions by catheters. Included are two superficially similar procedures, which differ in important respects. *Transluminal dilation* (Fig. 91-1) refers to the correction of stenotic lesions, not occlusions. *Transluminal recanalization* (Fig. 91-2) refers to the correction of vascular occlusion by the mechanical formation of an artificial lumen through the occluded segment, dilation playing an important but secondary role in the process. Both of the foregoing are nonoperative or, more accurately, "closed" procedures; they are percutaneous, image-guided alternatives to traditional surgical revascularization.

Rationale of Transluminal Angioplasty

The rationale of transluminal angioplasty resides in the physical and biologic properties of the obstructive process(es), and its outcome is influenced by such factors as the distribution, composition, and configuration of lesions in a given case [2–4]. In the ideal therapeutic situation, obstruction is due solely to a localized, primary, atheromatous transformation of the normal intima into a firm, mostly acellular, amorphous, collagenous core encroaching on the lumen and surrounded by a relatively normal outer arterial wall. This core, though often present in larger arteries, tends to obstruct locally at characteristic sites, such as the aortic and carotid bifurcations and the adductor hiatus segment of the superficial femoropopliteal artery—evidence that he-

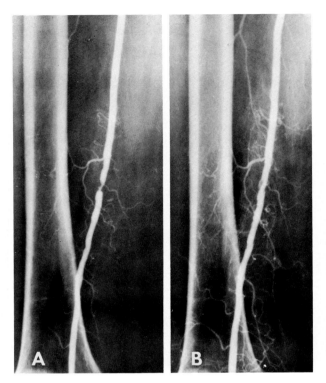

Figure 91-1. Transluminal dilation. (A) Before and (B) immediately after coaxial (12 French) dilation of a patent but severely narrowed lumen in the adductor hiatus segment of the superficial femoral artery of an elderly woman. Two pregangrenous toes healed, and the woman was free of ischemic pain until her death from heart failure 2 years later.

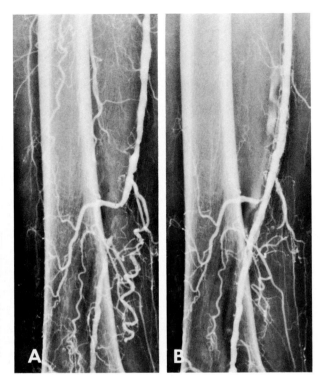

Figure 91-2. Transluminal recanalization. (A) Before and (B) after probe creation and coaxial catheter dilation of a neolumen through a 2-cm occlusion at the adductor hiatus segment of the superficial femoral artery in a 77-year-old woman. Arteriographically the lumen was patent after 3 years, and clinically it was still open after 9 years.

modynamic (as well as metabolic, dietary, inheritable, and other) factors play etiologic roles. Whatever the role of hydraulic stress, it is a fortunate fact that in the early, uncomplicated stages of the disease, arteries distal to local obstructions tend to be less heavily affected. To the extent that clinically significant luminal obstructions can be removed or bypassed, ischemia can be prevented and life and function preserved. Despite progress in the fibrinolytic removal of intraluminal clots [4, 5] we have yet to find a drug capable of resolving a mature primary atheromatous obstruction.

Transluminal angioplasty can do much in this direction by causing mechanical changes in the inelastic but compressible core and its surrounding mural remnants. At least two mechanisms appear to play roles, depending on the nature of the obstruction and the dilating force applied. The simpler of these mechanisms, wedge dilation, can be compared to the creation of a nail hole in a board by the compression of adjacent wood fibers. Poorly selected, ineptly placed or driven

nails can split boards; badly handled catheters can wreak their own kinds of clinical havoc. In simple dilation, the substance of the locally intruding core is forced peripherally against the remaining medial and adventitial outer arterial wall. The core is compressed, presumably with the release of fluid constituents. At the same time there occurs a local, in situ redistribution of atheromatous core substance, reducing the associated luminal irregularity. The desired result is the creation of an enlarged, rounder lumen surrounded by a compressed, inelastic cylindric transformation of the former core, and the relatively unchanged outer arterial wall (Fig. 91-3) [6]. Follow-up angiograms reveal that the remodeled lumen tends to retain its new shape. Experimental studies have shown that microscopic ablative changes occur in the lining surface of the core and that forcible balloon dilation can lead to intimal (core) cracks and separation between core [7] and media at the periatheromatous cleavage plane [8], a loose interface familiar to surgeons as the "plane of endarterectomy," to pathologists as

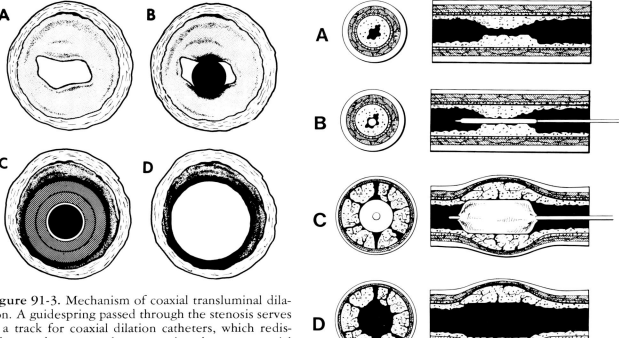

Figure 91-3. Mechanism of coaxial transluminal dilation. A guidespring passed through the stenosis serves as a track for coaxial dilation catheters, which redistribute and compress the core against the outer arterial wall. The lumen is enlarged without removal or detachment of the core (*stippled area*), much as a nail hole is made in wood. The diagrams are based on autopsy dilations. (From Dotter et al., Transluminal dilation of atherosclerotic stenosis. *Surg. Gynecol. Obstet.* 127:794, 1968.)

Figure 91-4. Balloon dilation, possible effects. The diagrams are based on animal studies of luminal enlargement by medial stretching with radial cracking of uncompressed atherosclerotic core. Comment: An enlargement exceeding that of the adjacent relatively normal lumen is useless and is most likely to occur with balloon overdistention. The nature of the lesion and the applied distending force determine the degree to which the differing mechanisms illustrated here and in Figure 91-3 are involved. (From Castaneda-Zuniga et al. [8]. Reproduced by permission of *Radiology*.)

a site of artifactual separation, and to angiographers as "subintimal" traps for ineptly manipulated guidewires or catheters (Fig. 91-4). Irreversible stretching of the outer arterial wall is unlikely in the absence of undue or continuing dilating force. This is fortunate, since medial recoil and integrity account for the rarity of false aneurysms following simple dilation. Luminal unevenness seen on postdilation angiograms is not necessarily ominous, since delayed follow-up studies often show its disappearance, with further improvement in the luminal contour (Fig. 91-5). Balloon overdistention can lead to arterial wall rupture and false aneurysm formation [9]. Simple tapered or coaxial dilation catheters, though not as likely to cause such complications, are generally limited to straightforward, antegrade use, as in the femoropopliteal system. Balloon dilators are required for pelvic and small branch arteries (renal and coronary), as well as contralateral, transbifurcation use, where tapered or coaxial catheter dilation is not feasible.

Transluminal dilation, by smoothing out the lumen, helps minimize the hemodynamic ill effects of turbulent flow. The roughness and obvi-

ous fragility of atheromatous cores observed during endarterectomy or at autopsy no more show that dilation generates fragmental embolization than scraps of limp rubber show the shape of the unburst balloon. In the intact catheterized artery, the dilated core, even when fenestrated and locally separated from the outer arterial wall, retains longitudinal continuity with the adjacent vascular lining, and thus does not embolize. In its simplest, least disruptive form, transluminal dilation brings about luminal enlargement and normalization of contour by in situ core compression—with or without splitting—not by reaming, drilling, or otherwise forcing solid material out of the artery. Except for the tools, the only thing removed from the artery is the obstruction. There are, of course, exceptions to the ideal. Blind-ended periatheromatous pockets, paralleling patent runoff lumens (especially

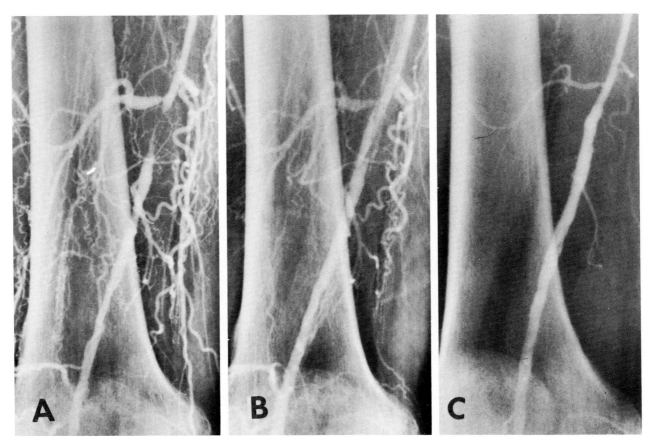

Figure 91-5. Delayed luminal improvement following transluminal recanalization in a 57-year-old surgeon with claudication. (A) Before and (B) immediately after recanalization. There is considerable neoluminal irregularity. (C) A 5-month follow-up angiogram shows a smoother, more normal lumen and the expected reduction in the no-longer-needed collateral arteries.

Figure 91-6. Transluminal angioplasty, recanalization pathways. Postmortem results. Transluminal recanalization of two occluded femoral arteries. (A) Trans- atheromatous pathway. (B) Periatheromatous pathway (X). It is not as likely to remain patent. (From Zeitler et al. [10]. Reproduced by permission of Springer.)

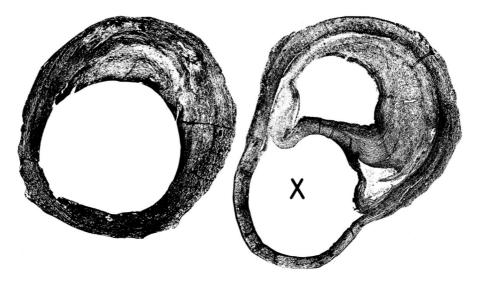

A   *B*

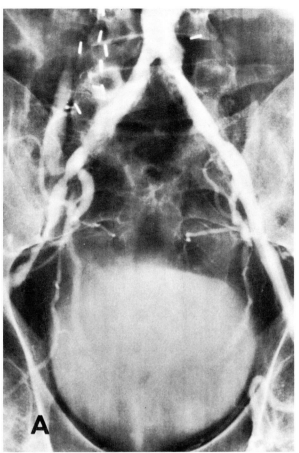
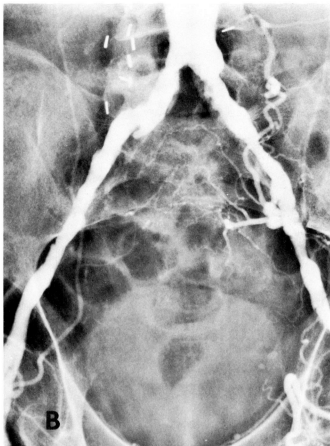

Figure 91-7. Periatheromatous neolumen, long-term patency. (A) Before and (B) 6½ years after caged balloon dilation of multiple right iliac artery stenoses in a 55-year-old man whose prior sympathectomy had not relieved severe claudication. As shown in (B), lasting good blood flow can occur through catheter-created periatheromatous pathways.

when unwisely dilated), can worsen distal ischemia. Periatheromatous lumen-to-lumen pathways are more prone to reclosure by virtue of the elasticity of the eccentrically stretched adjacent media (Fig. 91-6). Fortunately, even periatheromatous neolumens are capable of maintaining adequate blood flow for as long as 6 years in legs that might otherwise have been amputated (Fig. 91-7).

Spectrum of Atheromatous Obstruction

Atherosclerotic ischemia is caused by a spectrum of obstructive lesions [2, 3]. Arteriographically perceptible changes in the superficial femoral artery range from early, minimal luminal irregu-larity at the adductor hiatus segment to complete occlusion of the entire artery. Although the possible permutations of atheromatous obstructive disease approach infinity, certain morphologic patterns can be identified that bear importantly on the ease, technical approach, and prognosis of transluminal angioplasty (Fig. 91-8). Small, localized, noncircumferential luminal intrusions may represent immature atheromas or mural thrombi, which, being soft and relatively elastic, offer little resistance to and often are little changed by dilation. Redilation several months later is more likely to succeed. Localized, tight, centrally situated stenosis due to a mature, firm, primary atheromatous lesion is a more favorable therapeutic target. Its dilation often requires considerable force, a favorable prognostic factor. Severe atherostenotic luminal irregularity provides a more difficult technical problem, but, if

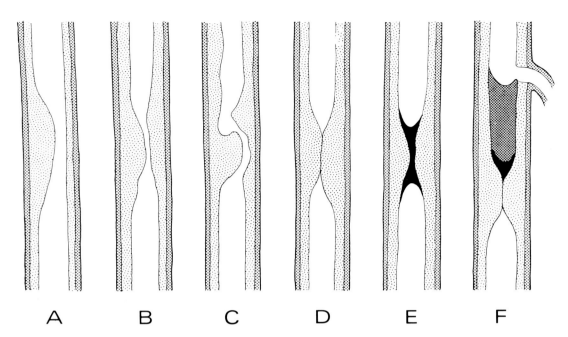

A   B   C   D   E   F

Figure 91-8. Pathologic spectrum of atherosclerotic obstruction in peripheral arteries. (A) Moderate, eccentric luminal narrowing. (B) Severe but simple stenosis—ideal for dilation. (C) Irregular stenosis with a luminal cul-de-sac (sometimes difficult to dilate). (D) Complete (virtual) luminal occlusion without clot, the easiest type to recanalize. (E) Secondary thrombosis of a narrowed lumen. (F) Propagated long-segment thrombotic occlusion above a primary lesion, the poorest indication for catheter therapy. (From Zeitler et al. [10]. Reproduced by permission of Springer.)

approached with caution and experience (and good luck), it should not compromise a good outcome. Advanced core thickening produces a gone-but-not-thrombosed virtual lumen. Guidewire passage, a necessary preliminary to dilation, is somewhat less certain than when patency permits visually controlled pathfinding. A funnellike proximal luminal termination helps point the guidewire in the right direction. The closure of atherostenotic lesions is commonly due to or associated with secondary thrombosis. Typically, the slow development of an atheromatous adductor hiatus narrowing leads to the development of collateral pathways from the deep femoral artery. Depending on the respective roles played by collateral vessels and the stenosed lumen, there may or may not be clinical repercussions when narrowing becomes occlusion. A small, fresh, central thrombus is unlikely to hinder guidewire passage across a short segmental occlusion; unfortunately, such clots soon begin to undergo organization, often propagating proximally to the origin of a functioning branch artery. This angiographically recognizable situation makes the procedure more difficult and its prognosis less certain. In general, the longer and older a propagated luminal obliteration, the more

difficult its penetration by a guidewire. Even though the best possible transocclusive route is found and dilated, the resulting rough-surfaced neolumen is more vulnerable to collapse and thrombosis than is the smooth, stable, partly endothelialized surface achieved by dilating a stenotic but patent lumen. Lineal mural calcification is not prejudicial to the safety or success of transluminal angioplasty in peripheral arteries. On the contrary, it suggests a stable adherence between core and media, and provides a useful guide to the location of the arterial wall during transluminal angioplasty.

Procedure for Peripheral Transluminal Angioplasty

The techniques and tools of transluminal angioplasty differ, depending on the location and nature of the target lesions, the feasible catheter access routes, and the preferences, skill, experience, and clinical judgment of the angiographer. Similarly requisite are the facilities, supplies, and highly trained personnel of a modern angiographic laboratory. If the foregoing are lacking, to attempt transluminal angioplasty would be to jeopardize the patient's chance for improvement and unfairly discredit a therapeutic technique of value.

The following views on how to do transluminal angioplasty reflect a personal series of over 800 treated cases of atherostenotic disease affecting the lower extremities. There is at least one larger series (Zeitler's) [10], but none covering a longer span of time. The past clearly shows that in most areas of medicine, including transluminal angioplasty, today's "state of the art" is likely to become tomorrow's antiquity. Furthermore, technical descriptions, including the following, are subject to bias, are often incomplete, and are potentially out of date by the time of publication; at best, they are partial substitutes for direct observation and the chance to cross-examine others already experienced in the area.

PREANGIOPLASTY MANAGEMENT

Some patients are referred on the basis of angiographic findings; others with a request for arteriography and, if indicated, transluminal treatment at the same session. The latter approach eliminates the possible need for repeating studies by ensuring that adequate, up-to-date arteriograms are available at the time of the intended angioplasty. Some patients are sent for help or seek help directly because positive surgical measures are unwarranted or unwanted or have been exhausted. Long-distance evaluation can sometimes be done on the basis of transmitted clinical data and arteriograms, averting useless travel and hospitalization for those who are clearly not candidates for the procedure.

At the University of Oregon Medical School, patients referred for possible transluminal angioplasty are admitted or are transferred to beds under the care of the diagnostic radiology staff. When needed, consultative support from medical, surgical, or other clinical services is obtained. Routine preliminary studies, in addition to history and physical examination, include noninvasive peripheral vascular appraisal, chest x-ray, electrocardiogram, urinalysis, complete blood count, hematocrit, coagulation tests, and blood typing and crossmatching. If the patient is taking anticoagulants, they are stopped. Currently, 0.5 gm of aspirin daily is recommended for 2 or 3 days before and forever after angioplasty.

The procedure and its prognosis and risks are explained to the patient, and the patient's informed consent is obtained for aortoperipheral arteriography and possible transluminal angioplasty. Peripheral (unlike coronary) transluminal angioplasty is no longer considered an experimental procedure, a position supported in Oregon by Blue Cross, Medicare, and other third-party payers. Premedication consists of mild sedatives and, in some instances, atropine.

PROCEDURAL STRATEGY AND TECHNIQUES

Procedural plans are based on what is already known about the individual on the angiographic table. It is prudent to prepare both femoral puncture sites, even though only one may be used. In most patients with leg ischemia, including those with probable iliac artery narrowing, conventional transfemoral arteriographic examination of the aorta, its renal and pelvic branches, and the arteries of both legs down to ankle level is a necessary starting point. Ordinarily, studies are done in the anteroposterior projection, with additional oblique views if needed to resolve doubts concerning possible hidden iliac artery or proximal deep femoral artery narrowing. In the presence of the patient, the findings are reviewed. If angioplasty is indicated, a plan of attack is formulated on the basis of the number, location, character, and clinical importance of the visualized lesions.

FEMOROPOPLITEAL LESIONS

Assume, for example, that no significant iliac artery narrowings are present in a patient whose claudication appears to be caused by a localized narrowing at the level of the adductor hiatus segment on the opposite, prepared, but yet uncatheterized side.

Although the narrowing might be accessible via the original puncture site to a long balloon catheter passed over the aortic bifurcation and downward [11], we prefer to introduce a second, downstream catheter into the proximal superficial femoral artery on the affected side. The injection of contrast agent through the previously placed diagnostic catheter permits fluoroscopically guided, one-stick, front-wall entry at the desired spot [12]. We use a 4.5-inch-long arterial needle to avoid exposure of our hands in such circumstances. Lacking such means for guided puncture, reference to an available arteriogram can aid direct entry into the superficial femoral artery rather than the common or deep femoral artery. Trauma to a patent common or deep femoral artery is more likely to make matters worse than trauma to a stenotic or occluded superficial femoral artery, already bridged by collateral vessels from the deep femoral artery. For those of us who are less than perfect, attempted downstream puncture of the superficial femoral artery will sooner or later result in inadvertent entry into the nearby deep femoral artery. When this happens, it is best not to remove the guidewire or catheter or to attempt to flip it over into the superficial femoral artery, lest local bleeding cause delay and further obscure the true target. Instead, reflux opacification from the deep femoral artery should be used to guide a separate puncture into the superficial femoral artery. If not already given, 2 to 3 cc of a 1:1,000 heparin solution is injected into the artery to be treated.

Whether the target lesion is stenotic or occlusive and whether coaxial [1], tapered [13, 14], or balloon catheters [15–18] are used to treat it, the next step is to reach the lesion and get a guidewire across it. It helps if 30 percent contrast agent is injected into the proximal superficial femoral artery for preangioplasty visualization. Next, a small diagnostic or 8 French Teflon dilating catheter is placed about an inch above the lesion, and through it, a 0.038-inch or a 0.045-inch straight-tip guidewire is advanced through the narrowed lumen (easy to do) or occluded lumen (not always easy to do). If, during attempted recanalization, the exploring guidewire enters the periatheromatous cleavage plane, its progress may be alongside rather than into the patent distal lumen. This unhappy situation can be suspected if there is continuing resistance to guidewire passage rather than the gratifying drop in resistance that signals that the guidewire has reached its patent target. Unless the distal lumen is entered within an inch or so beyond the lesion, the guidewire should be withdrawn and further attempts made to find a more direct lumen-to-lumen pathway. Under no circumstance should a blindending, paraluminal guidewire path be dilated at the potential expense of a previously open runoff lumen, since a serious reduction in the blood flow can result (Fig. 91-9). The foregoing technical problem is most often encountered in longsegment occlusions, especially if secondary intraluminal clots have undergone fibrotic organization. In such a situation, provided undue efforts by the radiologist have not impaired the runoff bed, bypass grafting offers an established, workable alternative. Its outcome and the patient's future

should not be jeopardized by repeated, unsuccessful efforts to recanalize.

Once a guidewire has traversed the stenosis or occlusion, creating a lumen-to-lumen pathway, all that remains is the actual dilation. It can be done using coaxial, tapered, or balloon catheters. Coaxial dilation, the originally described method, used successfully in hundreds of femoropopliteal obstructions, involves the passage of an 8 French Teflon tapered-tip catheter over the guidewire through the obstructed segment. Usually this is easy to do. Care should be taken that guidewires or catheters are not allowed to advance into small, easily damaged, distal branches of the popliteal artery while attention is focused on the site of treatment. During guidewire transit through occluded segments, contrast agent injected around the guidewire may help find or even create the intended lumen-to-lumen pathway. Horváth suggests the use of Rheomacrodex for this purpose [19].

Once the guidewire and the 8 French pilot catheter have reached the distal open lumen, it is safe to remove either (but not both!). Distal luminal catheter reentry is signaled by reflux blood flow, often sluggish and nonpulsatile due to collateral damping. Special attention should be given to the prevention of catheter clotting. Next, with the guidewire in place and protruding a safe distance beyond the 8 French catheter, the outer 12 French coaxial catheter is threaded over both and patiently is pushed through the obstruction. If proximal buckling prevents forced passage of the main dilating catheter through the obstruction, a stiffener consisting of a length of metal tubing passed over the guidewire and within but not all the way through the 8 French catheter can straighten things out and provide the needed authority. It is important that both the inner and the outer Teflon dilation catheters have smoothly tapered tips and fit together properly. If their tips are cut at a slight (20–30°) angle, catheter rotation and gentle advancement during introduction into the artery and passage through the lesion can minimize mural trauma and core disruption. When the large dilation catheter reaches the distal lumen, both catheters are pulled up together to a point above the obstruction, the guidewire is removed, and postdilation arteriography is done. If the results are satisfactory, a final 3 cc of heparin and a saline chaser are injected, the catheters are removed, and manual hemostatic pressure is applied over the puncture site.

Staple [13] and van Andel [14] have used

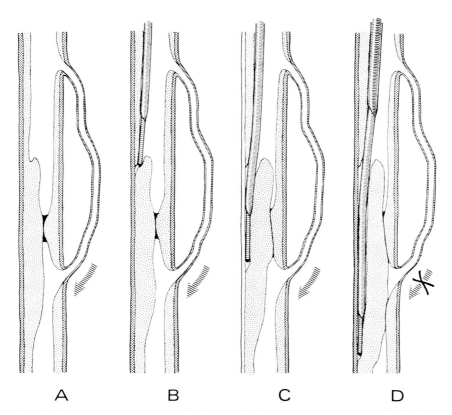

A   B   C   D

Figure 91-9. Transluminal angioplasty—an avoidable technical error. Once they are in the periatheromatous cleavage plane (A), guidewires and catheters tend to dissect further (B and C) rather than reenter the lumen. Periatheromatous paraluminal dissection and dilation distal to an occlusion (D) can make the patient worse rather than better and should be avoided—if necessary, by abandoning the effort.

one-piece tapered Teflon catheters that dilate by the same mechanism as coaxial catheters. Depending on the length of the narrowed end of these catheters, the dilation of low popliteal lesions can pose problems with respect to undesired entry into distal, best undisturbed, smaller branches.

Balloon dilation catheters à la Grüntzig [18] are currently in wide use. In femoropopliteal lesions, where dilation is both literally and figuratively straightforward, coaxial and tapered Teflon catheters have certain advantages. They can, in one pass, dilate multiple lesions, minimizing procedure time and the risk of fibrin cloaking or thrombus formation on the surface of balloons. Wedge dilation can often be accomplished in seconds or minutes, the entire procedure in as little as 10 minutes; balloon dilation is usually more time consuming. For use in the femoropopliteal system, tapered or coaxial Teflon dilation catheters offer other (though less important) advantages. They are durable and can often be reused. They are commercially available in well-made sets (Cook) at relatively low cost or

can be made up as needed from bulk Teflon tubing.* Unlike balloon catheters, they rarely cause overdistention and are incapable of bursting inside arteries.

If balloon catheters are to be used to treat severe narrowings and occlusions of leg arteries, the prior passage of Teflon dilation catheters may be required to make room for them. Balloon dilation is essential to the treatment of iliac [15–18], aortic [20, 21], and branch (renal [22] and coronary [23]) artery lesions. In femoropopliteal lesions, they can be highly effective and have certain advantages in addition to the smaller entry hole required and consequently lower risk of hematoma formation. Their flexibility allows contralateral dilation, though not recanalization; that is, up one femoral artery, across the aortic bifurcation, and down the other side to the

*Anyone sufficiently skilled in arterial catheterization to undertake transluminal angioplasty will realize that the relative lengths of coaxial catheters, guidewires, and stiffeners depend on the individual anatomic circumstances. Catheters can be shortened as needed, either before or after their insertion.

lesion [11]. This is the method of choice for dilating stenoses of the common or deep femoral artery and proximal femoropoliteal graft anastomoses, where nearby entry trauma or hematoma could imperil an otherwise successful outcome. The crossover route may also be of value in avoiding a dense surgical scar rather than trying to force a way through it.

ILIAC ARTERY AND AORTIC LESIONS

Iliac artery and aortic stenoses involve tortuous routes and luminal dimensions that demand the use of expanding rather than simple wedge dilation. The first iliac artery dilation, done with a Fogarty (latex) balloon catheter in 1965, is still patent (Fig. 91-10). Difficulties in later attempts

on other patients with iliac artery stenoses made it evident that unreinforced latex balloons lacked the authority required to dilate most atherosclerotic lesions. Porstmann's "Korset catheter" [16] provided the basic idea that led to the development of the caged balloon catheter system [17], in which the balloon, mounted on a guidewire-tip cannula, was expanded within a Teflon catheter at a site where longitudinal slits provided a cagelike reinforcement (Fig. 91-11A). This worked well in hundreds of iliac artery dilations (Fig. 91-12), but in 1974 was outmoded by Grüntzig's ingenious double-lumen catheter, which had a strong, preshaped, polyvinyl balloon [18]. Grüntzig's design permitted forceful dilation to chosen diameters using small, flexible balloon catheters (see Fig. 91-11B). These

---

Figure 91-10. First transluminal iliac artery dilation, 14-year patency. (A) Before and (B) after dilation by a Fogarty (latex) balloon catheter in 1965. (C) The lumen was arteriographically patent in 1979, 2 years after a redilation with a Grüntzig-type plastic balloon.

(D) Serial views of the latex balloon being pulled through a relatively unyielding stenosis. There was good symptomatic relief despite residual narrowing. (E) A polyvinyl balloon shows a similar deformity during the 1977 redilation.

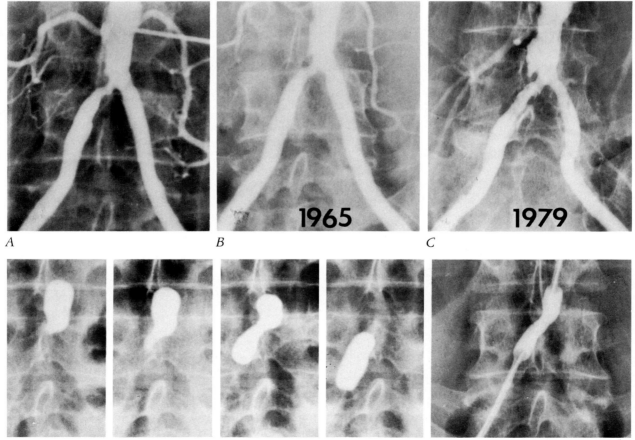

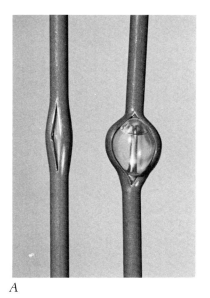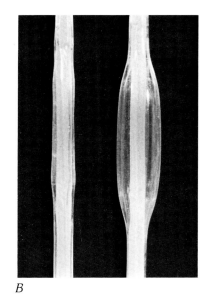

A   *B*

Figure 91-11. Balloon catheters for iliac artery dilation. (A) Caged balloon catheter (Porstmann, Dotter). (B) Polyvinyl balloon catheter (Grüntzig). The polyvinyl balloon catheter, properly handled, is less thrombogenic and easier to use; the caged balloon catheter can provide greater authority but is rarely required (see also Fig. 91-13).

Figure 91-12. Transluminal iliac artery dilation, caged balloon. (A) Predilation, a 95 percent stenosis (*arrow*) at the level of the bifurcation of the left common iliac artery. The internal iliac artery is occluded. (B) Following dilation. The lumen remained open, with no recurrence of the severe claudication. Ironically, had the patient not been successfully treated, he might not have drowned while swimming a year later.

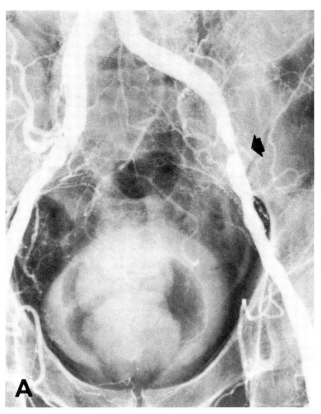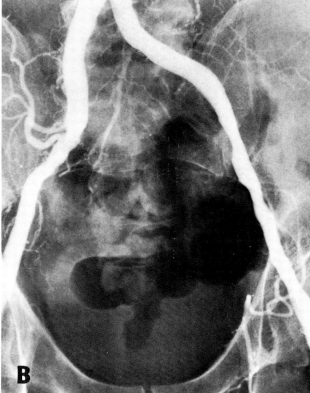

catheters and their derivatives (e.g., polyethylene balloons) [24] have a central lumen that allows their insertion and placement over various ordinary guidewires that can be changed or removed for such procedures as angiographic injections and pressure measurements. Balloon distention is achieved through a separate, smaller lumen running in the catheter wall. Instrumental variations on Grüntzig's theme make possible the transluminal dilation of small but important branches, such as the coronary and renal arteries. The expanding force, being hydraulic, can be exerted despite tortuous catheter routes. Their availability did much to stimulate today's widespread use of transluminal angioplasty.

Preformed polyvinyl or polyethylene balloons are designed to expand to certain diameters at specific inflating forces. Various sizes are available for various purposes. To control pressures in "calibrated" balloon dilators, we first tried an elaborate and costly ($1,000 +) device that produced preset, foot-controlled, instantly reversible pressures [25]. Except for coronary dilation, we found this device cumbersome and unnecessary. Next, we used simple gauges to monitor pressures. Accurately measured pressures are useful only to the extent that they produce specified responses in the balloons. Since each expansion inevitably modifies the future response characteristics of polyvinyl balloons, their calibration by manufacturers is both difficult and subject to change by user pretesting (necessary to prevent the insertion of defective units) and by repeated use. Balloon performance is also influenced by the configuration of the surrounding abnormal arterial wall.* Experience and common sense indicate that, for most purposes, the "feel" and the fluoroscopic appearance of balloons at various stages and sites of distention can provide safe, workable control. Balloons 8 mm in diameter and 1.5 cm long on 8 or 9 French catheters work well in the iliac arteries. Opinions vary as to how iliac artery dilation should be done. The description that follows is based on my own experience.

In a typical patient with unilateral claudication due to a localized narrowing of a common iliac artery, the distal femoral artery is punctured and a suitable guidewire is passed upward and, with care, though the stenosis. Base-line transstenotic

pressure gradients and, if needed, arteriograms are obtained using appropriate catheters. With the guidewire back in place, the diagnostic catheter is removed and the dilation catheter (its balloon tested and emptied) is inserted and passed until the balloon lies well above the stenosis. With a 10-cc syringe, the balloon is *partially* distended with dilute contrast agent and gently drawn down until its deformity and increased resistance to movement signal engagement with the stenosis. The plunger of the distending syringe is then released and the balloon, no longer under pressure, is drawn down into the stenosis. Manual fluoroscopically controlled balloon distention is then done. Undue force is avoided by limiting the distended balloon diameter to that of the prestenotic artery, by the feel of the force on the plunger, and by resistance to movement of the balloon at various stages and sites of distention. The use of a 10-cc distending syringe offers some protection against overdistention. Because of the hydraulic advantage, similar force on the plunger of a smaller-caliber syringe causes higher, possibly dangerous, balloon pressures. Relying on visual and manual feedback, we have yet to burst either a balloon or an artery [9], two reported complications likely to occur through overdependence on specified hydraulic pressures. Regardless of the distending force, a local eccentric enlargement of the balloon signals possible impending balloon failure, especially in balloons previously distended by testing or prior use.

Several balloon distentions at one or more locations may be needed to obtain an adequate lumen, as gauged by lowered resistance to balloon movement, the disappearance of visible balloon constriction, the arteriographic findings, and the reduction of transstenotic pressure gradients.

Transstenotic pressure measurement is a useful, objective indicator of the functional severity of the stenosis before the procedure and the success achieved by dilation (Fig. 91-13). Gradients of under 20 mm Hg during vasodilation are reportedly acceptable [27]. In inelastic, eccentric atheromas, dilation with ordinary balloon catheters may fail to provide the desired reduction in the pressure gradient, and the use of the more authoritative caged balloon catheter may be required. The objective of transluminal angioplasty is restoration of function, not a good-looking lumen. This is important, since postdilation angiograms are often not as impressive as might be hoped. To quote Thompson

---

*Blowing up a balloon the first and succeeding times is an exaggerated way of illustrating the point. Blowing up a balloon partly surrounded by a mailing tube gives an idea of what can happen inside diseased arteries.

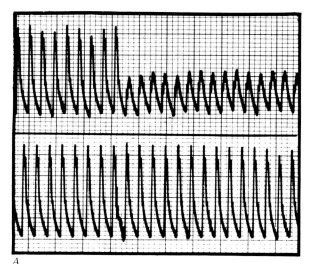

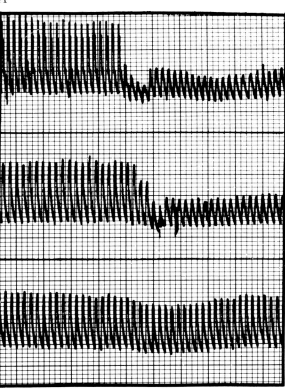

Figure 91-13. Pressure gradients, guides to successful transluminal dilation. (A) Two pullout pressure recordings show the satisfactory disappearance of a systolic pressure gradient of 50 mm Hg after iliac artery dilation. (B) Initial efforts in another patient using an 8-mm diameter polyvinyl balloon dilator failed to achieve a significant reduction in a pressure gradient of 80 mm Hg. Use of a caged balloon catheter produced the desired result, as shown in the lowest pullout pressure measurement (recorded at a slower paper speed than the first example).

and Goldin, "This is not cause for despair if the gradient has gone [28]." Postangioplasty luminal irregularities, presumably reflecting periatheromatous filling by blood and/or contrast agent, are often gone on follow-up arteriograms (see Fig. 91-5).

Because of the normally curved and frequently tortuous routes followed by the iliac arteries, iliac artery occlusions are not as easily or as safely traversed as occlusions in leg arteries. They nevertheless can be recanalized [15, 29], especially if they are short and are located in relatively straight segments. At present, long iliac artery occlusions are best managed surgically. In patients with unilateral iliac artery occlusions, for whom aortofemoral surgery poses an unusual risk (because of age or illness), transluminal dilation of a patent but stenotic opposite iliac artery can make possible the less hazardous femoral-femoral bypass grafting [30] (Fig. 91-14). Similarly, in patients with lengthy femoropopliteal occlusions, preliminary transluminal iliac artery dilation, by increasing inflow pressures, can substantially improve the prognosis of femoropopliteal bypassing [31].

In a patient with unilateral iliac artery stenosis as evidenced by grossly different femoral pulsations, a diagnostic catheter passed up the good side can provide angiofluoroscopic guidance for puncture and passage on the affected side. As mentioned, a long arterial puncture needle should be used to keep the operator's hands out of the fluoroscopic beam in this and similar situations. Concomitant contrast visualization from above can spell the difference between success and failure and can materially reduce the risk of arterial perforation during attempted retrograde guidewire passage through a tortuous, stenotic iliac artery lumen.

POSTANGIOPLASTY MANAGEMENT

A compression dressing is applied following the manual achievement of hemostasis. Incorporating half of a sponge-rubber ball, flat side down, may be of value. Patients are told that puncture site bleeding might occur and what to do about it (e.g., "Press here and call for a nurse") and are reassured about the possible appearance later of discoloration. Wherever possible, the patient is permitted to walk a few hours after the procedure. Heparin is not given after angioplasty unless the resulting lumen appears unusually rough and thrombus formation is a significant risk. In

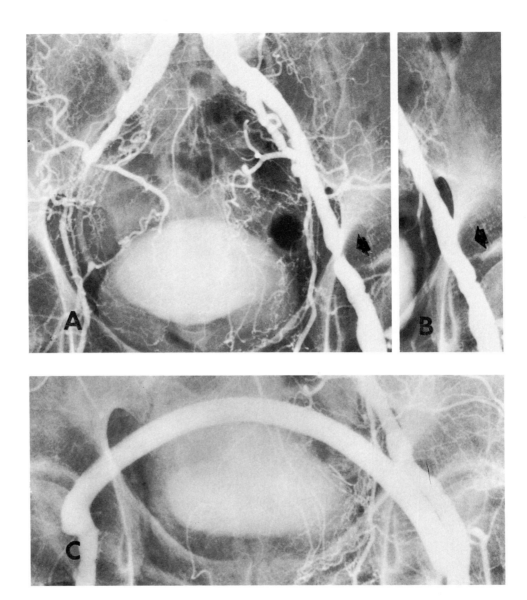

Figure 91-14. Transluminal dilation and vascular surgery, complemental, not competitive. This 70-year-old man with right external iliac artery occlusion had had three myocardial infarctions and was not a candidate for aortofemoral grafting. Bilateral claudication was relieved by the transluminal dilation of a severe left external iliac artery stenosis (*arrows*, A and B) that permitted successful, low-risk placement of a femoral-femoral graft (C). Five years later, the bilateral symptomatic improvement has persisted.

such cases, heparin is given for a few days. In the past, we rarely advised long-term anticoagulant therapy, but there is evidence that it favors lasting patency [32, 33]. Horváth recommends sodium pentosan polysulfate (SP 54, Benecheme), a drug said to promote fibrinolysis and to retard atherogenesis [34].

Transluminal angioplasty usually involves hospitalization for 1 or 2 days. Repeat noninvasive studies are done, and patients are advised not to smoke, to walk regularly, and to take 1 aspirin each day. Those with preexisting ischemic ulcers or toes are told what to do to facilitate healing. Before discharge, patients are given a phone number and are told to phone to report any sudden change in their condition. They and their referring physicians are informed (by telephone) about the immediate outcome and the long-range prognosis of angioplasty and are urged to provide follow-up information a year later (sooner if clini-

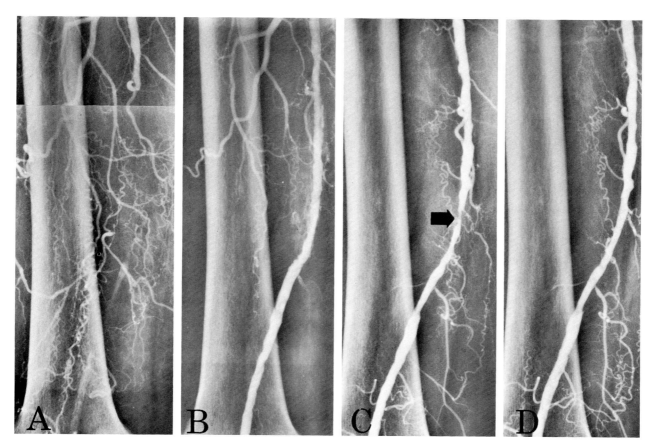

Figure 91-15. Transluminal retreatment. (A) Long-segment, femoropopliteal occlusion in an 80-year-old man. (B) The lumen is patent but irregular a week after a successful coaxial recanalization. As advised, the patient returned when symptoms began to recur 3 months later. (C) Stenosis (*arrow*) at the site of a prior recanalization. (D) Good lumen diameter was obtained by simple dilation, with persisting clinical relief at 2½ years. About 20 percent of successfully treated patients have required redilation. In progressive disease, the retreatment capability is a therapeutic advantage.

cally warranted). Long-term follow-up arteriograms are rarely done in the absence of recurrent symptoms. Occasionally, copies of preangioplasty and postangioplasty arteriograms are sent to the referring physician, who also gets a copy of the hospital discharge summary.

RETREATMENT

In about 1 of 5 successfully treated patients, symptoms due to recurrent obstruction at the treated site indicate the need for retreatment or a surgical alternative. Redilation several months or more following initially successful transluminal angioplasty seems to result in a more durable improvement, perhaps because with time, lesions tend to become firmer and are therefore more likely to stay open the second time around. Recurrent symptoms can also be caused by progres-

sive disease in untreated areas. Narrowing of a successfully recanalized segment can be relieved by simple dilation, which is easier to do and more likely to last (Fig. 91-15).

Successful transluminal angioplasty for unilateral claudication is often followed by the appearance of previously masked symptoms caused by lesions on the opposite, untreated side. For this reason, prophylactic dilation of symptomatically silent, contralateral stenoses should receive serious consideration at the time the "bad" side is treated. In 1 of our patients, three dilations were done before a stable lumen was achieved. Ironically, after 2 symptom-free years, the patient died of a myocardial infarction while mowing his lawn. Another patient, in her eighties, confined to bed by ischemic leg pain and thought incapable of withstanding aortofemoral surgery, successfully underwent right iliac artery dilation three times and left iliac artery dilation twice, giving her 5 relatively comfortable years and restoring her mobility to the time of her death. Repeated transluminal angioplasty can play a useful role in the continuing management of progressive peripheral atherosclerotic disease; fortunately, its use is not limited by the number of remaining leg veins or the hazard of surgery for the elderly patient.

Risks of Transluminal Angioplasty

Done properly in appropriate candidates, transluminal angioplasty involves procedural risks only slightly greater than those of the diagnostic studies required for surgical case selection.

Despite the advanced age, frequent presence of gangrene, and generally poor physical condition of many of the 800 patients treated since 1964 at the University of Oregon Medical School, only three lives were lost and numerous amputations were averted. Many of our early patients were referred for transluminal angioplasty only after conventional surgical revascularization had been considered and rejected because of the high risk and the poor chance of success (as, for example, in an elderly patient with a prior myocardial infarction, poor runoff arteries, rest pain, perhaps gangrene). Transluminal procedures undertaken as last-chance salvage efforts necessarily lead to lower overall success rates; but this was considered an acceptable trade-off for the help given to many who had nowhere else to turn.

MORTALITY

Two deaths were directly attributable to transluminal therapy, both from myocardial infarction. In each, the ultimately fatal complication was first evidenced the day following an apparently successful procedure marked by a period of significant hypotension. It is not clear whether the low blood pressure was the cause or a result of the infarction although the absence of electrocardiographic changes during the procedure gave reason to suspect the former. The restoration of blood flow into a previously underperfused leg can cause a sudden increase in the body's effective vascular capacity, as evidenced by the increased distal arterial caliber seen in postangioplasty arteriograms and the leg vein distention evident at the end of a successful procedure. In patients with diseased, diffusely narrowed, and poorly compliant arteries, impaired compensation in vascular tone can lead to hypotension and reduced coronary flow. The removal of a dilatation catheter following successful transluminal angioplasty is hemodynamically comparable to the removal of an aortic clamp in that both procedures may lead to sudden, profound hypotension requiring prompt counteraction. Thus, in older patients, especially where there is unusual blood loss, the means for preventing or combating hypotension must be on hand and can be lifesaving. Premedication with atropine, the use of intravenous fluids, and the availability of vasopressive drugs during the procedure are useful.

One patient died of pulmonary embolism and previously unsuspected gas gangrene several days following the successful reestablishment of the blood flow to his foot. He had been considered too gravely ill to undergo amputation, evidently a justified opinion. His death was not regarded as a result of transluminal angioplasty.

Considering the number of our patients with congestive heart failure, prior myocardial infarctions (three patients had had three each), diabetes (in about one-third), gangrene, and generalized arteriosclerosis, an overall series mortality of under 1 percent is gratifyingly low.

ARTERIAL PUNCTURE SITE PROBLEMS

Postpuncture hematomas developed after an estimated 5 to 8 percent of procedures. In at least 2 patients, initially successful catheter revascularization was negated by undue manual hemostatic efforts. In several cases, surgical exposure and suturing were required to control persistent bleeding or thrombosis at the site of the puncture. One patient suffered serious retroperitoneal bleeding from an unusually high puncture in the common femoral artery, another from an iliac artery perforation. Both complications were recognized in time for successful emergency surgery. To reduce the incidence of postpuncture bleeding or thrombosis, care is taken to ensure that arterial punctures are dilated rather than torn open to admit catheters. Dilating catheters must be smoothly tapered, and their tips rounded and obliquely terminated, to facilitate their nontraumatic insertion through the arterial wall. A flared tip on a dilation catheter or a burst or an incompletely emptied balloon can tear its way into or out of the artery. Blood loss during or following transluminal angioplasty, though it should be avoidable, can be severe enough to require transfusion. Entry site bleeding or hematomas are more frequent following angioplasty than diagnostic catheterization, probably because larger catheters and balloon dilators require larger holes. Though more heparin is given during transluminal angioplasty than in diagnostic catheterization, protamine sulfate is not given at the termination of angioplasty to neutralize the heparin effect. Entry site trauma and thrombosis leading to acute ischemia have required emergency surgery in several instances.

OTHER COMPLICATIONS, INCLUDING IMMEDIATE FAILURE

The immediate failure of transluminal angioplasty most often is the result of an inability to find a satisfactory lumen-to-lumen pathway through the narrowed or occluded segment. Although the conversion of a severe stenosis to an occlusion produces little worsening in symptoms, results can be catastrophic if previously patent runoff, collateral-fed arteries are lost. A serious, avoidable risk of transluminal angioplasty results from overly persistent efforts to effect reentry via a paraluminal path extending too far beyond the primary obstructing lesion.

In several cases, postangioplasty filling defects in distal arteries attributed to recent catheter clots would probably have escaped detection without immediate follow-up angiography. Small clots lodging in a previously narrowed segment can lead to thrombotic occlusion but also have been observed to undergo lysis in the course of a few days. Emboli, unseen in small, distal arteries, were probably responsible for transient episodes of local burning or hypoesthesia in the foot reported by several patients. In all of them, the benefit conveyed by the procedure overshadowed the transient symptoms attributed to minor emboli. Only 1 of our 800 treated patients was proved to have had significant downstream embolization by core fragments. No doubt such embolization occurs, but it is difficult to identify it. Excluding entry site complications, luminal loss is most often caused by subatheromic dissection or by the thrombosis of a rough-surfaced neolumen following angioplasty. As yet, there is no certain way of reducing the incidence of thrombosis other than by excluding all patients with complete occlusions, an unjustified way of bettering the overall statistics, since it would deny many patients the benefits of successful recanalization. In at least 4 treated cases, transluminal angioplasty either caused or hastened the need for amputation. That such unhappy results were confined mostly to earlier treated cases is attributed to better case selection and improved technique. As is often true of innovative procedures, especially surgical procedures, the accumulation of experience has been the necessary, sometimes painful, road to improvement.

Results of Transluminal Angioplasty

Ideally, all patients should have objective follow-up studies, including arteriography. Unfortunately, reliable follow-up information is often hard to get. The results of transluminal angioplasty could be objectively quantitated by a controlled comparison with other forms of therapy, but this approach is unlikely to be taken. An appraisal of a consecutive series of more recently treated cases would necessarily exclude long-term results. In any case, past experience provides the best currently available means of estimating the value of transluminal angioplasty in various types of lesions and in individual patients. The collective results of transluminal angioplasty in several large case series have been reported; they are similar to ours [32, 35–37].

In general, the patient with an iliac or femoropopliteal artery lesion suitable for *dilation* has a 70 to 80 percent chance of receiving long-term (2 or more years) benefit, though retreatment will be necessary in about 20 percent. As might be expected, the results of transluminal *recanalization* are not as good as those of transluminal dilation. An overall 2-year postrecanalization patency rate of about 50 percent does not provide a prognosis for the individual patient. The patient with a short segmental luminal occlusion has an outlook almost as good as that of someone with a severe local stenosis. At the opposite end of the occlusive spectrum, the patient with complete obliteration of the entire superficial femoropopliteal system with poor runoff vessels has a much poorer chance of receiving immediate or lasting benefit through transluminal recanalization.

Case Selection: Transluminal Angioplasty and Surgery

INDICATIONS FOR TRANSLUMINAL DILATION

In the treatment of localized or diffuse narrowing of the iliac or femoropopliteal arteries, transluminal dilation is indicated regardless of the state of the runoff arteries, the severity of symptoms, or the degree of tissue ischemia. Despite a somewhat higher incidence of minor complications, it is not much more hazardous to the patient than simple arteriography. Stated differently, transluminal dilation of pelvic and femoral arteries is indicated wherever it is physically possible and appears likely to convey benefit, present or future, to the patient. It can be used in patients with minimal symptoms. Its relative advantages over surgery are such that *if it can be done, it should be done, and until it has, surgery should not.*

INDICATIONS FOR TRANSLUMINAL RECANALIZATION

In patients with lengthy occlusions (20 cm or longer), transluminal recanalization is best reserved for those for whom surgery is for some reason impossible or contraindicated or has failed without precluding catheter recanalization. It is

Figure 91-16. Seven-year patency after transluminal angioplasty. Recanalization of the right and dilation of the left superficial femoral arteries in a 72-year-old man. Diagnostic arteriography and bilateral transluminal therapy were done in a single hour-long procedure. The 7-year follow-up arteriograms show continued patency.

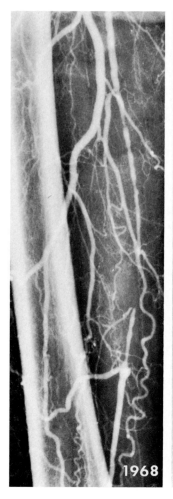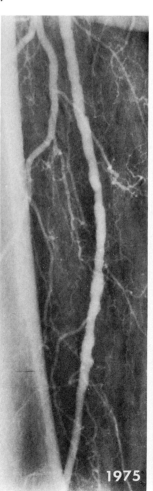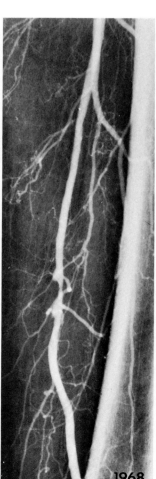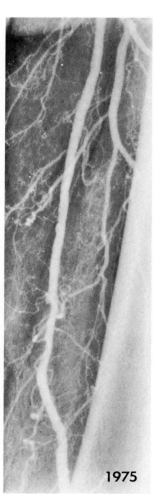

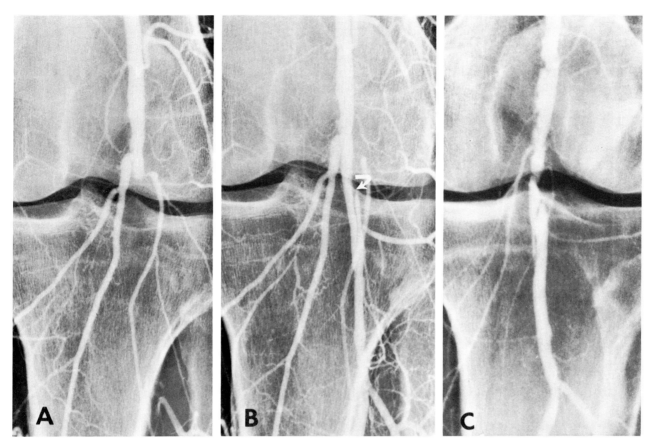

Figure 91-17. Nine-year patency following transluminal treatment of long-segment popliteal occlusion. (A) Popliteal occlusion from the knee to the origin of small, collateral-filled tibial branches. (B) Immediately after recanalization. The tibial branches are distended, and the collateral vessels are still filling. An intimal flap is evident (*arrow*). (C) The lumen is patent 9 years later. The collateral flow is markedly reduced. There are a persistent intimal flap and progressive atheromatous changes but good flow. Since the patient was symptom free, it was thought that retreatment was not indicated. (Magnification arteriography.)

nevertheless clear from many successes that transluminal recanalization offers a frequently effective alternative to operation and is capable of conveying equally impressive long-term benefits (Figs. 91-16, 91-17). In patients with short-segment occlusions of the superficial femoral or popliteal artery, an initial trial of transluminal recanalization is justifiable if it is done with care not to impair a surgical effort in the event of transluminal failure. If surgery is not a possibility, it is particularly important that attempted transluminal recanalization not leave the patient any worse for the effort. Although this is nearly always possible, it is not always achieved, especially by those lacking the experience to know when to abandon an unproductive effort before it becomes a dangerous one.

Last-chance, all-or-nothing salvage efforts are justifiable alternatives to an otherwise "inevitable" amputation and, as such, should always receive serious consideration. Here, there is little to lose and much to gain. In this series, an estimated 20 or more otherwise inevitable amputations, several of which had already been scheduled, were avoided by either transluminal recanalization or dilation. In some patients, transluminal therapy substantially lowered the level of required amputation. To illustrate the foregoing, successful transluminal recanalization of an occluded femoropopliteal artery, though too late to save a foot seriously affected by diabetic ischemic osteomyelitis, reestablished pulsatile blood flow though all three tibial arteries at the level of ankle resection (Fig. 91-18).

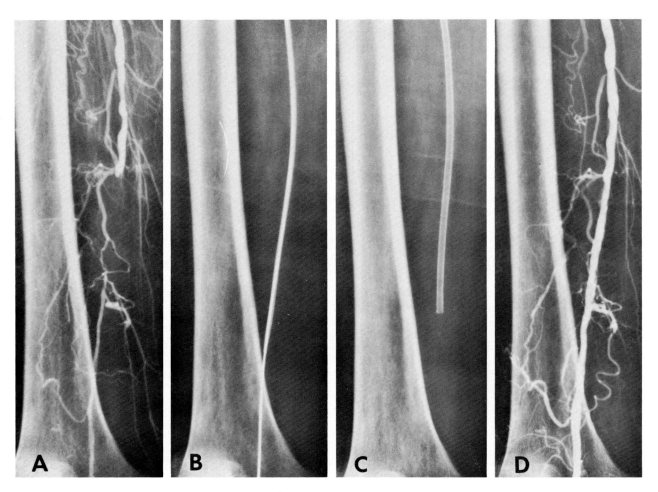

Figure 91-18. Transluminal coaxial recanalization. A 54-year-old woman with diabetic osteomyelitis in multiple bones of the foot. (A) There is segmental occlusion at the level of the adductor hiatus. (B) A guide and an 8 French Teflon catheter traverse the lesion. (C) An outer 12 French coaxial dilation catheter remains in place. (D) There is good restoration of the lumen, with resulting enlargement of the popliteal artery. After an unavoidable amputation of a foot, done a few days later, vigorous pulsatile blood flow was noted in all three major arteries. Recanalization had lowered both the level and the risk of amputation.

Transluminal Angioplasty and Surgery

Transluminal dilation is safer, swifter, easier; it involves less hospitalization, lower costs, and a shorter "down time" than conventional reconstructive arterial surgery (Fig. 91-19). It is as likely as surgery to succeed and can be considered whether the ischemic consequences of the basic disease are mild symptoms or severe gangrene. Unlike surgery, its chances of success are not seriously compromised by severe distal disease. Unlike aortoiliac surgery, transluminal angioplasty poses no risk to sexual potency (which it appears to have restored in 2 or 3 patients, perhaps by renewing their confidence or by allowing them to run fast enough to catch some-

one). Unlike bypass grafting, transluminal retreatment is not limited by the number of available veins, veins that might better be saved for possible future coronary surgery. Its failure need not compromise the patient's condition or chances for successful surgery. Although in the interest of safety we do not recommend it, we have dilated a severe iliac stenosis in an *outpatient*, with lasting relief of disabling claudication.

The foregoing, admittedly biased, comparison is based on experience in over 800 treated cases. In stressing the relative advantages and disadvantages of different approaches to the mechanical problem of arterial occlusive disease, it is possible to mislead by placing complementary methods in a seemingly competitive relationship. This position is unwarranted. The complications

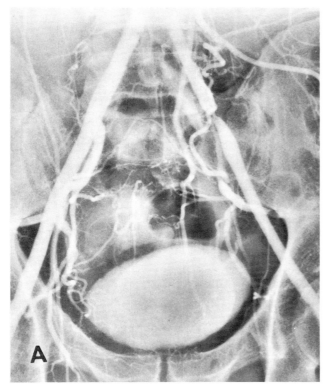

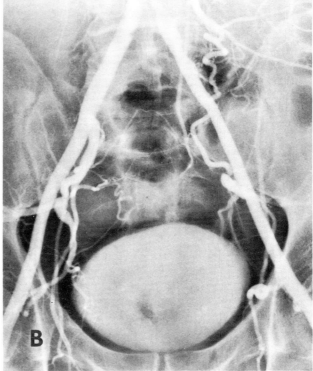

Figure 91-19. Transluminal iliac artery dilation in an outpatient. (A) Before and (B) two years after transluminal dilation of severe left iliac artery stenosis. Although outpatient angioplasty is rarely done, the re- sults invite comparison with its surgical equivalent. In localized iliac artery narrowing, transluminal dilation is indicated, surgery is not.

of transluminal angioplasty have often required emergency surgical salvage; its failures have often been followed by surgical success. Combined approaches have served where neither would have worked alone. Thus, transluminal dilation has made femoral-femoral or femoropopliteal grafting possible where aortoiliac surgery was technically not feasible, unsafe, or unacceptable to the patient (see Fig. 91-14). Despite the increasing professional awareness of transluminal angioplasty, many patients are still offered vascular surgery without being informed of an existing nonoperative alternative. Perhaps a future successful malpractice action will help put the "full" in "full disclosure."

Future Possibilities

A decade ago, the corresponding chapter in the second edition of this book concluded with hopeful predictions about the future of transluminal angioplasty [38]. The discussion looked ahead to (1) the eventual acceptance of trans- luminal angioplasty as an alternative to surgical revascularization, (2) its potential application to coronary, renal, and other arteries, and (3) improvements in tools and techniques that would result when the innovative efforts of others came on line. With respect to these predictions, the future is now.

Transluminal angioplasty has now become a respectable technique. There has been an upsurge in the scientific reporting of it (Fig. 91-20), and 2,500 procedures are done each month (estimated by the number of catheter dilators sold by one of several manufacturers). Other chapters in this book deal with coronary and renal artery angioplasty, techniques made possible by the innovations of others. Transluminal dilation has been used in carotid [39] and vertebral [40] arteries, in stenotic vein grafts [41, 42], in postrenal transplant stenosis [43], and in other nonatherosclerotic vascular obstructions [44–46].

What lies ahead? In a broad sense, the term *transluminal recanalization* refers to any real or conceptual means of removing vascular occlusions, and therefore could include embolectomy and endarterectomy. A feasible percutaneous ap-

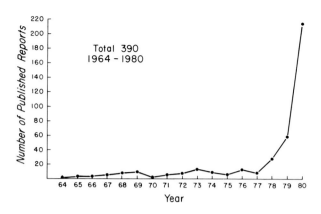

Figure 91-20. Scientific publications on transluminal angioplasty, 1964–1980, worldwide. ASCA computer scan figures include certain titles not listed in the quarterly *Index Medicus.*

proach to transluminal embolectomy has been worked out and awaits only the development of the needed catheter. A step toward percutaneous endarterectomy has already been taken by Gianturco's design of a lumen-following auger-type drill. A different step toward the same objective may lie in the use of transluminal fiberoptic lasers. A transluminal approach to the percutaneous creation of intrahepatic portosystemic shunts first explored in animals by Rösch in 1968 [47] is now being modified, using newly developed tools, and may soon be ready for clinical trials. If these hopeful extrapolations are fulfilled as well as were those of a decade ago, the future of transluminal angioplasty will be as exciting as its past has been.

References

1. Dotter, C. T., and Judkins, M. P.   Transluminal treatment of arteriosclerotic obstruction: Description of a new technic and a preliminary report of its application. *Circulation* 30:654, 1964.
2. Dotter, C. T.   Arteriosclerosis. *Semin. Roentgenol.* 5:228, 1970.
3. Dotter, C. T.   Transluminal Angioplasty—Pathologic Basis. In E. Zeitler, A. Grüntzig, and W. Schoop (eds.), *Percutaneous Vascular Recanalization.* Berlin, Heidelberg, New York: Springer, 1978. P. 3.
4. Dotter, C. T., Rösch, J., and Seaman, A. J.   Selective clot lysis with low-dose streptokinase. *Radiology* 111:31, 1974.
5. Martin, M., and Zeitler, E.   Percutaneous Transluminal Recanalization (PTR) and Fibrinolysis: Fibrinolytic Treatment of Femoral Reocclusions Subsequent to PTR Procedures. In E. Zeitler, A. Grüntzig, and W. Schoop (eds.), *Percutaneous Vascular Recanalization.* Berlin, Heidelberg, New York: Springer, 1978. P. 152.
6. Dotter, C. T., Judkins, M. P., Frische, L. H., and Rösch, J.   Nonoperative treatment of arterial occlusive disease: A radiologically facilitated technic. *Radiol. Clin. North Am.* 5:531, 1967.
7. Block, P. C., Baughman, K. L., Pasternak, R. C., and Fallon, J. T.   Transluminal angioplasty: Correlation of morphologic and angiographic findings in an experimental model. *Circulation* 61:778, 1980.
8. Castaneda-Zuniga, W. R., Formanek, A., Tadavarthy, M., Vlodaver, Z., Edwards, J. E., Zollikofer, C., and Amplatz, K.   The mechanism of balloon angioplasty. *Radiology* 135:565, 1980.
9. Schwarten, D. E., Yune, H. Y., Klatte, E. C., Grim, C. E., and Weinberger, M. H.   Clinical experience with percutaneous transluminal angioplasty (PTA) of stenotic renal arteries. *Radiology* 135:601, 1980.
10. Zeitler, E., Grüntzig, A., and Schoop, W. (eds.).   *Percutaneous Vascular Recanalization.* Berlin, Heidelberg, New York: Springer, 1978.
11. Bachman, D. M., Casarella, W. J., and Sos, T. A.   Percutaneous iliofemoral angioplasty via the contralateral femoral artery. *Radiology* 130:617, 1979.
12. Dotter, C. T., Rösch, J., and Robinson, M.   Fluoroscopic guidance in femoral artery puncture: Technical note. *Radiology* 127:266, 1978.
13. Staple, T. W.   Modified catheter for percutaneous transluminal treatment of arteriosclerotic obstructions. *Radiology* 91:1041, 1968.
14. van Andel, G. J.   *Percutaneous Transluminal Angioplasty. The Dotter Procedure. A Manual for the Radiologist.* Amsterdam and New York: Elsevier, 1976.
15. Dotter, C. T., Judkins, M. P., Frische, L. H., and Mueller, R.   The "non-surgical" treatment of ilio-femoral arteriosclerotic obstruction. *Radiology* 86:871. 1966.
16. Porstmann, W.   Ein neuer Korsett-Ballonkatheter zur transluminalen Rekanalisation nach Dotter unter besonderer Berücksichtigung von Obliterationen an den Beckenarterien. *Radiol. Diagn.* (Berl.) 2:239, 1973.
17. Dotter, C. T., Rösch, J., Anderson, J. M., Antonovic, R., and Robinson, M.   Transluminal iliac artery dilatation—nonsurgical catheter treatment of atheromatous narrowing. *J.A.M.A.* 230:117, 1974.
18. Grüntzig, A., and Hopff, H.   Perkutane Rekanalisation chronischer arterieller Verschlüsse mit einem neuen Dilatationskatheter. Modifikation der Dotter-Technik. *Dtsch. Med. Wochenschr.* 99:2502, 1974.
19. Horváth, L., Illes, I., and Varro, J.   Complications of the Transluminal Angioplasty Excluding the Puncture Site Complications. In E. Zeitler, A. Grüntzig, and W. Schoop (eds.), *Percutaneous Vascular Recanalization.* Berlin, Heidelberg, New York: Springer, 1978. P. 126.

20. Grollman, J. H., Del Vicario, M., and Mittal, A. K. Percutaneous transluminal abdominal aortic angioplasty. *AJR* 134:1053, 1980.
21. Velasquez, G., Castaneda-Zuniga, W., Formanek, A., Zollikofer, C., Barreto, A., Nicoloff, D., Amplatz, K., and Sullivan, A. Nonsurgical aortoplasty in Leriche syndrome. *Radiology* 134:359, 1980.
22. Grüntzig, A., Kuhlmann, U., Vetter, W., Lütolf, U., Meier, B., and Siegenthaler, W. Treatment of renovascular hypertension with percutaneous transluminal dilation of a renal artery stenosis. *Lancet* 1:801, 1978.
23. Grüntzig, A. Transluminal dilatation of coronary artery stenosis (letter to the editor). *Lancet* 1:263, 1978.
24. Abele, J. E. Technical considerations about balloon catheters and transluminal dilatation. *AJR* 155:901, 1980.
25. Grüntzig, A. *Die perkutane transluminale Rekanalisation chronischer Arterienverschlüsse mit einer neuen Dilatationstechnik.* Baden-Baden: Witzstrock, 1977.
26. Katzen, B. T., and Chang, J. Percutaneous transluminal angioplasty (PTA) with the Grüntzig balloon catheter: Technical problems encountered in the first forty patients. *Cardiovasc. Radiol.* 2:3, 1979.
27. Udoff, E. J., Barth, K. L., Harrington, D. P., Kaufman, S. L., and White, R. I. Hemodynamic significance of iliac artery stenosis: Pressure measurements during angiography. *Radiology* 132: 289, 1979.
28. Thompson, K. R., and Goldin, A. R. Angiographic techniques in interventional radiology. *Radiol. Clin. North Am.* 17:375, 1979.
29. Tegtmeyer, C. J., Moore, T. S., Chandler, J. G., Wellons, H. A., and Rudolf, L. E. Percutaneous transluminal dilatation of a complete block in the right iliac artery. *AJR* 133:532, 1979.
30. Eidemiller, E. R., Porter, J. M., Rösch, J., Dotter, C. T., and Krippaehne, W. W. Surgical treatment of bilateral iliac artery occlusive disease in high-risk patients. *Am. Surg.* 40:511, 1974.
31. Porter, J. M., Eidemiller, L. R., Dotter, C. T., Rösch, J., and Vetto, M. Combined arterial dilatation and femorofemoral bypass for limb salvage. *Surg. Gynecol. Obstet.* 137:409, 1973.
32. Wierny, L. R., Plass, R., and Porstmann, W. Long-term results in 100 consecutive patients treated by transluminal angioplasty. *Radiology* 112:543, 1974.
33. Zeitler, E. Leistungsfähigkeit der perkutanen Beseitigung arterieller Obliterationen mit der Dotter-Technik. In H. Ehringer (ed.), *Fortschritte der konservativen Therapie der peripheren arteriellen Verschlusskrankheit. Aktuelle Probleme in der Angiologie.* Berne, Stuttgart, and Vienna: Huber, 1974. Vol. 24, p. 70.
34. Horváth, L. Percutaneous transluminal angioplasty: Importance of anticoagulant and fibrinolytic drugs. *AJR* 135:951, 1980.
35. Schmidtke, I., Zeitler, E., and Schoop, W. Late Results of Percutaneous Catheter Treatment (Dotter's Technique) in Occlusion of the Femoropopliteal Arteries, Stage II. In E. Zeitler, A. Grüntzig, and W. Schoop (eds.), *Percutaneous Vascular Recanalization.* Berlin, Heidelberg, New York: Springer, 1978. P. 96.
36. Schoop, W., Levy, H., Cappius, G., Mansjoer, H., and Zeitler, E. Early and Late Results of PTD in Iliac Stenosis. In E. Zeitler, A. Grüntzig, and W. Schoop (eds.), *Percutaneous Vascular Recanalization.* Berlin, Heidelberg, New York: Springer, 1978. P. 111.
37. van Andel, G. J. Transluminal iliac angioplasty: Long-term results. *Radiology* 135:607, 1980.
38. Dotter, C. T. Transluminal Angioplasty. In H. L. Abrams (ed.), *Angiography* (2nd ed.). Boston: Little, Brown, 1971. P. 1287.
39. Mathias, K., Rohrbach, R., Neff, W., and Ensinger, H. Percutaneous Transluminal Dilatation (PTD) of Carotid Artery Stenosis. In E. Zeitler, A. Grüntzig, and W. Schoop (eds.), *Percutaneous Vascular Recanalization.* Berlin, Heidelberg, New York: Springer, 1978. P. 66.
40. Motarjeme, A. Percutaneous transluminal angioplasty of the vertebral arteries. *Radiology* 139:715, 1981.
41. Alpert, J. R., Ring, E. J., Berkowitz, H. D., Freiman, D. B., Oleaga, J. A., Gordon, R., and Roberts, B. Treatment of vein graft stenosis by balloon catheter dilation. *J.A.M.A.* 242:2769, 1979.
42. Ford, W., Wholey, M. H., Zikria, E. A., Miller, W. H., Samadani, S. R., Koimattur, A. G., and Sullivan, M. E. Percutaneous transluminal angioplasty in the management of occlusive disease involving the coronary arteries and saphenous vein bypass grafts. Preliminary results. *J. Thorac. Cardiovasc. Surg.* 79:1, 1980.
43. Sniderman, K. W., Sos, T. A., Sprayregen, S., Saddekni, S., Cheigh, J. S., Tapia, L., Tellis, V., and Veith, F. J. Percutaneous transluminal angioplasty in renal transplant arterial stenosis for relief of hypertension. *Radiology* 135:23, 1980.
44. Martin, E. C., Diamond, N. G., and Casarella, W. J. Percutaneous transluminal angioplasty in non-atherosclerotic disease. *Radiology* 135:27, 1980.
45. Furrer, J., Grüntzig, A., Kugelmeier, J., and Goebel, N. Treatment of abdominal angina with percutaneous dilatation of an arteria mesenterica superior stenosis. *Cardiovasc. Intervent. Radiol.* 3:43, 1980.
46. Mathias, V. K., Schlosser, V., and Reinke, M. Katheterrekanalisation eines Subklaviaverschlusses. *ROEFO* 132:346, 1980.
47. Rösch, J., Hanafee, W. N., and Snow, H. Transjugular portal venography and radiologic portacaval shunt: An experimental study. *Radiology* 92:1112, 1969.

2. Occlusive Techniques

Particulate Embolization Materials

DONALD P. HARRINGTON

Embolization therapy is one of the foundation stones of interventional radiology. The variety of materials employed (they range from biologic products, such as muscle slips and autologous clot, to the newest of the plastic particles and "super glue" [37]) is a tribute to the imagination of the large number of investigators in this area.

This chapter explores the characteristics of the largest group of materials used for embolization, those consisting of particles. While numerous particulate materials have been used, the focus of this chapter is on autologous clot, Gelfoam, polyvinyl alcohol, and Avitene. These four materials, which are the commonest particles in general clinical use, demonstrate the wide range of characteristic advantages and disadvantages of embolization with particulate material.

The origins of embolization therapy can be traced to the work of Brooks in the 1930s, who used muscle slips for the occlusion of a traumatic carotid-cavernous fistula [11]. The introduction of muscle slips via an arteriotomy was usually but not always followed by a surgical ligation of the internal carotid artery [51].

This embolization method was successfully utilized by others for the treatment of neurovascular arteriovenous malformations (AVMs) [6, 25, 40]. Lussenhop et al. were the first to use embolization as the primary method of therapy [57, 59, 60], employing silicone spheroids introduced directly into the carotid artery. In 1968 Doppman et al. successfully pioneered embolization via a percutaneously placed catheter when they embolized a spinal cord AVM with stainless steel pellets [28]. In 1977 Rösch et al., using autologous clot, were the first to use embolization therapy for the treatment of gastrointestinal tract bleeding [77]. These technical innovations were rapidly followed by therapeutic embolization of a renal AVM by Rizk et al., using fat [76], and an embolic therapy of hypersplenism by Madison, using autologous clot [61]. The clinical applications of embolic therapy are detailed in the other chapters in Section 2.

General Principles

While there is no ideal particulate material that can be used in all clinical situations, there are some characteristics that are shared by all the major particulate materials, as well as variable characteristics that must be considered in choosing one particulate material over another (Tables

Table 92-1. Determinants of Appropriateness of Embolic Materials

Availability[a]

Cost[a]

Ease of use[a]

Toxicity[a]

Longevity of occlusion[b]

Particle size[b]

Volume of injected material[b]

[a]Determinant is relatively uniform for particulate embolic materials.
[b]Determinant varies among the particles.

92-1, 92-2). In general, all the particulate materials are readily available, inexpensive, and not directly toxic. All the particulate materials except autologous clot produce a mild inflammatory reaction that is greatest with Avitene [46] and least with polyvinyl alcohol [83, 87]; the toxic reaction with Gelfoam is in the middle [4].

The longevity of the particles within the vascular system is an important variable to consider. Both experimental and clinical data indicate that autologous clots persist for hours to days within the vascular system [4, 9, 66, 73]. Both Gelfoam and Avitene are occlusive from days to weeks and are known to be totally resorbed after 3 to 6 months [4, 46, 87]. Polyvinyl alcohol is considered a permanent agent and can be demonstrated

Table 92-2. Particulate Embolic Material: Comparison of Properties

Embolic Materials	Availability	Ease of Use[a]	Longevity of Occlusion	Particle Size[b]
Biologic				
Muscle slips	Obtained via minor surgery	+++	Days to weeks	Intermediate to large
Fibrous and subcutaneous tissue	Obtained via minor surgery	+++	Days to weeks	Intermediate to large
Autologous clot	Readily available in hospital	++++[c]	Hours to days	Variable
Gelatin and fiber				
Gelfoam	Readily available in hospital	+++	Weeks	Intermediate to large
Oxycel	Readily available in hospital	++	Weeks	Intermediate
Avitene	Readily available in hospital	++++	Weeks	Small
Metallic				
Carbon microspheres	Not in common use; readily available on order	++	Permanent	Variable
Metal filings	Not in common use; readily available in hospital	++	Permanent	Variable
Stainless steel balls	Not in common use; readily available on order	+	Permanent	Large
Metal balls, Silastic coated	Not in common use; readily available on order	++	Permanent	Variable
Plastic				
Polyvinyl alcohol	In common use; readily available on order	++[d]	Permanent	Intermediate to large
Silastic spheres	In common use; readily available on order	++	Permanent	Variable
Sephadex particles	Not in common use; readily available on order	++	Permanent	Variable
Acrylic spheres	Not in common use; readily available on order	++	Permanent	Variable
Polystyrene spheres	In common use; readily available on order	++	Permanent	Variable

[a]++++ (easiest) to + (most difficult).
[b]Scale is based on size in commonest use.
[c]Ease of use in patients with poor clotting function: +.
[d]Ease of use in compressed form: +.

histologically to be present for months [15, 83, 87].

Particle size is also a variable in the choice of embolic material although in many cases size cannot be exactly established, as, for example, with autologous clot, which tends to fragment first within the catheter and then again as it passes through the circulation. The final particle size has not been accurately determined, even with histologic examination. Gelfoam and polyvinyl alcohol are sized at the table by the operator, usually into millimeter particles [22]. Polyvinyl alcohol does not break down further after injection. Gelfoam is fragmented with passage through the catheter, as has been documented by Greenfield et al. [38]. Gelfoam particles may be further compacted within the circulation after injection. Avitene has the smallest particle size, with single fibers in the 200-μ range, up to clumps of millimeter-sized particles. The ratio of small particles to large ones can be altered by vigorous mixing of the particles, which increases the numbers of smaller particles. Since Avitene particles, unlike other major particles, can penetrate to arteriolar levels where collateral supply is not possible because all the vessels are functioning as end-arteries, ischemic necrosis may result [12, 13, 46]. All the particulate materials are easy to inject, although polyvinyl alcohol has been considered somewhat more difficult than the other three particulate materials [82].

Avitene and Gelfoam are easily available because of their use in surgery. Polyvinyl alcohol is readily available on order from the supplier. The expense of these products is minimal compared to the overall expense of the procedure.

Autologous Clot

Autologous clot was the first widely used particulate material for catheter embolization [9, 73–75]. Gelfoam has subsequently become the more popular particulate material, although there remain some specific indications for and strong advocates of the continued use of autologous clot [17, 72, 78].

The advantages of autologous clot include its availability, ease of injection, low cost, and lack of toxicity, but even the most obvious advantage, the availability of blood, is not an advantage if the blood will not clot. Other characteristics of autologous clot that are advantageous include the

fragmentation that occurs with clot as it passes through the catheter and the arterial tree, which provides good distal penetration to the level of bleeding [74]. This penetration is augmented in the treatment of hemorrhagic lesions or AVMs by the so-called sump effect, a preferential flow of particles to the bleeding site or lesion [16, 35, 44, 89]. The sump effect is an advantage in all forms of particulate embolization. The limited incidence of ischemic necrosis with autologous clot suggests that penetration does not extend to below the level where collateral vessels prevent ischemic necrosis.

The intravascular persistence of autologous clot became a point of controversy because of the early experimental work performed using the renal artery in dogs. Bookstein et al. injected aliquots of autologous clot alone, and autologous clot modified by the addition of varying concentrations of Amicar (aminocaproic acid) [9]. (Amicar is an antifibrinolytic agent that is added to autologous clot to retard clot breakdown and to prolong its intravascular life.) The unmodified clot rapidly lysed and was cleared in 45 minutes, with minimal ischemic damage. When 0.24 percent Amicar was added, no difference was noted. The addition of 12.5 percent Amicar obstructed vessels longer than did the smaller amounts of Amicar or unmodified clot and resulted in somewhat slower lysis of clot, with complete clearing in 24 hours, as opposed to 45 minutes with clot alone. Despite experimental evidence of rapid lysis of clot, the clinical use of autologous clot in 9 patients with upper gastrointestinal tract bleeding was successful, with control of bleeding in all 9 patients [9]. The initial experimental and clinical work suggested that autologous clot could stop bleeding and then be lysed before ischemic injury occurred.

Chuang et al. controlled experimentally induced renal hemorrhage using both autologous clot alone and Amicar-modified autologous clot in the canine model [20]. Rebleeding occurred in 2 animals with autologous clot alone but was controlled with a second injection of clot. No rebleeding occurred from kidneys embolized with modified autologous clot. Follow-up arteriography 3 hours after embolization demonstrated more thrombosis in the kidneys embolized with the modified clot, but at the time of sacrifice, 6 to 10 weeks after embolization, the degree of scarring was the same in all embolized kidneys, indicating some degree of ischemic damage with all materials.

The results obtained using the canine model are controversial because of the very active fibrinolytic system of the dog as compared to that of man. Osterman et al. evaluated the short-term intravascular life of clot using the domestic swine, which has a fibrinolytic system similar to man's. With autologous clot, heat-treated autologous clot, and Amicar-modified autologous clot, total or partial occlusion persisted in all animals at 24 hours, and at 15 days 50 percent of vessels were recanalized [66]. In a long-term study of emboli in domestic swine, recanalization following autologous clot embolization was complete at 4 months [4]. The evidence for less rapid lysis of autologous clot in the domestic swine, coupled with the findings of Vlahos et al. [85], who demonstrated renal infarction after 1 hour of embolization in the canine renal artery irrespective of embolic material, overturns the early optimism that autologous clot could prevent bleeding without infarction.

Because of the relatively short life of autologous clot, its use cannot be recommended for tumor embolization or for any embolization requiring long-term occlusion [36].

A major disadvantage of autologous clot is apparent in patients with poor clot formation, which can result from prolonged bleeding or liver dysfunction. Methods of overcoming these defects in clotting include the addition of thrombin to blood in order to speed up clot formation and the addition of Oxacyl to the thrombus in order to provide a network for thrombosis [9]. Oxacyl, a cellulose product, tends to form a lattice-work for thrombosis. Oxacyl and blood are mixed, allowed to clot, and then injected. This technique was a forerunner to the use of Gelfoam, which, when used alone, is less complicated and provides the same results [9, 74]. Oxacyl-modified clot is longer lived than unmodified clot in the canine kidney in the short term [9]. Long-term studies indicate clearing by 4 months [4].

While autologous clot as an embolic agent still has avid supporters, it has been largely superseded by Gelfoam, which has a number of similar properties but is simpler to use, particularly in the patient with an altered hematologic system [17, 73].

Gelfoam

Gelfoam (Upjohn) is an absorbable gelatin sponge that was primarily used for surgical hemostasis prior to the advent of embolic

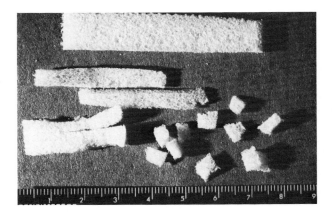

Figure 92-1. At the top of the photograph is shown the most common form of Gelfoam, the 2-×-6-mm strip. Such a strip can be cut to any size, as is shown below. The smallest particles are the easiest ones to work with and are the most common size. Since compaction and fragmentation occur with passage through the catheter, the ultimate size of the particle is smaller than illustrated.

therapy. The most widely used of all particulate embolic materials [23, 35, 36, 41, 42, 80], Gelfoam acts as a matrix for the formation of thrombus.

Gelfoam is readily available at low cost. Its popularity is, in part, due to its ease of use, particularly when compared to the preparation of autologous clot. The product is packaged in sheets that can be cut into small pledgets (Fig. 92-1). These pledgets can vary in size from 2 × 5 to 3 × 5 mm to large segments of 3 × 3 × 30 mm. The larger size is compressible and can be shaped so that the pledget is tapered at one end [22]. All sizes of this material are injected through the standard angiographic catheters (see Fig. 92-3). A powdered form of Gelfoam is used to control hemorrhage in the gastrointestinal tract but does not enjoy the widespread use of the individual pledgets [35].

Gelfoam induces a mild-to-moderate tissue reactivity, which enhances its thrombogenic effect. Gelfoam particles have been combined with a sclerosing agent, such as Sotradecol (sodium tetradecyl sulfate; Elkins-Sinn), in order to enhance its thrombotic effect by increasing the inflammatory reaction. This combination has been used for the embolization of gastric and esophageal varices in the treatment of bleeding associated with portal hypertension [68]. Studies of nonvascular tissue reactivity and absorption of particles in primates indicate peak tissue reactivity at 20 days, with clearing of tissue reactivity and Gelfoam in 45 days [54]. Short-term histologic changes (several days after Gelfoam embolization) indicate a panarteritis with a leukocyte infiltration into all vessel layers and disruption of the intimal and elastic layers [64, 79]. Gold and Grace established the intravascular longevity of Gelfoam in dogs, demonstrating its presence 24 to 48 hours after embolization of the left gastric artery. The Gelfoam was not present 7 to 10 days after injection, although thrombus was found in the small vessels of more than half of the experimental animals [33]. Long-term evaluation after Gelfoam embolization in the dog kidney demonstrated partial recanalization between 21 and 23 days and complete recanalization between 30 and 35 days [85]. Because of the very active fibrinolytic system in the dog, the study of the fate of Gelfoam emboli was repeated in the domestic swine. Embolized left gastric vessels and proximal renal vessels recanalized after 4 months. Residual Gelfoam was found in a single vessel, while organized thrombus was found in small end-arteries of the spleen and kidney. The vessel sizes were not specified [87].

Gelfoam has been used to advantage in conjunction with Gianturco coils and detachable balloons for tissue ablation in tumor therapy [22]. Particulate embolization with Gelfoam, which penetrates to the distal circulation, is followed by the introduction of Gianturco coils or detachable balloons for the occlusion of proximal vessels. The short intravascular life of Gelfoam is not a factor because of the permanent proximal occlusion, and the possible backflow of Gelfoam is minimized by the proximal coil or detachable balloon [32].

Polyvinyl Alcohol

Polyvinyl alcohol, also referred to as Ivalon (Unipoint), is a particulate embolic material that is like a sponge, an intriguing and important characteristic. (Nonmedical products composed of polyvinyl alcohol include the common household sponge.) Highly compressible, polyvinyl alcohol expands on contact with an aqueous medium, such as blood.

Polyvinyl alcohol was previously used as a prosthetic material in vascular surgery, but it was supplanted by Teflon and Dacron. Porstmann et al. have used polyvinyl alcohol for nonsurgical closure of patent ductus arteriosus [69]. Polyvinyl alcohol is supplied in a compressed and a noncompressed form, as well as in a powdered form.

It is readily available from the supplier but is not in common use in the hospital setting, as are Gelfoam and Avitene. The expansile capacity of the compressed form of the material has led to some difficulty in injecting it through standard angiographic catheters. This difficulty can be overcome, as discussed later in the chapter. The noncompressed form is slightly more difficult to inject than Gelfoam but less difficult to inject than the compressed form.

Polyvinyl alcohol is biologically inert, unlike other particulate embolic materials. This biologic property results in minimum inflammatory reaction within blood vessels and provides a permanently occlusive intravascular agent [13, 15, 52, 87].

Vlahos et al. demonstrated no angiographic evidence of recanalization 14 weeks after renal artery embolization in dogs [85]. Total occlusion was confirmed histologically. Castaneda-Zuniga et al. demonstrated long-term occlusion in the canine model using the splenic artery for embolization [15]. Animals were examined at 3 days, at 15 days, and after 9 months. At 3 days, thrombosis had formed around the polyvinyl alcohol fragments, which appeared to penetrate the vessel wall. At 15 days, multiple polymorphonuclear leukocytes were present in the media of the vessel, and at 9 months fibrotic scarring with permanent occlusion was present without evidence of inflammation. Vlahos et al. suggest that trauma from the penetration of the vessel wall could explain the inflammatory response [15]. White et al. demonstrated long-standing occlusion with polyvinyl alcohol at 4 months in the splenic and renal circulations of domestic swine, also without inflammation [87].

AVITENE

Avitene (microfibrillar collagen hemostat [MCH]; Avicon) is an embolic material that provides a matrix for thrombus formation. Since this material is widely used as a topical hemostatic agent, its ready availability is assured. Avitene is easily and quickly prepared by simply mixing the material with saline or contrast material, resulting in a mixture that has the consistency of applesauce (Fig. 92-2). An advantage of Avitene is the ease with which it can be injected through catheter systems as small as 3 French. Avitene provides good arterial penetration with particle sizes that range from 1-mm clumps of particles to single 200-μ fibers. As mentioned, the percentage of smaller particles is increased by mixing.

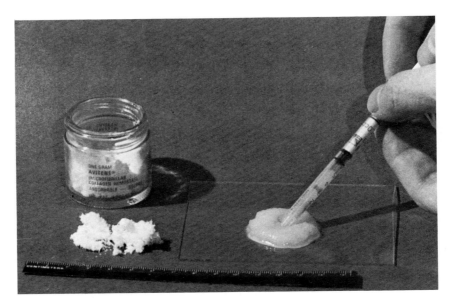

Figure 92-2. Avitene in the form obtained from the supplier is shown on the left. After it is mixed with saline or contrast material, Avitene has the consistency of applesauce and is easily drawn into the injection syringe.

Diamond et al. applied Avitene in cases in which marked degrees of ischemia were important, as in renal tumors and AVMs [26]. The small particle size can also be a two-edged sword and lead to unwanted necrosis, as was noted by Kaufman et al., who demonstrated gastric infarction in 2 animals after embolization of the gastrosplenic artery [46]. Small-vessel penetration is responsible for the ischemic effects of Avitene, and the possibility of tissue infarction is much higher than with the use of Gelfoam or polyvinyl alcohol. Theoretically, when Avitene is used in the treatment of AVMs, pulmonary embolization is possible with passage of small particles from the arterial into the venous and pulmonary circulations, although this has not been documented.

Recanalization occurs in as little as 2 weeks in large vessels, but thrombosis is present up to 3 months in smaller vessels [26, 46]. Despite the possible dangers of ischemia, the small particle size and the ease of passage of Avitene through small catheters make it highly desirable when superselective catheter placement is necessary or total ablation is required.

Individual Organ Embolization

The many successful examples of liver embolization attest to the safety and efficacy of the procedure [42–44, 86]. Theoretical support for the safety of embolization comes from surgical attempts at devascularization of the liver for treatment of neoplastic lesions, the results of which suggest that ischemic necrosis of the liver is difficult to achieve because of the diversity of the arterial blood supply and the rapid formation of collateral vessels [5, 9, 71]. Experimental studies of embolization provided the final link that established that the method was safe and effective within certain limits [12, 18, 24].

Cho et al. undertook experimental embolization of the liver to determine the effects on liver functions from a metabolic and histologic point of view. The experiment involved occlusion of the hepatic arterial circulation in dogs with Gelfoam pledgets measuring 2 to 3 mm. These pledgets were introduced under fluoroscopic control, and occlusion was confirmed angiographically. Alkaline phosphatase, serum glutamic pyruvic transaminase (SGPT), sulphobromophthalein retention (BSP), and serum bilirubin were measured. Serum alkaline phosphatase peaked in 24 hours at approximately 240 IU per liter, with a control of approximately 80 IU per liter, and returned to normal at 6 weeks. SGPT peaked at 3 days and was normal at 6 weeks. Serum bilirubin and BSP retention remained in the normal range throughout the experimental period. Anatomic and histologic study at 6 weeks demonstrated limited (2–3 cm in diameter) areas of infarction in the subcapsular region in 3 of 11 dogs. Overall, the liver sizes were normal.

The clinical and experimental data suggest the relatively benign nature of particulate embolization in the liver, but the work of Doppman et al. has modified that view and gives further insight into the physiology of particulate embolization [29]. Using silicone rubber, Doppman's group embolized the hepatic arteries of 6 rhesus monkeys; 2 rhesus monkeys used as controls had hepatic artery embolization with Gelfoam. Multiple small infarctions and bile cysts were noted histologically after the sacrifice of the animals. The silicone rubber embolization obstructed the entire hepatic arterial tree and was permanent, whereas in the controls Gelfoam lodged in more proximal vessels and was a temporary occlusive agent.

Bergener et al. reported similar extensive liver necrosis after embolization of hepatic arteries in rabbits with 175-μ polystyrene microspheres [12]. Particle size and the degree of penetration are the key factors in the ischemic changes in an organ such as the liver that is normally well vascularized and collateralized.

In a parallel work, Castaneda-Zuniga et al. used various combinations of embolization to the blood supply of the upper gastrointestinal tract in dogs [13]. In group 1, left gastric and splenic branches were embolized; in group 2, left gastric branches alone were embolized; and in group 3, splenic branches alone were embolized. The authors used polyvinyl alcohol particles smaller than 500 μ in diameter as the embolic material. Gastric ulceration resulted in 3 of 5 animals in group 1, 1 of 5 animals in group 2, and none of 5 animals in group 3. Only 1 animal in group 1 had three-vessel embolization (splenic artery, left gastric artery, and right gastric artery embolization); this animal suffered gastric infarction. Histologic examination indicated that in the animals without ulceration, the embolized vessels ranged from 0.44 mm to 1.86 mm in diameter, but in the animals with ulceration, embolized arteries as small as 0.22 mm in diameter were identified. This finding confirms the importance of particle size and collateral circulation in ischemic damage. The authors concluded that if necrosis is to be avoided, embolic particles should be greater than 300 μ in diameter.

The volume of embolization has been only partially studied, and the practical question of how much to inject does not have a clear answer at present. Bergener et al. in experimental embolization with rabbits demonstrated an exponential relationship between the volume of injected microspheres and the amount of tissue damage [12]. The volume of embolic material is not the major problem in the upper gastrointestinal tract, but it is recommended that lesions of the small bowel and colon be treated with a minimum volume of embolic material delivered superselectively [10]. The major clinical impact of volume of embolic material used is in the splenic circulation. Proximal splenic artery occlusion or large-particle embolization, which allows adequate collateralization of distal vessels, is well tolerated [39, 82]. The early therapy for hypersplenism involved the introduction of large volumes of small embolic particles into the distal splenic circulation, which led to numerous complications, including abscess formation, rupture of the spleen, and death [14, 36, 88]. Experimental embolization utilizing an animal model also resulted in multiple abscess formation [18]. Spigos et al. reevaluated the technique of particulate embolization and found that a smaller volume or partial embolization and a strict antibiotic regimen reduced the incidence of splenic abscess formation [80]. The role of antibiotic therapy is important in this process, but the clinical and experimental work suggests that the smaller volume of embolic material and the partial obliteration of the splenic circulation are the keys to safe and successful catheter therapy of hypersplenism. Similar results are reported by Owman et al., who confirmed the safety of the method in a canine model [67].

Other Particles

Although this chapter focuses on four major particulate materials, a large variety of other kinds of particles are also available for embolization. These fall into several broad categories, as discussed in the following paragraphs.

The first embolic particles were *biologic products*. Brooks et al. and others employed muscle slips [6, 11, 25]. Subcutaneous and fibrous tissues are two other sources of emboli, but, unlike muscle slips, they are usable for catheter-placed embolization [36]. Rizk et al. used fat particles as an embolic material [76]. These biologic particles were originally chosen because of their availability at a time when embolization was a surgical procedure. The present use of percutaneous catheter embolization makes the use of such biologic products obsolete, with the exception of autologous clots.

Metal-based embolic particles have been used because of their availability, radiopacity, and permanence. Carbon microspheres [63], stainless steel pellets [28], metal filings [30], and Silastic-containing steel balls [62] fall into this category.

The most versatile category of other particles is made up of the various forms of *plastic spheres* and *microspheres.* These products are invaluable when uniformity and exact sizing of particles are important. Applications are seen in the use of 175-μ polystyrene microspheres for the embolization of hepatic arteries in rabbits, by Burgener and Göthlin, and the embolization of the splenic artery, by Guilford and Scatliff, with silicone spheres [12, 39].

Most plastic particles can be made radiopaque. A difficulty in application is that residual particles are left in the catheter after embolization. At present, plastic particles are more frequently used for embolization of head and neck lesions, and are not generally used in the abdominal and peripheral vascular circulations. Other specific types of particles in this group include Sephadex particles [50], acrylic spheres [58], methyl-methacrylate spheres [60], and Silastic and silicone spheres [31, 55, 57].

Complications of Embolic Therapy and Their Avoidance

Complications of embolic procedures, real or hypothetical, are of major concern to interventional radiologists. I will not deal with the numerous individual reports of complications but instead will look at broad categories of complications, which, with few exceptions, are ischemic in nature. (A discussion of complications associated with catheter placement and manipulation is beyond the scope of this chapter but can be found elsewhere in this book.) Ischemia leading to some degree of tissue injury in the embolized circulation may occur to a varying degree in all embolization procedures. This ischemia with tissue destruction is the desired result of treatment of neoplastic processes [22, 34, 36, 41]. If embolic therapy is not aimed at the neoplastic process, any clinically evident ischemic event in the target circulation is a complication of embolization [1, 2, 13, 14, 46, 56, 70, 84, 88]; this unintentional ischemia is the most common complication. The second cause of complications from embolization is backflow of particles from the

target circulation to any nontarget circulation [27, 84, 90].

Avoiding ischemic complications is a rather imprecise process that involves decisions about particle size and volume of embolized materials, coupled with a knowledge of organ vascularity and collateral supply. As an example, the likelihood of infarction with particles larger than 300 μ in the upper gastrointestinal tract and liver is small, but the situation can be shifted in the other direction if the collateral circulation is altered by massive embolization of multiple vessels [74]. Alternatively, the collateral circulation can be reduced by pharmacologic means, such as with the vasoconstrictor vasopressin [19]. Such a reduction may be responsible for the complication reported by Prochaska et al. in which autologous clot embolization and prolonged vasopressin therapy were followed by ischemic necrosis of the stomach [70]. In less well-collateralized circulations, such as the small bowel, particle size larger than 300 μ in small volumes with superselective placement seems to protect the patient from ischemic damage [10]. In the renal circulation, which has many end-arteries, ischemic necrosis is inevitable but is limited by the volume of material, and it may be further limited if the material is rapidly cleared [21]. As previously discussed, partial embolization is the key to successful catheter treatment in hypersplenism [80].

The second major problem that causes complications, backflow of embolic particles into nontarget circulations, has a number of technical solutions involving methods of injecting particles. The phenomenon of backflow embolization has been well documented by Greenfield et al., who used cineangiography to define the extent of this phenomenon in the canine kidney [38]. Backflow embolization of Gelfoam particles occurred with continued injection of embolic material after the occlusion of segmental branches. Levin et al. confirmed this finding in canine renal vessels and demonstrated the backflow phenomenon with as few as 2 Gelfoam particles in the kidney and 15 particles in the superior mesenteric artery circulation [53]. The indications prior to backflow of particles were slow flow and/or stasis at the time of contrast injection in any of the tested circulations. Kerber described this same problem in the clinical situation and noted, as did the earlier authors, that test injections to determine the efficacy of embolization can also cause the backflow of embolic particles [47, 48]. Methods of controlling backflow include the use of a balloon occlusion catheter to block the backflow of particles into nontarget circulations [38]. Kerber suggested wedging the catheter in the artery to be embolized for control but noted that both the balloon-catheter and the wedged-catheter techniques modify the forward flow of blood, which, in turn, decreases the advantageous distal flow of embolic particles. Backflow of emboli can occur when occlusion is released. An alternative method described by both Kerber and Levin et al. consists of careful fluoroscopic monitoring of flow patterns of injected material to determine the precise end point of segmental occlusion [47, 48, 53]. Levin et al. further recommended injection of only single particles for the greatest control of embolization when Gelfoam pledgets are used.

Particulate Injection Techniques

The single-particle injection technique is practical and useful for the occlusion of small vessels, such as the left gastric artery and the gastroduodenal artery. The technique involves placing a single piece of tantalum-soaked Gelfoam at a time into a Luer-Lok stopcock with the stopcock in the closed position (Fig. 92-3A). A tuberculin syringe containing 1 cc of saline is attached to the Gelfoam-containing stopcock. The

stopcock is then turned to the open position and connected to the angiographic catheter. Injection is achieved with a slow, firm pressure, as illustrated in Figure 92-3B. A slow, careful increase in the injection pressure applied to the syringe is necessary to avoid explosive injection of particles as they leave the catheter tip. The major criticism of this technique is that it is very time consuming in larger circulations, in AVMs, and for the total occlusion of tumors. A widely accepted method for the injection of many particles of Gelfoam is to suspend 1- to-3-mm pledgets in a 1- to 5-cc contrast-filled syringe. The injection technique is the same as that for individual pledgets (Fig. 92-3B). An alternative technique is to place a reservoir in the system. Kricheff and Berenstein use an introducer system in which different types and sizes of particles can be stored and injected (Fig. 92-4) [49]. Figure 92-5 illustrates a similar technique, described by Bank and Kerber [3].

Polyvinyl alcohol in the compressed state is more difficult to inject than Gelfoam. Several techniques have been developed to solve this problem. Berenstein and Kricheff have suspended in contrast material hand-punched particles that are 0.038 to 0.089 cm (0.015–0.035 inches) in diameter and either have injected these particles with a standard syringe or have utilized the solid particle introducer system as illustrated in Figure 92-4 [7, 8, 49]. Kaufman has described a simpler approach using single particles of polyvinyl alcohol in which a pledget measuring 1

Figure 92-3. (A) The injection of single particles of Gelfoam as described by Levin et al. [53] involves placing single particles of saline-soaked Gelfoam into the distal portion of a two-way stopcock with the stopcock closed. (B) A 1-cc syringe filled with contrast material is then connected to the stopcock, and, after the stopcock is opened, a firm, controlled injection is performed in the manner illustrated. (Courtesy of David C. Levin, M.D.)

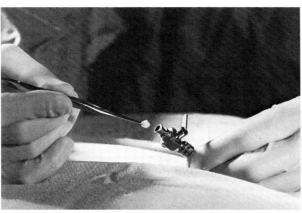

A

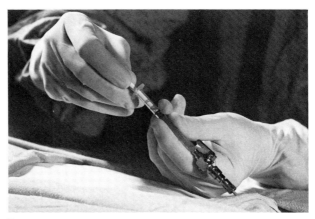

B

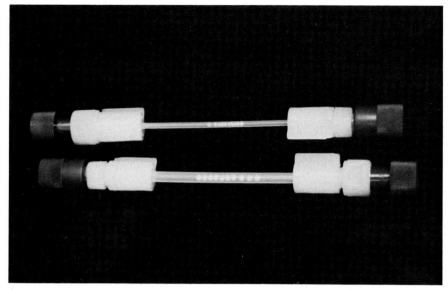

A

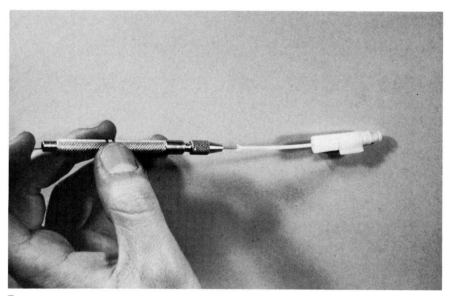

B

Figure 92-4. The NYU introducer system. (A) Two different sizes of introducers; they contain Silastic spheres. (B) With a catheter hole punch (*left*), plugs of polyvinyl alcohol are positioned directly into the introducer (*right*), which has one cap off. (C) The introducer (*middle*) is placed into the delivery system. The injection syringe is to the right, and the embolization catheter is to the left. The catheter tip loops to the top of the figure. (From Kricheff and Berenstein [49]. Reproduced by permission of *Radiology*.)

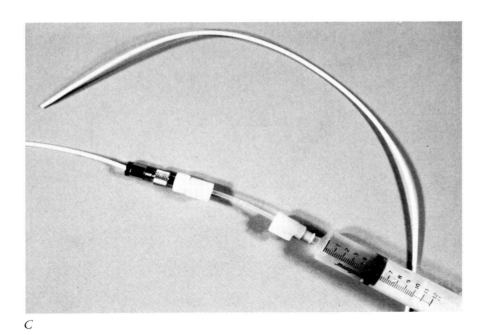

C

Figure 92-5. The injection system described by Kerber [48] consists of an injection syringe (*bottom*) and tubing connected to a three-way stopcock. The larger syringe (*top*) and the connecting tubing provide a reservoir for particles that can be easily transferred to the injection system.

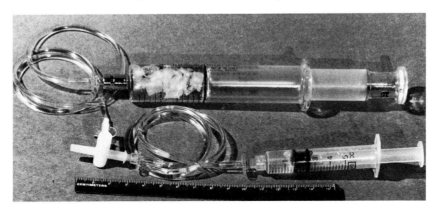

× 1 × 10 mm is soaked in saline and then introduced into the male end of a K-50 extension tube that had been preloaded with dilute contrast material [45]. Rapid, controlled injection followed.

Larger plugs of polyvinyl alcohol can be injected through the present catheter systems. But the method goes beyond the scope of this discussion.

Avitene is easily drawn up into a syringe and injected through a standard angiographic catheter, but care must be taken to clear completely the delivery systems of residual particles.

All the previously discussed methods of preventing backflow of particles can be used with the injection methods just described.

Other Techniques

Opacification of embolic materials as an aid to injection can be achieved by soaking non-radiopaque particles in tantalum [53, 77] or by mixing them with contrast materials as previously noted [47, 48]. Polyvinyl alcohol is available with barium impregnation. Another method of identifying therapeutic emboli is radionuclide labeling, which can be used to identify the final localization of the particle but is not useful at the time of injection [24].

In many cases of embolic therapy, extensive catheter manipulation, multiple catheter changes, or the use of nonstandard catheters can be anticipated, and the use of an Introducer Sheath (Cordis) at the puncture site can facilitate any of these maneuvers.

References

1. Anderson, J. H., VuBan, A., Wallace, S., Hester, J. P., and Burke, J. S. Transcatheter splenic arterial occlusion: An experimental study in dogs. *Radiology* 125:95, 1977.
2. Balsys, R., and Cross, R. Multiple aneurysm formation as a complication of interventive angiography. *Radiology* 126:91, 1978.
3. Bank, W. L., and Kerber, C. W. Gelfoam embolization: A simplified technique. *Am. J. Radiol.* 132:299, 1979.
4. Barth, K. H., Strandberg, J. D., and White, R. I. Long term follow-up of transcatheter embolization with autologous clot, Oxycel and Gelfoam in domestic swine. *Invest. Radiol.* 12:3, 1977.
5. Bengmark, S., and Rosengren, K. Angiographic study of the collateral circulation to the liver after ligation of the hepatic artery in man. *Am. J. Surg.* 119:620, 1970.
6. Bennett, J. E., and Zook, E. G. Treatment of arteriovenous fistulas in cavernous hemangiomas of face by muscle embolization. *Plast. Reconstr. Surg.* 50:84, 1972.
7. Berenstein, A., and Kricheff, I. I. Catheter and material selection for transarterial technical considerations: I. Catheters. *Radiology* 132:619, 1979.
8. Berenstein, A., and Kricheff, I. I. Catheter and material selection for transarterial embolization: Technical considerations: II. Materials. *Radiology* 132:631, 1979.
9. Bookstein, J. J., Chlosta, E. M., Foley, D., and Walker, J. F. Transcatheter hemostasis of gastrointestinal bleeding using modified autogenous clot. *Radiology* 113:277, 1974.
10. Bookstein, J. J., Naderi, M. J., and Walter, J. F. Transcatheter embolization for lower gastrointestinal bleeding. *Radiology* 127:345, 1978.
11. Brooks, B. The treatment of traumatic arteriovenous fistulas. *South. Med. J.* 23:100, 1930.
12. Burgener, F. A., and Göthlin, J. H. Angiographic, microangiographic and hemodynamic evaluation of hepatic artery embolization in the rabbit. *Invest. Radiol.* 13:306, 1978.
13. Castaneda-Zuniga, W. R., Jauregul, H., Rysavy, J., and Amplatz, K. Selective transcatheter embolization of the upper gastrointestinal tract: An experimental study. *Radiology* 127:81, 1978.
14. Castaneda-Zuniga, W. R., Hammerschmidt, D. E., Sanchez, R., and Amplatz, K. Nonsurgical splenectomy. *AJR* 129:805, 1977.
15. Castaneda-Zuniga, W. R., Sanchez, R., and Amplatz, K. Experimental observations of short and long-term effects of arterial occlusion with Ivalon. *Radiology* 126:783, 1978.
16. Chang, J., Katzen, B. T., and Sullivan, K. P. Transcatheter Gelfoam embolization of post-traumatic bleeding pseudoaneurysms. *AJR* 131:645, 1978.
17. Cho, K. J., and Reuter, S. R. Embolic control of superior mesenteric artery hemorrhage caused by abdominal abscesses. *AJR* 128:1041, 1977.
18. Cho, K. J., Reuter, S. R., and Schmidt, R. Effects of experimental hepatic artery embolization on hepatic function. *AJR* 127:563, 1976.
19. Chuang, V. P., Reuter, S. R., Cho, K. J., and Schmidt, R. W. Alterations in gastric physiology caused by selective embolization and vasopression infusion of the left gastric artery. *Radiology* 119:533, 1976.
20. Chuang, V. P., Reuter, S. R., and Schmidt, R. W. Control of experimental traumatic renal hemorrhage by embolization with autologous blood clot. *Radiology* 117:55, 1975.
21. Chuang, V. P., Reuter, S. R., Walter, J., Foley, W.

D., and Bookstein, J. J.   Control of renal hemorrhage by selective arterial embolization. *AJR*
125:300, 1975.

22. Chuang, V. P., Wallace, S., Swanson, D., Zornoza, J., Handel, S. F., Schwarten, D. E., and
Murray, J.   Arterial occlusion in the management
of pain from metastatic renal carcinoma. *Radiology*
133:611, 1979.

23. Chuang, V. P., Wallace, S., Zornoza, J., and
Davis, L. J.   Transcatheter arterial occlusion in
the management of rectosigmoidal bleeding.
Radiology 133:605, 1979.

24. Conroy, R. M., Lyons, K. P., Kuperus, J. H.,
Juler, G. I., Joy, I., and Pribram, H. F. W.   New
technique for localization of therapeutic emboli
using radionuclide labeling. *AJR* 130:523, 1978.

25. Cunningham, D. S., and Paletta, F. X.   Control
of arteriovenous fistulae in massive facial hemangioma by muscle emboli. *Plast. Reconstr. Surg.*
46:305, 1970.

26. Diamond, N. G., Casarella, W. J., Bachman, D.
M., and Wolff, M.   Microfibrillar collagen
hemostat: A new transcatheter embolization
agent. *Radiology* 133:775, 1979.

27. Doppman, J. L., and DiChiro, G.   Paraspinal
muscle infarction. *Radiology* 119:609, 1976.

28. Doppman, J. L., Dighird, G., and Ommaya, A.
Obliteration of spinal cord arteriovenous malformation by percutaneous embolization. *Lancet*
1:477, 1968.

29. Doppman, J. L., Girton, M., and Kahn, E. R.
Proximal versus peripheral hepatic artery embolization: Experimental study in monkeys. *Radiology*
128:577, 1978.

30. Fingerhut, A. G., and Alksne, J. F.   Thrombosis
of intracranial aneurysms. *Radiology* 86:342,
1966.

31. Fleischer, A. S., Kricheff, I., and Kansohoff, J.
Postmortem findings following the embolization
of an arteriovenous malformation. *J. Neurosurg.*
37:606, 1972.

32. Gianturco, C., Anderson, J. H., and Wallace, S.
Mechanical devices for arterial occlusion. *AJR*
124:428, 1975.

33. Gold, R. E., and Grace, D. M.   Gelfoam embolization of the left gastric artery for bleeding ulcer.
Radiology 116:575, 1975.

34. Goldin, A. R., Naude, J. H., and Thatcher, G. N.
Therapeutic percutaneous renal infarction. *Br. J.
Urol.* 46:133, 1974.

35. Goldman, M. L., Land, W. C., Jr., Bradley, E. L.,
III, and Anderson, J.   Transcatheter therapeutic
embolization in the management of massive upper
gastrointestinal bleeding. *Radiology* 120:513, 1976.

36. Goldstein, H. M., Wallace, S., Anderson, J. H.,
Bree, R. L., and Gianturco, C.   Transcatheter occlusion of abdominal tumors. *Radiology* 120:539,
1976.

37. Grace, D. M., Pitt, D. F., and Olo, R. E.   Vascu-

lar embolization and occlusion by angiographic
techniques and an alternative to operation. *Surg.
Gynecol. Obstet.* 143:469, 1976.

38. Greenfield, A. J., Athanasoulis, C. A., Waltman,
A. C., and LeMoure, E. R.   Transcatheter embolization: Prevention of embolic reflux using
balloon catheters. *AJR* 131:651, 1978.

39. Guilford, W. B., and Scatliff, J. H.   Transcatheter
embolization of the spleen for control of splenic
hemorrhage and in situ splenectomy: An experimental study using silicone spheres. *Radiology*
119:549, 1976.

40. Hamby, W. B., and Gardner, W. I.   Treatment of
pulsating exophthalmos with report of two cases.
Arch. Surg. 37:676, 1933.

41. Hlava, A., Steinhart, L., and Navratil, P.   Intraluminal obliteration of the renal arteries in kidney tumors. *Radiology* 121:323, 1979.

42. Jander, H. P., Laws, H. L., Kogutt, M. S., and
Mihas, A. A.   Emergency embolization in blunt
hepatic trauma. *AJR* 129:249, 1977.

43. Kadir, S., Athanasoulis, C. A., Jirisg, E., and
Greenfield, A.   Transcatheter embolization of
intrahepatic arterial aneurysms. *Radiology* 134:
335, 1980.

44. Katzen, B. T., Rossi, A., Passaniello, R., and
Simonett, G.   Transcatheter therapeutic arterial
embolization. *Radiology* 120:523, 1976.

45. Kaufman, S. L.   Simplified method of transcatheter embolization with polyvinyl alcohol foam
(Ivalon). *AJR* 132:853, 1979.

46. Kaufman, S. L., Strandberg, J. O., DumBarta, K.
H., and White, R. I., Jr.   Transcatheter emboli-
zation with microfibrillar collagen in swine. *Invest.
Radiol.* 13:200, 1978.

47. Kerber, C. W.   Catheter therapy: Fluoroscopic
monitoring of deliberate embolic occlusion.
Radiology 125:538, 1977.

48. Kerber, C. W.   Flow-controlled therapeutic embolization: A physiologic safe technique. *AJR*
134:557, 1980.

49. Kricheff, I. I., and Berenstein, A.   Simplified
solid-particle embolization with a new introducer.
Radiology 131:794, 1979.

50. Lalli, A. F., Peterson, N., and Bookstein, J. J.
Roentgen-guided infarctions of kidneys and
lungs. *Radiology* 93:434, 1969.

51. Lang, E. R., and Buch, P. C.   Treatment of
carotid-cavernous fistula by muscle embolization
alone: The Brooks method. *J. Neurosurg.* 22:387,
1965.

52. Latchaw, R. E., and Gold, L. H. S.   Polyvinyl
foam embolization of vascular and neoplastic lesions of the head, neck and spine. *Radiology*
131:669, 1979.

53. Levin, D. C., Beckmann, C. F., and Hillman, B.
Experimental determination of flow patterns of
Gelfoam emboli: Safety implications. *AJR* 134:
525, 1980.

54. Light, R. U., and Prentice, H. R. Surgical investigation of a new absorbable sponge derived from gelatin for use in hemostasis. *J. Neurosurg.* 2:435, 1945.

55. Lin, S. R., LaDow, C. S., Jr., Tatoian, J. A., and Go, E. B. Angiographic demonstration and silicone pellet embolization of facial hemangiomas of bone. *Neurosurgery* 7:201, 1974.

56. Lina, J. R., Jaques, P., and Mandell, V. Aneurysm rupture secondary to transcatheter embolization. *AJR* 132:553, 1979.

57. Longacre, J. J., and Unterthiner, R. A. Treatment of facial hemangioma by intravascular embolization with silicone spheres; case report. *Plast. Reconstr. Surg.* 50:618, 1972.

58. Loop, J. W., and Foltz, E. L. Applications of angiography during intracranial operation. *Acta Radiol.* [Diagn.] (Stockh.) 5:363, 1966.

59. Luessenhop, A. J., and Presper, J. H. Surgical embolization of cerebral arteriovenous malformations through internal carotid and vertebral arteries; long-term results. *J. Neurosurg.* 42:443, 1975.

60. Luessenhop, A. J., and Spence, W. T. Artificial embolization of cerebral arteries; report of use in a case of arteriovenous malformation. *J.A.M.A.* 172:1153, 1960.

61. Maddison, F. E. Embolic therapy of hypersplenism (abstract). *Invest. Radiol.* 8:280, 1973.

62. Mahalley, M. S., and Boone, S. C. External carotid cavernous fistula treated by arterial embolization. *J. Neurosurg.* 40:110, 1974.

63. Miller, F. J., Jr., Rankin, R. S., and Gliedman, J. B. Experimental internal iliac artery embolization evaluation of low viscosity silicone rubber, isobutyl 2-cyanoacrylate and carbon microspheres. *Diagn. Radiol.* 129:51, 1978.

64. Miller, M. D., Johnsrude, I. S., and Jackson, D. C. Improved technique for transcatheter embolization of arteries. *AJR* 130:183, 1978.

65. Ohta, T., Nishimma, S., Kikuchi, H., and Toyama, M. Closure of carotid-cavernous fistula with polyurethane foam embolus: Technical note. *J. Neurosurg.* 38:107, 1973.

66. Osterman, F. A., Bell, W. R., Montali, R. J., Novak, G. R., and White, R. I. Natural history of autologous blood clot embolization in swine. *Invest. Radiol.* 2:267, 1976.

67. Owman, T., Lunderquist, A., Alwmark, A., and Borjesson, B. Embolization of the spleen for treatment of splenomegaly and hypersplenism in patients with portal hypertension. *Invest. Radiol.* 14:457, 1979.

68. Pereiras, R., Viamonte, M., Jr., Russell, E., LePage, J., White, P., and Hutson, D. New techniques for interruption of gastroesophageal venous blood flow. *Radiology* 124:313, 1975.

69. Porstmann, W., Wierny, L., Warnke, H., Gerstberger, G., and Romaniek, P. A. Catheter closure of patent ductus arteriosus. *Radiol. Clin. North Am.* 9:203, 1971.

70. Prochaska, J. M., Flye, N. W., and Johnsrude, I. S. Left gastric artery embolization for control of gastric bleeding. A complication. *Radiology* 107:521, 1973.

71. Redman, S. R., and Reuter, S. R. Arterial collaterals in the liver hilus. *Radiology* 94:575, 1970.

72. Reuter, S. R. Embolization of gastrointestinal hemorrhage (editorial). *AJR* 133:557, 1979.

73. Reuter, S. R., and Chuang, V. P. Control of abdominal bleeding with autogenous embolized material. *Radiology* 14:86, 1974.

74. Reuter, S. R., Chuang, V. P., and Bree, R. J. Selective arterial embolization for control of massive upper gastrointestinal bleeding. *AJR* 125:119, 1975.

75. Ring, E. J., Athanasoulis, C., Waltman, S. C., et al. Arteriographic management of hemorrhage following pelvic fracture. *Radiology* 109:65, 1973.

76. Rizk, G. K., Atallah, N. K., and Bridi, G. I. Renal arteriovenous fistula treated by catheter embolization. *Br. J. Radiol.* 46:222, 1973.

77. Rösch, I., Dotter, C. T., and Brown, M. I. Selective arterial embolization: New method for control of acute gastrointestinal bleeding. *Radiology* 102:303, 1972.

78. Rosen, R. J., Feldman, L., and Wilson, A. R. Embolization for postbiopsy renal arteriovenous fistula: Effective occlusion using homologous clot. *AJR* 131:1072, 1978.

79. Sniderman, K. W., Franklin, J., and Sos, T. A. Successful transcatheter Gelfoam embolization of a bleeding cecal vascular ectasia. *AJR* 131:157, 1978.

80. Spigos, D. G., Jonasson, O., Mozes, M., and Capek, V. Partial splenic embolization in the treatment of hypersplenism. *AJR* 132:777, 1979.

81. Stanley, R. J., and Cubillo, E. Nonsurgical treatment of arteriovenous malformations of the trunk and limb of transcatheter arterial embolization. *Radiology* 115:609, 1975.

82. Tadavarthy, S. M., Knight, L., Ovitt, T. W., Snyder, C., and Amplatz, K. Therapeutic transcatheter arterial embolization. *Radiology* 111:13, 1974.

83. Tadavarthy, S. M., Moller, J. H., and Amplatz, K. Polyvinyl alcohol (Ivalon)—a new embolic material. *AJR* 125:609, 1975.

84. Tegtmeyer, C. J., Smith, T. H., Shaw, A., Barwick, K. W., and Kattwinkel, J. Renal infarction: A complication of Gelfoam embolization of a hemangioendothelioma of the liver. *AJR* 128:305, 1977.

85. Vlahos, L., Karatzas, G., Papaharalambous, N., and Pontifex, G. R. Percutaneous arterial embolization in the kidneys of dogs: A comparative

study of eight different materials. *Br. J. Radiol.* 53:289, 1980.

86. Walter, J. F., Paaso, B. T., and Cannon, W. B. Successful transcatheter embolic control of massive hematobilia secondary to liver biopsy. *AJR* 127:847, 1976.

87. White, R. I., Strandberg, J. V., Gross, G. S., and Barth, K. H. Therapeutic embolization with long-term occluding agents and their effects on embolized tissues. *Radiology* 125:677, 1977.

88. Wholey, M. H., Chamorro, H. A., Rao, G., and Chapman, W. Splenic infarction and spontaneous rupture of the spleen following therapeutic embolization. *Cardiovasc. Radiol.* 1:249, 1978.

89. Wolpert, S. M., and Stein, B. M. Factors governing the course of emboli in the therapeutic embolization of cerebral arteriovenous malformations. *Radiology* 131:125, 1979.

90. Woodside, J., Schwarz, H., and Bergreen, P. Peripheral embolization complicating bilateral renal infarction with Gelfoam. *AJR* 126:1033, 1976.

Steel Coil Embolus and Its Therapeutic Applications

SIDNEY WALLACE
VINCENT P. CHUANG
JAMES H. ANDERSON
CESARE GIANTURCO

The materials available for embolization include autologous clot and tissue; clot that has been modified (e.g., with thrombin, heat, or Amicar); Gelfoam; Oxycel; Ivalon (polyvinyl alcohol foam); cyanoacrylates; Silastic and metallic spheres; silicone and silicone rubber; Ethibloc, Avitene, and Sotradecol; lyophylized porcine dura mater; balloon catheters and detachable balloons; and metallic devices, such as brushes and stainless steel coils, with attached wool and Dacron strands [8, 18, 19, 32, 57]. The majority of these materials act as peripheral emboli that become trapped at various levels in the vascular bed into which they are injected. The use of many of these materials often gives a variable degree of occlusion not only because of their inhomogeneous distribution but also because of their nature. Blood clot and Gelfoam, for example, are biodegradable and readily recanalized. The need for a consistently reliable device that could be precisely placed for a more permanent central occlusion of larger vessels and could serve as an internal ligature was satisfied by the stainless steel spring coil embolus that Gianturco et al. devised [5, 15, 23, 53]. The attributes just mentioned are especially important in the occlusion of the major blood supply for the production of ischemia of neoplasms and the interruption and obliteration of vascular abnormalities and arteriovenous communications.

Coil Construction

ORIGINAL COIL

The original coil occluding device was made from a 5-cm curled segment of 0.038-inch stainless steel guidewire. Wool strands were attached to the proximal tip of the coil to facilitate thrombosis [23]. The coil was used with a nontapered-tip 7 French Teflon catheter. It was inserted into the catheter with a special, relatively stiff introducer stylet and then passed through the catheter with a modified guidewire (Fig. 93-1).

Increased utilization of the original coil created the necessity and demand for design modification. The wool attached to the coil was replaced with Dacron and the long, stiff introducer stylet was reduced in length to avoid inadvertent perfo-

Animal investigations supported in part by the John S. Dunn Research Foundation and the George A. Cook Memorial Fund.

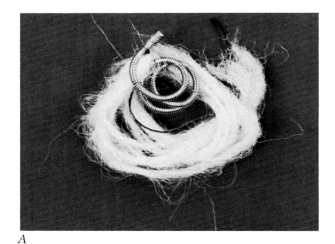

A

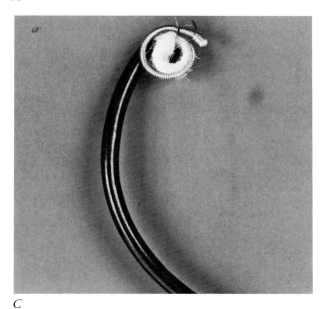

C

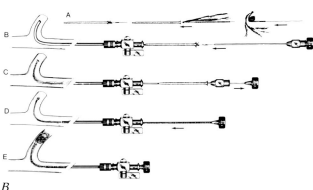

B

Figure 93-1. Original coil. (A) The stainless steel coil with attached wool strands. It has a 5-mm helix diameter. (B) The sequence of events in coil insertion. (C) The coil as it emerges from a 7 French Teflon nontapered-tip catheter.

Figure 93-2. Mini-Coil. Stainless steel coil (A) with attached Dacron strands. It has a 3-mm helix diameter, and passes through a 5 French polyethylene nontapered-tip catheter. The original coil (B) is shown for purposes of comparison.

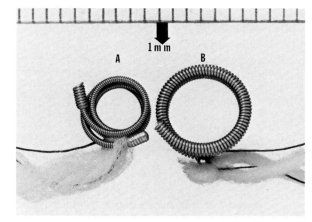

ration of the catheter when in a tortuous vessel. The conventional 0.038-inch soft-tip guidewire was found adequate and safer for propelling the coil through the catheter.

"MINI" COIL

It soon became apparent that the 7 French Teflon catheter was too rigid and too large for use in the occlusion of small tortuous vessels. The mini-coil differed from the original coil in that the mini-coil (1) was made from 5-cm segments of 0.021-inch stainless steel guidewire, (2) had a 3-mm section of 0.032-inch guidewire attached to its proximal tip as an adapter, (3) had a reduced amount of Dacron, and (4) was designed for use

5 cm

A

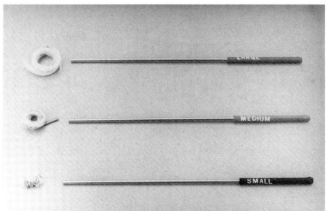

B

Figure 93-3. Newer coil. (A) Centipede appearance. (B) The coils are available in 3-mm, 5-mm, and 8-mm helix diameters. (C) The Dacron strands are dispersed through the length of the coil.

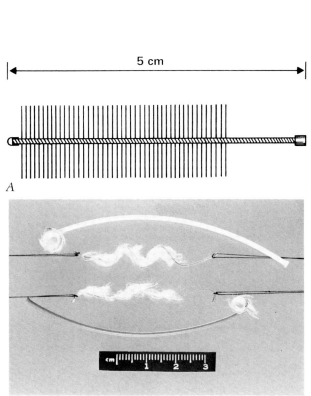

C

with a 5 French polyethylene catheter with a nontapered tip (Fig. 93-2).

The use of a guidewire with a smaller diameter (0.021 inch) reduced the force exerted by the coil against the internal wall of the catheter. A reduction in the amount of Dacron decreased the friction between the coil and the catheter wall [5].

NEWER COIL

The demand for a coil that could be used with the tapered-tip catheters ordinarily used for angiography stimulated the development of the presently available model of coil [15]. The adaptation that was made eliminated the necessity for catheter exchange, which was frequently required with the nontapered-tip catheter. The newer coil differs from the others in that the Dacron strands have been removed from the distal tip of the coil and replaced by multiple shorter strands evenly distributed throughout the first 4 cm of the 5-cm wire segment. This gives the coil the appearance of a centipede (Fig. 93-3). The coil is constructed of a 0.028-inch guide-

wire with a 3-mm 0.032-inch adapter at the tip. Unlike previous coils, the newer coil does not require a special introducer and can be inserted and passed through the catheter with the use of a standard 0.038-inch guidewire. The newer coils are designed for use with the 5 French polyethylene and 6.5 French Torcon catheters tapered to a 0.038-inch guidewire. The coils (Cook) are available in helix diameters of 3 mm, 5 mm, and 8 mm, to permit better selection of the size coil appropriate to the diameter of the vessel to be occluded. It is strongly recommended that before the procedure, the newer coil be used in other types of catheters and in in vitro tests through the specific catheter.

Factors Governing Use

Several factors that govern the use of the coil should be emphasized. The ease of passage through a given catheter is a function of (1) the catheter material (e.g., Teflon, polyethylene); (2) the internal diameter of the catheter relative to the size of the guidewire used in making the coil; (3) the amount of Dacron and the manner in which the Dacron is attached; (4) the size of the guidewire used to push the coil through the catheter; (5) the helix diameter of the curled coil, which influences the tension of the coil against the inner wall of the catheter; and (6) the size of the tapered-tip catheter and the shape of the curve at the catheter tip.

These factors influence the coefficient of friction and, therefore, the ease of passage of the coil through the catheter. It is essential to use the recommended combination of sizes of coil, catheter, and guidewire. Failure to do so may result in the coil's becoming wedged within the lumen of the catheter or jammed between the guidewire used to push it through the catheter and the wall of the catheter. Special precautions should be taken with a Torcon catheter, because the inner diameter of this catheter changes near the tip, at the junction of the internal wire mesh and the soft distal section.

Embolization Technique

The use of a combination of particulate emboli for the peripheral vascular bed and central occlusion of the major supplying vessel is superior to the use of a single component. This conclusion is based on the results of laboratory experimentation in the occlusion of renal and splenic arteries in dogs [2, 3]. It was impossible to infarct totally either the spleen or the kidney. The viable areas were most numerous at the periphery of the organ, presumably supplied by capsular or collateral vessels. The viscera were initially engorged, enlarged, and edematous for a few days to a week, but after 3 to 9 weeks, there was marked atrophy.

Gelfoam (surgical gelatin) serves as a framework for additional thrombus formation. Histologic sections of arteries occluded by Gelfoam show an intense acute arteritis characterized by polymorphonuclear cells infiltrating the vessel wall and the immediate perivascular tissues. Presumably, the arteritis is a direct reaction to intravascular Gelfoam. If occlusion is the desired result, the inflammatory reaction is probably advantageous.

The use of the coil alone decreases the diameter of the available lumen, but, unless the vessel is small enough, the coil does not obstruct flow. Endothelial proliferation takes place at the points of contact with the vessel wall. The wool or Dacron threads serve as the nidus for thrombosis. Dacron evokes an inflammatory process in the vessel wall that is less severe than that resulting from wool. The steel coil and the threads create a fairly consistent occlusion [22].

Balloon catheters have not been employed by us in peripheral embolization utilizing particulate material. The Gelfoam particles are cut into approximately 2-to-3-mm cubes (Fig. 93-4). Once the peripheral branches are embolized, the flow slows considerably. Gelfoam segments 3 × 3 × 20 mm or larger are then injected. A 1-cc syringe is best suited for this task, allowing greater control of the emboli. Five to 10 Gelfoam particles or one segment is placed in the syringe at a time. The syringe is filled with saline or contrast mate-

Figure 93-4. Gelfoam (surgical gelatin). Particles consisting of approximately 3-mm cubes and 3 × 3 × 20-mm segments injected with a 1-to-2 cc syringe. Five to 10 particles or 1 segment is injected at a time.

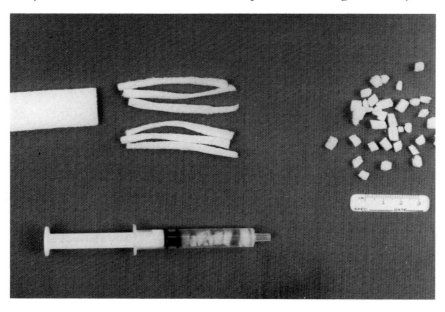

rial, the latter especially when the flow slows. No attempt is made to fill the central vessels completely with emboli, which lessens the need for a balloon catheter and minimizes unintentional embolization.

The original stainless steel coils with a 5-mm helix diameter require a 7 French nontapered-tip Teflon catheter. A renal infarction is accomplished by delivering the Gelfoam through a 6.5 French polyethylene catheter tapered to a 0.045-inch wire, which better accommodates the Teflon catheter during an exchange and allows a more secure placement. A 7 French dilator is initially passed over the 0.045-inch wire to ease the passage of the Teflon catheter. Because of the relative rigidity of the Teflon catheter, the tip of the catheter is constantly observed during the installation of the coils.

The "mini"-coil with a 3-mm helix diameter must be used with a 5 French nontapered-tip polyethylene catheter. This catheter is used alone or through an 8 French Teflon catheter as a coaxial system.

The newer coils can be used with catheters tapered to a 0.038-inch guidewire, either 5 French polyethylene or 6.5 French torque-controlled catheters. These coils, which have 3-mm, 5-mm, and 8-mm helix diameters, can be used through the same catheter, depending on the diameter of the vessel to be occluded. At times, a combination of sizes, or multiple coils, is necessary for the occlusion.

The coil, if smaller than the diameter of the vessel, is carried with the flow. Gentle passage of a J or C guidewire is used to push the coil peripherally when so desired. If the helix diameter is too large for the diameter of the vessel, the coil will uncoil or elongate. A Gelfoam segment may be injected between coils to ensure a better occlusion.

The configuration of the catheter should be such that it comfortably conforms to the vascular anatomy. Catheter exchange may be necessary to accomplish a better placement. Occlusion of smaller vessels (e.g., the left gastric, gastroduodenal, or lumbar artery) is undertaken only when good catheter placement is achieved. Gelfoam and, more recently, Ivalon particles are usually employed, and, if possible, a 3-mm coil is added.

In the presence of massive shunts, such as those seen occasionally in renal neoplasms and more frequently in arteriovenous fistulas, occlusion is accomplished with coils alone or with Gelfoam segments followed by coils.

Clinical Experience and Applications

Arterial embolization and occlusion have been effective in the management of patients with hemorrhage (especially from the gastrointestinal and genitourinary tracts), neoplastic disease, aneurysm, arteriovenous malformation, and fistula. Our experience now includes the clinical use of more than 1,200 coils.

The neoplasms successfully treated by this transcatheter approach include renal carcinoma, primary and secondary hepatic neoplasms, and benign and malignant tumors of bone. Arterial embolization of neoplasms is done (1) to control hemorrhage; (2) preoperatively, to facilitate resection by decreasing blood loss and operating time; (3) to inhibit tumor growth; (4) to relieve pain; and, perhaps, (5) to stimulate an immune response to the ischemic neoplasm.

HEMORRHAGE

Transcatheter intraarterial embolization is particularly efficacious in the management of acute bleeding of benign or malignant etiology, especially in patients who are often poor surgical candidates [8, 25, 28, 44]. The control of hemorrhage in such patients is often lifesaving and may enable the patient to tolerate better more specific therapy (surgery, radiation therapy, or chemotherapy).

Gastrointestinal Tract Bleeding

Vasopressin infusion has been successfully utilized to control gastrointestinal bleeding unresponsive to conservative medical management [6, 7]. Intravenous vasopressin is the preferred treatment for venous bleeding, especially from esophageal varices. It has also been effective at times for the treatment of diffuse gastrointestinal bleeding as seen in patients with leukemia. Intraarterial vasopressin is effective for the management of arterial hemorrhage due to stress ulcers, gastritis, and superficial mucosal tears. The frequent failure to control hemorrhage from duodenal ulcers is due to the chronicity of peptic ulceration or dual blood supply originating from the celiac and superior mesenteric arteries [8]. Intraarterial infusion of vasopressin is quite successful in the treatment of colonic bleeding in benign conditions, diverticulosis, and postbiopsy.

Vasopressin is usually ineffective in the management of gastrointestinal tract bleeding in patients with malignant neoplasms. The necessarily prolonged presence of an infusion catheter is fraught with an increased incidence of such adverse factors as thrombosis, hemorrhage, and infection in the artery infused as well as at the puncture site. This is especially critical in patients receiving chemotherapy, who may be pancytopenic or immunosuppressed.

Gastrointestinal tract bleeding in cancer patients has been controlled by embolization of the left gastric, gastroduodenal, superior and inferior pancreaticoduodenal, inferior mesenteric, or internal iliac artery [25, 27, 28]. Obviously, selective catheterization is essential for embolization and occlusion.

Left Gastric Artery. In a group of patients with gastric bleeding associated with gastric carcinoma, lymphoma, chronic myelogenous leukemia, and agnogenic myeloid metaplasia, emergency selective left gastric artery catheterization and embolization with Gelfoam alone or in combination with 3-mm coils have been successful. Left gastric artery embolization has also been effective in the management of bleeding of benign etiology (e.g., mucosal tears and ulcerations). Bleeding from ulceration in the gastric remnant of a previous partial gastrectomy and gastrojejunostomy has also been adequately managed by left gastric artery occlusion [25, 51].

Hepatic Artery. Hemorrhage associated with trauma, biopsy, aneurysm, fistula, and neoplasm has been managed by intraarterial embolization. The technical aspects, risks, and rewards are discussed in greater detail later in this chapter.

Gastroduodenal Artery. Embolization of the gastroduodenal artery and its branches is the preferred approach in duodenal hemorrhage [28, 56]. The multiplicity of the vascular supply to the duodenum via the gastroduodenal and pancreaticoduodenal branches adds to the technical difficulty in controlling bleeding or in occluding the tumor vascular supply.

Illustrative Case
A 19-year-old man with stage IVB Hodgkin's disease, with hepatosplenomegaly, jaundice, ascites, and peripheral edema developed intermittent massive hematemesis and melena while undergoing chemotherapy. Endoscopic examination revealed a bleeding site in the proximal portion of the duodenum. The man's poor physical condition precluded surgical intervention.

Selective arteriography demonstrated that the superior pancreaticoduodenal and gastroduodenal arteries originated separately from the hepatic artery supplying the bleeding ulcer in the duodenum. The superior pancreaticoduodenal artery was embolized with Gelfoam, and the gastroduodenal artery was occluded with a coil, controlling the hemorrhage. Two weeks later, an upper gastrointestinal tract examination disclosed a large benign ulcer in the second portion of the duodenum (Fig. 93-5). There has been no recurrence of bleeding since the occlusion.

Superior Mesenteric Artery. Bleeding from branches of the superior mesenteric artery is usually controlled by vasopressin infusion. Successful embolization of these branches with clot and Gelfoam has been reported in diverticulitis and angiodysplasia. On occasion, bleeding from neoplasms has been treated by Gelfoam embolization. This requires greater selective catheterization of the bleeding vessel and even more careful and cautious embolization. Gelfoam is more frequently employed for this purpose. The potential complications of bowel ischemia and necrosis are greater.

Inferior Mesenteric Artery. The collateral circulation to the left colon is derived from two major sources: the first source, more widely known, is the superior mesenteric artery through the middle colic or accessory middle colic arcade (Riolan) and the marginal artery (Drummond); the second source, less recognized, is the internal iliac artery. The middle and inferior hemorrhoidal arteries originate from the internal iliac arteries and readily form collateral channels with the superior hemorrhoidal artery from the inferior mesenteric artery. Thus the rectum is not as vulnerable to ischemic colitis as is the descending colon, which depends on the marginal artery as the sole source of collateral supply. Occlusion of the superior hemorrhoidal artery is not as critical as was previously thought [17]. Patients with bleeding from carcinoma of the sigmoid colon and invasion of the colon by ovarian carcinoma were treated successfully by inferior mesenteric artery embolization. Bleeding from radiation enteritis has been controlled by this approach. Gelfoam is usually adequate for this purpose, but coils might be used in conjunction with Gelfoam.

Internal Iliac Artery. It should be stressed that hemorrhoidal vessels originate from the internal iliac artery, and rectal bleeding may respond to embolization of this vessel, especially postresec-

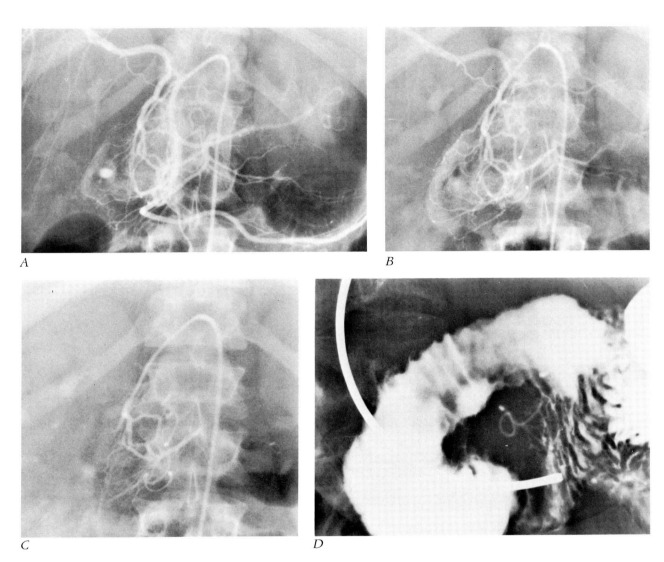

Figure 93-5. (A) A selective gastroduodenal angiogram demonstrates the bleeding site in the duodenum. The superior pancreaticoduodenal artery is visualized. (B) A selective superior pancreaticoduodenal angiogram with a 4 French catheter passed through a 7 French catheter again shows the bleeding site. Note the wire coils in the completely occluded gastroduodenal artery. (C) An injection of contrast material into the superior pancreaticoduodenal artery after occlusion with Gelfoam. (D) An upper gastrointestinal series 2 weeks later shows a benign duodenal ulcer. Note the wire coil from a previous gastroduodenal occlusion.

tion of the sigmoid colon where collateral vessels originate from the internal iliac artery [17].

Genitourinary Tract. Bleeding originating from pelvic trauma, postradiation changes, and neoplasms of the bladder or cervix are readily controlled by embolization of one or both internal iliac arteries [9, 34, 43]. This embolization has been accomplished with Gelfoam particles and segments and with steel coils [46].

RENAL CARCINOMA

Our most extensive experience with intravascular occlusion has been in the management of patients with renal carcinoma [1, 26, 36, 51]. One hundred patients with renal carcinoma were managed in part by transcatheter intraarterial embolization of the neoplasm [52]. Of these 100 patients, 26 had localized disease, embolized prior to nephrectomy to facilitate the surgical procedure. Forty-nine patients had metastases usually limited to the lung or bone and treated by embolization, nephrectomy, and hormonal therapy. Infarction alone was the palliative treatment for another 25 patients, whose disease was more extensive.

When it is technically feasible, the patient with a renal carcinoma is treated by a transabdominal radical nephrectomy. Embolization is not yet recommended as an adjunct in the removal of small or moderate-size tumors localized within the capsule (stage I) since it is not considered advantageous to subject these patients to the morbidity associated with embolization. Removal of larger stage I tumors (> 7 cm in diameter), which are frequently hypervascular, is facilitated by renal artery occlusion. The 5-year survival rate of patients with stage I disease is approximately 60 percent.

Stage II neoplasms include those extending through the capsule into the perinephric fat. The presence of regional lymph node metastases or a tumor thrombus in the renal vein or inferior vena cava signifies stage III disease. The 5-year survival for patients with stage II or stage III renal carcinoma is 30 to 35 percent. In cases involving these advanced tumors, especially if they are hypervascular, dilated tortuous veins usually cover the surface of the neoplasm and the renal hilum. Regional lymph node metastases and a tumor thrombosis in the renal vein or inferior vena cava may impede access to the renal artery.

Preoperative renal artery occlusion with Gelfoam and stainless steel coils can help facilitate nephrectomy (Fig. 93-6). In the presence of tumor thrombus, the hazards of tumor embolization are reduced and thrombectomy is facilitated. With the decrease in the arterial inflow, the veins collapse. The occluded renal artery, containing the steel coils and manifesting an associated inflammatory response, is readily palpated in the hilus and is, in essence, preligated. The major hilar renal veins are approached and ligated first. The infarcted neoplasm and kidney are edematous, creating a more definable plane between the kidney and the renal bed. These factors decrease blood loss and reduce the time required for surgery.

Approximately 25 to 40 percent of patients with renal carcinoma present with metastatic disease, stage IV. Spontaneous remission of metastases after nephrectomy has been widely publicized, but only 40 to 60 cases have been reported, with an incidence of 0.8 percent [39]. In a review of 642 cases of renal carcinoma at M. D. Anderson Hospital (MDAH), Houston, only 5 cases (less than 1%) were found with spontaneous remission of metastases after nephrectomy [47]. The median survival of 5.9 months with pulmonary metastases was not statistically altered by nephrectomy or hormonal therapy. With osseous metastases, the median survival following nephrectomy was extended from 10 to 16 months. However, it must be appreciated that patients undergoing nephrectomy usually have less extensive disease. Patients with hepatic or cerebral metastases were not subjected to nephrectomy because of their 3-month and 2½-month median survival, respectively.

Localized Disease: Embolization with Nephrectomy
Twenty-five patients had regionally advanced tumors without metastases and were treated by embolization 1 to 6 days prior to surgery to facilitate the operative procedure. Twenty-four to (preferably) 72 hours yielded optimal conditions for the operative procedure. Fifteen patients are alive, with a median follow-up of 24 months and a range of 11 to 61 months. The 10 patients who died had a median survival of 13 months, with a range of 3 to 47 months.

Limited Metastases: Embolization, Nephrectomy, Depo-Provera
Of the 100 patients in our series, 49 presenting with metastases were treated by occlusion, nephrectomy, and hormonal therapy. The time interval between occlusion and nephrectomy was usually 4 to 7 days, with 10 months being the longest interval. The response to this combined regimen is usually observed within 4.5 months.

In this group of 49 patients with limited metastases, the median cumulative survival thus far is 14 months, in contrast to 6 months for a control group treated by nephrectomy alone. A response was noted in 18 (36%) of the 49 patients. Seven responses were complete, with the disappearance of metastases for 9 to 15 months (Fig. 93-7). Of the 7 patients, 4 are alive after 7 to 44 months and 3 died 14 to 19 months after nephrectomy. Five patients had a partial response (50% or more reduction). Of these 5 patients, 1 is still alive after 41 months while 4 died after 12 to 24 months. Six patients experienced a measurable regression of less than 50 percent or stabilization for longer than 12 months. Of these 6 patients, 5 are alive after 15 to 44 months and 1

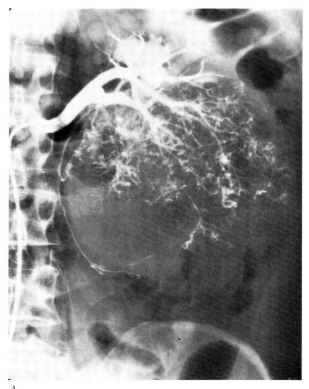

A

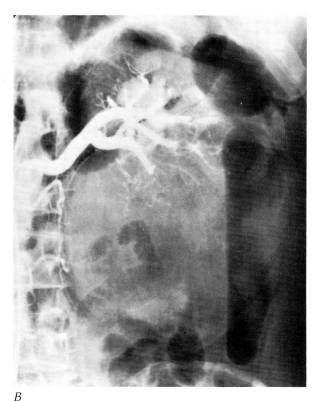

B

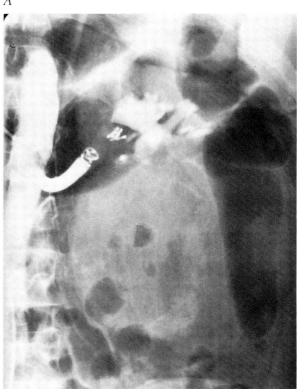

C

Figure 93-6. (A) Hypervascular carcinoma of the left kidney. (B) The initial embolization with Gelfoam particles. (C) Occlusion of the renal artery with coils.

died 17 months after nephrectomy. In view of the survival statistics, stabilization of the disease was considered a response. Of the 18 responders, 9 are still alive, with a median follow-up of 25 months.

Extensive Metastases: Embolization Alone

Twenty-six patients were treated by embolization without nephrectomy. These patients were not candidates for surgery because of their general medical condition or the extent of tumor involvement. One patient with apparent contiguous growth of tumor into the liver underwent infarction without nephrectomy and is still alive without demonstrable metastases 56 months later. He had immediate and permanent relief of pain. In retrospect, the vessels to the neoplasm originating from the hepatic artery most probably represented parasitization rather than invasion. One other patient is alive with progressive disease 14 months after infarction. The remaining 24 patients survived 1 week to 11 months, with a median survival of 4 months.

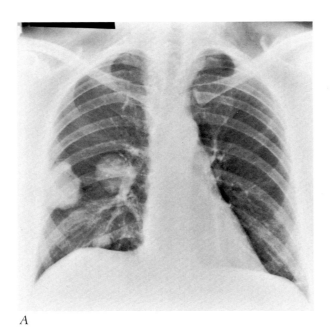

A

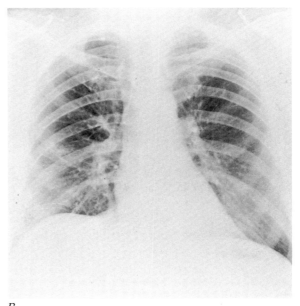

B

Figure 93-7. Complete response to embolization, nephrectomy, and Depo-Provera therapy. (A) A chest admission examination shows multiple pulmonary metastases. (B) A chest examination 6 months later no longer demonstrates metastases.

Complications

Although the complications discussed here are those seen with renal artery embolization, they do occur to varying degrees with embolization in general. Virtually all patients undergoing renal artery occlusion experience *flank pain* that lasts 24 to 48 hours and that requires narcotics for relief. The narcotics are given intravenously in aliquots of 25 mg of Demerol during embolization. *Fever* of up to 40° C almost always accompanies the pain, lasting as long as 5 days, but antibiotics are seldom needed. *Anorexia, nausea,* and *vomiting* may occur for 3 to 5 days, requiring symptomatic management. In a few patients, *paralytic ileus* required nasogastric suction and intravenous fluids. *Hypertension* occurs in many patients during embolization and lasts 2 to 4 hours. No patient has experienced persistent hypertension.

Major complications have been relatively few. *Renal failure* occurred in 2 patients, in 1 of whom it was irreversible. It was believed to be related to the large volume of contrast material (300 cc) and to the infarction that was performed at the same time. These two events have been separated by at least 24 hours without another episode of failure. *Renal abscess* complicated occlusion in 1 patient, and another patient had gas in the retroperitoneal space, presumably due to tumor necrosis. In the presence of a urinary tract infection or calculi, antibiotics are given before and after embolization.

Unintentional embolization of the Gelfoam and steel coils is always a potential complication [58, 59]. Loss of a coil into the aorta occurred in 2 patients. Chuang [11] has extracted an errant steel coil with a Dormier basket (Fig. 93-8), while Habighorst [29] used a Fogarty catheter. Surgery was reported necessary for the removal of a coil that migrated to the opposite renal artery after the occlusion of a renal carcinoma.

BONE TUMORS

Arterial embolization of tumors of bone was suggested for the relief of pain by Feldman et al. in the management of a patient with metastases to the ilium from an unknown primary neoplasm [20].

Metastases

Bone metastases from renal carcinoma occur in 30 to 45 percent of patients and are more frequently hypervascular. The lack of vascularity of the neoplasm does not influence management. The lumbar spine and pelvis are the most common sites of skeletal metastases. In a series of 10 patients at MDAH [16] who failed to respond

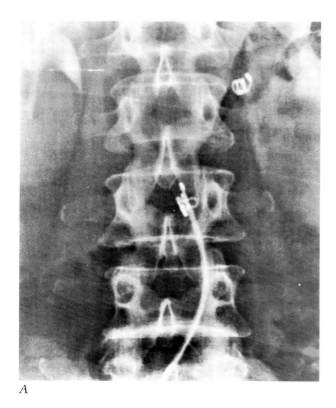

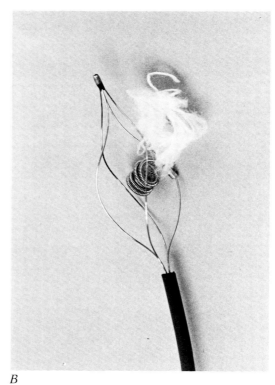

A   *B*

Figure 93-8. Unintentional embolization. (A) Retrieval of the coil from the aorta with a Dormier basket. (B) An in vitro demonstration.

to conventional treatment, embolization was not undertaken until at least 6 weeks after radiotherapy. In pelvic metastases, the appropriate internal iliac arteries were occluded. This is sometimes best accomplished by puncture of the contralateral femoral artery and subsequent passage of the catheter through the aortic bifurcation to the ipsilateral internal iliac artery, especially when the coils are used. In our use of this procedure in the spine, we have embolized no higher than the third lumbar arteries for fear of occluding the anterior spinal artery.

Arterial occlusion effectively controlled pain in 7 patients who failed to obtain relief from conventional therapy (Fig. 93-9). The mechanism of pain relief following occlusion is not obvious; however, it is postulated, especially in hypervascular neoplasms, that occlusion decreases the size of the tumor and slows its progression. This, in turn, decreases the pressure of expansion or stretching of the periosteum containing the nerve fibers that are, in part, responsible for pain. None of the osteolytic metastases showed evidence of healing; none showed obvious progression after embolization. Pain was alleviated for 1 to 6

months. The temporary and palliative nature of this pain relief may be related to the completeness of the occlusion and the availability of collateral circulation. In any event, the ability to control pain by this approach makes it a viable therapeutic alternative.

Preoperative embolization of the arterial supply to hypervascular metastases of the proximal femur and proximal humerus has made a significant contribution to the therapeutic management. The medial and lateral humeral and femoral circumflex vessels were occluded with Gelfoam and, when possible, with steel coils just prior to the operative procedure. Internal fixation or prosthetic replacement of a pathologic fracture of renal carcinoma metastases is usually associated with the loss of 1 to 3 liters of blood, which was minimized by this approach. After embolization, 500 cc was the maximum replacement necessary in these patients.

Benign Neoplasms of Bone
Stimulated by the 6-year remission of a sacral aneurysmal bone cyst (ABC) after bilateral internal iliac artery ligation, transcatheter arterial em-

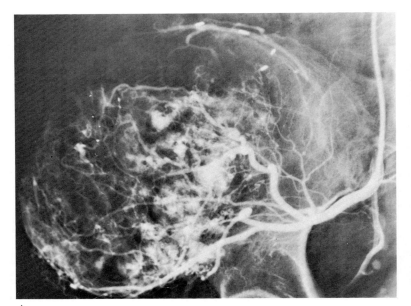

A

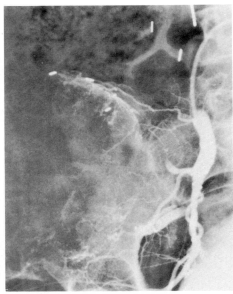

B

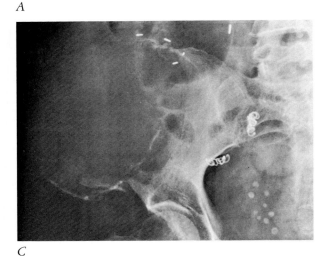

C

Figure 93-9. Metastatic renal carcinoma. (A) Hypervascular metastasis in the right ilium. (B) Embolization with Gelfoam and coils. (C) The pain from the metastases was relieved for 6 months though the lytic lesion failed to change.

bolization was evaluated as an alternative method of treating benign bone tumors [54]. From 1975 to 1979, 10 patients with giant cell tumor (GCT) and/or ABC were treated by embolization. There were 9 females and 1 male, ranging in age from 13 to 46. Seven of the neoplasms were in the sacrum, extending to or exclusively in the innominate bone, 3 in the lumbar spine, and 1 in the humerus. Eight of the tumors were GCT, 1 was an ABC, and 1 had elements of both. Six of the patients had previously failed to respond to chemotherapy and/or radiotherapy. All 10 patients complained of pain and were considered for embolization for symptomatic relief.

Technique of Embolization. Arteriography of the involved area was initially carried out to define the vascular supply. For tumors of the pelvis, the contralateral femoral artery was usually catheterized, which allowed ready access to the branches of the ipsilateral internal iliac artery. Embolization was performed utilizing small particles and segments of Gelfoam and stainless steel coils.

Complications. Complications were related to the vessels embolized and the materials employed. Recanalization of the artery occurred in 1 patient, whose pain recurred 1 month after embolization. Reexamination and reembolization occluded the vessel and relieved the pain.

Transient paresthesia in the buttock and lateral aspects of the foot occurred in 1 patient following embolization. Complete recovery was noted in a few weeks. This response may be related to occlusion of the perineural vascular plexus. Persistent progressive foot drop complicated internal iliac artery embolization of a malignant GCT in another patient. This patient had an aggressive neoplasm associated with pulmonary metastases. However, the foot drop was temporally related to the embolization.

Results. The patients were evaluated clinically for pain relief and radiographically for increased calcification. The pain was alleviated in 7 (70%) of the 10 patients and there was increased calcification in 5 (50%) of the 10 patients. One patient who had had marked pain relief for 4 months was then lost to follow-up. Five of the 9 remaining patients responded to arterial embolization. One of these had a surgical resection of the tumor 13 months after embolization. The patient had a reduction in tumor size of approximately 20 percent with shell-like calcification of the margin of the tumor. This lesion was easily resected, without recurrence for 2 years. The other 4 patients had healing of the lesion as demonstrated by calcification at the periphery and became asymptomatic for 14 to 55 months. The remaining 3 patients were considered failures although one did have transient pain relief for 2 months.

In general, arterial embolization yielded a 56 percent success rate in the treatment of GCT and ABC and is a valuable alternative method, especially when surgery is impossible.

Illustrative Case
A 13-year-old girl with a GCT of L4 had been treated by surgery, a laminectomy, followed by radiation therapy. The tumor responded slightly, as defined by CT scanning, but for only a few months. Embolization was considered a last resort when the patient showed progressive disease, became bedridden, and experienced unrelenting back pain, bilateral lower extremity numbness, and weakness.

Selective angiography of the right and left fourth lumbar arteries and the third right lumbar artery revealed a hypervascular neoplasm. Each of these lumbar arteries was embolized with Gelfoam particles and small stainless steel coils with attached Dacron delivered through a 5 French nontapered-tip polyethylene catheter (Fig. 93-10).

Twenty-four hours later, there was almost complete subsidence of back pain. The numbness gradually disappeared. The patient was discharged with a back brace. Her progressive clinical improvement was accompanied by calcification and marked reduction of the size of the neoplasm. Two years after vascular occlusion, the lesion was almost completely calcified. The young lady is actively participating in athletic activities with no complaints, and she is neurologically intact.

LIVER

The liver is the major organ most frequently involved by metastatic disease. The patient's hepatic metastases rather than the primary neoplasm usually govern the course of the disease as well as the survival. The median survival for patients with untreated liver metastases from carcinoma of the colon is 150 days; from the stomach, 60 days; and from the pancreas, 50 days. In view of this ominous prognosis, an aggressive therapeutic approach is justified. Surgery is still the preferred treatment of primary or secondary neoplasms of the liver localized to resectable segments. The transcatheter management of hepatic neoplasms, whether primary or secondary, includes arterial infusion and occlusion [13]. The transcatheter approach necessitates a familiarity with the hepatic vascular anatomy.

Anatomic variations of the hepatic arteries have been divided into 10 types by Michels [38]. The classic distribution of the artery originating from the common hepatic branch of the celiac artery occurs in approximately 55 percent of the population. An aberrant hepatic artery is one that arises from a source other than the celiac-hepatic artery. In Michels' study of 200 cadavers, 41.5 percent had an aberrant artery. An accessory hepatic artery is one that is in addition to the one normally present. A replaced hepatic artery is one that substitutes for the normal hepatic artery that is absent. The incidence of aberrant right hepatic artery is 26 percent and the incidence of aberrant left hepatic artery is 28 percent. These aberrant arteries can originate from the left gastric artery, the superior mesenteric artery, or branches from both.

Redistribution of Hepatic Flow

Redistribution of the hepatic arterial flow is accomplished by selective occlusion of certain of the multiple hepatic arteries so that the entire supply originates from one artery [13, 14]. This facilitates the technical aspects of hepatic arterial infusion and allows for delivery of the chemotherapeutic agent to the entire liver (Fig. 93-11). The site of the occlusion should be proximal to the first bifurcation of the hepatic artery, which enables the intrahepatic collateral vessels to develop as the primary arterial supply. This is best achieved by using stainless steel coils with attached Dacron strands. The development of intrahepatic collateral vessels is instantaneous in most cases [42]. Following hepatic arterial redistribution, the catheter is repositioned into the nonembolized artery, and the infusion of the chemotherapeutic agent is begun. The efficacy of the intrahepatic collateral arterial infusion has been demonstrated by the regression of neoplasm in both the lobe receiving the native circu-

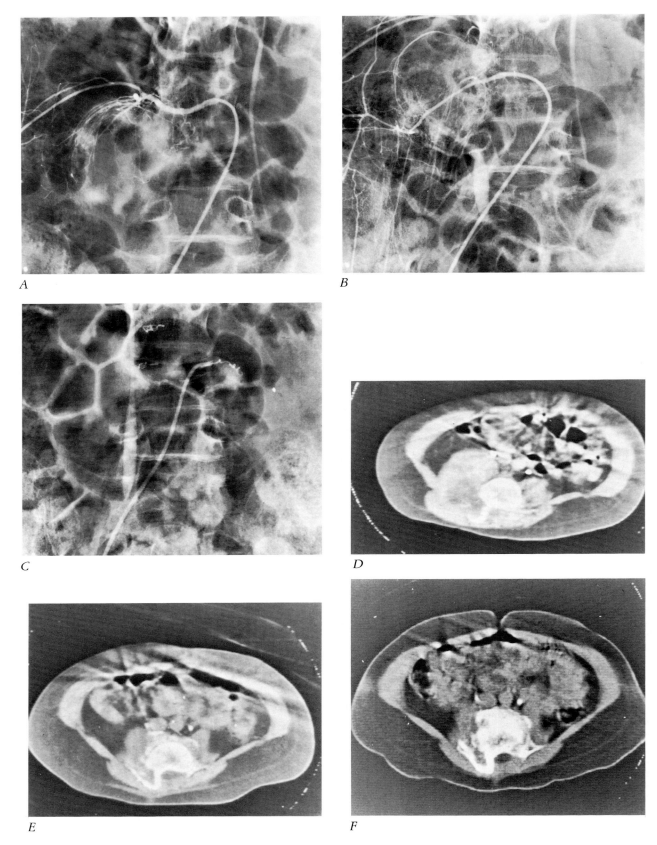

A

B

C

D

E

F

Figure 93-10. Giant cell tumor at L4. (A) Arteriography of L3 and (B) L4 arteries revealed a hypervascular neoplasm. (C) Embolization of right L3 and L4 and left L4 arteries with Gelfoam and minicoils. (D) Computed tomography of the giant cell tumor prior to embolization. (E) Computed tomography of the tumor 6 months after the occlusion. (F) Computed tomography 1½ years later.

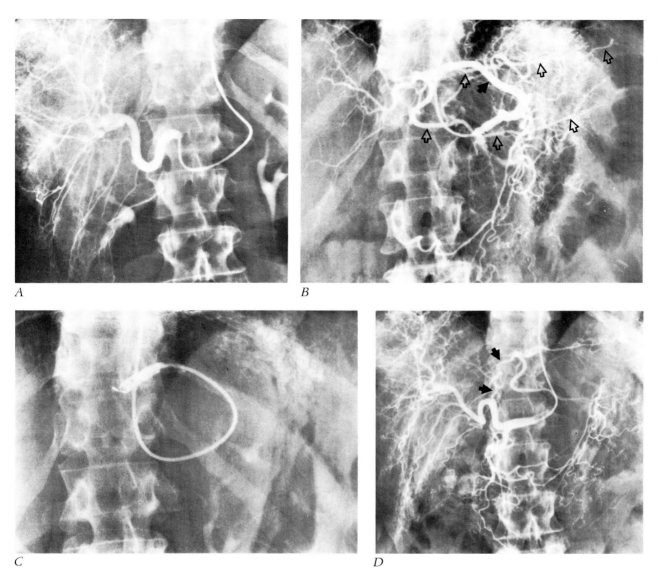

Figure 93-11. Redistribution of the hepatic arterial supply. (A) The right hepatic artery originated from the celiac artery. (B) The left hepatic artery (*solid arrow*) originated from the left gastric artery before its branching (*open arrows*). (C) Occlusion of the left hepatic artery with new coils. (D) The entire hepatic supply was opacified from the common hepatic artery through intrahepatic collaterals (*arrows*), allowing an infusion of a chemotherapeutic agent to the entire liver through one vessel.

lation and the lobe receiving the collateral circulation. The response in the lobe receiving the collateral circulation might be due to either the effect of chemotherapy or the reduced flow through the collateral vessels.

Illustrative Case

A 56-year-old woman was seen at MDAH for consideration of transcatheter intraarterial hepatic infusion for the treatment of metastases from a carcinoma of the sigmoid colon.

Angiography demonstrated a replaced right hepatic artery from the superior mesenteric artery, a left hepatic artery originating from the aorta, and an anomalous vessel communicating between the left hepatic artery and the gastroduodenal arteries, which, with the splenic artery, constituted the celiac axis. The multiplicity of vessels negated maximum single-vessel chemotherapy infusion. The replaced right hepatic artery and the gastroduodenal arteries were occluded with small wire coils. Intrahepatic collateral circulation developed so that the entire liver was eventually infused through the left hepatic artery. This patient responded to the hepatic artery infusion of 5-fluoro-2'-deoxyuridine and mitomycin C, and she is alive 2½ years later (Fig. 93-12).

Hepatic Devascularization—Transcatheter Embolization

Normal hepatic parenchyma receives approximately 20 to 25 percent of its nourishment from the hepatic artery and 75 to 80 percent from the portal vein. Ninety to 95 percent of the blood supply to a hepatic neoplasm, primary or secondary, originates from the hepatic artery. Approximately 20 percent of normal liver is necessary for survival. Hepatic devascularization is undertaken only if less than 70 percent of the liver is replaced by tumor, the remainder of the liver is normal, and the portal vein is patent. Surgical ligation has resulted in a decrease in the size of the hepatic lesions and subjective improvement of complaints [21, 37, 40].

A review of 72 hepatic arterial embolizations performed in MDAH suggests that hepatic tumor devascularization by arterial embolization is an effective method in the management of primary and secondary hepatic neoplasms. Our experience also indicates that combined peripheral and proximal occlusion of hepatic arteries is more effective in tumor devascularization than proximal occlusion alone. Devascularization of a hepatic neoplasm can be achieved percutaneously by combined peripheral embolization with particulate material (Gelfoam) and central occlusion with a stainless steel coil. More recently, Ivalon has become commercially available in particulate form and is a relatively easy and an effective agent for embolization [12, 32, 48]. Transcatheter hepatic artery embolization can be used (1) in patients with unresectable primary hepatic neoplasms; (2) preoperatively, to facilitate surgery of a resectable neoplasm; (3) in metastatic neoplasms that fail to respond to chemotherapy; (4) as the initial management of certain metastases usually refractory to chemotherapy; and (5) to control pain and/or hemorrhage of a hepatic neoplasm.

Illustrative Case

A 32-year-old woman was referred to MDAH with hepatosplenomegaly and a radionuclide scan demonstrating a localized defect in the left lobe of the liver. At laparotomy, multiple nodules were found, particularly in the lateral segment of the left lobe. Biopsy of this lesion revealed a cholangiocarcinoma of the liver. The artery supplying the left lobe of the liver was surgically ligated.

Selective proper hepatic arteriography, 2 weeks later, opacified the right hepatic artery. The arteries to the lateral segment of the left lobe were visualized via intrahepatic collateral channels. Multiple moderately vascular lesions were demonstrated (Fig. 93-13).

Hepatic artery embolization was performed utilizing Gelfoam. One stainless steel coil was introduced into the proper hepatic artery, producing complete occlusion. Hepatic devascularization was associated with right upper quadrant pain, fever, nausea, and vomiting for 3 days. Liver function studies worsened for 3 weeks, gradually returning to preocclusion levels. The treatment was supplemented with chemotherapy.

One year later, reevaluation by angiography delineated an extensive collateral network in the region of the porta hepatis, originating primarily from the gastroduodenal artery. Occlusion of the gastroduodenal artery was accomplished by employing 3 wire coils. Hepatic dearterialization in conjunction with systemic chemotherapy resulted in 20 months of productive life, but the patient finally succumbed to diffuse metastatic disease 2 years after the initial occlusion.

Comment. Michels [38] found 26 different extrahepatic collateral pathways in cadavers. Koehler et al. [35] demonstrated angiographically intrahepatic and extrahepatic collateral channels after hepatic artery ligation. These originated from the replaced hepatic, inferior phrenic, omental, pancreaticoduodenal, and gastroduodenal arteries along the porta hepatis, as well as from recanalization of the ligated hepatic artery. The vasa vasorum of the occluded vessels most probably contributed to the collateral supply. The origin and level of collateral vessels depend on the site of the occlusion and the vascular anatomy.

ARTERIOVENOUS FISTULAS

The stainless steel coil is ideal for transcatheter vascular occlusion of arteriovenous fistulas. The coil length and helix diameter must be tailored to the fistulous tract. Fistulas were surgically created between the carotid artery and the jugular vein in dogs [4]. Angiographic studies performed prior to, immediately after, and 4 weeks after occlusion demonstrated (1) the patency of the fistula, (2) the successful occlusion of the fistula from either the arterial or the venous approach, and (3) the continued patency of the major arterial and venous components after the fistula was occluded.

Renal Fistulas

More than 125 renal arteriovenous fistulas have been reported since the initial description by

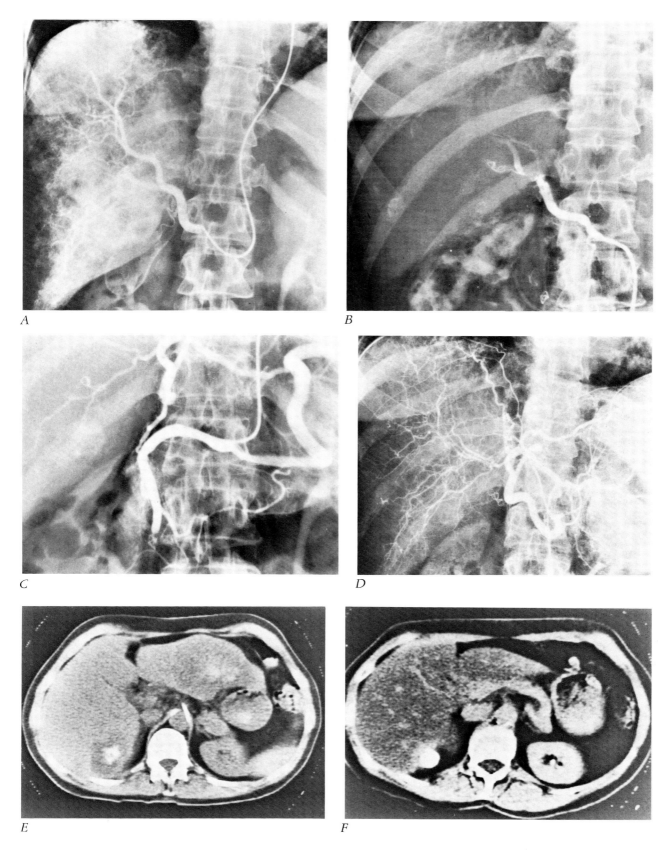

A

B

C

D

E

F

Figure 93-12. Redistribution of the hepatic flow. (A) The replaced right hepatic artery originated from the superior mesenteric artery. (B) Occlusion of the right hepatic artery with coils. (C) The gastroduodenal artery was occluded. (D) The entire hepatic supply originated from the left hepatic artery, which arose separately from the aorta. (E) Computed tomography of the liver prior to a hepatic artery infusion. Metastases were seen in each lobe; some of them contained calcium. (F) The response of the metastases to the hepatic artery infusion.

2167

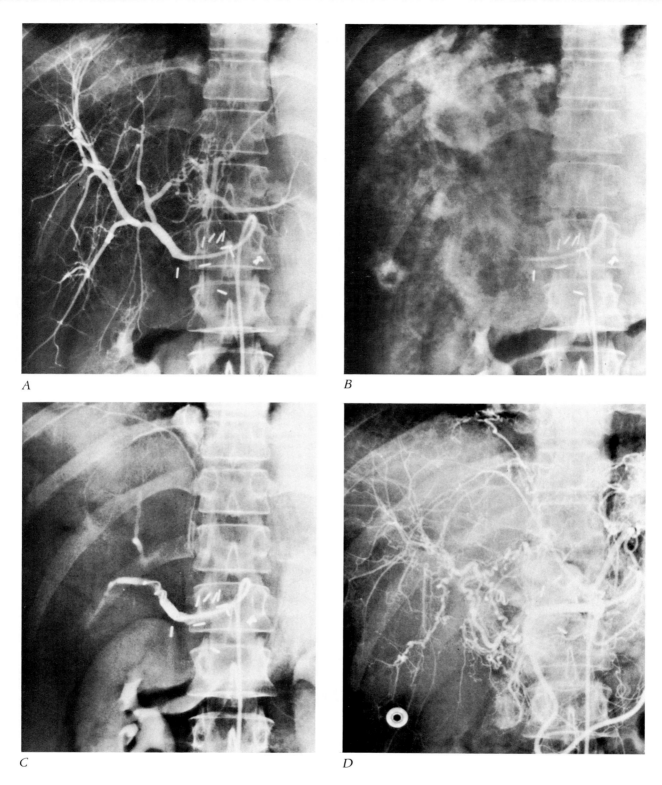

A

B

C

D

Figure 93-13. Hepatic artery occlusion. (A) A selective hepatic arteriogram after surgical ligation of the left lateral hepatic artery reveals hepatic collateral circulation to the left lateral segment via the left medial segmental branches. (B) Multiple hypervascular neoplastic masses are opacified throughout the liver. (C) The hepatic artery was occluded initially with Gelfoam and then by a single coil. (D) A selective gastroduodenal arteriogram 1 year later shows extensive collateral vessels originating from the gastroduodenal artery supplying the intrahepatic arteries. (E) The hypervascular masses are smaller. (F) The gastroduodenal artery was occluded with 3 coils.

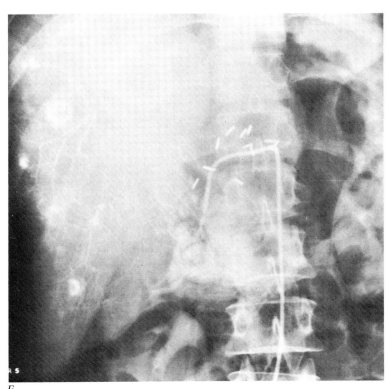

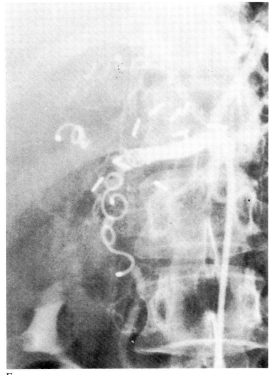

E   F

Varela [50] in 1923. These fistulas have been classified according to (1) their location, that is, whether they are intrarenal or extrarenal, and (2) whether they are congenital, acquired, or idiopathic. The congenital, or cirsoid, variety is usually a fistula composed of multiple communicating vessels, in contrast to the single communication more frequently seen in the acquired type.

Acquired arteriovenous fistulas may be due to such causes as accidental trauma (blunt or penetrating), an operation (usually nephrectomy), neoplasm, inflammation, or rupture of an aneurysm. Following needle biopsy, the incidence of arteriovenous fistulas is approximately 16 percent. Most of these fistulas respond spontaneously, with 4 percent persisting. This variety of arteriovenous fistula frequently is a single intrarenal communicating channel between the artery and the vein. Rupture of a renal artery aneurysm can result in an arteriovenous fistula. Aneurysmal dilatation with dissection of the renal artery may be a complication of fibromuscular hyperplasia. Renal artery aneurysm may be congenital or secondary to such factors as ar-

teriosclerosis, infection, trauma, and polyarteritis nodosa.

The size and anatomic configuration of the vascular components (feeding artery, fistula, and draining veins) of the intrarenal arteriovenous fistula dictate the therapeutic approach. Small fistulas can be managed by the transcatheter embolization of a variety of particulate materials. With larger fistulous tracts, the potential complications of pulmonary emboli limit their use. Successful nonsurgical management of these large intrarenal communications has been accomplished by cyanoacrylates, balloons, brushes, Gelfoam segments, and stainless steel coils with attached strands [24, 33].

Aside from pulmonary emboli, the reported complications are related to the organ and vascular bed occluded. If sufficient tissue is infarcted when the feeding artery is occluded, occlusion is almost invariably associated with severe pain and fever for 2 to 5 days.

Illustrative Case
A 60-year-old woman with known polycystic disease was examined by renal angiography because of un-

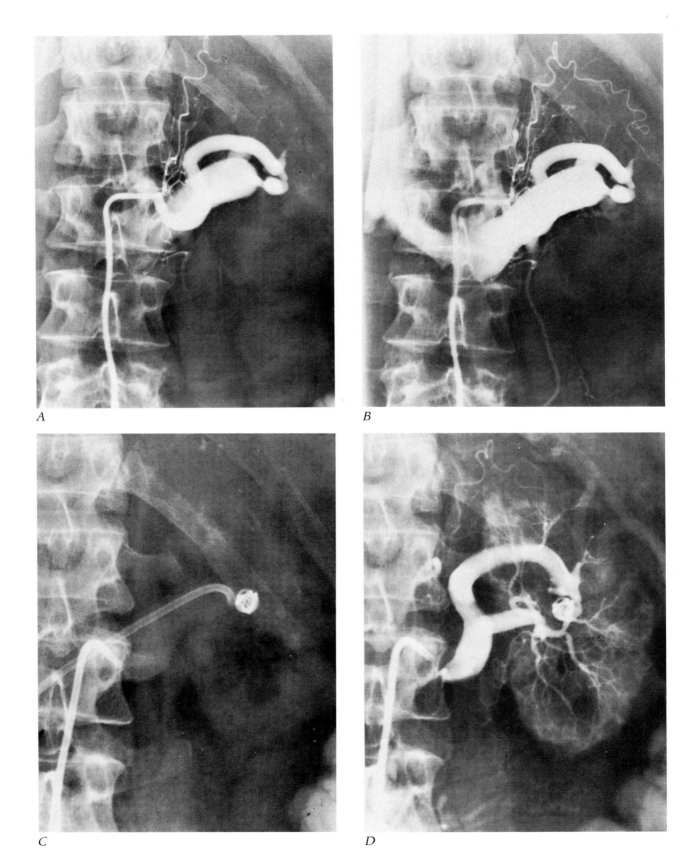

A

B

C

D

Figure 93-14. Renal arteriovenous fistula. (A) This arteriovenous fistula was a complication of a needle biopsy. (B) Opacification of the renal vein and the inferior vena cava with little perfusion of the left kidney. (C) Catheter in the renal artery. Second catheter in the fistula through the renal vein. Two coils were deposited in the fistula. (D) A left renal arteriogram immediately after the embolization shows an occlusion of the fistula. (E) Nephrogram demonstrates the cystic nature of the disease and a normal renal vein.

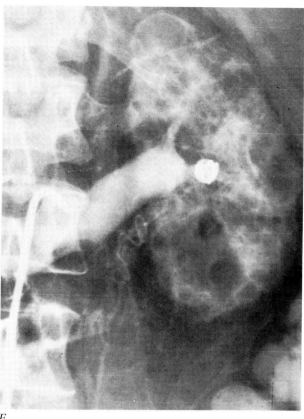

E

controlled persistent hypertension and a bruit over the left flank. Multiple cysts were demonstrated in the right kidney. The origin of the left renal artery was narrowed, presumably secondary to atherosclerosis. An arteriovenous fistula was opacified in the left kidney with little perfusion of the renal parenchyma (Fig. 93-14). The fistula was considered to have resulted from a needle biopsy 1 year previously.

In view of the bilateral renal disease and impaired renal function, an alternative to nephrectomy for the treatment of the arteriovenous fistula seemed advisable. Three days after the arteriogram, the intravascular occlusion procedure was performed. Because the fistula could not be catheterized from the arterial side, the left renal vein was traversed and the tip of the catheter was placed into the single fistulous tract. Two coils were placed into the communicating segment. Repeat left renal arteriography demonstrated that the fistula had been occluded, with significant improvement in the perfusion through the polycystic left kidney [55].

Follow-up examination 17 months later revealed no evidence of a bruit, and the hypertension was relieved by medication.

Transcatheter occlusion of arteriovenous fistulas (postnephrectomy, renal, vertebral artery

to jugular vein, carotid artery to jugular vein, pulmonary, gastroduodenal, brachial, and internal iliac) has been successfully accomplished with the use of stainless steel coils [10, 49]. Arterial aneurysms have also been managed by the transcatheter deposition of coils in the aneurysm and feeding vessels [30, 31]. Ivalon plugs have been used in the closure of patent ductus arteriosus [41, 45].

Conclusion

The stainless steel coil is only one of the materials available to the interventional radiologist. Prior to its use, experience with the technique should be gained in the laboratory or in in vitro trials. It is stressed that in the management of a specific problem, the interventional radiologist should take the approach he is most familiar with that will achieve the desired result.

ACKNOWLEDGMENTS

I would like to thank Mr. Eugene Szwarc for providing the prints that illustrate this chapter. Shirley Anne Davis, Susan Davis, and Portia Bartonico also deserve recognition for their assistance in the preparation of this manuscript.

References

1. Almgard, L. E., Fernstron, I., Haverling, M., and Ljungqvist, A. L. Treatment of renal adenocarcinoma by embolic occlusion of the renal circulation. *Br. J. Urol.* 45:474, 1973.
2. Anderson, J. H., Chica, G., Wallace, S., and Johnson, D. E. Experimental Studies with Transcatheter Vascular Occlusion. In D. E. Johnson, and M. L. Samuels (eds.), *Cancer of the Genitourinary Tract.* New York: Raven, 1979. Pp. 57–65.
3. Anderson, J. H., VuBan, A., Wallace, S., Hester, J. P., and Burke, J. S. Transcatheter splenic arterial occlusion: An experimental study in dogs. *Radiology* 125:95, 1977.
4. Anderson, J. H., Wallace, S., and Gianturco, C. Transcatheter intravascular coil occlusion of experimental arteriovenous fistulas. *AJR* 129:795, 1977.
5. Anderson, J. H., Wallace, S., Gianturco, C., and Gerson, L. P. "Mini" Gianturco stainless steel coils for transcatheter vascular occlusion. *Radiology* 132:301, 1979.

6. Athanasoulis, C. A., Baum, S., Waltman, A. C., Ring, E. J., Imbembo, A., and Vander Salm, T. J. Control of acute gastric mucosal hemorrhage. Intra-arterial infusion of posterior pituitary extract. *N. Engl. J. Med.* 290:597, 1974.

7. Baum, S., and Nusbaum, M. The control of gastrointestinal hemorrhage by selective mesenteric arterial infusion of vasopressin. *Radiology* 98:497, 1971.

8. Bookstein, J. J., Chlosta, E. M., Foley, D., and Walter, J. F. Transcatheter hemostasis of gastrointestinal bleeding using modified autogenous clot. *Radiology* 113:277, 1974.

9. Bree, R. L., Goldstein, H. M., and Wallace, S. Transcatheter embolization of the internal iliac artery in the management of neoplasms of the pelvis. *Surg. Gynecol. Obstet.* 143:597, 1976.

10. Castaneda-Zuniga, W., Epstein, M., Zollikofer, C., Nath, P. H., Formanek, A., Ben-Shacher, G. and Amplatz, K. Embolization of multiple pulmonary artery fistulas. *Radiology* 134:309, 1980.

11. Chuang, V. P. Nonoperative retrieval of Gianturco coils from abdominal aorta. *AJR* 132:996, 1979.

12. Chuang, V. P., Soo, C. S., and Wallace, S. Ivalon embolization in abdominal neoplasms. *AJR* 136:729, 1981.

13. Chuang, V. P., and Wallace, S. Current status of transcatheter management of neoplasm. *Cardiovasc. Intervent. Radiol.* 3:256, 1980.

14. Chuang, V. P., and Wallace, S. Hepatic arterial redistribution for intraarterial infusion of hepatic neoplasms. *Radiology* 135:295, 1980.

15. Chuang, V. P., Wallace, S., and Gianturco, C. A new improved coil for tapered tip catheter for arterial occlusion. *Radiology* 135:507, 1980.

16. Chuang, V. P., Wallace, S., Swanson, D., Zornoza, J., Handel, F., Schwarten, D. E., and Murray, J. Arterial occlusion in the management of pain from metastatic renal carcinoma. *Radiology* 133:611, 1979.

17. Chuang, V. P., Wallace, S., Zornoza, J., and Davis, L. J. Transcatheter arterial occlusion in the management of rectosigmoid bleeding. *Radiology* 133:605, 1979.

18. Doppman, J. L., Zapol, W., and Pierce, J. L. Transcatheter embolization with a silicone rubber preparation: experimental observations. *Invest. Radiol.* 6:304, 1971.

19. Dotter, C. T. Selective instant arterial thrombosis with isobutyl cyanoacrylate. Work in progress at the 59th Scientific Assembly and Annual Meeting of the Radiological Society of North America, Chicago, Ill., Nov. 25–30, 1973.

20. Feldman, F., Casarella, W. J., Dick, H. M., and Hollander, B. A. Selective intra-arterial embolization of bone tumors. A useful adjunct in the management of selected lesions. *AJR* 123:130, 1975.

21. Fortner, J. G., Mulcar, R. J., Solis, A., et al. Treatment of primary and secondary liver cancer by hepatic artery ligation and infusion chemotherapy. *Am. Surg.* 178:162, 1973.

22. Ghaveri, H. S., Gerlock, A. J., Jr., and Ekelund, L. Failure of steel coil occlusion. A case of hypernephroma. *AJR* 130:556, 1978.

23. Gianturco, C., Anderson, J. H., and Wallace, S. Mechanical devices for arterial occlusion. *AJR* 124:428, 1975.

24. Goldman, M. L., Fellner, S. K., and Parrott, T. S. Transcatheter embolization of renal arteriovenous fistula. *Urology* 6:386, 1975.

25. Goldstein, H. M., Medellin, H., Ben-Menachem, Y., and Wallace, S. Transcatheter arterial embolization in the management of bleeding in the cancer patient. *Radiology* 115:603, 1975.

26. Goldstein, H. M., Medellin, H., Beydoun, M. T., Wallace, S., Ben-Menachem, Y., Bracken, R. B., and Johnson, D. I. Transcatheter embolization of renal cell carcinoma. *AJR* 123:557, 1975.

27. Goldstein, H. M., Wallace, S., Anderson, J. H., Bree, R. L., and Gianturco, C. Transcatheter occlusion of abdominal tumors. *Radiology* 120:539, 1976.

28. Granmayeh, M., Wallace, S., and Schwarten, D. Transcatheter occlusion of the gastroduodenal artery. *Radiology* 131:59, 1979.

29. Habighorst, V. L. V., Kreutz, W., Klug, B., et al. Spiralembolization der Nierenarterie nach Gianturco. *ROEFO* 128:47, 1978.

30. Jonsson, K., Bjernstad, A., and Eriksson, B. Treatment of a hepatic artery aneurysm by coil occlusion of the hepatic artery. *AJR* 134:1245, 1980.

31. Kadir, S., Athanasoulis, C. A., Ring, E. J., and Greenfield, A. Transcatheter embolization of intrahepatic arterial aneurysm. *Radiology* 134:335, 1980.

32. Kerber, C. W., Bank, W. O., and Horton, J. A. Polyvinyl alcohol foam: Prepackaged emboli for therapeutic embolization. *AJR* 130:1193, 1978.

33. Kerber, C. W., Freeny, P. C., Cromwell, L., Margolis, M. T., and Correa, R. J., Jr. Cyanoacrylate occlusion of a renal arteriovenous fistula. *AJR* 128:663, 1977.

34. Kobayashi, I., Kusano, S., Matsubayashi, T., and Uchida, T. Selective embolization of the vesical artery in the management of massive bladder hemorrhage. *Radiology* 136:345, 1980.

35. Koehler, R. E., Karobkin, M., and Lewis, F. Arteriographic demonstration of collateral arterial supply to the liver after hepatic artery ligation. *Radiology* 117:49, 1975.

36. Lalli, A. F., Peterson, N., and Bookstein, J. J. Roentgen guided infarction of kidney and lung—a potential therapeutic technic. *Radiology* 93:434, 1969.

37. Markowitz, J. The hepatic artery. *Surg. Gynecol. Obstet.* 95:644, 1952.

38. Michels, N. A. *Blood Supply and Anatomy of the Upper Abdominal Organs.* Philadelphia: Lippincott, 1955.

39. Montie, J. E., Stewart, B. H., Straffon, R. A., Banowsky, L. H., Hewitt, C. B., and Montague, D. K. The role of adjunctive nephrectomy in patients with renal cell carcinoma. *J. Urol.* 117:272, 1977.

40. Nilsson, L. A. Therapeutic hepatic artery ligation in patients with secondary liver tumors. *Rev. Surg.* 23:374, 1966.

41. Portsmann, W., Hieronymi, K., Wierny, L., and Warnke, H. Nonsurgical closure of oversized patent ductus arteriosus with pulmonary hypertension: Report of a case. *Circulation* 50:376, 1974.

42. Reuter, R. S., and Redman, R. H. *Gastrointestinal Angiography.* Philadelphia: Saunders, 1977. P. 308.

43. Ring, E. J., Athanasoulis, C., Waltman, A., Margulis, M. N., and Baum, S. Arteriographic management of hemorrhage following pelvic fracture. *Radiology* 109:65, 1973.

44. Rösch, J., Dotter, C. T., and Brown, M. J. Selective arterial embolization. A new method for control of acute gastrointestinal bleeding. *Radiology* 102:303, 1972.

45. Sato, K., Fujino, M., Kozuka, T., Naito, Y., Kitamura, S., Nakano, S., Ohyama, C., and Kawashima, Y. Transfemoral plug closure of patent ductus arteriosus. Experiences in 61 consecutive cases treated without thoracotomy. *Circulation* 51:337, 1975.

46. Schwartz, P. E., Goldstein, H. M., Wallace, S., and Rutledge, F. N. Control of arterial hemorrhage using percutaneous arterial catheter technique in patients with gynecologic malignancy. *Gynecol. Oncol.* 3:2760, 1975.

47. Sternberg, J. Personal communication, 1976.

48. Tadavarthy, S. M., Moller, J. H., and Amplatz, M. Polyvinyl alcohol (Ivalon)—a new embolic material. *AJR* 125:609, 1975.

49. Taylor, B. G., Cockerill, E. M., Manfredi, F., and Klatte, E. C. Therapeutic embolization of the pulmonary artery in pulmonary arteriovenous fistula. *Am. J. Med.* 64:360, 1978.

50. Varela, M. E. Aneurisma arterivenso de los vaso renales y asistolia consecutiva. *Rev. Med. Lat.-Am.* 14:3244, 1923.

51. Wallace, S. Interventional radiology. *Cancer* 37:517, 1976.

52. Wallace, S., Chuang, V. P., Swanson, D. A., Brackery, B., Hersh, E. M., Ayala, A., and Johnson, D. Embolization of renal carcinoma —experience with 100 patients. *Radiology* 138: 563, 1981.

53. Wallace, S., Gianturco, C., Anderson, J. H., Goldstein, H. M., Davis, L. J., and Bree, R. L. Therapeutic vascular occlusion utilizing steel coil technique: Clinical applications. *AJR* 127:381, 1976.

54. Wallace, S., Granmayeh, M., De Santos, L. A., Murray, J. A., Romsdahl, M. M., Bracken, R. B., and Jonsson, K. Arterial occlusion of pelvic bone tumors. *Cancer* 43:322, 1979.

55. Wallace, S., Schwarten, D. E., Smith, D. C., Gerson, L. P., and Davis, L. J. Intrarenal arteriovenous fistulas: Transcatheter steel coil occlusion. *J. Urol.* 120:282, 1978.

56. White, R. I., Jr., Giargiana, F. A., Jr., and Bell, W. Bleeding duodenal ulcer control: Selective arterial embolization with autologous blood clot. *J.A.M.A.* 229:546, 1974.

57. White, R. I., Jr., Kaufman, S. L., Barth, K. H., DeCaprio, V., and Strandberg, J. D. Therapeutic embolization with detachable silicone balloons. *J.A.M.A.* 241:1257, 1979.

58. Wirthlin, L. S., Gross, W. S., James, T. P., and Sadiq, S. Renal artery occlusion from migration of stainless steel coils. *J.A.M.A.* 243:2064, 1980.

59. Woodside, J., Schwartz, H., and Bergreen, P. Peripheral embolization complicating bilateral renal infarction with Gelfoam. *AJR* 126:1033, 1976.

Selective Tissue Ablation by Therapeutic Pharmacoangiography

KYUNG J. CHO
WILLIAM D. ENSMINGER
JAMES J. SHIELDS
DOUGLASS F. ADAMS

Developments in angiographic technique have made it possible to deliver a variety of agents into defined regional vascular beds. Progress in the technique of selective catheterization has improved our ability to identify and diagnose diseased areas and then to treat such areas by delivery of therapeutic agents into the appropriate specific vasculature [6, 7, 18, 46]. The latter, therapeutic, role will be the major emphasis of this chapter, especially as it applies to neoplastic disease.

To the degree that selective catheterization is achieved, it is possible to deliver regionally effective concentrations of appropriate agents with diminished systemic effects. Direct regional infusion can be amplified by taking advantage of the well-recognized difference in response of normal vessels and tumor vessels to vasoactive agents. The regional delivery of certain antineoplastic agents has been widely practiced with the same rationale. Manipulations of the flow rate and the distribution of blood through tumor-bearing regions have only recently been attempted as means to selectively enhance the exposure of tumors to drugs.

Various embolic agents have been administered through selectively placed catheters in order to disrupt blood flow and thereby to destroy tissue. However, attempts at total obliteration of the diseased tissue may fail because vessels previously constricted in the vascular bed may subsequently dilate and because rapid development of collateral vessels generally occurs following such proximal occlusion.

Combinations of the above approaches, all of which depend crucially on selective catheterization, play a major role in current and projected therapeutics. This chapter reviews the development of pharmacoangiographic tissue ablation and emphasizes the recent clinical and laboratory investigations in this rapidly expanding field.

Historical Background

The development of therapeutic pharmacoangiography for tissue ablation has largely stemmed from experiences during diagnostic angiography and preclinical animal studies. With improvements in selective percutaneous angiographic technique, angiography has not only provided precise localization of tumors but also helped to investigate the vascular responses of both normal vessels and tumor vessels to various intraarte-

2175

rially administered vasoactive substances. Tumor vessels devoid of elastic tissue and muscles are less responsive to vasoactive agents than are normal vessels. Because of this, epinephrine has been one of the most common agents used for diagnostic pharmacoangiography. Abrams et al. [1] demonstrated the diagnostic value of intraarterial epinephrine to enhance angiographic demonstration of renal cell carcinoma. The lack of tumor response to epinephrine was observed in a patient with renal cell carcinoma, and it was suggested that therapeutic application of the drug in cancer chemotherapy by redistributing blood flow to the organ containing tumor might be attempted. The redistribution of blood flow—that is, the selective vasoconstriction of normal vessels in the presence of nonresponsive tumor vessels—may allow the selective perfusion of the cytotoxic agent into the tumor bed. Recently, Iwaki et al. [37] demonstrated a relative increase in the tumor to liver ratio of mitomycin C concentration when mitomycin and epinephrine were administered concurrently in the rabbit VX2 carcinoma.

Epinephrine has short-lived (minutes-long)

vasoconstrictive effects, particularly on the celiac circulation [48]. Its constrictive effect on the mesenteric circulation is less prominent because of the greater dilatation effect mediated through beta receptors. The dilatation effect can be blocked by the simultaneous administration of the beta-blocker propranolol. Owing to both its alpha and beta effects, the prolonged infusion of epinephrine may be deleterious to the elderly patient with atherosclerotic heart disease. Owing to its vasoconstrictive effect, epinephrine was initially used to control gastrointestinal hemorrhage [48]. The prolonged infusion of epinephrine can generate ischemic problems. In a preclinical animal study by Cho et al. [17], a 3-hour infusion of epinephrine or vasopressin used to arrest experimental splenic hemorrhage was noted to cause massive splenic infarction in 3 of 15 dogs (Fig. 94-1). This reaction suggests that the infusion of vasoconstrictors into the splenic artery might be useful in the nonsurgical management of hypersplenism in poor-risk surgical patients. Clinical trials have yet to be undertaken.

The injurious effects of contrast medium on tissue and vascular endothelium have been well

Figure 94-1. Splenic infarction after a 3-hour splenic arterial infusion of a vasoconstrictor in a dog. (A) Longitudinal section of a grossly infarcted spleen. Approximately 80 percent of the spleen is infarcted. The darker part of the spleen is the normal residual spleen (*arrow*). (B) Histologic section of a splenic infarct demonstrates a broad subcapsular zone of old infarct with an attached omentum. (From Cho and Schmidt [17]. Reproduced by permission from *Invest. Radiol.*)

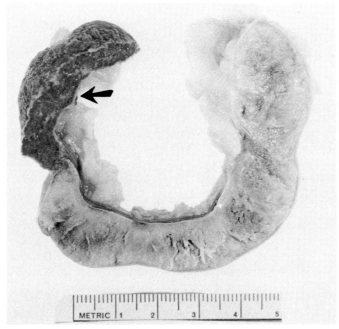

A

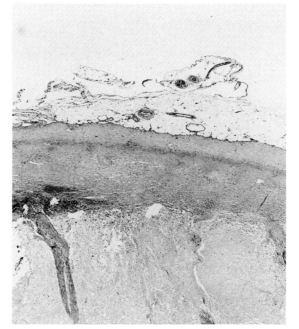

B

documented. Unintentional intraadrenal extravasation of contrast medium with subsequent adrenal insufficiency is one of the complications that could occur during adrenal venography (Fig. 94-2) [11, 22, 28, 29]. Hemorrhage is likely to occur when contrast medium is injected forcefully through a wedged catheter. Extravasation of contrast medium during peripheral venography has also been known to cause skin necrosis [52]. This initial experience with contrast medium has led to its utilization in attempts to ablate hormone-producing tissue or tumor, as will be described below.

Regional infusions of cytotoxic agents for localized cancer using percutaneous angiography for catheter placement have been used for nearly 3 decades [4, 13, 55, 56]. The regional tumors emphasized have included cancer of the head and neck [10, 38], pelvic region [60], extremities [53], and liver [4, 13, 55]. Owing largely to the relative lack of effective systemically administered agents and to advances in angiographic technique, there has been a recent upsurge of interest in regional chemotherapy. The majority of regional chemotherapy studies have had as a major focus the treatment of primary and metastatic tumors in the liver. By direct hepatic arterial infusion of appropriate agents, it is possible to increase the exposure of tumor fed from the hepatic artery from twofold to several hundredfold, depending on the agent [19, 26]. With the fluorinated pyrimidines, 5-fluorouracil (FU) and 5-fluoro-2'-deoxyuridine (FUDR), response rates of 50 to 80 percent have been achieved in the treatment of hepatic tumors by direct hepatic arterial infusion. This is in contrast to the usual response rates of 10 to 20 percent achieved by systemic infusion [4, 13, 25, 55]. Despite these response rates, enthusiasm for direct hepatic arterial infusion has been tempered by the associated morbidity and the technical problems of maintaining a continuous arterial infusion [14, 19]. As described in detail in Chapter 100, the problems can be surmounted and effective programs developed, especially under circumstances in which the radiologist, the medical oncologist, the surgical oncologist, and the other specialists bring their talents to bear in drawing up cooperative protocols.

The dependence of hepatic tumors on the hepatic artery with the ability of normal hepatic parenchymal tissue to survive on the portal blood supply has provided a basis for hepatic arterial ligation. Certainly this procedure has produced tumor necrosis and regression in many instances [3, 44]. However, durable tumor control has not generally been obtained, because proximal hepatic arterial occlusion is rapidly circumvented by collateralization [38]. As will be discussed below, more distal and/or intermittent occlusion may be able to generate the same degree of tumor ischemic necrosis without stimulating collateralization and thus be a more durable treatment modality.

Tissue Ablation by Contrast Staining

Transcatheter embolization to create ischemic necrosis has been used successfully to reduce the mass or the function of splenic, adrenal, and renal tissue and of parathyroid adenomas. The initial popularity of splenic embolization for the treatment of hypersplenism has sharply declined because of the development of splenic abscesses. Recently, Spigos et al. [51] reported that partial, rather than complete, splenic embolization with rigorous aseptic technique and concurrent an-

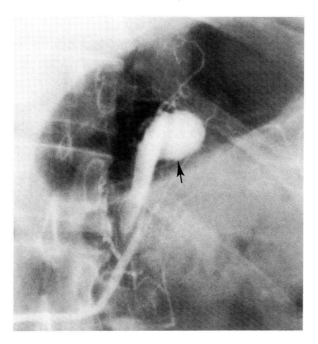

Figure 94-2. Unintentional medical adrenalectomy. A left adrenal venogram demonstrates a large extravasation of contrast medium (arrow). Extravasation of contrast medium also occurred in the right adrenal gland during the venogram. Subsequently, the patient developed adrenal insufficiency.

tibiotic therapy can significantly reduce the anticipated high incidence of complications [45, 51]. The embolic method has also been used to control the nephrotic syndrome and severe hypertension in patients with end-stage renal disease by producing embolic renal infarcts [2, 36, 43, 47].

Doppman et al. [21] embolized two mediastinal adenomas and one intrathyroidal adenoma in three patients who had had unsuccessful neck explorations. Only the mediastinal adenomas were infarcted. Hyperparathyroidism recurred in one patient; the others were still normocalcemic 8 months after embolization. Catheter perfusion of chemical agents has been attempted in a limited number of circumstances in an effort to destroy adrenal and renal tissue and parathyroid adenomas. Contrast medium itself has played a major role in tissue destruction. Since the introduction of angiography, it has been recognized that cellular injury may result from prolonged exposure of tissue to a high concentration of contrast medium [16, 50]. Unintentional prolonged exposure of tissue to contrast medium can occur during diagnostic angiography in the presence of catheter-induced proximal vascular occlusion.

Unintentional intraadrenal extravasation of contrast medium with subsequent adrenal insufficiency has accidentally occurred during adrenal venography. Forceful injection through a wedged catheter disrupts vascular integrity and is the primary factor in the creation of extravasation. Basing their approach on these observations, Zimmerman et al. [61, 62] used transvenous extravasation of a mixture of nitrogen mustard and contrast medium to ablate adrenal function. Their initial clinical trial in six patients with metastatic carcinoma was promising, and the technique has been advocated as an alternative to surgical adrenalectomy in poor-risk patients. Further clinical trials with long-term follow-up are needed to determine the safety, completeness, and duration of this method of adrenalectomy.

More recently, Doppman et al. [20], using the wedged-catheter technique, reported a method of ablating hyperfunctioning parathyroid adenomas. Initially, they unintentionally created interstitial permeation of contrast agent ("contrast stain") in the parathyroid adenoma during diagnostic angiography, and they found that the stain resulted in the reduction of hypercalcemia in three patients. In these patients, who received small volumes of dilute contrast medium, ele-

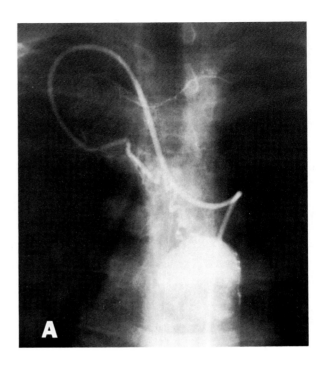

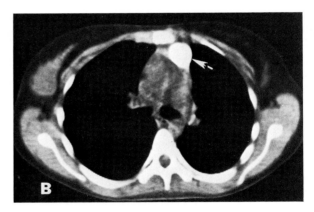

Figure 94-3. Angiographic ablation of mediastinal adenoma in a 21-year-old woman with persistent hypercalcemia after a negative neck exploration. (A) Angiogram taken during intentional infusion of contrast medium (Renografin-76) in the right thymic artery. A 3-cm adenoma is stained. Left thymic artery, which also supplied the adenoma, was perfused with contrast medium. (B) Computed tomography of the upper mediastinum, 24 hours after contrast staining, demonstrates dense accumulation of contrast medium in the adenoma (*arrow*). The patient subsequently became normocalcemic.

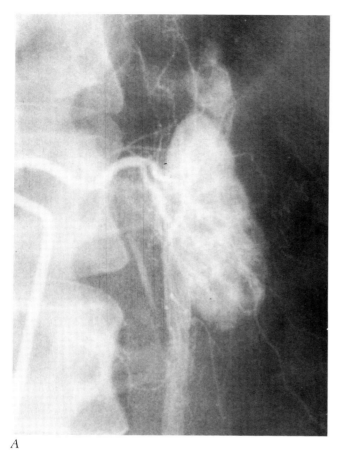

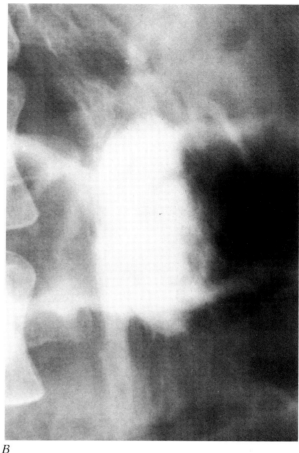

A

B

Figure 94-4. Therapeutic contrast stain of an end-stage kidney. (A) A selective left renal angiogram obtained during an intraarterial injection of contrast medium in a patient with atrophy of the kidney that caused hypertension. (B) Note the intense renal staining by contrast medium due to the catheter occlusion of the renal artery. In subsequent studies the renal volume was shown to be decreased.

vated serum calcium levels returned in 3 to 6 months. In their later three patients, adenomas were intentionally stained with large amounts of concentrated contrast medium; these patients remained normocalcemic for 2 to 18 months after staining (Fig. 94-3). Doppman et al. also described the feasibility of staining the tumor via a transvenous route. The duration of control of hyperfunctioning parathyroid adenomas utilizing contrast stain technique has not yet been established.

To ablate renal tissue, one of us deliberately stained an end-stage kidney with contrast medium, injecting the contrast medium through the wedged catheter (Fig. 94-4). Follow-up indicated that the renal parenchyma was substantially reduced in volume and that only a collecting system remained viable. In another patient, this technique, supplemented by the use of Gianturco coils, reduced renal functioning enough to alleviate the cosmetic problem of a fistula of the ureter in a patient who had terminal cancer.

More Recent Techniques and Agents Used for Tissue Ablation

In this section, several promising recently developed infusion methods for selective destruction of tissue are described, and illustrations are given of our ongoing clinical and experimental studies.

The arterial circulation to organs that are abnormal must be controlled before a chemical infusion for ablation is performed. Although selective placement of an infusion catheter into the desired vessel can be achieved by either surgical methods or percutaneous catheterization, the percutaneous technique is preferred because of its technical ease and its low morbidity when short-term treatments are involved.

The two angiographic methods of controlling the arterial circulation involve (1) wedging the angiographic catheter into the feeding artery and (2) using an occlusion balloon catheter. The usefulness of the catheter-wedging method is limited since only vessels smaller than the catheter can be occluded. Thus this method allows for ablation of only part of an organ or a tumor that has a small feeding artery. The balloon catheter, on the other hand, is useful for controlling flow through larger arteries and thus for destruction of a large bulk of tissue in the arterial watershed. With the recent advances in balloon-catheter technology, together with the development of the percutaneous catheterization technique, balloon occlusion of the second- or third-order branches of the major arteries is also possible. The purpose of balloon occlusion proximal to chemical infusion is to reduce the blood flow that dilutes the agent and thus to deliver higher concentrations of the drug for a given dose. This maximizes exposure to the toxic agent in the treated area per set amount of systemic exposure and hence improves the therapeutic selectivity.

The advantages of infusion techniques are that (1) infusions may permit the total tissue destruction of the infused organ with diminished systemic toxicity owing to rapid dilution of the toxic agent on the venous side, (2) an infusion may be repeated, and (3) infusions can be done with standard angiographic techniques.

The therapeutic perfusion method is still in the experimental stage, and further pilot clinical experience is needed before it can be broadly applied to patients in a safe and effective way. The following contrast agents and chemical substances have been tested in our laboratory for the ablation of renal parenchymal tissue (medical nephrectomy).

BARIUM SUSPENSION

Barium particles are small enough to occlude arteriolar capillary beds, thereby preventing the development of collateral circulation and subsequently resulting in complete tissue death (Fig. 94-5). Barium particles as small as 0.5 to 1.5 mμ do not appear to pass through capillaries when injected into the renal artery in vivo because rapid vascular spasm develops immediately after the injection. Obviously, barium should not be used in an organ with a vascular neoplasm and an arteriovenous shunt because of the possibility of pulmonary, or even systemic, embolization. A balloon catheter may be used to prevent reflux of

---

Figure 94-5. Renal infarction by barium suspension. (A) The entire left renal vascular bed is filled with the barium suspension. (B) The embolized left kidney, 10 weeks after the embolization, had shrunk uniformly, while the contralateral kidney showed compensatory hypertrophy. Microscopic examination demonstrated a complete infarction with no viable glomeruli.

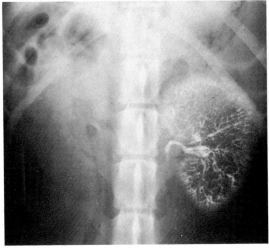

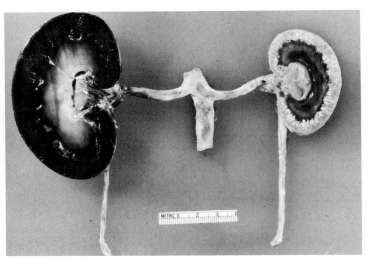

A

B

the barium particles into the aorta. Histologic examination of the kidneys embolized with barium in our laboratory revealed uniform infarcts and a marked granulomatous reaction around the extravasated barium. The long-term effect of intravascularly administered barium is not known, and its use as a perfusing agent should be limited to patients with end-stage kidney disease and segmental stenosis that cannot be treated otherwise. The use of barium infusion has been reported in two patients, one with end-stage renal disease with severe hypertension, and one with hemodynamically significant segmental renal artery stenosis [33, 47].

CONTRAST MEDIA

The toxicity of contrast medium is increased with high concentrations of the contrast medium and concomitant obstruction of the vascular bed. The mechanism of the contrast toxicity is not clearly understood, but hyperosmolarity and, perhaps, chemotoxicity leading to destruction of the vascular bed are probably responsible for subsequent ischemic necrosis. It is essential to inject contrast agent into an obstructed vascular bed to produce interstitial permeation of the contrast agent, which is likely to cause tissue death. In one such case, the kidney was stained by a pressure injection of 24 cc of Renografin-76 for 3 seconds (Fig. 94-6A). The extravasated contrast agent persisted for several hours. Nonuniform staining requires a repeat injection of contrast agent to secure complete infarction. A follow-up angiogram done 5 days after the initial staining revealed severe cortical and perinephric edema (Fig. 94-6B). A repeat angiogram done 10 weeks after the initial staining revealed a marked shrinking of the kidney (Fig. 94-6C).

ALCOHOL

Intraarterial injection of absolute alcohol can cause immediate thrombosis of the arteries and subsequent tissue necrosis. In our experiments, intraarterial injection of 3 to 5 cc of absolute alcohol into the canine renal artery reproducibly produced total occlusion of the renal arteries resulting in a massive infarct (Fig. 94-7). Other investigators have also demonstrated the efficacy of intraarterial alcohol for medical nephrectomy in both animals and humans [23, 42]. The systemic levels of ethyl alcohol from therapeutic infusion remain far below the toxic levels [23]. The local

pharmacologic mechanism for alcohol-produced injury was felt to be due to the precipitation and dehydration of cells [34]. This injurious action is directly related to the alcohol concentration. Therefore, the obstruction of the circulation should greatly enhance the cytotoxicity of the alcohol.

SCLEROSING AGENTS

Sclerosing agents produce endothelial damage, thrombosis, and an inflammatory response with subsequent vascular obliteration. They have been used in the treatment of varicose veins of the extremities, hemorrhoids, oral hemangiomas, and esophageal varices [8, 54, 58]. Quinine and urea hydrochloride, sodium morrhuate, and sodium tetradecyl sulfate are the commonly available agents. Sodium morrhuate, the soap (morrhuate sodium injection, NF; Eli Lilly), is the sodium salt of the fatty acid of cod-liver oil. It is supplied as a 5 percent solution, and an intravenous injection may cause a hypersensitivity reaction. Sodium tetradecyl sulfate (Sotradecol; Elkins-Sinn), an alkyl sulfate, is a strong sclerosing agent; it is 1.5 to 4.0 times as effective as sodium morrhuate [54]. It is available in a 1 or 3 percent aqueous solution. Quinine and urea hydrochloride is a solution of a double salt; its 5 percent solution has been used to obliterate varicose veins.

Experimental studies have demonstrated that recanalization of sclerosed vein occurs less frequently when high concentrations of the agent are injected. Therefore, intraarterial or intravenous injection of sclerosant into an obstructed vascular bed will mix less with blood and so will result in a more permanent obliteration of the vascular bed.

In our experiment, 3 percent sodium tetradecyl sulfate was injected into the canine renal arteries through an occlusion balloon catheter. This technique produced rapid thrombosis of the entire renal vascular bed. Persistent occlusion of the renal artery was confirmed by an angiogram 4 weeks after the Sotradecol infusion (Fig. 94-8). The kidneys were diffusely infarcted on gross and histologic examinations. These preliminary animal studies suggest that transcatheter infusion of a sclerosing agent may be useful for organ or tumor infarction, control of hemorrhage, and obliteration of vascular malformations.

The potential complications of the perfusion method utilizing the above-mentioned agents are

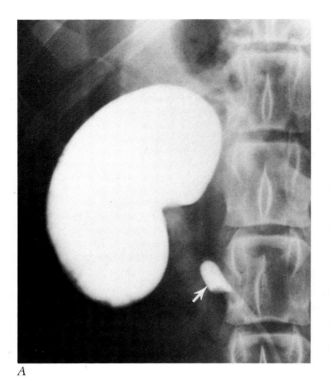

A

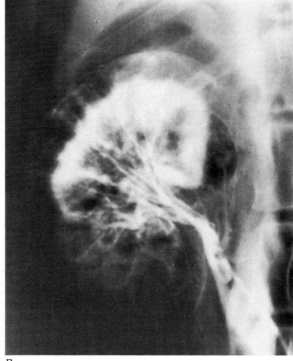

B

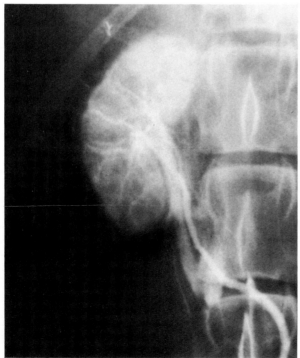

C

Figure 94-6. Renal infarction by contrast stain. (A) Note the diffusely intense staining of the entire kidney by a selective renal arterial perfusion of 24 cc of Renografin-76 using an occlusion balloon catheter (*arrow*). (B) A repeat renal arteriogram 6 days after an initial contrast staining demonstrates severe cortical and perinephric edema. (C) A repeat angiogram 10 weeks after the contrast staining demonstrates a severe shrinking of the kidney.

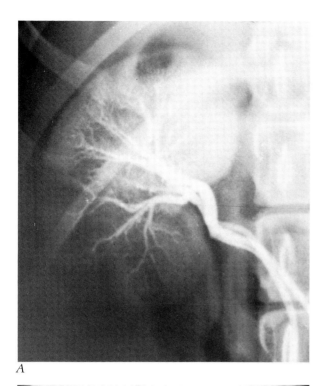

A

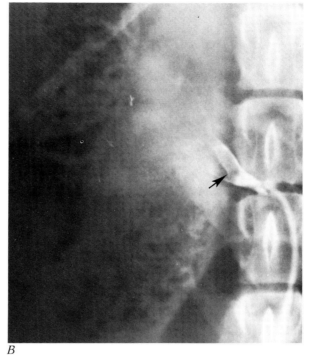

B

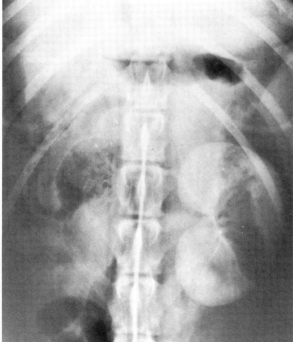

C

Figure 94-7. Experimental renal infarction by intraarterial ethanol infusion. (A) A control right renal angiogram shows a normal kidney. (B) A repeat angiogram 2 weeks after an infusion of 5 cc of absolute ethanol demonstrates an occlusion of the main renal artery (*arrow*). (C) The nephrographic phase of an aortogram 4 weeks after the infusion demonstrates a nonfunctioning right kidney.

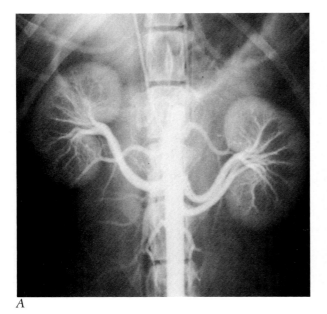

A

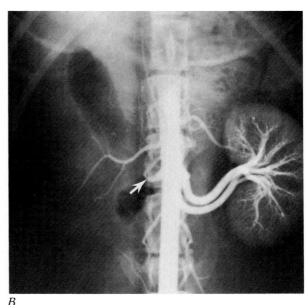

B

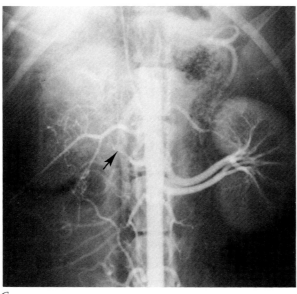

C

Figure 94-8. Experimental renal infarction with intraarterial perfusion of a sclerosing agent. (A) A control abdominal aortogram demonstrates normal kidneys bilaterally. (B) An aortogram 3 days after an intraarterial perfusion of 6 cc of 3 percent sodium tetradecyl sulfate (Sotradecol) demonstrates a complete occlusion of the right renal artery (*arrow*). (C) An aortogram 4 weeks after the perfusion demonstrates a persistent occlusion of the right renal artery (*arrow*) and a nonfunctioning right kidney.

not clearly defined since most experience has been limited to experimental animals.

INTERNAL ORGAN HYPERTHERMIA

There is evidence from a variety of preclinical models and preliminary clinical studies that cancer cells are often more sensitive than normal cells to heat and that temperature elevations of 42 to 44° C for several hours may selectively destroy malignant cells, with subsequent regression of the cancer [15, 32]. It has also been shown that hyperthermia can potentiate the effect of ionizing radiation and chemotherapeutic agents [35, 41].

A number of techniques have been described for systemic and local hyperthermia in cancer therapy. In recent investigations, we have demonstrated that internal organ temperatures can be reproducibly and predictably elevated by a controlled perfusion technique using occlusion balloon catheters. The percutaneous introduction of an occlusion balloon catheter into a renal artery and the subsequent perfusion of heated blood raised the renal temperature to 43° C. The temperatures of the liver could be changed significantly with portal venous perfusion, but the hepatic arterial perfusion caused only minimal temperature changes. An infusion into the lobar portal vein raised the temperature of one lobe selectively while the nonperfused lobe remained unchanged. With the use of a superselective catheterization technique, the temperature of part of an internal organ or a tumor can be selectively elevated. The technique may have a therapeutic role in cancer management, or it can be used as an adjunct to radiation therapy and chemotherapy.

Use of Degradable Starch Microspheres for Temporary Occlusion of the Vascular Bed—Alone and with Antineoplastic Agents

Recently, starch microspheres (Spherex; Pharmacia) of uniform (40-μ) size that are digested by serum amylase so that a 10-to-20-minute half-life pertains in the bloodstream have become available for clinical investigation [5, 49]. Although the microspheres initially occlude the microcirculation of the arteriolar level, digestion by serum amylase proceeds from within the central core so that contraction occurs with the subsequent movement of the spheres into the capillary bed prior to complete dissolution. In preclinical studies, temporary occlusion (for 10–20 minutes) of the vascular bed of the rat kidney and the rat splanchnic bed was demonstrated to occur with appropriate intraarterial injection [59]. No significant tissue damage occurred from the temporary ischemia. However, the temporary regional hypoxemia allowed a doubling of the tissue tolerance for radiotherapy, suggesting a role for such treatment when abdominal radiotherapy is to be given [30]. In such an instance, selective temporary obstruction of blood flow by intraarterially injected microspheres would be used to protect normal gut and renal tissue but not tumor.

The ability of the starch microspheres temporarily to occlude blood flow through the arterial vasculature of tumor-bearing liver has recently come under clinical study [5, 24]. With progressive dose increases in microspheres injected into the hepatic artery, there is progressive partial occlusion of the arteriolar vasculature and the hepatic arterial flow. With sufficiently large doses, complete occlusion and blockage of the arterial flow can be effected (Fig. 94-9). With time, the microspheres are degraded by serum amylase, and the arterial flow resumes. It appears that temporary blockage of the arterial flow can lead to infarction of the tumor nodules without significant liver damage (Fig. 94-9D), confirming that the tumor is dependent on the arterial blood supply whereas the portal vein supply suffices for the normal liver parenchyma.

The starch microspheres have also been used to entrap the rapidly acting, short half-life drug bischlorethylnitrosourea (BCNU) in the arterial vasculature of tumor-bearing liver in patients. It was hypothesized that entrapment of BCNU in the temporarily occluded vasculature might lead to a reduced spillover of the drug into the systemic circulation and thus to a reduction in its systemic toxicity (myelosuppression). Previous clinical pharmacologic studies had suggested a six- to sevenfold increase in regional hepatic BCNU exposure with short-term BCNU infusions into the hepatic artery [27]. The studies to date suggest a 70 to 90 percent reduction in systemic exposure to BCNU when microspheres are used to entrap the drug in tumor-bearing liver in patients [24]. Such entrapment could potentially increase hepatic tumor exposure by 20- to 70-fold while decreasing systemic exposure by the 70 to 90 percent previously indicated. Preclinical studies with other active chemotherapeutic agents (e.g., actinomycin D) suggest that bolus hepatic arterial injection of drug with microspheres may markedly increase the hepatic regional uptake of other agents as well. As will be discussed below, the ability to use bolus drug injections markedly diminishes the catheter-induced morbidity associated with prolonged infusions. Hence the starch microspheres, as well as balloon catheterization, will certainly play a prominent role in future experimental investigations of regional cancer treatment.

Prolonged catheterization for chemotherapy infusions using percutaneous angiography for catheter placement is a well-established technique, especially as it is applied to hepatic arterial infusions [4, 19, 55]. However, the morbidity with this technique is appreciable and increases with the duration of the infusion [19]. Unless the arterial configuration is especially favorable, the relatively rigid catheters needed for guided placement and their thrombogenic properties lead to hepatic arterial perforation and thrombosis after 4 to 6 weeks. With time, the stability of the catheter-tip position and the variable regions of liver infused present other problems that have been recognized only recently [39, 40]. A final major problem with continuous infusion techniques has been the need to use a pumping system for the constant delivery of drug solutions. A reliable and easily tolerated totally implantable subcutaneous pump (Infusaid; Infusaid Corp.) has recently been marketed [12, 25]. This pump can be connected to angiographically percutaneously placed catheters. However, the use of Silastic catheters and surgical placement at laparotomy is probably preferable when constant prolonged (longer than 3 weeks) infusion is con-

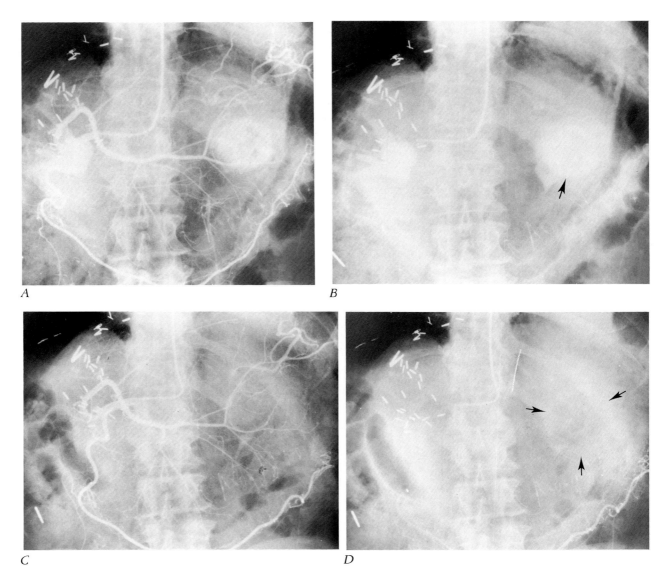

A

B

C

D

Figure 94-9. Temporary occlusion of hepatic arterial circulation with degradable starch microspheres in a 55-year-old man with metastases in the left hepatic lobe. A right hepatic lobectomy for a hepatoma had been performed 1 year earlier. (A) A selective hepatic angiogram (midarterial phase) from the transaxillary approach showing a vascular mass in the left lobe of the liver. (B) The capillary phase of the same angiogram showing a homogeneous tumor stain with central lucency (*arrow*). (C) A repeat angiogram (arterial phase) 24 hours later reveals nearly complete recanalization of the hepatic arterial branches that had become occluded immediately after the injection of 20 cc of starch microspheres. (D) The capillary phase of (C) shows a decreased tumor stain and a large central lucency (*arrows*).

sidered desirable [25]. In many instances, if the right catheter system were available for percutaneous placement, such placement for prolonged infusions would be associated with a lower morbidity and would be more convenient. Until such a placement system becomes available, it is perhaps best to use percutaneous angiography with bolus or short-term (shorter than 3 weeks) drug infusions in programs with appropriate agents.

Value and Limitations of Regional Approaches in Cancer Treatment

The major value of regional approaches to cancer treatment lies in the treatment of significant and symptomatic tumors of vital organs. Such treatment is often palliative, but it may ultimately be curative in regionally confined malignancies, such as high-grade brain tumors, some hepatomas, and a small group of hepatic metastases. The techniques and experimental approaches described in this chapter take advantage of the ability of angiography to define selected (abnormal) regions as well as to deliver agents that in themselves display further (antineoplastic) selectivity. Often, the control of tumor in one area may only be palliative; although it may prolong life, it may not cure. However, the development of effective approaches applicable to tumor in many regions is a step in the right direction. When combined with effective treatment for microscopic disease systemically, ablation of bulk regional tumor may be curative. Furthermore, in tumor that has a propensity to spread to specific regions, adjuvant treatment of such regions with angiographic approaches may be curative in many more patients [57].

References

1. Abrams, H. L.   The response of neoplastic renal vessels to epinephrine in man. *Radiology* 82:217, 1964.
2. Adler, J., Einhorn, R., McCarthy, J., Goodman, A., Solangi, K., Varanasi, U., and Thelmo, W. Gelfoam embolization of the kidneys for treatment of malignant hypertension. *Radiology* 128:45, 1978.
3. Almersjö, O., Bengmark, S., Engevik, L., Hafström, L. O., and Nilsson, L. A. V. Hepatic artery ligation as pretreatment for liver resection of metastatic cancer. *Rev. Surg.* 23:377, 1966.
4. Ansfield, F. J., Ramirez, G., Davis, H. L., Wirtanen, G. W., Johnson, R. O., Bryan, G. T., Manalo, F. B., Borden, E. C., Davis, T. E., and Esmaili, M. Further clinical studies with intrahepatic arterial infusion with 5-fluorouracil. *Cancer* 36:2413, 1975.
5. Aronsen, K. F., Hellekant, C., Holmberg, J., Rothman, U., and Teder, H. Controlled blocking of hepatic artery flow with enzymatically degradable microspheres combined with oncolytic drugs. *Eur. Surg. Res.* 11:99, 1979.
6. Athanasoulis, C. A., Baum, S., Rösch, J., Waltman, A. C., Ring, E. J., Smith, J. C., Sugarbaker, E., and Wood, W. Mesenteric arterial infusions of vasopressin for hemorrhage from colonic diverticulosis. *Am. J. Surg.* 129:212, 1975.
7. Athanasoulis, C. A., Baum, S., Waltman, A. C., Ring, E. J., Imbembo, A., and Vander Salm, T. J. Control of acute gastric mucosal hemorrhage: Intraarterial infusion of posterior pituitary extract. *N. Engl. J. Med.* 290:597, 1974.
8. Baurmash, H., and Mandel, L.   The nonsurgical treatment of hemangioma with Sotradecol. *Oral Surg.* 16:777, 1963.
9. Bengmark, S., Rosengren, K. Angiographic study of the collateral circulation to the liver after ligation of the hepatic artery in man. *Am. J. Surg.* 119:620–624, 1970.
10. Bertino, J. R., Mosher, M. D., DeConti, R. C. Chemotherapy of cancer of the head and neck. *Cancer* 31:1141, 1973.
11. Bookstein, J. J., Conn, J., and Reuter, S. R. Intra-adrenal hemorrhage as a complication of adrenal venography in primary aldosteronism. *Radiology* 90:778, 1968.
12. Buchwald, H., Grage, T. B., Vassilopoulos, P. P., Rohde, T. D., Varco, R. L., and Blackshear, P. J. Intraarterial infusion chemotherapy for hepatic carcinoma using a totally implantable infusion pump. *Cancer* 45:866, 1980.
13. Burrows, J. H., Talley, R. W., Drake, E. H., San Diego, E. L., and Tucker, W. G. Infusion of fluorinated pyrimidines into hepatic artery for treatment of metastatic carcinoma of the liver. *Cancer* 20:1886, 1967.
14. Cady, B.   Hepatic arterial patency and complications after catheterization for infusion chemotherapy. *Ann. Surg.* 178:156, 1973.
15. Cavaliere, R., Ciocatto, E. C., Giovanella, B. C., Heidelberger, C., Johnson, R. O., Margottini, M., Mondovi, B., Moricca, G., and Rossi-Fanelli, A. Selective heat sensitivity of cancer cells: Biochemical and clinical studies. *Cancer* 20:1351, 1967.
16. Chien-Hsing, M., Adler, J., and Elkin, M.   Early renal vein opacification during selective renal angiography. Trueta phenomenon or technical artifact? *Radiology* 112:61, 1974.
17. Cho, K. J., and Schmidt, R. W.   Selective arterial infusion of vasoconstrictors for control of traumatic splenic hemorrhage. *Invest. Radiol.* 13:67, 1978.
18. Cho, K. J., and Stanley, J. C.   Non-neoplastic congenital and acquired renal arteriovenous malformations and fistulas. *Radiology* 129:333, 1978.
19. Clouse, M. E., Ahmed, R., Ryan, R. B., Oberfield, R. A., and McCaffrey, J. A. Complications of long-term transbrachial hepatic arterial infusion chemotherapy. *AJR* 129:799, 1977.
20. Doppman, J. L., Brown, E. M., Brennan, M. F., Spiegel, A., Marx, S. J., and Aurbach, G. D. Angiographic ablation of parathyroid adenomas. *Radiology* 130:577, 1979.
21. Doppman, J. L., Marx, S. J., Spiegel, A. M., Mallette, L. E., Wolfe, D. R., Aurbach, G. D., and Geelhoed, G. Treatment of hyperparathyroidism by percutaneous embolization of a mediastinal adenoma. *Radiology* 115:37, 1975.
22. Eagan, R. T., and Page, M. I.   Adrenal insufficiency following bilateral adrenal venography. *J.A.M.A.* 215:115, 1971.

23. Ellman, B. A., Green, C. E., Eigenbrodt, E., Garriott, J. C., and Curry, T. Renal infarction with absolute ethanol. *Invest. Radiol.* 15:318, 1980.
24. Ensminger, W. D., Dakhil, S., Cho, K. J., Niederhuber, J., Doan, K., and Wheeler, R. Improved regional selectivity of hepatic arterial BCNU with degradable starch microspheres. *Cancer* 50:631, 1982.
25. Ensminger, W. D., Niederhuber, J., Dakhil, S., Thrall, J., and Wheeler, R. A totally implanted drug delivery system for hepatic arterial chemotherapy. *Cancer Treat. Rep.* 65:393, 1981.
26. Ensminger, W. D., Rosowsky, A., Raso, V., Levin, D. C., Glade, M., Come, S., Steele, G., and Frei, E., III. A clinical-pharmacologic evaluation of hepatic arterial infusion of 5-fluoro-2'-deoxyuridine and 5-fluorouracil. *Cancer Res.* 38:3784, 1978.
27. Ensminger, W. D., Thompson, M., Come, S., and Egan, E. M. Hepatic arterial BCNU: A pilot clinical-pharmacologic study in patients with liver tumors. *Cancer Treat. Rep.* 62:1509, 1978.
28. Fellerman, H., Dalakos, T. G., and Streeten, D. H. P. Remission of Cushing's syndrome after unilateral adrenal phlebography. *Ann. Intern. Med.* 73:585, 1970.
29. Fisher, C. E., Turner, F. A., and Horton, R. Remission of primary hyperaldosteronism after adrenal venography. *N. Engl. J. Med.* 285:334, 1971.
30. Forsberg, J. O., and Jung, B. Abdominal radiation response modified by hypoxia after intraaortal injection of starch microspheres. Experiments in the rat. *Acta Radiol. Oncol.* 17:353, 1978.
31. Garnick, M. D., Ensminger, W. D., and Israel, M. A clinical-pharmacological evaluation of hepatic arterial infusion of adriamycin. *Cancer Res.* 39:4105, 1979.
32. Giovanella, B. C., Stehlin, J. S., Jr., and Morgan, A. C. Selective lethal effect of supranormal temperatures on human neoplastic cells. *Cancer Res.* 36:3944, 1976.
33. Goldin, A. R., Naude, J. H., and Thatcher, G. N. Therapeutic percutaneous renal infarction. *Br. J. Urol.* 46:133, 1974.
34. Goodman, L. S., and Gilman, A. *The Pharmacological Basis of Therapeutics* (5th ed.). New York: Macmillan, 1975.
35. Hahn, G. M., Braun, J., and Har-Kedar, F. Thermochemotherapy: Synergism between hyperthermia and adriamycin or bleomycin in mammalian cell inactivation. *Proc. Natl. Acad. Sci. U.S.A.* 72:937, 1975.
36. Henrich, W. L., Goldman, M., Dotter, C. T., Rösch, J., and Bennett, W. M. Therapeutic renal arterial occlusion for elimination of proteinuria. *Arch. Intern. Med.* 136:840, 1976.
37. Iwaki, A., Nagasue, N., Kobayoshi, M., and Inokuchi, K. Intraarterial chemotherapy with concomitant use of vasoconstrictors for liver cancer. *Cancer Treat. Rep.* 62:145, 1978.
38. Jesse, R. H., Goepfert, H., Lindberg, R. D., and Johnson, R. H. Combined intraarterial infusion and radiotherapy for the treatment of advanced cancer of the head and neck. *AJR* 105:20, 1961.
39. Kaplan, W. D., D'Orsi, C. J., Ensminger, W. D., Smith, E. H., and Levin, D. C. Intraarterial radionuclide infusion: A new technique to assess chemotherapy perfusion patterns. *Cancer Treat. Rep.* 62:699, 1978.
40. Kaplan, W. D., Ensminger, W. D., Come, S. E., Smith, E. H., D'Orsi, C. J., Levin, D. C., Takvorian, R. W., and Steele, G. D., Jr. Radionuclide angiography to predict patient response to hepatic artery chemotherapy. *Cancer Treat. Rep.* 64:1217, 1980.
41. Kim, J. H., Hahn, E. W., Tokita, N., and Nisce, L. Z. Local tumor hyperthermia in combination with radiation therapy: I. Malignant cutaneous lesions. *Cancer* 40:161, 1977.
42. Klatte, E. C., Bendick, P., Donohue, J. P., Holden, R. W., Yune, H. Y., and Gilmor, R. L. Intraarterial chemical surgery. Presented at the 80th Annual Meeting of the American Roentgen Ray Society, Las Vegas, Nevada, April 21–25, 1980.
43. McCarron, D. A., Rubin, R. J., Barnes, B. A., Harrington, J. T., and Millan, V. G. Therapeutic bilateral renal infarction in end-stage renal disease. *N. Engl. J. Med.* 294:652, 1976.
44. Nilsson, L. A. Therapeutic hepatic artery ligation in patients with secondary liver tumors. *Rev. Surg.* 23:374, 1966.
45. Owman, T., Lunderquist, A., Alwmark, A., and Borjesson, B. Embolization of the spleen for treatment of splenomegaly and hypersplenism in patients with portal hypertension. *Invest. Radiol.* 14:457, 1979.
46. Reuter, S. R., Chuang, V. P., and Bree, R. L. Selective arterial embolization for control of massive upper gastrointestinal bleeding. *AJR* 125:119, 1975.
47. Reuter, S. R., Pomeroy, P. R., Chuang, V. P., and Cho, K. J. Embolic control of hypertension caused by segmental renal artery stenosis. *AJR* 127:389, 1976.
48. Rösch, J., Dotter, C. T., and Antonovic, R. Selective vasoconstrictor infusion in the management of arteriocapillary gastrointestinal hemorrhage. *AJR* 110:279, 1972.
49. Rothman, U., Arfors, K. E., Aronsen, K. F., Lindell, B., and Nylander, G. Enzymatical degradable microspheres for experimental and clinical use. *Microvasc. Res.* 11:421–430, 1976.
50. Sidd, J. J., and Decter, A. Unilateral renal dam-

age due to massive contrast dye injection with recovery. *J. Urol.* 97(1):30, 1967.

51. Spigos, D. G., Jonasson, O., Mozes, M., and Capek, V. Partial splenic embolization in the treatment of hypersplenism. *AJR* 132:777, 1979.

52. Spigos, D. G., Thane, T. T., and Capek, V. Skin necrosis following extravasation during peripheral phlebography. *Radiology* 123:605, 1977.

53. Stehlin, J. S., Jr., and Clark, R. L. Melanoma of the extremities: Experiments with conventional chemotherapy and perfusion in 339 cases. *Am. J. Surg.* 110:366, 1965.

54. Steinberg, M. H. Evaluation of Sotradecol in sclerotherapy of varicose veins. *Angiobiology* 6: 519, 1955.

55. Sullivan, R. D., Norcross, J. W., and Watkins, E. Chemotherapy of metastatic liver cancer by prolonged hepatic artery infusions. *N. Engl. J. Med.* 270:321, 1964.

56. Sullivan, R. D., Watkins, E., Jr., Oberfield, R., and Khazei, A. Current status of protracted arterial infusion chemotherapy. *Surg. Clin. North Am.* 47:769, 1967.

57. Taylor, I., Rowling, J., and West, C. Adjuvant cytotoxic liver perfusion for colorectal cancer. *Br. J. Surg.* 66:833, 1979.

58. Terblanche, J., Northover, J. M. A., Bornman, P., Kahn, D., Silber, W., Barbezat, G. O., Sellars, S., Campbell, J. A. H., and Saunders, S. J. A prospective controlled trial of sclerotherapy in the long-term management of patients after esophageal variceal bleeding. *Surg. Gynecol. Obstet.* 148: 323, 1979.

59. Tuma, R. F., Forsberg, J. O., Schosser, R., and Arfors, K. E. The use of degradable microspheres in producing transient ischemia for drug and radiation therapy. *Fed. Proc.* 37:876, 1978.

60. Watkins, E., Jr., Hering, A. C., Luna, R., and Adams, H. D. The use of intravascular balloon catheters for isolation of the pelvic vascular bed during pump-oxygenator perfusion of cancer chemotherapeutic agents. *Surg. Gynecol. Obstet.* 111:464, 1960.

61. Zimmerman, C. E., Eisenberg, H., Spark, R., and Rosoff, C. B. Transvenous adrenal destruction: Clinical trials in patients with metastatic malignancy. *Surgery* 75(4):550, 1974.

62. Zimmerman, C. E., Kettyle, W. M., Eisenberg, H. R., Spark, R., Rosoff, C. B., and Cohen, R. B. Transvenous adrenalectomy. *J. Surg. Res.* 12:124, 1972.

Bucrylate, Silicones, and Ivalon as Agents for Intravascular Embolization

MARTIN L. GOLDMAN

Why More Embolic Agents?

Considerable experience has been gained with transcatheter embolization techniques, particularly those using Gelfoam and coils. These techniques are not without risk [1, 17]. The main complications of embolization include ischemia and infection of the embolized region. Gastric necrosis and duodenal and jejunal ischemia have all been reported, as have hepatic and splenic infarction and abscess. Passage of the embolic material out of the vessel that is being occluded into other vessels has also resulted in hepatic infarction, hepatic abscess, splenic abscess, renal infarction, spinal cord paralysis, and gangrene of the lower extremities. In attempts to avoid these complications, other embolic agents have been investigated in the laboratory and in clinical situations. As a result of studies with bucrylate (Ethicon), silicone (Dow-Corning), and Ivalon (Unipoint), the therapeutic role of transcatheter embolization has increased.

BUCRYLATE

Bucrylate (isobutyl 2-cyanoacrylate) belongs to a class of adhesives of the alkyl 2-cyanoacrylates (Fig. 95-1) [33]. The adhesive nature of these compounds was discovered by accident. A drop of the highly purified alkyl 2-cyanoacrylate was placed between the prisms of a refractometer in order to obtain its refractive index for comparison to that of a previously prepared sample. When an attempt was made to open the refractometer, the prisms could not be pulled apart. Since then, the adhesive nature of these compounds has been studied extensively.

The alkyl 2-cyanoacrylates are converted from the liquid to the solid state by polymerization when pressed into a thin film between two adherents. This polymerization occurs at room temperature and does not require the use of a solvent or an added catalyst. The bonding action is the result of anionic polymerization. The polymerization is catalyzed by the action of minute amounts of water on weak bases present on the adherent surfaces and is a highly exothermic reaction. The polymerization of the alkyl 2-cyanoacrylates occurs without appreciable change in volume, and as a result these compounds cannot be used as space fillers. The setting time ranges from a few seconds to a few minutes and varies with the inhibitor content and viscosity, the nature of the adherents, and the temperature

2191

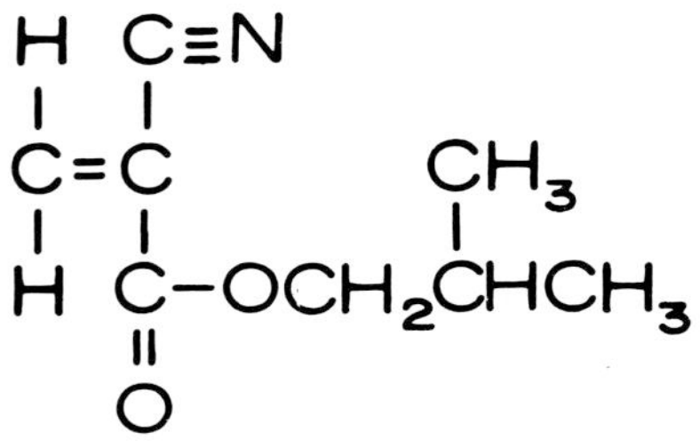

H   C≡N
| |
C=C   CH₃
| | |
H   C—OCH₂CHCH₃
‖
O

Figure 95-1. Chemical structure of bucrylate, an isobutyl ester of 2-cyanoacrylate.

and humidity. When an alkyl 2-cyanoacrylate comes in contact with moist animal tissue, a good bond can be obtained if the tissues are approximated quickly. In many instances, however, the time needed to approximate tissues and apply pressure is such that the extremely rapid polymerization of the monomer results in a poor bond. Also, the viscosity is so low that it is difficult to keep the monomer in the area desired. As a result, even though the adhesive can be used in patching vascular anastomoses, its clinical use is certainly limited.

Eastman 910, a methyl 2-cyanoacrylate, was the first tissue adhesive available for application. The product was not sterile, and there was some indication that it was carcinogenic in cancer-prone rats, but that was not substantiated in dogs. Ethicon was able to produce in sterile form a methyl 2-cyanoacrylate that did not contain additives. Although this material has not been shown to be carcinogenic, it does produce an acute reaction with inflammatory exudate and necrosis of cells that are in direct contact with the adhesive. The extent of the necrosis is directly related to the quantity of the adhesive. By using higher molecular-weight homologues of the methyl 2-cyanoacrylate, the histotoxicity that had been seen with the methyl 2-cyanoacrylate is markedly reduced. This reduction in histotoxicity is accomplished without impairing the unique tissue properties of the 2-cyanoacrylates. Isobutyl 2-cyanoacrylate, or bucrylate, has been used both in laboratory animals and in humans to apply dry dura mater over arterial punctures; to reinforce ruptured intracranial aneurysms; to achieve hemostasis in the aorta, liver, kidney, lung; to close fistulas of the intestinal tract; and to seal lung parenchyma [32]. There has been no experimental or clinical evidence to indicate that bucrylate is carcinogenic [1, 3, 16]. Only in studies involving pigs [45] has there been evidence of bucrylates producing a chronic inflam-

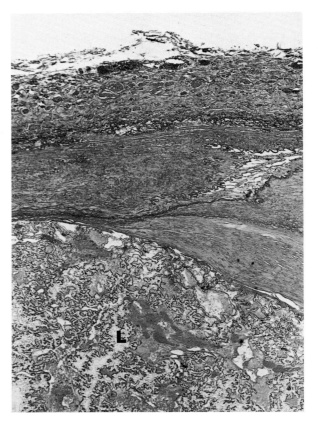

Figure 95-2. Cross-section of the iliac artery in a patient 1 month after a bucrylate embolization shows a complete occlusion of the vessel lumen (*L*) by an organizing thrombus of bucrylate and blood cells. There is no evidence of inflammation in the vessel wall. (H&E ×53.)

matory reaction. This finding, however, has not been substantiated in the arterial system of other animals or of humans (Fig. 95-2).

The transcatheter administration of bucrylate for abdominal use was introduced by Dotter et al. [15]. Bucrylate has several unique characteristics that make it desirable as an embolic agent. As a monomer it has a low viscosity, and so it can be injected easily through 2 and 3 French catheters to allow highly selective catheterization and embolization [17]. The monomer mixes easily with Ethiodol, Pantopaque, or tantalum powder [11, 17]. As a result, fluoroscopic control during the embolization procedure is easily accomplished. When the monomer comes in contact with the ions in blood, it undergoes polymerization. The polymerization occurs within seconds, and during the process the bucrylate incorporates within it the blood elements, resulting in approximately a

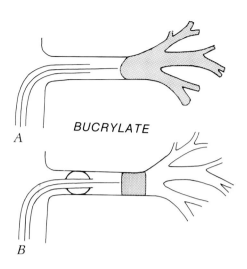

BUCRYLATE

A

B

Figure 95-3. Diagrammatic representation of coaxial catheter techniques of administering bucrylate. (A) A cast of the entire vascular bed can be obtained, or (B), with an outer balloon occlusion catheter, a localized vascular occlusion that mimics a surgical ligation of the vessel can be accomplished.

doubling of the size of the embolic cast. As the polymerization continues, the bucrylate becomes adherent to the blood vessel wall, and the lumen of the vessel can be completely and permanently occluded. By varying the catheter techniques (Fig. 95-3)—for example, by using coaxial catheters and balloon occlusion catheters—as well as by varying the concentration of Pantopaque or Ethiodol mixed with the bucrylate, the angiographer can obtain peripheral or proximal vascular occlusions or can even obtain a cast of almost the entire vascular system of an organ or area that is being embolized.

The main disadvantages of bucrylate are that its proper use requires considerable experience as well as an investigational exemption from the Food and Drug Administration (IND). But by taking advantage of the unique properties of bucrylate, we have used transcatheter embolization with bucrylate to occlude vessels in over 60 patients with various clinical problems.

Silicones

Silicones [4, 7, 37] are man-made organosilicon compounds that consist of long-chained polymers of alternating silicon and oxygen atoms with organic groups attached. The R group can be almost any organic group, but the most common one is

the methyl group (CH_3). The individual unit is called a methylsiloxane. The polymer is a polydimethylsiloxane (Fig. 95-4), and the number of units (n) determines the physical characteristics of the silicone [46]. The higher the value of n, the greater the viscosity of the silicone. If n is 2, the silicone is volatile and will cause a severe inflammatory reaction if injected subcutaneously. If n is approximately 100, the viscosity of the silicone is similar to that of No. 35 oil. When n approaches 1,000, no tissue reaction is noted, and the silicone is more viscous. When n is 10,000, the silicone is inert and is almost a solid. Because their chemical nature and physical properties can be varied so extensively, silicones can be very reactive chemicals or they can be liquids, gels, greases, defoamers, waxes, rubbers, and resins [37]. But most silicones, like their ancestor, quartz (SiO_2), are inert [4].

Because industrial-grade silicones contain additives that may be toxic and perhaps even carcinogenic when used in patients, only properly prepared medical-grade silicones should be used for clinical applications [7, 46]. Silastic is the trademark for Dow-Corning's medical-grade silicone rubber. Medical-grade silicone rubber is made from high-viscosity dimethylpolysiloxanes.

There are two basic types of material available for medical use. A heat-vulcanizing type and a room-vulcanizing type (RVT) [4, 7, 37, 46]. The heat-vulcanizing material is prepared with an extremely high viscosity fluid, with silicon dioxide as a filler and with dibenzylperoxide as a catalyst. With the addition of heat, vulcanization takes place by the breakdown of the peroxide and the subsequent cross-linkage of polydimethylsiloxane chains. The higher the viscosity of the basic fluid, the harder the end product.

The RVT material is basically a fluid of relatively low viscosity, with a filler of diatomaceous earth. With the addition of the catalyst stannous

Figure 95-4. Chemical structure of a silicone polymer. To each silicon atom an organic group is attached. When the group is a methyl radical, the result is a polydimethylsiloxane.

$$\begin{array}{c} CH_3 \\ | \\ Si-O \\ | \\ CH_3 \end{array} \left[\begin{array}{c} CH_3 \\ | \\ Si-O \\ | \\ CH_3 \end{array} \right]_n \begin{array}{c} CH_3 \\ | \\ Si-O \\ | \\ CH_3 \end{array}$$

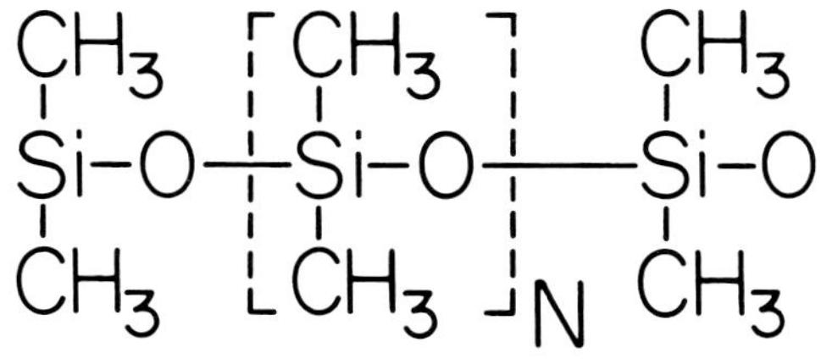

octoate, a rubbery material is formed in a few minutes. The process does not require heat nor does it produce heat [36]. Generally, the RVT rubbers are weaker and more likely to tear than are the heat-vulcanized products.

Extensive experimental studies have been performed to evaluate the local and systemic responses to solid silicone rubber and to injected fluid silicone plus catalyst with in vivo vulcanization. Animal and human studies [4, 14, 36, 37, 46] have shown that silicone as a prosthetic material has less toxicity than virtually any other foreign material placed in the body. The silicone is essentially histologically inert, it is not phagocytized or metabolized, and it has no antigenic or carcinogenic properties in animal studies. There is no evidence that the body can cause disintegration of the silicone, and there is no evidence of malignant tumor formation secondary to the use of medical-grade silicone. Silicone prostheses have been used without systemic or local reaction in an estimated 100,000 patients with ventriculovascular shunts or in patients undergoing plastic surgery, orthopedic surgery, or cardiovascular surgery [36].

There are two forms of silicone that can be used as an embolic agent: (1) Dow-Corning's Silastic 382, a medical-grade liquid silicone preparation [36], and (2) silicone rubber spheres (Heyer-Schulte). The medical-grade dimethylpolysiloxane (Silastic 382; Dow-Corning) is too viscous for injection through an angiographic catheter [14]. Viscosity may be reduced to acceptable levels with silicone fluid 360. Vulcanization takes place by mixing these solutions with catalysts, Dow-Corning M (stannous oxide) and tetraethylsilicate, a colinker. By varying the ratio of elastomer 382 to silicone fluid 360 and by altering the amount of catalyst used, the vulcanization time from a liquid to a hard rubber substance can be controlled to range from less than a minute to 20 minutes [3, 25, 36].

The advantages of liquid silicone as an embolic agent are that (1) it is inert and so the vessels show only intimal hyperplasia; (2) it can be injected through catheters as small as 1 French [34], allowing superselective catheterization and embolization; (3) it can be mixed with tantalum powder, which adds to the safety of embolization by permitting fluoroscopic control; (4) it does not cross an intact vascular system and is trapped within small ($40\text{-}\mu$) vessels; and (5) prior to embolization, vulcanization time can be accurately assessed by taking a sample of the substance that is to be injected and stirring it within a vial.

The disadvantages of liquid silicone are that (1) it is difficult to use (the injecting material may transform very rapidly from a liquid to a thick viscous material, making injection through the catheter difficult); (2) if arteriovenous shunts are present, the silicone may pass through the abnormal shunts and cause embolization to the heart and lungs [36]; (3) occlusion of $40\text{-}\mu$ vessels may produce unwanted ischemia and infarction of the organ embolized or vital structures within the region embolized; and (4) an IND is necessary for its use.

The other form of silicone that has been used as an embolic agent is Silastic spheres [3, 23, 25], which are available in sizes varying from 0.5 to 3.0 mm in diameter and can be purchased radiopaque, having been impregnated with barium. This material was first used as an embolic agent by Luessenhop in 1962 [31], to occlude inoperable cerebral arteriovenous malformations.

An 8 or 9 French nontapered catheter is necessary for injection of the spheres [29]. Because many central nervous system lesions are inaccessible to direct catheterization, embolization of the Silastic spheres relies on the so-called sump effect. Once the spheres are injected into the vascular system, they cannot be controlled but in a flow-guided manner go to the area of highest vascularity. Initially, embolization of the vascular mass is done with the smallest spheres that can be trapped within the vascular lesion [25]. As the smaller vessels are occluded, progressively larger and larger spheres are injected in an attempt to occlude completely the vascular abnormality that is being embolized. Because the spheres follow the direction of flow, it is possible that the smaller microspheres may cross the vascular abnormality and embolize to the lung. It is also possible that when the flow within the vascular abnormality is slowed or stopped, inadvertent embolization to other than the vascular abnormality may occur. Silastic spheres have had wide applicability in the central nervous system [25] in embolization of glomus jugulare tumors, dural arteriovenous malformations, vascular tumors of the base of the skull, arteriovenous malformations of the subtemporal and pterygoid fossas, and vascular lesions of the vertebral bodies.

There are several drawbacks to the use of these spheres. Because the spheres tend to cling together in the injection syringe and in the connecting tubing, they are difficult to inject [43]. Special mechanical injection devices have been designed to facilitate injection [25]. The spheres have the drawback of being a particulate embolic agent. When flow within the vessel that is being embolized is slowed, other vessels may become occluded. When the splenic artery in dogs was embolized to control splenic bleeding, as flow within the splenic artery slowed, left gastric and pancreatic branches were occluded with the spheres [23]. Furthermore, embolization with spheres is time consuming and expensive [28]. Forty particles cost about $18 (in 1980), and a patient may require 200 to 400 spheres. In addition, Silastic spheres do not promote thrombosis of the lesion embolized, and complete occlusion of an embolized lesion is the exception rather than the rule [3]. For these reasons and because of the need to use large nontapered catheters that do not allow superselective catheterization, Silastic spheres have little applicability in general abdominal angiography.

Ivalon

Ivalon is a polyvinyl alcohol that has been converted into a spongelike material [5, 43]. It is produced by foaming the polyvinyl alcohol resin by beating air into it. The froth from the foaming is poured into a mold that is hardened over a period of 24 hours by washing it separately with sulfuric acid and/or formaldehyde [24, 43]. As a result of this hardening process, polyvinyl alcohol is made insoluble. The polymer structure of methyl radicals attached to hydroxyl groups (Fig. 95-5) gives Ivalon the property of being soft and resilient when wet yet hard and rigid when dry. It is heat stable to 120° C, but above 95° C it is thermoplastic, meaning that even in its dry state Ivalon remains flexible. Ivalon was first used commercially as a domestic sponge, but it was replaced by the less expensive cellulose. Ivalon industrial sponges are still widely used—for example, as wicking agents in the production of

Figure 95-5. Chemical structure of Ivalon, a polymer of methyl radicals attached to hydroxyl groups.

$$-CH_2-CH-CH_2-CH-CH_2-CH-CH_2$$
$$\quad\ \ \ OH \qquad\ \ OH \qquad\ \ OH$$

cardboard cartons. Ivalon has also been used as an ion exchange resin because the foam is a negatively charged colloid and so strongly absorbs cations [43]. Because of its ability to absorb water, Ivalon is used in electroplating and photography.

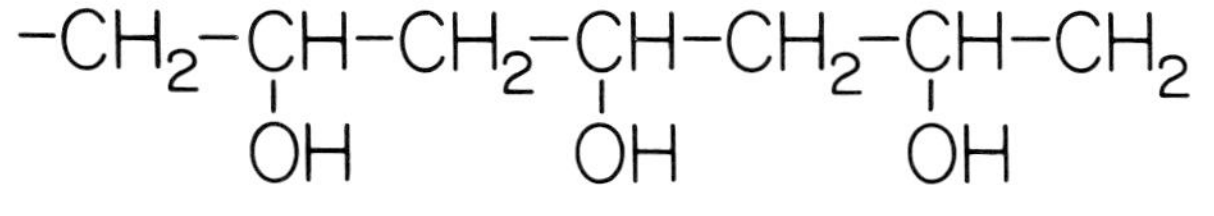

In animal studies it was shown that the Ivalon sponge structure is invaded by fibrocytes and that the Ivalon serves as a framework for this fibrocytic infiltration. With time, the Ivalon becomes an integral part of the body [43]. Because of this incorporation, Ivalon was used as a synthetic prosthesis and it was introduced experimentally in 1949 as a prosthesis in the hemothorax following a pneumonectomy [22, 24]. In the early days of cardiac surgery, Ivalon was used in the closure of septal defects, in reconstruction of the mitral valve, and as a graft for the repair of abdominal aortic aneurysms [2, 10, 24, 43]. It has also been used as a tissue substitute for bone, as dura mater, and as a subcutaneous implant in reconstructive surgery [2]. However, because they became increasingly rigid in time and broke down, the Ivalon [24, 43] patches formerly used to repair cardiac defects, have in most instances now been replaced by Dacron, Teflon, and silicone prostheses.

Ivalon as an embolic agent was introduced in 1966 by Porstmann [38]. With the use of Ivalon plugs, Porstmann was able to close patent ductus arteriosus in young children. The advantages of using Ivalon as an embolic agent [29, 43] are:

1. It is readily available commercially.
2. It can be obtained or prepared in small granular size.
3. It can be injected through standard angiographic catheters, allowing selective catheterization to be done.
4. It can completely occlude the lumen of the vessel.
5. It is relatively inert (but it does produce a mild inflammatory reaction in the early postembolization period). This reaction is thought to be due to disruption of the vessel wall by Ivalon particles (Fig. 95-6) [10].
6. It provides permanent vascular occlusion.
7. It does not fragment and thus does not cause more distal embolization that could occlude undesired terminal vessels.
8. It can be purchased radiopaque [28], having been mixed with barium. This increases fluoroscopic control during the embolization procedure.

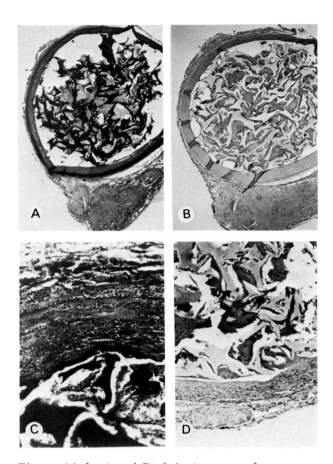

Figure 95-6. (A and B) Splenic artery after a recent embolization. Plastic fragments fill the lumen. Note the blood clot between fragments. The wall of the artery is unaltered. (C and D) The artery 15 days after embolization showing disruption of the intima of the artery, disarranged elastic tissue, and wall with marked inflammatory infiltrate. In (A) and (C), the plastic stains black with van Gieson's stain. (×40, 40, 250, and 100, respectively.) (From Castaneda-Zuniga et al. [8]. Reproduced by permission from *AJR*.)

The main disadvantage of Ivalon is that it is difficult to use. A dry compressed fragment of Ivalon may enlarge to several times its original size soon after it has been soaked in saline or contrast agent [27]. This property of Ivalon, along with its high coefficient of friction [28], makes it difficult to inject through catheters. Various investigators, however, have been able to overcome this difficulty [3, 27–29]. Ivalon also is a particulate embolic agent. As a result, as flow slows in the vessel being occluded, other collateral vessels may be occluded or embolic material may escape into the general circulation [8, 9, 43].

Techniques of Embolization

In embolization procedures, the catheter should be placed as close as possible to the area of abnormality. This positioning allows selective delivery of the embolic agent without unnecessary occlusion of collateral vessels. The catheter must be in a stable position that is unaffected by respiratory motion. Also, it should not occlude the vessel that is to be embolized. By having the embolic material carried by the vessel flow distal to the placement of the catheter, there is less possibility of reflux of embolic material out of the vessel that is being occluded.

High-quality fluoroscopy, when coupled with opacification of the embolic agent, adds greatly to the safety of the embolization procedure. Bucrylate is easily made radiopaque by mixing it with Ethiodol and Pantopaque. These contrast agents, however, slow the rate of polymerization of the bucrylate [11]. Tantalum powder of the 5-μ size does not slow polymerization and it gives good opacification, but it is difficult to obtain. The larger (50-μ) tantalum powder tends to precipitate rapidly and it gives uneven opacification of the embolic material. Silicone also is made radiopaque by mixing it with tantalum powder. Ivalon can be obtained commercially already radiopaque, having been mixed with barium.

In embolization of a vessel, a slow injection of embolic material is favored over a rapid injection. A rapid injection of bucrylate can cause the adhesive to pass through the capillaries and occlude venules, thus increasing the possibility of infarction [15]. With particulate embolic material such as Ivalon, a rapid injection may cause recoil of the catheter, with inadvertent embolization of particulate matter out of the embolized vessel and into the general circulation.

Coaxial catheter techniques are another aid to embolization (see Figs. 95-9A, 95-12C). One may be able to advance the smaller inner catheter into a more selective position. Also, when using bucrylate, one can inject the adhesive through the coaxial catheter, remove the inner catheter, and then do a follow-up angiogram through the outer catheter. This is a technique that we have often used with bucrylate. Coaxial catheters can also be passed through balloon occlusion catheters (see Fig. 95-10C). The use of balloon occlusion catheters is particularly helpful when one wants to confine the embolic agent. These catheters may be used with bucrylate or silicone in embolizing an arteriovenous malformation or with bucrylate in effecting a localized vascular occlusion.

Considerations in Embolization

A region or an organ that is having its vascular supply occluded may undergo infarction. Infarction may be desirable in embolization of a renal tumor or a parathyroid adenoma, but, if infarction occurs in embolization of the stomach, intestines, or pelvis, the results may be disastrous. The development of infarction following embolization depends a great deal on the collateral vessels within the organ following the embolic procedure. The number of collateral vessels available depends on prior surgery in the region, the degree of arteriosclerosis, the presence of shock, and the use of vasoconstrictors, such as pitressin.

The embolic material used for occlusion may also affect the collateral supply to variable degrees. For example, in the control of bleeding it

Figure 95-7. Diagrammatic representation of transcatheter embolization done to control bleeding. (A) When vessels are occluded with particulate embolic material, such as Gelfoam or Ivalon, multiple collateral vessels may become occluded. (B) With bucrylate, however, a localized vascular occlusion can be achieved with sparing of collateral vessels.

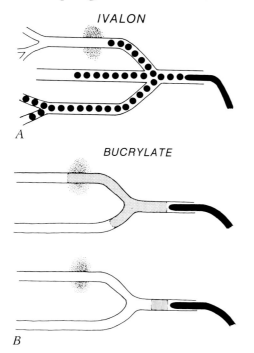

IVALON

A

BUCRYLATE

B

has been our experience that when particulate embolic material (such as Gelfoam) is used during the initial phase of the embolic procedure, the fragments go to the point of least resistance, directly to the bleeding branch. If the embolic procedure is stopped at that point, rebleeding is likely to occur. In order to obtain a more stable thrombus within the vessel, additional embolic material is injected into the feeding vessel. It is during this phase of embolization that multiple collateral branches become occluded with the particulate embolic material (Fig. 95-7A). As a result, if a region has its collateral flow reduced by embolic material it may become ischemic [18]. Because of this, when we embolize to control bleeding we use bucrylate and generally attempt to obtain a localized occlusion of the vessel as close to the bleeding site as possible (Fig. 95-7B). If elective surgery (e.g., gastrectomy) is to be performed after embolization, one must consider that a prior occlusion of collateral vessels by the emboli may jeopardize the viability of the gastric stump or its anastomosis [18].

In addition, one must not occlude the vasculature to an organ that is already infected. The few renal abscesses that have developed following embolization were in kidneys that were infected prior to embolization [21].

Clinical Applications

CONTROL OF HEMORRHAGE

The aim of embolization for the control of arterial hemorrhage from any region or organ is to stop the bleeding yet preserve organ function and viability. To accomplish this, we prefer to effect a localized vascular occlusion of the bleeding vessel, which does not compromise the collateral vessels. Such occlusion can be effectively accomplished with bucrylate. We have used bucrylate successfully to control gastric, intestinal (Fig. 95-8), renal, and pelvic hemorrhage [17, 39]. Ischemia of the embolized region did not develop. Because silicone is extremely difficult to confine to the bleeding vessel without its leaking from the bleeding site, it has no value in the control of hemorrhage. There have been a few reported cases in which Ivalon was used to control hemorrhage. Ivalon is essentially a substitute for Gelfoam, but it results in a permanent vascular occlusion. Our main concern about the use of Ivalon to control hemorrhage is that since this material

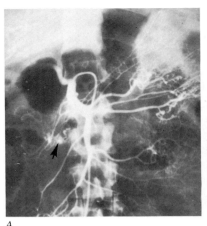 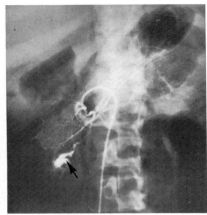 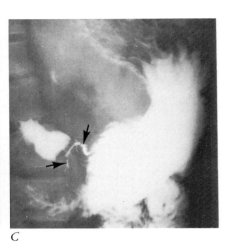

A   *B*   *C*

Figure 95-8. Successful control of a bleeding duodenal ulcer with bucrylate in a 28-year-old man with an infected renal transplant. (A) A superior mesenteric artery angiogram showing extravasation of contrast medium (*arrow*) in the duodenum. (B) The bleeding (*arrow*) is from a branch of the inferior pancreaticoduodenal artery. (C) An upper GI series done 3 years after embolization shows a persistent cast of bucrylate-tantalum mixture (*arrows*) in the proximal branches of the inferior pancreaticoduodenal artery.

does not adhere to the blood vessel wall, additional Ivalon fragments have to be injected to obtain a stable thrombus within the embolized vessel. As a result, collateral vessels can be occluded (see Fig. 95-7A). Also, as flow within the vessel slows, there is increased risk that any additional embolic material injected may escape from the vessel that is being embolized and enter the general circulation.

When using embolic therapy for the control of hemorrhage, one must also consider that although the bleeding vessel may be successfully occluded, rebleeding may develop at the site of embolization from collateral vessels. Such rebleeding has been observed in the stomach, duodenum [17], and pelvis.

MEDICAL NEPHRECTOMY

Total and permanent obliteration of the renal vasculature is a useful therapeutic modality that warrants further clinical investigation. We have used bucrylate successfully in the management of patients with severe uncontrolled hypertension, protein-losing nephropathy, and ureterocutaneous fistula and as an adjunct to preoperative surgery of renal tumors [39]. Because in the production of a medical nephrectomy it is necessary to obliterate as much of the intraparenchymal vascular bed as possible, bucrylate is an excellent embolic agent. By varying the catheterization techniques, the use and placement of coaxial catheters, and the use of balloon occlusion catheters, as well as by varying the rate of polymerization (by varying the percentage of Ethiodol or Pantopaque that the bucrylate is mixed with), the very small intrarenal vessels can be obliterated (Fig. 95-9).

Liquid silicone is also an effective embolic agent for producing a medical nephrectomy [14, 36]. Pathologic studies with the liquid silicone Microfil (Canton Bio-Medical Products) have shown that small 40-μ arterioles can be occluded [1, 11]. Liquid silicone has been successfully used to produce a nephrectomy in dogs. The main limitation to the use of silicone for nephrectomy would be the presence of arteriovenous shunts within the embolized kidney, such as occur in many patients with renal cell carcinoma.

In embolization, Ivalon does not occlude vessels as small as those that can be occluded with bucrylate or silicone. As a result, Ivalon has a more limited role in producing a medical nephrectomy than has bucrylate or silicone.

MEDICAL SPLENECTOMY

Although splenectomy has been performed for various conditions almost with impunity, it is being increasingly recognized that splenectomy is associated with increased susceptibility to overwhelming bacterial infection not only in infants and children, but also in adults. Because of this, preservation of functioning splenic tissue in pa-

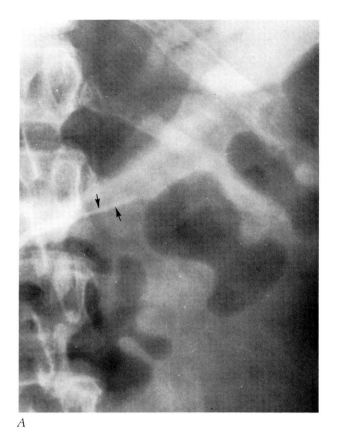

A

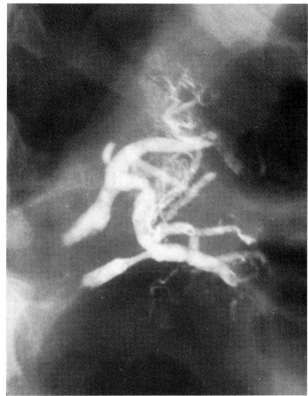

B

Figure 95-9. Successful medical nephrectomy with bucrylate in a 30-year-old man with a renal transplant and uncontrolled hypertension. (A) A coaxial catheter technique for the delivery of bucrylate consists of an inner 3 French Teflon catheter (*arrows*) passed through an outer 6.5 French catheter. (B) A selective injection of bucrylate-tantalum mixture into the two renal arteries of the native left kidney shows that almost the entire intraparenchymal renal vascular bed is filled with the bucrylate.

tients who would ordinarily undergo splenectomy is desirable. Although animal studies and the early reported cases of splenic artery embolization by Gelfoam were successful, several patients have developed splenic abscess. Most angiographers have thus felt that the spleen should not be embolized. Spigos [41, 42] introduced a technique of partial splenic artery embolization in which not more than 60 percent of the spleen was embolized at any one time. The Gelfoam used was soaked in antibiotics, and the patients received antibiotics prophylactically. In 33 patients, the technique proved successful in reversing the leukopenia seen in patients undergoing chronic renal dialysis or after renal transplantation. Only one patient developed an abscess.

We have been interested in another group of patients, those with cirrhosis [19], whose livers are impaired in their ability to clear the blood of circulating bacteria. Because of this impairment,

it is extremely important to preserve functioning splenic tissue in people who have cirrhosis and who need a splenectomy. Since a splenorenal shunt operation may become necessary in the event of recurrent variceal bleeding, it is also necessary for the spleen to be preserved.

Surgical ligation of the splenic artery in both animals and humans has been shown to be well tolerated and, in selected patients, to reverse the symptoms of hypersplenism and to maintain patency of the splenic vein. We have been investigating the therapeutic role of producing a localized vascular occlusion of the splenic artery by transcatheter embolization with bucrylate. In 13 patients with alcoholism and cirrhosis, splenic artery occlusion was done primarily for the control of variceal hemorrhage. In 12 of these patients, we were able to obtain a relatively localized ligation of the splenic artery (Fig. 95-10). Collateral vessels from the left gastric

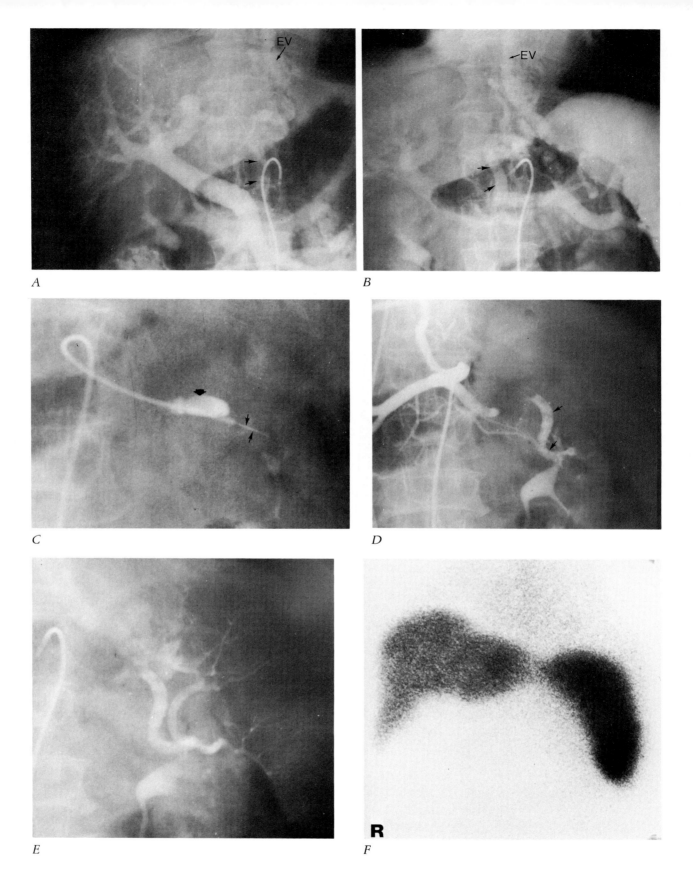

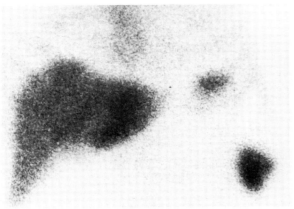

G

Figure 95-10. Successful control of bleeding esophageal varices by splenic artery occlusion with bucrylate in a 78-year-old man. (A and B) Venous phases of a superior mesenteric artery angiogram (A) and a splenic artery angiogram (B) show generalized portal hypertension with filling from both the splenic and the superior mesenteric artery injections of the coronary vein (*arrows*) and esophageal varices (*EV*). (C) The catheter system for the production of a localized occlusion of the splenic artery consists of an outer 7 French balloon occlusion catheter (*broad arrow*) and an inner 3 French Teflon coaxial catheter (*thin arrows*). (D and E) An immediate follow-up celiac artery angiogram. Early arterial phase (D) shows a localized occlusion of the splenic artery by a cast of bucrylate-Ethiodol mixture (*arrows*). (E) The late venous phase shows reconstitution of almost the entire intrasplenic arterial bed. These collateral vessels are from the left gastric, dorsal pancreatic, and gastroepiploic arteries. (F and G) ^{99m}Tc sulfur colloid liver–spleen scans performed prior to embolization (F) and 10 days after embolization (G) show that there has been splenic infarction but with preservation of functioning splenic tissue.

artery and the gastroduodenal artery reconstituted the intrasplenic arteries (Fig. 95-10E). In these patients, nuclear scans revealed preservation of functioning splenic tissue (Fig. 95-10G). In the one remaining patient, we were unable to confine the bucrylate to the splenic artery, and the material embolized distally to occlude small intrasplenic arteries. This patient developed a splenic abscess.

If a localized occlusion of the splenic artery can be obtained without distal embolization to the spleen, an abscess probably can be avoided. We are currently investigating this therapeutic technique. In patients with bleeding gastric varices secondary to splenic vein thrombosis, localized splenic artery occlusion may be the therapy

of choice (although most workers still favor splenectomy). In selected patients with generalized portal hypertension, splenic artery occlusion may be helpful in acutely controlling esophageal variceal bleeding. The rationale is that the splenic arterial contribution to portal hypertension is reduced and that with the splenic vein remaining patent, there is a reservoir other than the esophageal varices for the portal blood to pool in. Furthermore, although most patients with cirrhosis tolerate thrombocytopenia, a marked rise in the platelet count may decrease the tendency to recurrent bleeding [19].

Ivalon has been used in both the animal and the clinical situation for embolization of the splenic artery. In animals, its use has resulted in pancreatitis and gastric ischemia. In humans, pancreatitis and splenic hemorrhage have been reported [8].

ADJUNCT TO NONRESECTIVE THERAPY OF ABDOMINAL AORTIC ANEURYSMS

Elective aneurysmectomy with placement of an interposition graft is the treatment of choice for abdominal aortic aneurysm. In patients with concomitant renal, cardiac, or pulmonary disease, however, this form of surgery has a mortality of 20 to 60 percent. An alternative mode of therapy in such high-risk patients is desirable. We have been evaluating the nonresective treatment of abdominal aortic aneurysms [20, 30]. This treatment is directed toward producing thrombosis within the aneurysm. This goal is accomplished by first constructing an axillobifemoral bypass graft, thus preserving flow to the lower extremities. The outflow vessels from the aneurysm (the hypogastric and the external iliac arteries) are then surgically ligated (Fig. 95-11A). In 17 of 21 patients treated by this approach, thrombosis of the aneurysm was successfully achieved. In four patients, however, because of the surgeon's inability to ligate the hypogastric arteries successfully, persistent flow within these vessels maintained the patency of the abdominal aortic aneurysm. Using an axillary approach, we advanced the catheter to the distal abdominal aorta and injected bucrylate. In our first patient, because of incomplete occlusion of the iliac artery, the aneurysm did not undergo thrombosis, and the patient was readmitted to the hospital with rupture of his aneurysm. In our next three patients, however, we were able to occlude completely the outflow from the aneurysm by em-

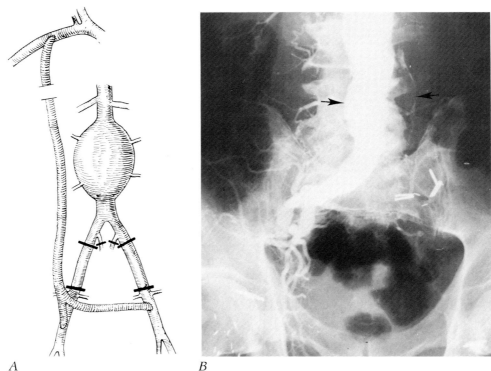

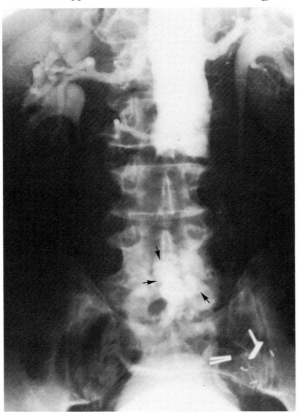

A

B

C

Figure 95-11. Successful nonresective therapy of an abdominal aortic aneurysm in a 70-year-old man. (A) Diagrammatic representation of nonresective therapy of an abdominal aortic aneurysm. An axillobifemoral bypass graft is performed with surgical ligation of the outflow vessels from the aneurysm. (B) An abdominal and pelvic angiogram following surgery shows persistent patency of the right hypogastric artery with flow within the abdominal aortic aneurysm (*arrows*). (C) An abdominal aortogram 20 minutes after a transcatheter injection of bucrylate-Ethiodol mixture shows a localized cast of the bucrylate (*arrows*) in the distal abdominal aorta, with thrombosis of the abdominal aortic aneurysm. (From Goldman et al. [20]. Reproduced by permission from *AJR*.)

bolizing either the distal abdominal aorta (Fig. 95-11C) or the iliac arteries. Within 20 minutes, embolization in these three patients resulted in a thrombosis of the abdominal aortic aneurysm up to the neck of the aneurysm. The renal arteries have remained patent. One of these patients was alive at 11 months after the procedure, and one was alive at 18 months after the procedure.

In the situation just described, bucrylate is the ideal embolic agent. Owing to its rapid polymerization, a localized vascular occlusion of even the abdominal aorta can be achieved. It is possible to use other embolic agents. A single plug of Ivalon that can swell to occlude a vessel that is 9 mm in diameter [47] can be advanced through the catheter. Similarly, coils can perhaps occlude the outflow within an iliac artery. Silicone presents definite risks in embolization of the hypogastric arteries. When the hypogastric artery of pigs has been embolized, hind limb paralysis has resulted. Because silicone has been seen within the arteriole-venule level of the vasa nervosa of the sciatic nerve in these animals, it is presumed that the hind limb paralysis is secondary to sciatic nerve ischemia [35].

ARTERIOVENOUS MALFORMATIONS

Congenital arteriovenous malformation is a therapeutic enigma. The abnormality consists of multiple feeding arteries to a large network of abnormal arteriovenous communications. Surgical cure can be accomplished only by total excision of the lesion. The excision requires radical surgery, such as might be performed for a malignancy, which may result in marked disfigurement and even amputation. Surgery frequently consists only of ligation of the feeding arteries. The surgeon may not be able to decide which arteries are feeding the abnormal communication and so may unnecessarily ligate vessels that are unrelated to the arteriovenous malformation. Transvascular therapy allows one to position the catheter directly in the feeding arteries. As a result, occlusion of the appropriate feeding vessels can be accomplished. The use of Ivalon plugs, coils, and detachable balloons and localized occlusion with tissue adhesive can accomplish what is essentially a surgical ligation of the feeding vessel. But unless the abnormal network of vessels is obliterated, other feeding vessels will resupply the arteriovenous malformation.

It was hoped that liquid silicone would be the ideal agent for injection into a feeding vessel and that it would produce obliteration of the entire malformation [14]. Liquid silicone has been used successfully in a few cases of small arteriovenous malformations of the spinal cord, but worsening of symptoms following embolization of spinal arteriovenous malformations has also been reported [26]. The worsening may have been secondary to occlusion of the main draining vein of the malformation by the silicone without obliteration of all the feeding arteries and the abnormal venous plexuses. As a result, venous hypertension developed, with subsequent enlargement of the arteriovenous malformation and further compression of the spinal cord.

The role of liquid silicone is also limited in

larger arteriovenous communications because it is extremely difficult to confine the liquid silicone to the abnormal vascular communications without inadvertent embolization to the lung. Some catheter techniques had theoretically seemed to hold promise for confining the liquid silicone, but clinically they have not been useful. Balloon occlusion catheters [3] or prior injection of the embolized vessels with vasoconstrictors, such as epinephrine [14], may aid in confining the injected silicone. Furthermore, it is possible that the silicone can be injected just prior to the time of complete vulcanization, when the silicone has a viscosity similar to that of toothpaste [14]. The continuous column of partially vulcanized material may then undergo complete vulcanization, leading to vascular occlusion of the arteriovenous abnormality. Another technique of confining the injected silicone to the embolized region is to mix the liquid silicone with carbonyl iron microspheres. A powerful superconducting electromagnet can then be applied over the target area [12, 36]. The injected material is held in place by means of this magnet during the period of vulcanization. This could prevent distal embolization in small arteriovenous malformations, but it is not likely to be useful in lesions with larger and more rapid abnormal shunting. These techniques, although possible, are not always available, and they are difficult to use and require extensive laboratory experience. Furthermore, use of the silicone in two patients with vascular meningiomas was complicated with facial nerve paralysis thought to be secondary to occlusion of the small arterioles to the facial nerve, with resultant ischemia of the facial nerve [6].

Bucrylate at present is the best embolic agent for the angiographic management of arteriovenous malformations. The polymerization time of bucrylate can be varied from 1 to 8 seconds by the appropriate dilution with Pantopaque [11]. As a result, one can occlude not only the feeding artery but also the abnormal plexus of vessels within the malformation without inadvertent escape of the embolic material to the lung. We have successfully utilized this principle in one patient with a congenital arteriovenous malformation (Fig. 95-12) and in another patient with a traumatic arteriovenous malformation.

THROMBOSIS OF TRUE AND FALSE ANEURYSMS

The principles of embolization of true and false aneurysms are similar to those for embolization of

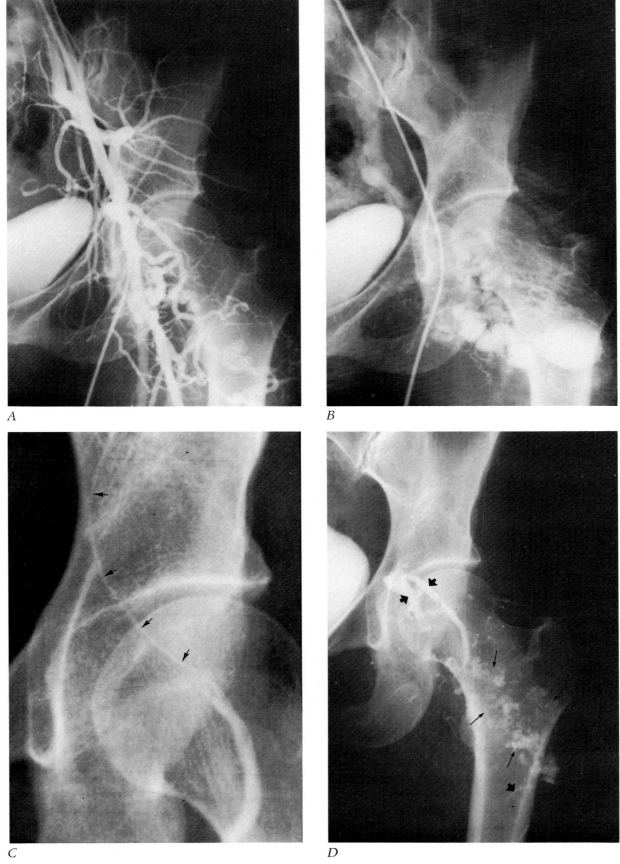

A

B

C

D

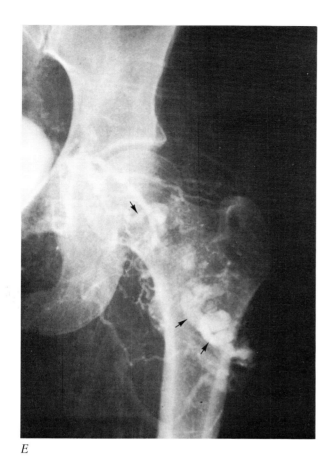

E

Figure 95-12. Successful embolization with bucrylate of a congenital arteriovenous malformation in a 38-year-old woman. (A and B) A common iliac artery injection, arterial phase (A) and venous phase (B), shows filling of a large arteriovenous malformation. The main feeders are from the hypogastric and the profunda femoris arteries. (C) With a coaxial catheter system, a 3 French Teflon catheter (*arrows*) is advanced deep into a branch of the hypogastric artery. (D) A plain film shows bucrylate-Pantopaque mixture within the three main feeding arteries (*broad arrows*) and also within the abnormal vascular plexuses (*thin arrows*). (E) An immediate follow-up common iliac artery angiogram shows thrombosis of most of the arteriovenous malformation. There is still some residual vascular supply (*arrows*), but there is no evidence of draining veins.

arteriovenous malformations. The aim is not only to occlude the feeding vessel but also to fill the lumen of the aneurysm. We have found bucrylate to be extremely effective in occluding true and false aneurysms (Fig. 95-13).

SUMMARY OF EMBOLIC AGENTS

Bucrylate has unique properties that make it an excellent embolic agent. The rate of polymeriza-

tion can be varied so as to obtain (1) a localized occlusion for control of bleeding or for production of a medical splenectomy or (2) a distal embolization for obliteration of arteriovenous malformations or for organ ablation. Injection of the bucrylate through coaxial catheters and balloon occlusion catheters allows for highly selective and localized vascular occlusions. Because of its wide versatility, I have favored bucrylate in almost all circumstances that require embolization.

Silicone is an intriguing embolic substance. Its main value is in the embolization of an intact vascular bed (Fig. 95-14) for organ ablation. One must be aware, however, that ischemic complications can develop because of distal vessel occlusion. Ischemia of the facial and sciatic nerves [6, 35] has been reported. Hepatic infarcts with biliary cysts have developed in the liver of primates [13]. Trapping the silicone by means of an external electromagnet presents exciting possibilities [6, 36]. Another role of silicone liquid may be the therapeutic management of tumor. Particles of beta-ionizing radiation, such as yttrium 90 or phosphorus 32, can be mixed with the liquid silicone and then injected into the tumor [44]. These particles provide a source of internal radiation that can be trapped within the tumor.

Ivalon is an alternative embolic material to Gelfoam. It has the disadvantages of other particulate embolic agents. Its advantages over Gelfoam are that it provides a permanent vascular occlusion and can be purchased radiopaque. As techniques develop for easier injection of the material, Ivalon probably will have wide applicability.

Conclusion

Rösch was the first to use therapeutic embolization in the abdomen to control intestinal hemorrhage [40]. This therapeutic modality has rapidly grown and is now useful in the management of a wide spectrum of difficult clinical problems. A randomized prospective controlled study, however, is needed to compare therapeutic embolization with other, more standard, therapeutic modalities. At present, embolization therapy should be performed when it is likely that it can correct the clinical problem as well as surgery can but with less risk. The decision to embark on embolic therapy should be made by a team that includes an angiographer, a surgeon, and, often, an internist of the appropriate subspecialty. For

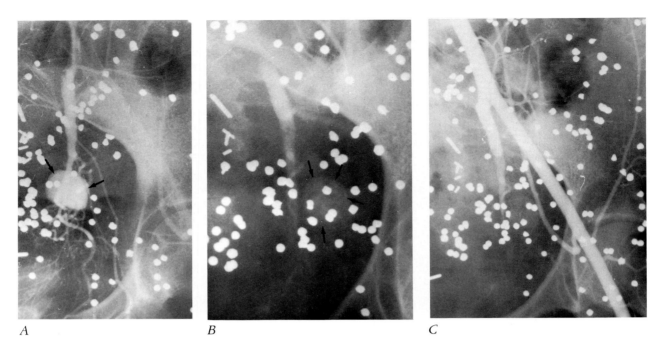

A   *B*   *C*

Figure 95-13. Successful control with bucrylate of a massive pelvic hemorrhage in a 35-year-old woman following a shotgun injury. (A) A hypogastric artery angiogram shows the presence of a false aneurysm (*arrows*). (B) A plain film of the pelvis shows a cast (*ar-* *rows*) of bucrylate-Ethiodol completely filling the lumen of the aneurysm and a portion of the main hypogastric artery. (C) An immediate follow-up common iliac artery angiogram shows complete obliteration of the false aneurysm by the bucrylate.

most embolic procedures, the usually available embolic materials, such as Gelfoam and coils, work well. But in the management of many other clinical situations—such as permanent nephrectomy, rapid occlusion of the splenic artery for the control of variceal bleeding, therapy adjunctive to nonresective therapy of abdominal aortic aneurysms as well as thrombosis of traumatic false and true branch vessel aneurysms, and control of arteriovenous malformations—other embolic agents are necessary. Bucrylate has proved to be clinically effective in a wide variety of clinical situations. It is not difficult to use, but one must become familiar with its properties and its safe use before he can apply it clinically.

When one is choosing any embolic agent, he must consider what agent he has had the most experience with and what agent he can use most safely to obtain the best therapeutic result. And before embarking on embolic therapy, the physician must obtain informed consent. He must discuss fully with the patient and his family not only the risks of the angiographic procedure but also the increased risks of embolization, which include ischemia of the embolized organ as well as infection of the embolized organ and inadvertent occlusion of vessels.

ACKNOWLEDGMENT

Figures 95-8, 95-9B, 95-10, 95-12, and 95-13 are from M. L. Goldman, Transcatheter embolization maneuver with bucrylate (in 100 patients). *Radiographics* 2(3), 1982. They are reproduced here with the permission of the editor and publisher.

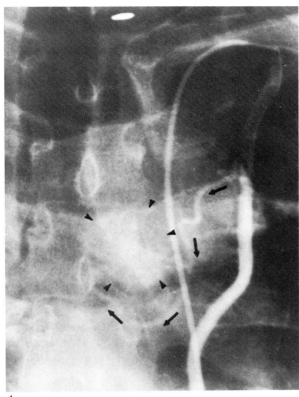

A

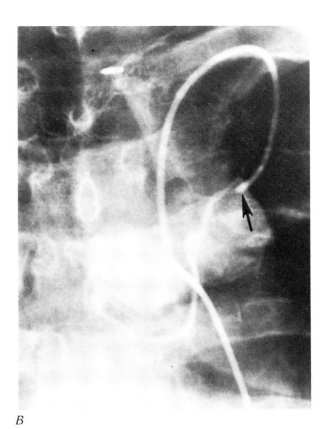

B

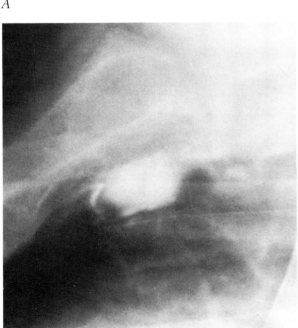

C

Figure 95-14. Successful infarction of a parathyroid adenoma by liquid silicone. (A) A selective left internal mammary artery angiogram shows a diffuse blush (*arrowheads*) of an anterior mediastinal parathyroid adenoma and a feeding vessel (*arrows*). (B) A selective injection of the feeding vessel with silicone shows a dense stain of silicone mixed with tantalum within the adenoma (*arrow*). (C) A lateral film made 1 hour after the embolization shows that the entire parathyroid adenoma is densely opacified with the silicone. (Courtesy of John Doppman, M.D.)

References

1. Athanasoulis, C. A. Therapeutic applications of angiography. *N. Engl. J. Med.* 302:1117, 1980.
2. Barnard, C. N., and Schrire, V. Ivalon baffle for posterior leaflet replacement in the treatment of mitral insufficiency: A follow-up study. *Surgery* 63:727, 1968.
3. Berenstein, A., and Kricheff, I. I. Catheter and material selection for transarterial embolization: Technical considerations: II. Materials. *Radiology* 132:631, 1979.
4. Bradley, S. Symposium on synthetics in maxillofacial surgery: I. The silicones in maxillofacial surgery. *Laryngoscope* 78:549, 1968.
5. Brown, J. B., Fryer, M. P., and Ohlwiler, D. A. Study and use of synthetic materials such as silicones and Teflon, as subcutaneous prostheses. *Plast. Reconstr. Surg.* 26:264, 1960.
6. Calcaterra, T. C., Rand, R. W., and Bentson, J. R. Ischemic paralysis of the facial nerve: A possible etiologic factor in Bell's palsy. *Laryngoscope* 86:92, 1976.
7. Calderwood, R. G. Polydimethyl siloxane implants in oral surgery. *J. Oral Surg.* 26:33, 1968.
8. Castaneda-Zuniga, W. R., Hammerschmidt, D. E., Sanchez, R., and Amplatz, K. Nonsurgical splenectomy. *AJR* 129:805, 1977.
9. Castaneda-Zuniga, W. R., Jauregui, H., Rysavy, J., and Amplatz, K. Selective transcatheter embolization of the upper gastrointestinal tract: An experimental study. *Radiology* 127:81, 1978.
10. Castaneda-Zuniga, W. R., Sanchez, R., and Amplatz, K. Experimental observations on short- and long-term effects of arterial occlusion with Ivalon. *Radiology* 126:783, 1978.
11. Cromwell, L. D., and Kerber, C. W. Modification of cyanoacrylate for therapeutic embolization: Preliminary experience. *AJR* 132:799, 1979.
12. Djindjian, R. Superselective internal carotid arteriography and embolization. *Neuroradiology* 9:145, 1975.
13. Doppman, J. L., Girton, M., and Kahn, E. R. Proximal versus peripheral hepatic artery embolization: Experimental study in monkeys. *Radiology* 128:577, 1978.
14. Doppman, J. L., Zapol, W., and Pierce, J. Transcatheter embolization with a silicone rubber preparation. Experimental observations. *Invest. Radiol.* 6:304, 1971.
15. Dotter, C. T., Goldman, M. L., and Rösch, J. Instant selective arterial occlusion with isobutyl 2-cyanoacrylate. *Radiology* 114:227, 1975.
16. Freeny, P. C., Mennemeyer, R., Kidd, C. R., and Bush, W. H. Long-term radiographic-pathologic follow-up of patients treated with visceral transcatheter occlusion using isobutyl 2-cyanoacrylate (bucrylate). *Radiology* 132:51, 1979.
17. Goldman, M. L., Freeny, P. C., Tallman, J. M., Galambos, J. T., Bradley, E. L., Salam, A., Oen, K. T., Gordon, I. J., and Mennemeyer, R. Transcatheter vascular occlusion therapy with isobutyl 2-cyanoacrylate (bucrylate) for control of massive upper-gastrointestinal bleeding. *Radiology* 129:41, 1978.
18. Goldman, M. L., Land, W. C., Jr., Bradley, E. L., III, and Anderson, J. Transcatheter therapeutic embolization in the management of massive upper gastrointestinal bleeding. *Radiology* 120:513, 1976.
19. Goldman, M. L., Philip, P. K., Sarrafizadeh, M. S., Gordon, I. J., Sarfeh, J. I., Smith, R. P., Salam, A., Galambos, J. T., and Powers, S. R. Medical splenectomy by transcatheter arterial embolization with bucrylate. *Radiology.* In press.
20. Goldman, M. L., Sarrafizadeh, M. S., Philip, P. K., Karmody, A. M., Leather, R. P., Parikh, N., and Powers, S. R. Bucrylate embolization of the distal abdominal aorta: An adjunct to nonresective therapy of abdominal aortic aneurysms. *AJR* 135:1195, 1980.
21. Goldstein, H. M., Wallace, S., Anderson, J. H., Bree, R. L., and Gianturco, C. Transcatheter occlusion of abdominal tumors. *Radiology* 120:539, 1976.
22. Grindlay, J. H. A plastic sponge prosthesis for use after pneumonectomy: Preliminary report of an experimental study. *Mayo Clin. Proc.* 24:538, 1949.
23. Guilford, W. B., and Scatliff, J. H. Transcatheter embolization of the spleen for control of splenic hemorrhage and in situ splenectomy: An experimental study using silicone spheres. *Radiology* 119:549, 1976.
24. Hawe, A., and Rastelli, G. C. Late deterioration of intracardiac Ivalon sponge patches. *J. Thorac. Cardiovasc. Surg.* 58:87, 1969.
25. Hilal, S. K., and Michelsen, J. W. Therapeutic percutaneous embolization for extra-axial vascular lesions of the head, neck, and spine. *J. Neurosurg.* 43:275, 1975.
26. Hilal, S. K., Sane, P., Michelsen, W. J., and Kosseim, A. The embolization of vascular malformations of the spinal cord with low-viscosity silicone rubber. *Neuroradiology* 16:430, 1978.
27. Kaufman, S. L. Simplified method of transcatheter embolization with polyvinyl alcohol foam (Ivalon). *AJR* 132:853, 1979.
28. Kerber, C. W., Bank, W. O., and Horton, J. A. Polyvinyl alcohol foam: Prepackaged emboli for therapeutic embolization. *AJR* 130:1193, 1978.
29. Latchaw, R. E., and Gold, L. H. A. Polyvinyl foam embolization of neoplastic lesions of the head, neck, and spine. *Radiology* 131:669, 1979.
30. Leather, R. P., Shah, D., Goldman, M. L., Rosenberg, M., and Karmody, A. M. Non-resective treatment of abdominal aortic aneurysms. Use of

acute thrombosis and axillofemoral bypass. *Arch. Surg.* 114:1402, 1979.

31. Luessenhop, A. J., and Spence, W. T.   Artificial embolization of cerebral arteries. Report of use in a case of arteriovenous malformation. *J.A.M.A.* 172:1153, 1960.

32. Matsumoto, T.   *Tissue Adhesives in Surgery.* Flushing, N.Y.: Medical Examination, 1972.

33. Medical Research Department, Ethicon, Inc. *Methyl 2-Cyanoacrylate Monomer. A Biodegradable Plastic Tissue Adhesive Review* (rev. ed.), 1966.

34. Miller, F. J., Jr., Nakashima, E. N., Mineau, D. E., and Osborn, A. G.   Delivery system for low viscosity silicone rubber through small co-axial catheters. *Radiology* 131:538, 1979.

35. Miller, F. J., Rankin, R. S., Gliedman, J. B., and Nakashima, E.   Experimental internal iliac artery embolization: Evaluation of low viscosity silicone rubber, isobutyl 2-cyanoacrylate, and carbon microspheres. *Radiology* 129:51, 1978.

36. Mosso, J. A., and Rand, R. W.   Ferromagnetic silicone vascular occlusion: A technic for selective infarction of tumors and organs. *Ann. Surg.* 178:663, 1973.

37. Mullison, E. G.   Silicones as artificial internal tissue and organ substitutes. *Ann. N.Y. Acad. Sci.* 120:540, 1964.

38. Porstmann, W., Wierny, L., Warnke, H., Gerstberger, G., and Romaniuk, P. A.   Catheter closure of patent ductus arteriosus: 62 cases treated without thoracotomy. *Radiol. Clin. North Am.* 9:203, 1971.

39. Rivard, D. J., Goldman, M. L., and Bennett, A. H.   Indications for medical nephrectomy employing transcatheter renal artery embolization. *J. Urol.* In press.

40. Rösch, J., Dotter, C. T., and Brown, M. J. Selective arterial embolization. A new method for control of acute gastrointestinal bleeding. *Radiology* 102:303, 1972.

41. Spigos, D. G., Jonasson, O., Mozes, M., and Capek, V.   Partial splenic embolization in the treatment of hypersplenism. *AJR* 132:777, 1979.

42. Spigos, D. G., Tan, W. S., Mozes, M., and Capek, V.   Splenic embolization. Scientific exhibit presented at the 65th Annual Meeting of the Radiological Society of North America. Atlanta, Ga., Nov. 1979.

43. Tadavarthy, S. M., Moller, J. H., and Amplatz, K.   Polyvinyl alcohol (Ivalon)—a new embolic material. *AJR* 125:609, 1975.

44. Turner, R. D., Rand, R. W., Bentson, J. R., and Mosso, J. A.   Ferromagnetic silicone necrosis of hypernephromas by selective vascular occlusion to the tumor: A new technique. *J. Urol.* 113:455, 1975.

45. White, R. I. Jr., Strandberg, J. V., Gross, G. S., and Barth, K. H.   Therapeutic embolization with long-term occluding agents and their effects on embolized tissues. *Radiology* 125:677, 1977.

46. Zarem, H. A.   Silastic implants in plastic surgery. *Surg. Clin. North Am.* 48:129, 1968.

47. Zollikofer, C., Castaneda-Zuniga, W. R., Galliani, C., Rysavy, J. A., Tadavarthy, M., Formanek, A., and Amplatz, K.   A combination of stainless steel coil and compressed Ivalon: A new technique for embolization of large arteries and arteriovenous fistulas. *Radiology* 138:229, 1981.

Embolotherapy with Detachable Balloons

ROBERT I. WHITE, JR.

For the past 20 years, balloon catheter techniques have played an important role in diagnostic and therapeutic cardiovascular radiology. Prominent among therapeutic cardiovascular balloons was the one developed by Rashkind for enlarging the intraarterial communication and improving mixing of arterial and venous blood in infants with transposition of the great arteries [1]. As a result of this technique, 90 percent of infants with transposition of the great arteries are alive rather than dead at the end of the first year of life. Nondetachable balloons have also been used to occlude the aorta before aneurysm resection, to treat carotid-cavernous fistulas, and to control hemorrhage [2–4].

The potential for detachable balloon occlusion techniques as part of the larger discipline of embolotherapy in vascular radiology was first recognized in Europe. Serbinenko developed detachable and perfusion balloons to assist in superselective angiography and to aid in the embolization of neurovascular arteriovenous malformations (AVMs) [5]. Shortly thereafter, Debrun and his colleagues developed a coaxial balloon system for treating neurovascular malformations based on a design different from Serbinenko's [6, 7].

Our interest in developing and extending these techniques throughout the cardiovascular system was stimulated largely by our earlier laboratory investigations of particulate material embolization [8–12]. It was realized that the potential for complications from inadvertent embolization of particulate material was great. Also, the non-reversibility of embolization once the particles were injected led to an "all-or-none" phenomenon. After selective catheterization of the artery, the blood flow carried the embolic material distally, producing the desired occlusion. Unfortunately, as the circulation became obliterated and stasis occurred, the risk of inadvertent embolization increased. Furthermore, in the application of these techniques, superselective catheterization was always required before safe injection of particulate material was possible. As clinical experience with the cardiovascular system increased, it was apparent that what was needed was the ability to produce localized arterial occlusion, have it reversible up to a certain point, and have it associated with the minimal risk of inadvertent embolization.

Biomedical engineers at Becton-Dickinson Company were already developing prototype perfusion and detachable balloons for use in neuroradiology [13]. Convinced of the potential importance of detachable balloons in cardiovascular radiology, we began a long-term study of balloons both in vitro and in animals [14–16]. After having made several modifications and gained a thorough understanding of balloon techniques, we began our clinical studies with the Mini-Balloon at the Johns Hopkins Hospital, January 1, 1978 [17, 18].

We also gained experience with the French technique developed by Debrun; this technique and the Mini-Balloon technique are discussed and compared in this chapter. Perfusion balloons used in combination with tissue adhesives or superselective angiography had less applicability in cardiovascular radiology than in neuroradiology and were subsequently dropped from our investigations.

Methodology and Techniques

DEBRUN TECHNIQUE

The balloon developed by Debrun and his colleagues is made of latex rubber. It is hand tied by the angiographer and advanced coaxially through an introducer catheter to the site of the occlusion. Three catheters are used coaxially. The inner catheter is a 110-cm 2 French clear Teflon catheter to which the balloon is tied (Fig. 96-1). This catheter is advanced through a 100-cm 5 French radiopaque polyethylene catheter tapered to the Teflon catheter. These catheters are as-

Figure 96-1. Steps in making a Debrun balloon. A 2 French Teflon catheter (B) is advanced into a latex sleeve (A). Latex ligature is tied around the neck of the balloon (C) and the rest of the sleeve is trimmed away (D). The balloon is inflated with contrast media via a Touhy-Borst adapter on the end of the Teflon catheter. A 5 French catheter (E) is advanced over the 2 French Teflon catheter before both of them are placed through the 9 French introducer catheter.

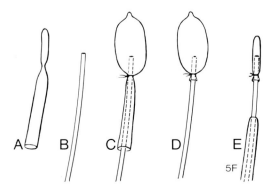

sembled under sterile conditions on the morning of the catheterization. Thin-wall 80- or 90-cm 9 French nontapered polyethylene catheters to which a steam shape has been added are advanced through indwelling vascular sheaths. For selective catheterization, 5 French selective catheters or Swan-Ganz–type catheters are advanced through the larger introducer catheter. Once the desired vessel is entered, the larger introducer catheter is advanced over the inner catheter, which serves only as a stent to guide the larger catheter. The inner catheter is withdrawn and the introducer catheter flushed. The previously matched and assembled 5 French and 2 French coaxial catheter system with a latex balloon at its end is advanced through the 9 French introducer catheter. Filled with radiopaque contrast material, the balloon is observed fluoroscopically and final positioning is confirmed by contrast injections through the introducer catheter (Fig. 96-2).

Early deflation of the balloon occurs unpredictably as contrast material leaks out of the balloon. In order to prevent early deflation, the contrast material is completely aspirated from the balloon and the balloon is filled with liquid silicone. At body temperature, the silicone mixture hardens, usually within 10 minutes. Hardening is determined by placing a similar silicone mixture in a waterbath at 37° C and observing for solidification.

Once the silicone has hardened within the balloon, detachment is accomplished by advancing the 5 French catheter over the 2 French Teflon catheter. The balloon is left in place, occluding the artery (Fig. 96-3).

SILICONE MINI-BALLOON TECHNIQUE

As in the Debrun technique, the vessel to be occluded is first catheterized with an introducer catheter sufficiently large to permit passage of the balloon through the end hole of the catheter.

Introducer Catheters for 1-mm Mini-Balloon

Prototype nontapered 6.5 French reinforced-wall polyethylene catheters with "Cobra," "sidewinder," and "H1H" shapes were developed. For pediatric use, a 5 French polyethylene nontapered catheter is employed and different shapes are formed with steam prior to catheterization. The only differences between these introducer catheters and the standard angiographic catheters are the nontapered end holes of 0.043 inch or

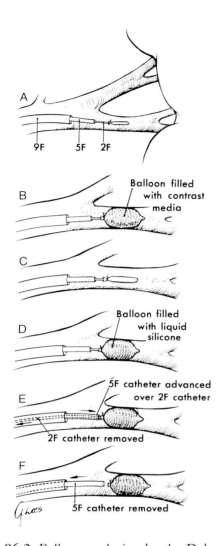

Figure 96-2. Balloon occlusion by the Debrun technique. The 9 French catheter has been advanced into the renal artery (A) (see text). Next, the 5 French and 2 French catheters are advanced through the 9 French catheter. Care must be taken that the 5 French catheter does not advance over the 2 French catheter and inadvertently detach the balloon. The balloon is test inflated with contrast media (B); if good positioning and occlusion are confirmed by test injections through the 9 French catheter, the balloon is ready for detachment. All the contrast material is aspirated and replaced by liquid silicone (C and D) (see text). Once the silicone has hardened, the balloon is detached by advancing the 5 French catheter over the 2 French catheter (E). The inner catheters are removed and a postocclusion angiogram is performed through the 9 French catheter (F).

greater in these introducer catheters. The 1-mm balloon measures 0.040 inch in diameter, and it will pass easily through the end hole of these introducer catheters (Fig. 96-4). This is an extremely important aspect of the procedure since it is desirable in some instances to aspirate the balloon completely and remove it altogether from the body if safe detachment or positioning cannot be achieved.

All introducer catheters are placed percutaneously through indwelling 7 French femoral artery or vein sheaths. We have favored sheaths with sidearms that permit flushing if a catheter is not in the body. The 1-mm silicone Mini-Balloon can predictably occlude vessels up to 4 mm in diameter. The Mini-Balloon is attached to a 2 French bismuth-loaded polyurethane catheter. Polyurethane was selected for the catheter material because of its inherent strength and acceptable flexibility. Introducer catheters of polyethylene are preferable to those made of other materials because they are easy to shape and because the coefficient of friction between the polyurethane balloon catheter and the polyethylene introducer catheter is favorable.

Introducer Catheters for 2-mm Mini-Balloon

Since it was soon realized that larger balloons were necessary to occlude vessels up to 9 mm in diameter, the 2-mm silicone Mini-Balloon was developed (Fig. 96-4). The 2-mm balloon requires a nontapered catheter with an 0.080-inch end hole for safe introduction and withdrawal. A thin-wall 9 French polyethylene introducer catheter was developed, similar to the one used for the Debrun technique. Steam shapes are placed in the introducer catheter, and it is advanced coaxially with a 5 French preformed, reinforced-wall, polyethylene catheter or a Swan-Ganz catheter leading it. Once the vessel to be embolized is selectively catheterized, the 9 French introducer catheter is shimmied over the Swan-Ganz or polyethylene catheter. Next, the inner catheter is removed, and the introducer catheter is flushed clear with heparinized saline. The 2-mm balloon is introduced through the 9 French catheter distal to the site of occlusion.

Balloon Preparation

Following diagnostic angiography, an assistant prepares the balloon catheter by purging it of air with an isoosmotic contrast agent (50% iodipamide meglumine with 50% sterile water).

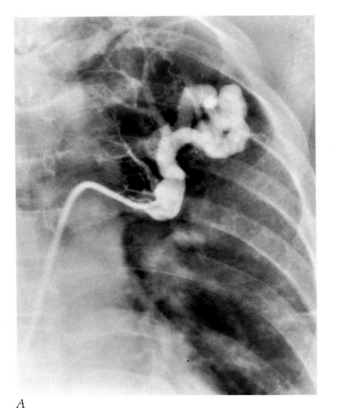

A

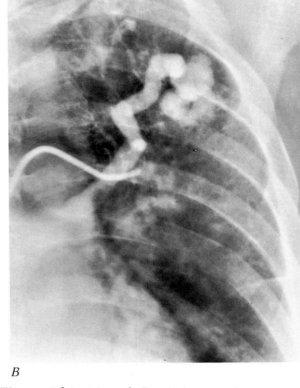

B

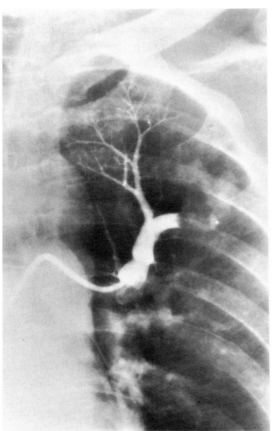

Figure 96-3. (A and B) A large pulmonary arteriovenous malformation in a patient with recurrent hemoptysis from the left upper lobe. The arterial and venous phases of the angiogram demonstrate a direct communication between the pulmonary artery and vein without intervening capillary bed. (C) The Debrun balloon is seen after detachment. A silver clip on the end is noted, and proximal, overlying the hardened silicone, is a small residual cap of contrast media. The normal branches to the left upper lobe are still preserved. No further hemoptysis has occurred for the past 2½ years of follow-up.

C

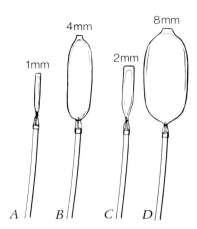

Figure 96-4. Uninflated 1-mm and 2-mm Mini-Balloons (A and C). With inflation, the 1-mm balloon reaches a maximum diameter of 4 mm (B), and the 2-mm balloon distends to 8 mm and sometimes to 9 mm (D).

In countries in which metrizamide is approved for intravascular use, this contrast material can also be used quite successfully. Since previous experiments demonstrated that silicone was semipermeable, prolonged balloon inflation was possible only using isoosmotic radiopaque balloon fillers [14–16]. This represents an important departure from the Debrun and Serbinenko techniques, in which predictable long-term balloon inflation was possible only with a balloon filler that hardened after injection.

Once purged of air, the balloon catheter is loaded into a coiling chamber through a coaxial catheter valve (Fig. 96-5). The coiling chamber permits smooth injection of the balloon catheter without knotting. At the proximal end of the coiling chamber is a Tuohy-Borst adapter, which secures the proximal portion of the balloon catheter. This is necessary because in high-flow AVMs, the entire balloon catheter could be injected into the patient were it not for the anchoring Tuohy-Borst adapter on the coiling chamber.

A small bolus injection of saline through the sidearm of the coaxial catheter valve propels the

Figure 96-5. Mini-Balloon catheter delivery system. The coiling chamber facilitates injection of the balloon catheter through the introducer catheter without knotting. Final manipulations are done with the coaxial catheter valve. The position of the balloon is confirmed by injections of contrast media through the sidearm of the valve into the introducer catheter. The balloon is inflated and deflated with measured amounts of isoosmotic iodipamide meglumine injected with a tuberculin syringe.

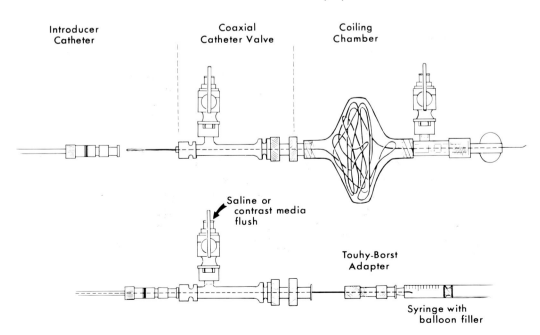

Mini Balloon Catheter Delivery System

balloon catheter through the introducing catheter into the circulation. Heparinized flushing solution and contrast material are injected through the sidearm of the coaxial valve during final manipulation of the balloon catheter (Fig. 96-5).

Final Balloon Positioning

Since the polyurethane balloon catheter is radiopaque, the position of the catheter (balloon) is readily visualized before the balloon is inflated (Fig. 96-6). The catheter is injected beyond the desired site of occlusion and gently pulled back under fluoroscopic guidance. The diagnostic angiogram provides a roadmap, and test injections through the introducer catheter assist in final positioning. The coiling chamber can be discarded at this point; or, if additional positioning is necessary, the chamber may be left in tandem with the coaxial catheter valve. A Tuohy-Borst adapter is

Figure 96-6. Diagrammatic representation of occlusion of a branch of the renal artery. After catheterization of the renal artery (A), the balloon catheter is injected through the introducer catheter (B) and the balloon is filled with isoosmotic iodipamide meglumine (C). Test injections of contrast media through the introducer catheter confirm that the balloon is in good position, completely occluding the artery. The balloon is detached (D) and a postocclusion angiogram is obtained (E).

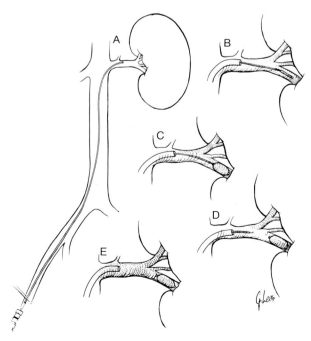

always attached to the balloon catheter to allow injection and withdrawal of isoosmotic radiopaque media from the balloon. After the balloon is filled, test injections are performed through the introducer catheter to confirm complete occlusion of the vessel by the balloon. Occlusion may be further documented by gentle tugging on the balloon catheter with the coaxial valve open; the balloon will not move if it is firmly occluding the vessel. These two confirmatory steps are important before the balloon is detected. Videotape recording of fluoroscopy is extremely useful for monitoring test injections and for documenting the position and occlusion by the balloon. Angiograms may also be obtained to confirm the balloon's position and occlusion before detachment.

At any point up to this time in the procedure, the balloon can be deflated and removed or repositioned. This measure of reversibility is an extremely important safety feature of both the Debrun and the Mini-Balloon techniques; it had not previously been available with particulate material or tissue adhesive embolization (Fig. 96-6).

Balloon Detachment

When the balloon is finally positioned for detachment, the coaxial valve is opened and the introducer catheter is straightened without being removed from its selective position. Then while a small additional amount of isoosmotic contrast material is injected into the balloon, a sharp tug is given to the balloon catheter. The force for detachment varies from 30 to 50 gm. The final volume of contrast material injected into the balloon depends on whether the 1- or the 2-mm balloon is used. Inflation of the balloon beyond the recommended volumes leads to a high incidence of balloon rupture and recanalization of vessels within the first 30 days. To prevent early balloon rupture, it is important to stay within the volume constraints determined experimentally for the 1- and 2-mm balloons. If the introducer catheter has an extremely tortuous course, the force of detachment may be dissipated along the course of the introducer catheter and not applied to the balloon. It may be necessary to tug gently on both catheters for successful balloon detachment in this instance.

There is no substitute for several hours of practice in vitro with one or two balloons before beginning clinical studies with these occlusion techniques. In this way, the subtleties of these techniques are better appreciated and so they can be performed more expeditiously in patients.

Clinical Experience

Occlusion techniques with detachable balloons have been applied in three general settings: (1) hemorrhage (posttraumatic, postneoplastic, or spontaneous), (2) preoperative occlusion of vascular neoplasms for "dry-field" surgery, and (3) vascular malformations. Balloon techniques may be used alone or in combination with particulate material embolization. Decisions about the choice of embolic material are based on whether the occlusion is to be distal or proximal, and whether it is to be short, intermediate, or long term, as well as on general considerations about the type of circulation to be occluded and the natural history of the disease.

HEMORRHAGE

While hard to prove experimentally, it is generally accepted that if posttraumatic or spontaneously occurring hemorrhage is controlled for 2 to 10 days, permanency of control is assured unless a new bleeding site develops. Many short- or intermediate-term agents have been used successfully in various types of hemorrhage. The paradigm of traumatic hemorrhage is the renal arteriovenous fistula or false aneurysm (Fig. 96-7) [17]. After penetrating trauma to the kidney, initial gross hematuria may subside, only to recur 24 to 72 hours after the injury. Diagnostic angiography reveals a single feeding artery to a false aneurysm, and in the case of an arteriovenous fistula, an early draining vein with caval opacification. Particulate agents are generally contraindicated because they can pass through the fistula to the lungs. Superselective catheterization and temporary balloon occlusion may control hemorrhage, but inconvenience and potential complications of an indwelling catheter left in place are associated with this approach [19, 20]. Detachable balloon catheters are carried by the blood flow quite readily to the fistula, and the occlusion is quite selective without the risks of inadvertent embolization. Detachable balloon techniques are probably the method of choice for occluding traumatic arteriovenous fistulas wherever they arise.

Other forms of traumatic hemorrhage without fistulas are also easily managed by detachable balloon occlusion. The choice of occluding material in hemorrhage without fistula is partly a function of the circulation and partly a function of superselective catheterization. In the pelvis, because of extensive collateral vessels, selective occlusion is not as important as it is in the kidney, where selective occlusion of only the bleeding artery is extremely important because of the lack of collateral circulation. Ideally, the more selective the occlusion, the better, since complications due to nonselective occlusions have occurred in the pelvis [21, 22]. If superselective catheter positioning cannot be achieved, detachable balloon techniques are even more desirable since the occluding balloon can be manipulated at some distance from the introducing catheter.

PREOPERATIVE OCCLUSION OF NEOPLASMS

Because of their highly vascular nature and their propensity to invade the renal veins and the inferior vena cava, malignant renal neoplasms are often occluded prior to resection. Preoperative occlusion is generally accomplished with Gelfoam peripherally and a permanent long-term occluding agent (e.g., Dacron coils) proximally [23, 24]. Detachable balloons have no real advantage over these other materials for proximal occlusion of large renal cell carcinomas.

Preoperative occlusion prior to liver resection is also desirable, and detachable balloons are easily introduced selectively in branches of the right or left hepatic artery from a position proximal in the common hepatic artery. In this way there is no need for superselective catheterization beyond the common hepatic artery (Fig. 96-8).

Combinations of peripheral embolization with Gelfoam or Avitene (microfibrillar collagen hemostat) and proximal balloon occlusion are also well suited for preoperative management of highly vascular head and neck tumors, such as carotid body tumors and/or angiofibromas. The combination of slurries of microfibrillar collagen and detachable balloons allows the radiologist to use less of the particulate material and to secure final placement of all particulate material with the detachable balloon.

VASCULAR MALFORMATIONS

Congenital systemic artery-to-vein malformations are among the most difficult ones to treat. Bal-

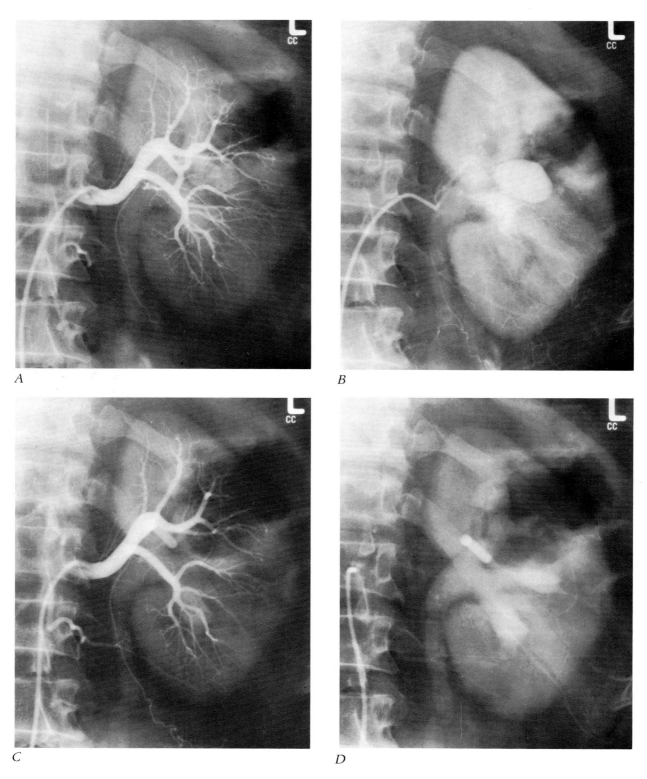

Figure 96-7. (A to D) Selective renal angiogram in a patient with recurrent hematuria after a stab wound. (A) Early phase and (B) late phase of the angiogram reveal large false aneurysm from an upper pole branch. (C and D) Following balloon occlusion, the aneurysm no longer fills. The hematuria cleared, and the patient was discharged 3 days later.

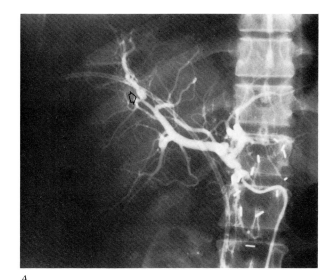

A

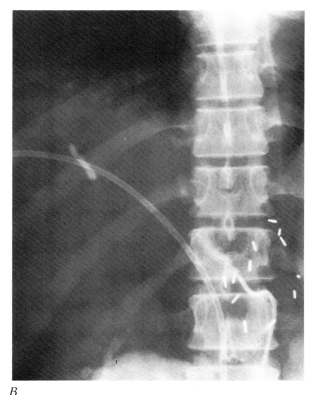

B

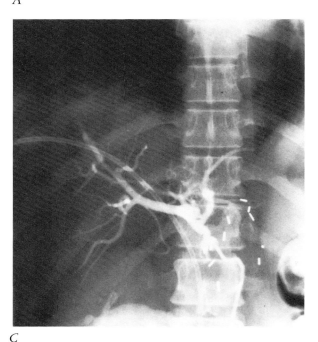

C

Figure 96-8. Encasement of the hepatic artery due to radiation and/or adenocarcinoma of the stomach. (A) The patient had received a percutaneous stent for obstructive jaundice due to metastatic nodes in the porta hepatis. Hemobilia developed 3 weeks later. A selective hepatic arteriogram demonstrates a false aneurysm of the right hepatic artery (*arrow*) adjacent to the stent. (B) A balloon was introduced. (C) A postocclusion angiogram reveals occlusion of the aneurysm. The patient's hemobilia did not recur for the remaining 6 months of his life. The encasement of the hepatic artery would have made superselective catheterization and embolization of the aneurysm with particulate materials quite difficult.

loons or coils blocking proximal branches produce the same effect as surgical ligation. A temporary reduction in the blood flow may occur, but the so-called sump effect of a low-resistance AVM leads to the development of collateral vessels. The blood flow soon returns to preembolization levels, only now the major access routes to the interstices of the AVM are occluded. Modified liquid tissue adhesives or silicone offers the best opportunity to obliterate the interstices of the AVM, leading to a more effective palliation. Larger occluding devices are still used

preoperatively to allow dry-field surgery, much as they are used before resection of vascular neoplasms.

Pulmonary AVMs are quite different in their response to proximal occlusion [25–28]. In most instances, a single low-pressure pulmonary artery branch enters a large AVM that connects directly to a pulmonary vein. The AVM usually is nonseptated, connecting directly with the vein. Occasionally the feeding artery divides into a serpiginous pattern of vessels before connecting with the pulmonary vein. In the nonseptated AVM, particulate materials are contraindicated since they may pass directly through the AVM into the left side of the heart, leading to systemic embolization. In the serpiginous type, particulate materials may hold up in the branching pattern of the AVM, but still there is a risk of systemic embolization.

Balloon techniques are particularly advantageous in both types of AVM. Balloons can be precisely placed beyond all normal branches to the lung, thus avoiding the potential for pulmonary infarction. Additionally, test injections of contrast material before the release of the balloon are used to confirm occlusion, thus minimizing the risk of systemic embolization. While coils and other particulate materials have been used successfully for occluding pulmonary AVMs, the

risk of systemic embolization generally precludes their use.

A third, more common, congenital vascular malformation is testicular varicocele. It is estimated that 50 percent of the male population have absent or incompetent valves in the testicular vein but only 5 to 10 percent have clinical varicocele [29–31]. Varicocele is associated with male infertility, and surgical ligation of the testicular vein is reported to reverse infertility in 50 percent of patients.

A variety of transcatheter occluding agents have been used to block the testicular vein with short-term good results [30]. Anatomic variations commonly include collateral veins branching to reenter the testicular vein proximally or small parallel veins ascending with the main channel

Figure 96-9. Internal spermatic venogram (A) before and (B) after occlusion with detachable balloon. The balloon was placed just above the iliac crest and the left colic branch of the testicular vein, which commonly gives off collateral vessels to a varicocele.

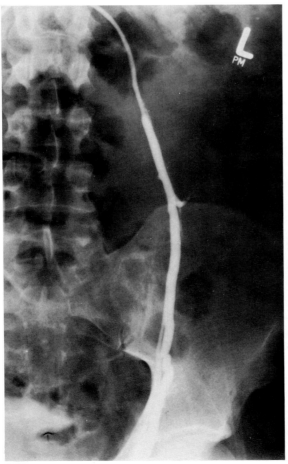

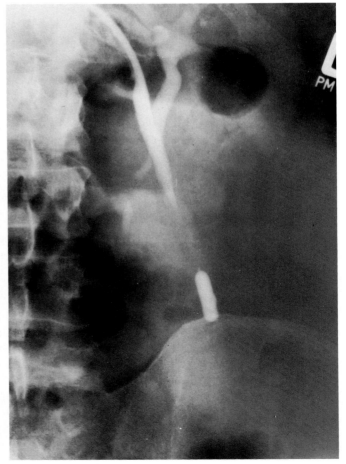

A

B

Table 96-1. Comparison of Detachable Balloon Techniques

	Debrun Technique	Mini-Balloon Technique
Material	Latex	Silicone
Diameter of occlusion	1–12 mm	1–9 mm
Balloon fillers	Silicone	Isoosmotic contrast material
Preparation of balloons	Difficult	Easy
Introduction catheters	Nontapered	Nontapered
Introduction techniques	3-catheter system, manual advancement	Coiling chamber and coaxial valve, flow directed
Indwelling vascular sheaths	Required	Required
Detachment	Easy	Easy unless excessive tortuosity of vessel
Reversibility	Possible until liquid silicone introduced	Possible at any time up to detachment
Balloon longevity	Silicone filler prevents deflation	6 months unless overinflated initially
Cost	Moderate	Expensive

from the pampiniform plexus entering the testicular vein just above the inguinal ring. These variations may account for recurrences after surgery and after transcatheter occlusion techniques. Balloon occlusion of the testicular vein is performed on an outpatient basis utilizing percutaneous techniques from the right femoral vein. A 7.3 French nontapered catheter is advanced through a 9 French indwelling femoral vein sheath into the renal vein. A Valsalva maneuver performed during test injections of contrast material in the renal vein identifies the orifice of the testicular vein. The catheter is placed in the proximal testicular vein, and a venogram using a single exposure closely collimated to the course of the testicular vein, but not including the scrotum, is obtained. This technique identifies important anatomic variations that occur in up to 40 percent of patients. If the testicular vein is less than 4 mm in diameter, a 1-mm Mini-Balloon is selected for occlusion. If the vein is larger, a 0.045-inch straight guidewire is advanced through the 7.3 French catheter deep into the testicular vein. The guidewire serves as a stent that permits exchange of the 7.3 French catheter for the 9 French polyethylene introducer catheter, and the 2-mm Mini-Balloon is used for occlusion (Fig. 96-9).

Routine use of gonadal shielding has proved very effective in limiting the radiation dose to the testes [31]. Patients are discharged 2 to 4 hours after the procedure. Balloon occlusion of the testicular vein has the potential to become the most acceptable technique for varicocele occlusion. The major advantage of this approach over others is its ability to place the balloon precisely above any collateral veins that could be involved in a recurrence.

Summary

Table 96-1 outlines the advantages and disadvantages of the Debrun and the Mini-Balloon techniques. Both techniques require thorough familiarization before use, and both require modification of the standard catheterization techniques. Both are considered intravascular implants, but, unlike heart valves and pacemakers, after 20 days there is no need for continued function since the vessel is occluded by organized thrombus antegrade and retrograde to the first branch point. While these techniques are considered more complicated than other embolization techniques, that disadvantage is outweighed by the preciseness of placement and the potential reversibility of detachable balloon occlusion. Ongoing modification of both techniques should lead to further simplification of each of them.

ACKNOWLEDGMENT

Figures 96-1, 96-2, and 96-4 to 96-8 appeared in S. E. Kadir, S. L. Kaufman, K. H. Barth, and R. I. White, Jr., *Selected Techniques in Interventional Radiology.* Philadelphia: Saunders, 1982. They are reproduced with the permission of the authors and the publisher.

References

1. Rashkind, W. J., and Miller, W. W. Creation of an atrial septal defect without thoracotomy. A palliative approach to complete transposition of the great arteries. *J.A.M.A.* 196:191, 1966.

2. Heimbecker, R. O. An aortic tampon. For emergency control of ruptured abdominal aneurysm. *Can. Med. Assoc. J.* 91:1024, 1964.

3. Prolo, D. K., and Handberry, J. W. Intraluminal occlusion of a carotid-cavernous fistula with a balloon catheter. *J. Neurosurg.* 35:237, 1971.

4. Wholey, M. H., Stockdale, R., and Hung, T. K. A percutaneous balloon catheter for immediate control of hemorrhage. *Radiology* 95:65, 1970.

5. Serbinenko, F. A. Balloon catheterization and occlusion of major cerebral vessels. *J. Neurosurg.* 41:125, 1974.

6. Debrun, G., Lacour, P., Caron, J. P., Hurth, M., Comoy, J., Keravel, Y., and Laborit, G. Experimental approach to the treatment of carotid-cavernous fistulas with an inflatable and isolated balloon. *Neuroradiology* 9:9, 1975.

7. Debrun, G., Lacour, P., Caron, J. P., Hurth, M., Comoy, J., and Keravel, Y. Detachable balloon and calibrated-leak balloon techniques in the treatment of cerebral vascular lesions. *J. Neurosurg.* 49:635, 1978.

8. Osterman, F. A., Jr., Bell, W. R., Montali, R. J., Novak, G. R., and White, R. I., Jr. Natural history of autologous blood clot embolization in swine. *Invest. Radiol.* 11:267, 1976.

9. Barth, K. H., Strandberg, J. D., and White, R. I., Jr. Long term follow-up of transcatheter embolization with autologous clot, Oxycel and Gelfoam in domestic swine. *Invest. Radiol.* 12:273, 1977.

10. White, R. I., Jr., Strandberg, J. V., Gross, G. S., and Barth, K. H. Therapeutic embolization with long-term occluding agents and their effects on embolized tissues. *Radiology* 125:677, 1977.

11. Barth, K. H., Strandberg, J. D., Kaufman, S. L., and White, R. I., Jr. Chronic vascular reactions to steel coil occlusion devices. *AJR* 131:455, 1978.

12. Kaufman, S. L., Strandberg, J. D., Barth, K. H., and White, R. I., Jr. Transcatheter embolization with microfibrillar collagen in swine. *Invest. Radiol.* 13:200, 1978.

13. Pevsner, P. H. Micro-balloon catheter for superselective angiography and therapeutic occlusion. *AJR* 128:225, 1977.

14. White, R. I., Jr., Ursic, T. A., Kaufman, S. L., Barth, K. H., Kim, W., and Gross, G. S. Therapeutic embolization with detachable balloons. Physical factors influencing permanent occlusion. *Radiology* 126:521, 1978.

15. Kaufman, S. L., Strandberg, J. D., Barth, K. H., Gross, G. S., and White, R. I., Jr. Therapeutic embolization with detachable Silastic balloon: Long-term effects in swine. *Invest. Radiol.* 14:156, 1979.

16. Barth, K. H., White, R. I., Jr., Kaufman, S. L., and Strandberg, J. D. Metrizamide, the ideal radiopaque filler for detachable Silastic balloon embolization. *Invest. Radiol.* 14:35, 1979.

17. White, R. I., Jr., Kaufman, S. L., Barth, K. H., DeCaprio, V., and Strandberg, J. D. Embolotherapy with detachable silicone balloons. Technique and clinical results. *Radiology* 131:619, 1979.

18. White, R. I., Jr., Barth, K. H., Kaufman, S. L., DeCaprio, V., and Strandberg, J. D. Therapeutic embolization with detachable balloons. *Cardiovasc. Intervent. Radiol.* 3:229, 1980.

19. Wholey, M. H. The technology of balloon catheters in interventional angiography. *Radiology* 125:671, 1977.

20. Dunnick, N. R., Doppman, J. L., and Brereton, H. D. Balloon occlusion of segmental hepatic arteries. Control of biopsy-induced hemobilia. *J.A.M.A.* 238:2524, 1977.

21. Braf, Z. F., and Koontz, W. W., Jr. Gangrene of bladder. Complication of hypogastric artery embolization. *Urology* 9:670, 1977.

22. Hietala, S. O. Urinary bladder necrosis following selective embolization of the internal iliac artery. *Acta Radiol.* [*Diagn.*] (Stockh.) 19:316, 1978.

23. Gianturco, C., Anderson, J. H., and Wallace, S. Mechanical devices for arterial occlusion. *AJR* 124:428, 1975.

24. Goldstein, H. M., Wallace, S., Anderson, J. H., Bree, R. L., and Gianturco, C. Transcatheter occlusion of abdominal tumors. *Radiology* 120:539, 1976.

25. Taylor, B. G., Cockerill, E. M., Manfred, F., and Klatte, E. C. Therapeutic embolization of the pulmonary artery in pulmonary arteriovenous fistula. *Am. J. Med.* 64:360, 1978.

26. White, R. I., Jr., Barth, K. H., Kaufman, S. L., and Terry, P. B. Detachable silicone balloons: Results of experimental study and clinical investigations in hereditary hemorrhagic telangiectasia. *Ann. Radiol.* 23:338, 1980.

27. Terry, P. B., Barth, K. H., Kaufman, S. L., and White, R. I., Jr. Balloon embolization for treatment of pulmonary arteriovenous fistulas. *N. Engl. J. Med.* 302:1189, 1980.

28. Jonsson, K., Hellekant, C., Olsson, O., and Holen, O. Percutaneous transcatheter occlusion of pulmonary arterio-venous malformation. *Ann. Radiol.* 23:335, 1980.

29. Walsh, P. D. A new cause of male infertility (editorial). *N. Engl. J. Med.* 300:253, 1979.

30. Zeitler, E., Jecht, E., Richter, E.-I., and Seyferth, W. Selective sclerotherapy of the internal spermatic vein in patients with varicoceles. *Cardiovasc. Intervent. Radiol.* 3:166, 1980.

31. Walsh, P. C., Barth, K. H., Kaufman, S. L., and White, R. I., Jr. Technic and long-term results of percutaneous occlusion of varicocele with detachable silicone balloons. *J.A.M.A.* 246:1701, 1981.

Therapeutic Interventional Radiologic Procedures in Neuroradiology

SADEK K. HILAL
PAUL SANE
MICHEL E. MAWAD
W. JOST MICHELSEN

Percutaneous therapeutic vascular procedures have developed significantly during the last 2 decades. The methodology for managing neurologic lesions actually started with the open surgical approach to the carotid artery in the operating room. Initially, the neurosurgeons injected such materials as pieces of muscle, fascia, cotton, gauze, and surgical clips. With the progress in the manufacture of catheters and catheter materials and with the increased skills of the neuroradiologists in selectively reaching the extracranial and intracranial vessels as well as the spinal intercostal vessels, the safe and reliable embolization of vascular lesions of the head, neck, and spine has come within the reach of the angiographer [1, 9, 10, 11, 13]. The performance of these procedures requires an excellent knowledge of the vascular anatomy and the hemodynamics of the vascular bed under management. The importance of conducting these procedures under radiographic control with image intensification cannot be sufficiently emphasized. It appears, therefore, that the skills required for the selective manipulation of catheters into small peripheral vessels and intracranial vessels and for safe radiologic monitoring are best demonstrated by an experienced radiologist. Nevertheless, it is crucial that all interventional neuroradiologic procedures be performed by a team that includes a neurosurgeon in attendance. These procedures are truly interdisciplinary efforts of the neurosurgeon and the neuroradiologist. Decisions about the extent of embolization and priority of the vessels to be embolized must be made jointly by the neurosurgeon and the neuroradiologist. The total management of a patient very frequently requires a combined effort of embolization and surgery. In such a case, the embolization procedure has the primary objective of facilitating surgery. Such an objective can be properly achieved only by continuous consultation during the procedure between neuroradiologist and neurosurgeon.

Embolization Catheters and Balloons

COAXIAL CATHETER SYSTEMS

Coaxial catheter systems are used in practically every interventional procedure. These systems require both sufficient dilatation of the arterial puncture before introduction and maintenance of 2223 a clot-free space between the various catheters. A continuous irrigation of the catheter space with heparinized saline is achieved by maintaining the saline reservoir under a constant pressure that is somewhat higher than the arterial pressure.

The coaxial catheter system may be made up of 2, 3, or even 4 catheters. The first (outermost) catheter may be a mylar sheath inserted at the site of the puncture and used to ease the introduction and frequent exchange of other tapered or nontapered catheters into the artery. The second catheter is usually a nontapered long catheter intended to reach the extracranial cerebral vessels or the intercostal vessels; it may be used to inject pellet emboli or to guide a softer inner catheter to its destination. This nontapered catheter may also be a multilumen catheter with a balloon to permit the temporary obliteration of an extracranial vessel during the injection of embolic materials and to prevent reflux of these materials into those segments of the arterial system that are not intended to be embolized. Interventional procedures in the external carotid artery provide a good example of the importance of balloon obliteration of the external carotid artery during embolization to protect the internal carotid artery.

The third (innermost) catheter may be a torque-controlled catheter. (Preshaped torque-controlled catheters are very useful in selectively reaching the extracranial vessels or the intracostal vessels.) It is used as a guide to the untapered second catheter. Used initially in the procedure, it may be replaced by another catheter (a multilumen balloon catheter or the coaxial detachable balloon catheter of Debrun [5] once the untapered second catheter has reached the desired position. Soft catheter systems, such as those featuring a controlled-leak balloon or a magnetic tip, must be introduced through a nontapered catheter that is positioned as closely as possible to the destination of the soft catheters.

MULTILUMEN CATHETERS WITH FIXED BALLOONS

With the progress that has been made in plastic technology and catheter materials, it has been possible to develop multilumen catheters as small as 2.5 French in caliber (0.8 mm in diameter). Double-lumen catheters of this type, described by Hilal and Michelsen in 1975 [10], have been used routinely in most embolization procedures at our institution that require the injection of liquid emboli. In these catheters, the balloon is made of latex and communicates with one of the channels in the catheter. The second, and larger, lumen opens distally to the balloon and is used to deliver contrast medium and the sometimes more viscous silicone rubber without influencing the inflation of the balloon. The complete independence of the balloon inflation from the injection of contrast media or embolization material is a safe, reliable, and highly desirable arrangement. Triple-lumen balloon catheters of this size have been manufactured on an experimental basis; they still have the drawback that the septa between the various channels may break down, thus establishing a communication between the injection lumen and the balloon lumen. Since these breakdowns can be quite dangerous, triple-lumen catheters should be considered experimental devices.

SOFT SINGLE-LUMEN CATHETERS

Soft single-lumen catheters are used in vessels in the distal arterial system, where multiple curves and branching points have to be negotiated. They are usually made of silicone rubber or very soft polyvinyl acetate. They were first used as flow-guided catheters by Dotter [7, 8]. Later they were used as magnetically guided catheters by Hilal et al. [9]; recently they have been used as balloon-guided catheters by us [2] (see Fig. 97-4). In the last case, the balloon is an integral part of the catheter and is used as a sail to generate enough pull on the catheter to permit its forward progression in the vascular system with the flow.

CONTROLLED-LEAK BALLOON CATHETERS

These catheters, developed by Kerber [12], consist primarily of a soft silicone rubber single-lumen tube that measures less than 1 mm in diameter and that has a permanently fixed balloon at its tip. The balloon has a small leak, which allows the delivery of contrast material or liquid embolic material after the balloon has been sufficiently inflated to permit the leak from its tip. The balloon is employed as a sail to pull the catheter in the direction of the blood flow, and therefore the catheter can reach distally in the vascular bed, such as within the sylvian fissure or on the cerebral convexity.

The balloon inflation and the delivery of the liquid from its tip are interdependent functions. To achieve a certain rate of injection, the balloon must reach a size that allows the aperture at the tip of the balloon to open sufficiently to permit the injection of the material. The size to which the balloon must distend to achieve the required rate of injection depends on the flexibility of the balloon, the size of the aperture, and the viscosity of the liquid being injected. With great skill, one could possibly control these variables, but uncertainty will always remain, adding to the risk of the procedure. The size of the balloon for a given injection rate of a given material cannot be predicted and overinflation of some of these balloons has occurred, causing intracranial vessels to tear. Recently Debrun [5] replaced the silicone balloons of Kerber with a latex balloon presumably increasing its reliability.

DETACHABLE BALLOONS

The first detachable balloons were reported in 1974 by Serbinenko [16], who used them intracranially to obliterate arterial branches supplying cerebral vascular malformations and to occlude carotid-cavernous fistulas from a percutaneous approach. Serbinenko's precise method of detaching the balloon and the material from which the balloon is made have not been revealed. But several groups working in Western countries have developed their own methods to achieve a very similar goal. In the United States, there are two available detachable balloon systems. The first one was developed by Debrun [2–4], who uses a latex balloon attached to a very fine polyethylene catheter measuring approximately 0.5 mm in diameter. The balloon is attached to the catheter by a thin latex thread wound around the base of the balloon over the tip of the catheter. The system has a second outer catheter that fits closely around the inner catheter carrying the balloon. The two catheters reach to the outside and can be controlled independently. When the balloon is to be detached after its inflation to the proper size, the outer catheter is pulled from the inner catheter, until it reaches the bottom of the balloon and thus causes its detachment. The latex thread wound around the base of the balloon maintains the seal needed to keep the balloon size. The advantage of the system is that the detachment of the balloon and the degree of its inflation are independent variables. Specifically,

one could detach the balloon when it is only partially inflated. Unlike other systems, balloon detachment does not require inflation to a degree that causes a certain amount of friction between the balloon and the vascular wall.

The second system available in the United States is that developed by the Becton-Dickinson Company. It features a Silastic balloon attached to a single-lumen catheter by a small valve mechanism. The catheter is constructed of flexible polyethylene tubing. In this system, when the balloon reaches a certain size, the valve mechanism between the balloon and the catheter permits the balloon to be loosened from the catheter and to be easily detached with a slight pull on the catheter. A certain amount of friction between the balloon and the vascular wall is necessary to allow this separation.

A major question regarding detachable balloons is, how long do they remain inflated after the detachment in the vascular system; that is, how long do they maintain the occlusion of the vessel? If the balloon is inflated with hypertonic contrast agent, it is possible that it will attract water from the surrounding blood, causing further distention of the balloon initially, but with time, the molecules of the contrast agent start to diffuse through the wall of the balloon to the outside and thus cause deflation of the balloon, a phenomenon that has been observed by many investigators. The deflation of the balloon results in the recanalization of the vessel or the fistula it was intended to occlude. At present, probably the best material to use for balloon inflation is low-viscosity silicone rubber, which polymerizes within the balloon without diffusing through its wall. The most commonly used substance for balloon inflation is a water-soluble radiopaque material with a decreased osmolarity (Cholangiografin). Water-soluble contrast agents are safe to use, particularly when there is leakage through the seal of the balloon. Silicone rubber may embolize distally in case of leakage, and therefore it should be used in the cerebral vascular system with great caution.

The catheters of these two types of detachable balloons are somewhat more rigid than the silicone catheter used with the controlled-leak balloon. The two systems of detachable balloons therefore cannot reach as far distally in the vascular system as can Kerber's catheters. It is believed that Serbinenko's detachable balloon system has a silicone rubber catheter, but there is no way of obtaining a precise description of Serbinenko's system.

Embolization Materials

Embolization materials can be classified into two categories, particulate emboli and liquid emboli.

PARTICULATE EMBOLI

The most commonly used particulate emboli in neuroradiology are the silicone rubber spheres, developed by Lussenhop and Spence [14]. These spheres come packaged in a variety of sizes, ranging from 3 or 4 mm in diameter down to 1 mm in diameter. The silicone spheres incorporate barium sulfate powder, which makes them radiopaque. They are faintly visible when viewed with an image intensifier and are very clearly seen on plain films. Localization radiographs must be used frequently during the embolization procedure to ascertain the location of the injected spheres. They are released in the internal carotid artery or the vertebral artery using a nontapered catheter. They reach their destination guided by the blood flow and the geometry of branching of the vessels. Silicone spheres are ideally suited for intracranial embolization. They are stable in size and offer a relatively smooth surface, features that are helpful in preventing the pellet from lodging in the wrong vessel. Some embolic materials (e.g., polyvinyl alcohol sponge) swell on their way to the lesion, thus increasing the risk of a premature occlusion of a large artery, such as an internal carotid artery or a basilar artery. Irregular emboli also have the added risk of getting stuck in a vessel at a branching point before reaching their destination. Silicone spheres act by mechanically blocking the flow in the vessel. They do not stimulate thrombus formation, a feature that may be desirable in brain lesions, in which retrograde thrombus propagation may have an adverse effect on the normal brain surrounding the region. The lack of thrombogenicity is viewed by some investigators as a disadvantage because it is felt that a thrombogenic material is likely to produce a more lasting effect. This concept has not been substantiated; and we think, on the contrary, that the risk may be more significant than the benefit.

For the management of intracranial arteriovenous malformations (AVMs), the silicone pellets are released in the carotid or vertebral arteries in the neck. Several factors affect their destination. The most important of these factors is the geometry of branching of the vessels leading to the arteriovenous malformation. As a rule, the silicone pellet will follow the branch that is in the most direct continuity with the parent artery. A silicone pellet in the suprachoroid internal carotid will almost always end in the middle cerebral artery because this branch is more in line with the internal carotid than is the anterior cerebral artery. This preferential flow of the pellets into the middle cerebral artery will take place even in cases where the anterior cerebral artery is larger than the middle cerebral artery [14, 19, 20]. Similar applications of this concept can be made in the case of deep vascular malformation supplied by the striate arteries. Newer techniques involving the use of single-lumen balloon catheters for the temporary occlusion of an intracranial vessel have been used recently by Hilal et al. [11] to aid the guidance of the pellets to an abnormal arterial branch that is arising at a difficult angle from the parent vessel. A lesser factor than the geometry of branching is the volume of blood flow to the malformation.

Gelfoam slurry or particles have been used for the embolization of vascular lesions in the brain, head, and neck. Gelfoam has the advantage of allowing the use of a small tapered catheter, and the material promotes temporary thrombosis. Recanalization is common because of the reabsorption of both the clot and the Gelfoam itself. Another important drawback of Gelfoam is the lack of a suitable permanent radiopaque marker that permits repeated follow-up by radiographic examinations.

Ivalon (polyvinyl alcohol) sponge is another type of particulate emboli that is frequently used. Like Gelfoam, Ivalon sponge can be injected through a tapered catheter and it expands further when it exits from the catheter on the way to the lesion. In our opinion, this expansion is suitable for extracranial and/or extracerebral lesions but may be dangerous for the nonguided embolization of intracranial lesions, because the material may get stopped on the way to the malformation to be treated. Ivalon sponge particles provide a more permanent obliteration than Gelfoam. Also, like Gelfoam, Ivalon sponge is not sufficiently radiopaque by itself and is customarily injected suspended in a solution of radiopaque water-soluble contrast medium. Like Gelfoam, it also promotes thrombosis, which may be somewhat more permanent than Gelfoam. Extreme care must be taken in using Gelfoam or Ivalon sponge in the extracranial vessels because of the danger of reflux of the substances in the internal carotid circulation during the procedure or even several hours afterward.

LIQUID EMBOLI

Two liquid embolic materials are now commonly used for therapeutic percutaneous embolization: low-viscosity silicone rubber and bucrylate. The advantages and disadvantages of each are discussed separately.

Low-Viscosity Silicone Rubber

This liquid embolization material was developed and adapted to practical application by Hilal and Michelson [10]. The decrease in the viscosity of the silicone rubber liquid achieved by these authors was a key factor in making this material injectable through small catheters, a prerequisite for selective embolization.

Low-viscosity silicone rubber is an inert liquid that polymerizes on the addition of a catalyst (stannous octoate). Polymerization occurs within an adjustable period of time, which may vary from 30 seconds to 7 or 8 minutes. The length of the polymerization period depends on the amount of catalyst used and the type and amount of cross-linker. The cross-linker by itself does not precipitate the polymerization of the silicone elastomer; it merely facilitates the process of polymerization when the high-viscosity elastomer is diluted with the inert silicone liquid.

The formulation commonly used is as follows:

Dow Corning elastomer-382	4 cc
Dow Corning silicone fluid-360 (20 cp)	30 cc
Cross-linker (tetraethyl silicate)	0.5 cc

The mixture is steam autoclaved before it is mixed with the particulate contrast agent, such as tantalum powder, the radiopaque substance of choice for this material. (The catalyst is, of course, autoclaved in a separate container but simultaneously with the silicone rubber mixture.) The mixture has a viscosity of approximately 60 cp.

Lower viscosity materials have been achieved on an experimental basis using a silicone fluid that has a viscosity of about 5 cp instead of the Dow Corning silicone fluid-360, which has a viscosity of 20 cp. The low-viscosity silicone rubber mixtures (< 50 cp) have been used for injection through multilumen balloon catheters in extracranial lesions and in detachable balloons. The silicone rubber has the advantage of being inert, and permits easy separation of the catheter from the vascular cast produced by the injection. It is not an adhesive substance and therefore does not attach itself firmly to the catheter or to the vascular wall. Its major limitation is that it takes at least 30 seconds to polymerize, which makes its use in rapid-flow situations (e.g., arteriovenous fistulas and high-speed shunting lesions) difficult. In the polymerized state, the cast is soft and rubbery, which avoids the drawbacks of a hard mass, particularly when used in soft tissues that are subject to a wide range of motion, such as those in the neck. Also, the soft cast allows easier surgical dissection subsequent to the embolization [15].

Silicone rubber of high viscosity (approximately 200–300 cp) may be injected directly in an external carotid artery branch supplying a large malformation or a large vascular tumor. In such a case, the material is deposited as large droplets that are carried by the blood flow to their destination. The method uses a less-selective injection approach than that used in multilumen balloon catheters inserted in the small branches of the external carotid artery. It should perhaps be limited to those cases in which superselective catheterization is not feasible.

During injection of the extracranial vessels, extreme care should be taken not to embolize a small vascular bed that supplies the skin of the face, where ischemic ulcerations could occur. To protect the skin when vascular malformations of the face are being embolized, an initial injection of small pellets or other particulate materials (e.g., Ivalon sponge) could be used to prevent the low-viscosity silicone rubber from reaching the small capillary vascular beds supplying the skin. The extent of preembolization with particulate emboli can be verified by angiography before the injection of silicone rubber.

As a rule, low-viscosity silicone rubber is ideally suited for extracerebral lesions, such as dural malformations and extracranial vascular tumors. Low-viscosity silicone rubber has also been used extensively in the embolization of spinal cord malformations and neoplasms of the spine. It has not generally been used for intracerebral vascular malformations. A foaming low-viscosity silicone rubber is currently being developed for use in intracerebral lesions. The material expands to almost twice its size on polymerization by releasing hydrogen gas, which initiates the foaming process.

Isobutyl 2-Cyanoacrylate

Isobutyl 2-cyanoacrylate (bucrylate; Ethicon) is a tissue adhesive that on contact with blood polymerizes into a hard mass within a few seconds [7]. The polymerization is precipitated by the electrolytes dissolved in the blood; glucose solutions do not initiate the polymerization process. Before the injection of bucrylate, an isotonic solution of dextrose is used during the procedure to flush the catheters and maintain their patency. (If salt solutions and radiopaque water-soluble contrast agents are present in the catheter, they will precipitate the premature polymerization of bucrylate in the catheter system.) The long-range biologic safety of bucrylate has not been completely established. There are some sporadic reports based on animal tests that suggest that it may have a carcinogenic effect. That observation has not been made in man, and the data on which the suspicion is based are not definitive. A limitation of bucrylate is its very fast polymerization time, which does not allow a complete filling of the vascular bed in a tumor. The addition of Pantopaque (a myelographic contrast agent) to bucrylate prolongs the polymerization time. Also, bucrylate sets as a hard mass that may be difficult to dissect surgically. Another limitation of bucrylate is that it may glue the tip of the catheter to the vascular wall. That complication may be avoided by coating the tip of the catheter with silicone jelly, thus preventing adhesion of the bucrylate to the catheter.

Bucrylate is most commonly used for intracerebral embolization. It can be delivered through a controlled-leak balloon catheter. It is not clear, however, whether in intracerebral lesions bucrylate has an advantage over silicone pellets. When liquid emboli are injected into the cerebral vascular system, they must be delivered very close to the malformation, to avoid obliterating the vessels that supply normal brain tissues surrounding the lesion. Liquid embolic material injected at a distance from the lesion obliterates the normal vessels before it reaches the malformation, clearly an undesirable effect since it adds to the ischemia of brain tissue around the lesion. Bucrylate has also been used for the obliteration of carotid-cavernous fistulas; it is injected directly into the cavernous sinus, where it solidifies. This approach has been reasonably successful but is less safe than the alternative, which involves the detachment of a Debrun balloon into the sinus. The direct contact of bucrylate with the intracavernous nerves and vessels may raise the question of its long-term safety.

PREREQUISITES FOR EMBOLIZATION MATERIALS

Embolization materials must be relatively inert substances devoid of short- or long-term adverse effects on the surrounding tissues. A slight thrombogenicity is desirable in most cases, except perhaps in intracerebral use. All embolizable substances must be radiopaque, visible by radiographic image intensification, which should be carried out during the procedure. Only in this fashion can absolute control of the quantity and rate of injection of these substances be achieved. An excessively high rate of injection could result in the escape of these materials into normal vascular beds, thus causing damage to tissues not involved by the lesion. It is also desirable that the embolized material retain its radiopacity for as long as it remains in the body, to permit follow-up radiography to determine whether any migration of the embolized substance occurred.

Embolic materials should be easily sterilized, and great care should be taken to avoid contamination during the sterilization procedure. A breach in sterile technique during embolization is more likely to result in complications than one during angiography. In most cases, it is desirable that embolic materials be nonbiodegradable, maintaining their obliteration capability for long periods of time. Only when surgery is contemplated soon after the embolization could one use a biodegradable or resorbable substance like Gelfoam.

RADIOPAQUE TAGS OF EMBOLIC MATERIALS

The following radiopaque substances are used to tag embolized materials:

(1) *Barium sulfate.* Barium sulfate powder is used during the manufacture of Silastic pellets. In this form, barium sulfate is inert and does not seem to produce tissue reaction. It is not recommended, however, for use with liquid emboli because it could result in granulomatous formation.

(2) *Tantalum powder and tantalum oxide powder.* These two radiopaque media are used in conjunction with silicone rubber and bucrylate. They

are available in particles whose average size is approximately 1 μ. (Larger particles tend to conglomerate and obliterate small catheters.) These substances are virtually inert and have been used in neurosurgical procedures for a long time. Some care should be exercised in handling these fine powders, because they are flammable. Tantalum powder is black and so should be avoided when one is managing a lesion near the face of a fair-skinned patient. As a rule, tantalum powder is preferred to tantalum oxide powder because of its smaller particle size. Tantalum oxide powder is white, which allows one to avoid the discoloration caused by tantalum powder. In any case, during the sterilization procedure the tantalum powder should be packaged separately and should be mixed with the silicone rubber just before the injection of the embolic material into the patient.

(3) *Water-soluble iodinated contrast agents.* Water-soluble iodinated contrast agents are injected with small particulate substances, such as Ivalon or Gelfoam suspensions. Under image intensification, it is possible to evaluate the reflux of the embolic material around the catheter during the injection, thus permitting proper control of the injection rate. Water-soluble iodinated contrast agents do not permit follow-up radiographic evaluation to determine the precise location of the injected embolic material and to establish whether migration occurred.

(4) *Pantopaque.* Pantopaque is used as a tag for Gelfoam and bucrylate. It is not a permanent tag with either substance, but it tends to remain somewhat longer with bucrylate. With bucrylate, Pantopaque has the added advantage of delaying the speed of polymerization of the tissue adhesive. This feature may be quite useful in filling the angioarchitecture of a complex malformation or tumor. Pantopaque is reactive with tissue and tends to promote thrombosis.

Embolization of Arteriovenous Malformations of the Brain

Embolization of AVMs of the brain is done for the following purposes:

(1) To reduce the blood flow through the AVM and so to diminish the chances of bleeding and promote thrombosis of the malformation.
(2) To facilitate surgery by reducing the intracranial pressure and by obliterating feeding ves-

sels that are difficult to reach at surgery. Vascular malformations supplied by the posterior cerebral and middle cerebral arteries provide a good example of this situation. The preoperative embolization of the posterior cerebral arteries could limit the surgical exposure to the middle cerebral arteries and may allow the surgery to be carried out from the cerebral convexity aspect without having to explore the tentorial surface of the brain. Similarly, the embolization of the striate arteries supplying the deeper part of an AVM of the cerebral convexity greatly aids resection.

(3) Occasionally, to obliterate the entire bed of the vascular malformation. Although uncommon, this goal is usually achievable in small vascular malformations. When done in larger malformations, the risk of the procedure tends to increase. The risks associated with embolization of the intracranial vascular malformations can be categorized as follows:

1. Risks that are related to the angiographic procedure itself, which is an inevitable part of the embolization technique. These risks include trauma to the artery and contrast reaction.
2. Risks that are caused by stray emboli resulting in the occlusion of vessels supplying normal brain-blood supply.
3. Risk of bleeding from an AVM as consequence of a complete or near-complete occlusion of a large vascular malformation. In these cases the sudden stop of the shunt may subject the cerebrovascular bed to a hemodynamic stress that cannot be accommodated by vessels that have lost their autoregulation ability. Another cause of intracranial hemorrhage is lodgment of embolic material in the venous outflow before the obliteration of the arterial supply. Such a complication is most likely to occur with bucrylate glue.

For descriptive purposes, cerebral vascular malformations are classified according to the vascular territory that supplies them. This classification also permits an easier discussion of the rationale and the feasibility of embolization in each kind of malformation.

MIDDLE CEREBRAL ARTERY MALFORMATIONS

Vascular malformations supplied primarily by the middle cerebral artery can be classified morphologically into three groups: (1) superficial vas-

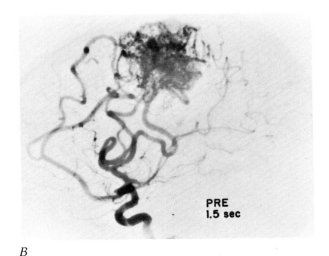

A

B

C

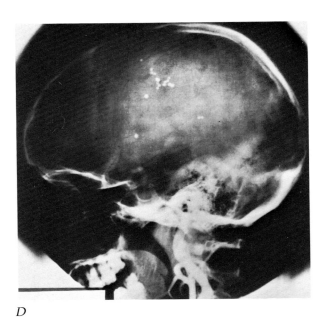

D

Figure 97-1. Embolization of a high convexity frontoparietal arteriovenous malformation (AVM). (A, B, and C) Preembolization internal carotid arteriogram shows a high convexity AVM supplied by the middle and anterior cerebral arteries. (D) A plain film of the skull shows the radiopaque emboli in the middle cerebral territory. The Silastic pellets were released in the internal carotid artery in the neck, using an open-tip catheter. (E, F, and G) Postembolization angiogram shows the malformation to have decreased in size; more important, it shows also that the middle cerebral supply to the malformation has been obliterated. Surgery was facilitated by reducing the flow to the malformation and limiting the surgery to control of arterial feeders to the branches of the anterior cerebral artery as a result of embolization of the middle cerebral branches.

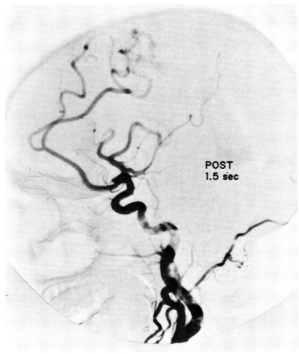

POST
1.5 sec

E

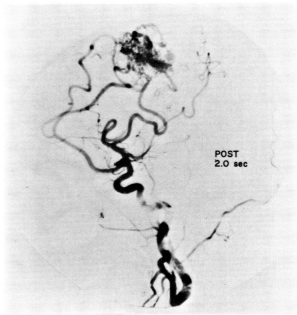

POST
2.0 sec

F

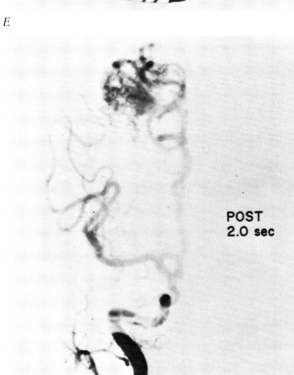

POST
2.0 sec

G

cular malformations supplied primarily by the leptomeningeal vessels, (2) deep malformations supplied primarily by the striate arteries, and (3) AVMs supplied by both leptomeningeal vessels and striate vessels.

The superficial vascular malformations of the middle cerebral artery territory are usually embolized easily by the injection of pellets or other particulate substances into the internal carotid artery. Recently, attempts at selectively catheterizing middle cerebral artery branches using a variety of techniques with balloon catheters have resulted in the successful obliteration of parts of the malformation. The risk of these selective catheterization techniques is substantial, because they may be associated with vascular tears or excessive obliteration of vessels before the malformation is reached, thus adversely affecting normal brain around the lesion.

Superficial middle cerebral malformations are, as a rule, easily embolizable because the leptomeningeal branches of the middle cerebral artery are in direct continuity with the main trunk of the middle cerebral artery. The deep malformations supplied primarily by the striate arteries are very difficult to embolize because injected particulate material tends to travel in the middle cerebral artery with the main blood flow to the superficial leptomeningeal branches of the mid-

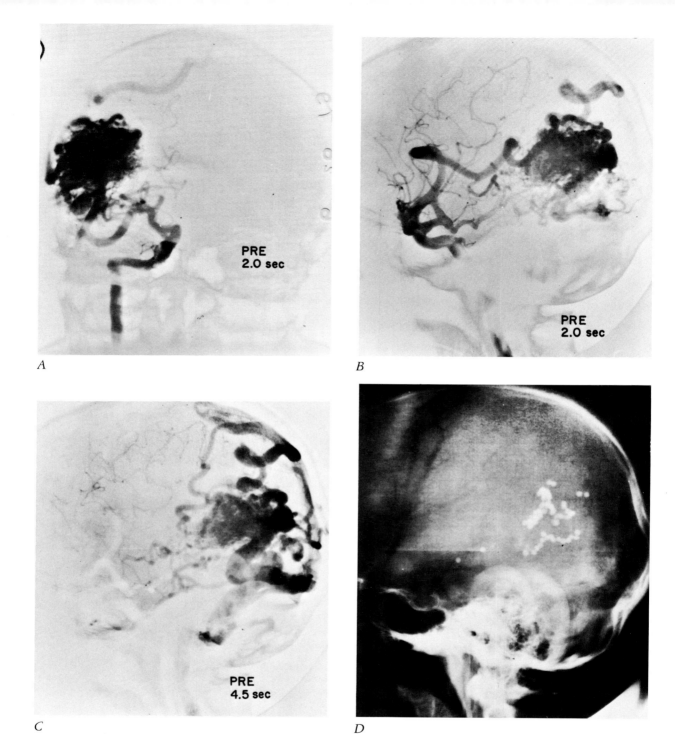

A

B

C

D

Figure 97-2. Embolization of a parietotemporal malformation. (A and B) An internal carotid angiogram at 2 seconds shows a large posterior temporal AVM supplied by the middle cerebral artery. The anterior cerebral artery fills from the opposite side and does not contribute to the AVM. Note the early venous filling at this stage. (C) At 4.5 seconds, more venous drainage of the AVM is seen into the lateral sinus and the superior sagittal sinus through a large cortical vein. (D) Lateral films after embolization with Silastic spheres into the internal carotid artery show the emboli in the AVM having reached the lesion through the middle cerebral artery branches. (E) Postembolization angiogram at 2 seconds shows a significant delay in the filling of the AVM. (F and G) Postembolization angiogram at 4.5 seconds shows the Silastic spheres situated in the center of the AVM. Compared to the preembolization frame obtained at the corresponding time, there is no evidence of filling of veins, indicating a significant slowing of the circulation through the AVM.

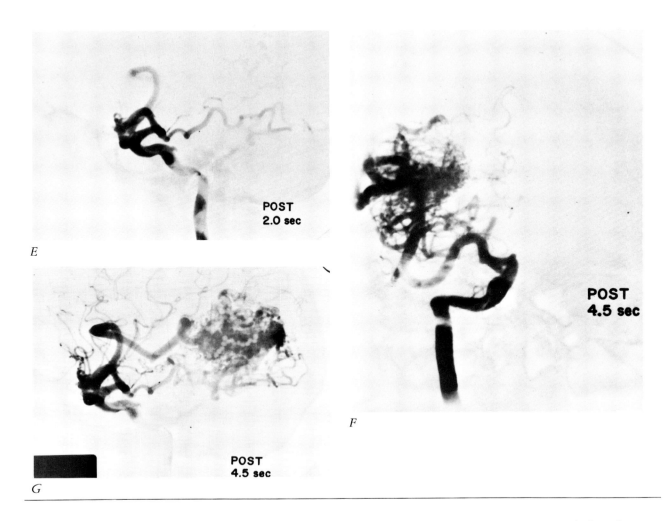

E

POST
2.0 sec

POST
4.5 sec

F

POST
4.5 sec

G

dle cerebral artery rather than make the sharp turn required to enter the striate vessels.

Figure 97-1 demonstrates a vascular malformation supplied primarily by the superficial branches of the middle cerebral artery and the branches of the anterior cerebral artery. Embolization carried out in the internal carotid artery resulted in the pellets lodging in the branches of the middle cerebral artery. There was a decrease in the abnormal vasculature, primarily as a result of the blockage of the middle cerebral feeders to the malformation. There was also a prolongation of the circulation time through the lesion, as determined from the two angiographic series. The subsequent surgical approach was concerned primarily with the control of the branches of the anterior cerebral artery that constituted the dominant source of the blood supply.

The patient whose case is illustrated in Figure 97-2 has a vascular malformation of the middle cerebral artery in the posterior temporal region. Embolization has resulted in a remarkable slow-ing of the circulation. It is assumed that the prolongation of the circulation time reflects a decrease in the blood flow through these abnormal vessels and, with it, a decreased chance of bleeding. A decrease in the blood flow results in a drop in the intracranial pressure. Both hemodynamic effects are beneficial and facilitate surgery (if surgery is indicated).

The patient whose case is illustrated in Figure 97-3 has a deep vascular malformation supplied primarily by the lenticulostriate branches of the middle cerebral artery. Embolization of pellets has resulted in the obliteration of the normal superficial middle cerebral vessels. The lack of penetration of the deep malformation by the emboli is due primarily to the geometry of branching of the striate arteries from the middle cerebral artery; the striate arteries arise at a rather sharp angle to the main trunk of the middle cerebral artery. The injected emboli tend to continue in a straight line in the leptomeningeal branches of the middle cerebral artery and to be distrib-

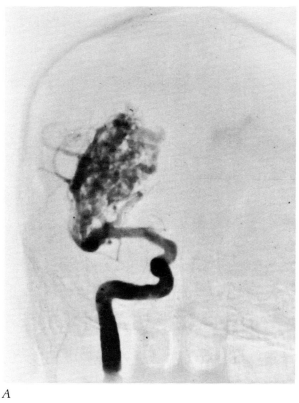

A

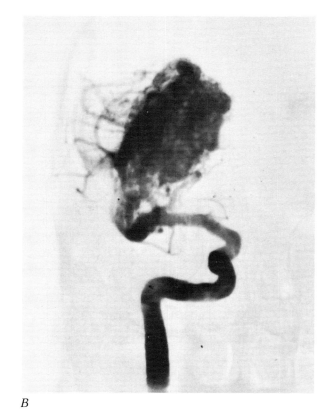

B

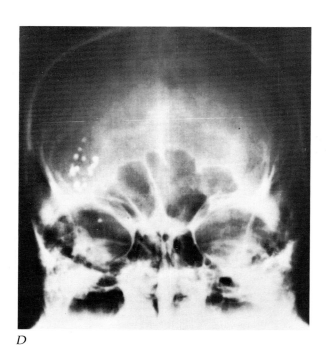

C

D

Figure 97-3. Vascular malformation of the basal ganglia and thalamus. (A and B) Preembolization arteriogram shows a deep vascular malformation supplied primarily by the lenticulostriate arteries. The rest of the middle cerebral artery supplies the malformation to a lesser extent. (C and D) Anteroposterior and lateral views of the skull after embolization show the pellets in the superficial middle cerebral artery. (E and F) Repeat internal carotid angiogram postembolization shows the pellets lodged in the normal superficial branches of the middle cerebral artery, with lack of penetration in the deep malformation due to the geometry of branching of the striate arteries. Further embolization would tend to occlude more of the normal branches. In this type of malformation, embolization is not effective.

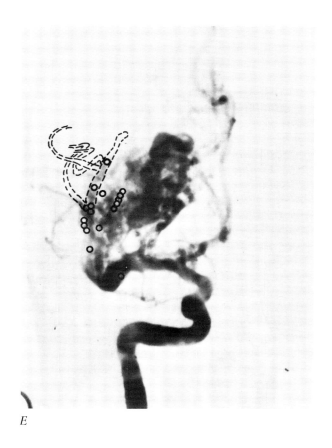

E

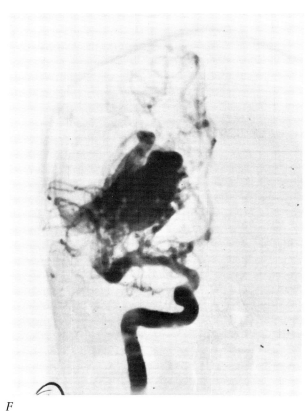

F

uted in the sylvian fissure and over the cerebral convexity. The result of the embolizations in this case was an undesirable blockage of normal cerebral vessels; the deep malformation itself was affected to a very limited degree.

Recently a new method was developed by Hilal and others for the selective embolization of the striate arteries using small single-lumen balloon catheters (2 French) advanced into the middle cerebral artery distal to the origin of the striate vessels feeding the malformation. The balloon then is inflated, temporarily obliterating the middle cerebral artery. Small silicone pellets (1.5 mm in diameter) then are released into the internal carotid artery. These pellets will reach the striate vessels selectively and cause either a complete obliteration of the deep part of the malformation or a substantial decrease of this lesion. This approach to the management of the deep malformation has greatly expanded the utility of this method in the control of otherwise untreatable deep vascular malformations and in facilitating surgery on superficial AVMs with a deep vascular supply. The example of Figure 97-4 is a good illustration of this approach.

Embolization of intracranial vascular malfor-

mations with particulate emboli should be carefully monitored by frequent radiographs of the skull and angiograms made during the procedure. This precaution is particularly important in malformations that are unlikely to be successfully treated with embolization, such as those arising from the anterior cerebral artery and the deep striate branches of the middle cerebral artery.

VASCULAR MALFORMATIONS OF THE POSTERIOR CEREBRAL ARTERY

Embolization of the posterior cerebral artery territory with particulate emboli is performed by introducing a nontapered catheter into the origin of a vertebral artery. Because of the anatomy of the posterior circulation, an embolus injected into the vertebral artery tends to travel through the intracranial portion of the vertebral artery and the basilar artery without entering any of their branches until it reaches the tip of the basilar artery, where it may lodge in an enlarged thalamoperforate artery or one of the posterior cerebral arteries. All proximal branches arising from the basilar artery or the intracranial segment of the vertebral artery tend to be avoided by a

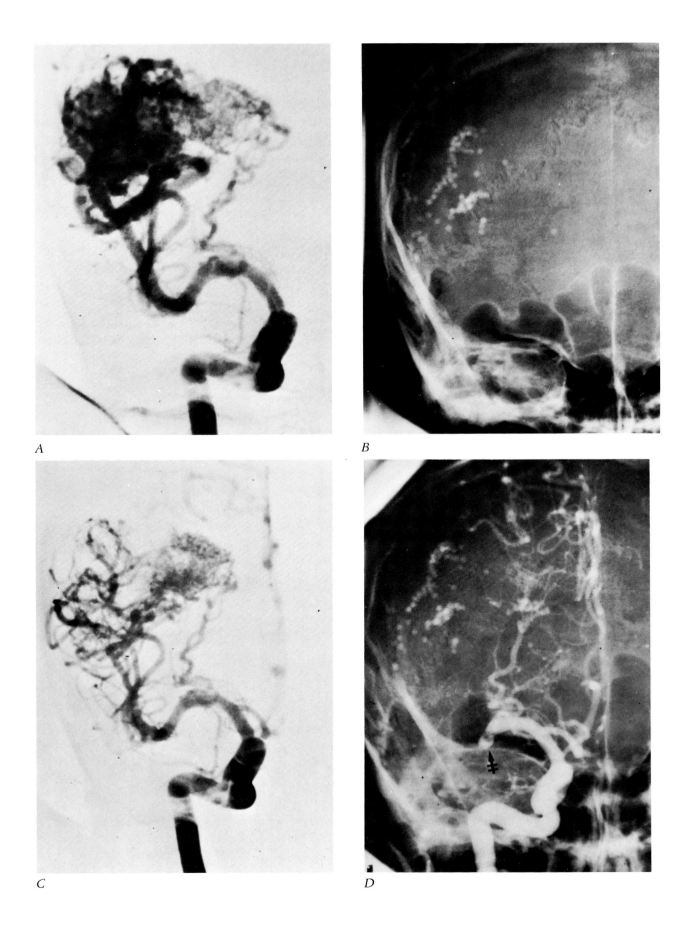

A

B

C

D

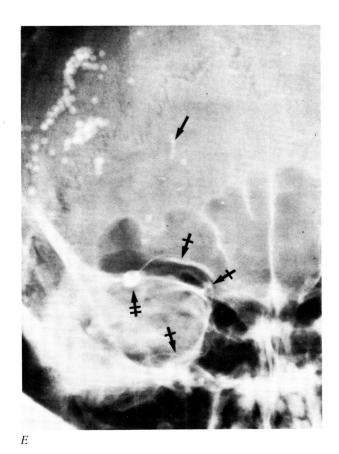

E

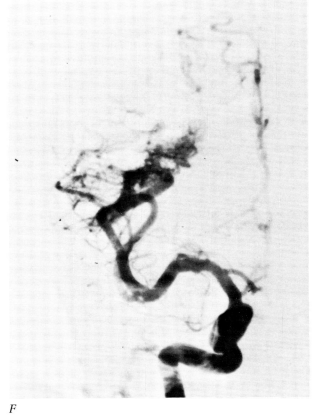

F

Figure 97-4. AVM involving the cerebral convexity and basal ganglia. The lesion is supplied by the superficial and deep branches of the middle cerebral artery and illustrates the recently developed technique of embolizations with a combination of *silicone pellets and temporary occlusion with an intracranial balloon catheter.* (A) Anteroposterior view of a right carotid arteriogram showing the vascular malformation of the frontoparietal operculum reaching deep to the wall of the ventricle. The AVM is supplied by large superficial branches of the middle cerebral artery in their course in the sylvian fissure and after reaching the surface of the brain. There is also a prominent lenticulostriate artery feeding the deeper part of the vascular malformation. (B) Approximately 60 silicone pellets (2-mm) were embolized in the internal carotid artery and reached as expected the superficial branches of the middle cerebral artery in the sylvian fissure and on the surface of the cerebral convexity. (C) Angiogram taken after the embolization of the superficial branches of the middle cerebral artery shows the reduction of the superficial component of the AVM. The prominent lenticulostriate artery supplying the deep part of the malformation is still visualized without change. No pellets entered this vessel. Because of the reduction of the AVM, the anterior cerebral artery is better visualized on this injection than was demonstrated initially on the angiogram illustrated in (A), where it did not fill with contrast. (D) Angiogram performed after the introduction of a balloon catheter, in the middle cerebral artery distal to the origin of the lenticulostriate artery. The balloon is partially filled with contrast medium and air (*arrow*). The lenticulostriate artery arising proximal to the balloon is well demonstrated on this injection and fills the deeper part of the malformation. The balloon temporarily has occluded all the distal branches of the middle cerebral artery beyond the origin of the enlarged lenticulostriate branch. (E) With the balloon inflated (*double-barred arrow*), small (1-mm) silicone pellets were embolized and are seen to have reached the deeper part of the vascular malformation supplied by the enlarged lenticulostriate artery. The newer pellets (*regular arrow*) are recognized by comparing this radiograph with the radiograph illustrated in (B). The temporary occluding balloon (*double-barred arrow*) and the fine catheter leading to it (*single-barred arrows*) can be recognized readily. (F) Angiogram obtained after the embolization of the deeper part of the malformation and after retraction of the temporary occluding balloon catheter. There is a remarkable decrease in the size of the remaining malformation and a complete occlusion of the deep lenticulostriate artery supplying this lesion. As compared to (A), the anterior cerebral artery is well filled because of the reduction of the AVM.

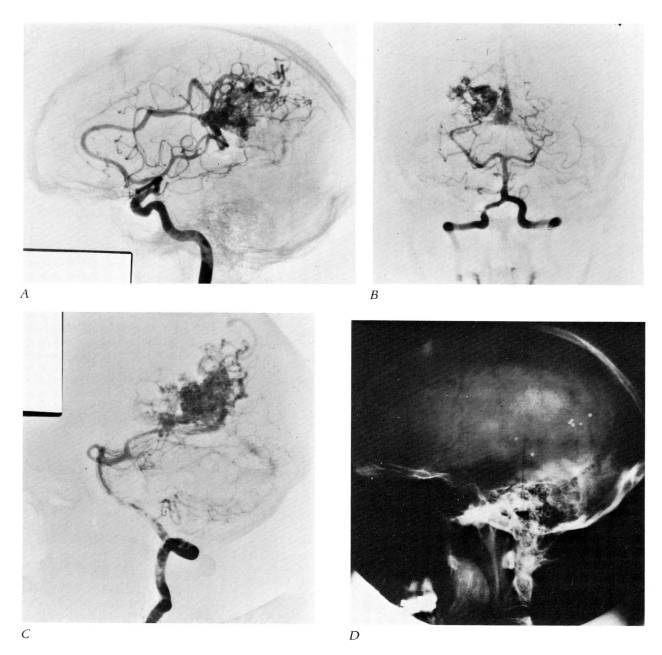

A

B

C

D

Figure 97-5. Deep AVM with a dual supply from the anterior and the posterior cerebral arteries. (A) Lateral view of the internal carotid arteriogram demonstrates the supply from the anterior cerebral artery. The middle cerebral branches did not supply the AVM. (B and C) Vertebral angiogram shows the AVM supplied by the posterior cerebral artery. (D) After embolization of the vertebral artery, Silastic spheres are seen in the AVM and in the posterior cerebral branches. (E and F) Postembolization angiography of the vertebral artery shows a remarkable reduction in the size of the AVM—to almost complete obliteration. This embolization has facilitated surgery by primarily limiting it to branches of the anterior cerebral artery.

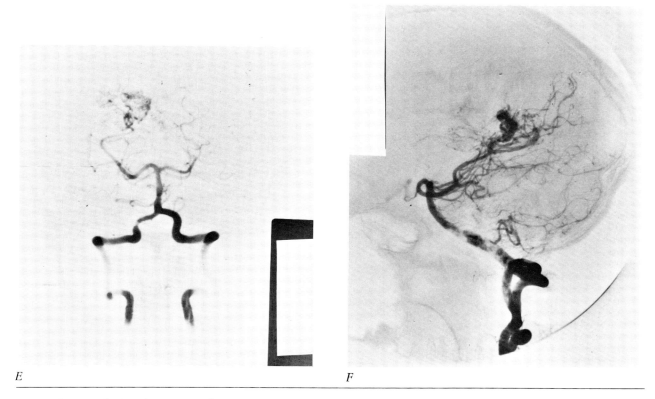

E

F

particulate embolus because of the rather sharp angle at which these branches arise from the parent vessel. It is extremely difficult to embolize a malformation in the posterior inferior cerebellar artery in spite of the fact that the vessel may be quite large and may supply a substantial vascular malformation. The angle at which the posterior inferior cerebellar artery arises from the vertebral artery is acute and does not lend itself to ready entry by a particulate embolus traveling in the vertebral artery. The same statement may be made about the anterior inferior cerebellar artery and the superior cerebellar artery. In all these cases, if the embolus is to enter one of these branches, it will have to reverse its direction of forward flow.

A pellet injected into the vertebral artery tends to enter the larger of the two posterior cerebral arteries, which is, as a rule, the vessel leading to the malformation. Occasionally, however, the geometry of branching of the vertebral artery into the two posterior cerebral arteries allows a preferential flow of the embolus to the smaller of the two posterior cerebral arteries. Because of this possibility, an anteroposterior radiograph of the skull in the Towne's view should be taken after the injection of the first 2 or 3 pellets in order to localize the injected emboli and ascer-

tain that the pellets reached the abnormal side. Great care should be taken to ensure that the pellets are smaller than the lumen of the basilar artery so that an inadvertent block of this important vessel does not occur. Also, one should avoid using substances such as Gelfoam or, possibly, Ivalon sponge for the embolization of posterior cerebral vascular malformations, because these sponge materials may get stuck in the basilar artery.

The embolization of malformations supplied by the posterior cerebral arteries and the thalamoperforate arteries in almost 200 patients in our own experience did not result in a single complication from the inadvertent embolization of vertebral and basilar artery branches other than the posterior cerebral arteries. A few transient complications did occur in this series as a result of embolization of posterior cerebral malformations; the complications were primarily transient visual field defects, and they disappeared in 2 or 3 days. In our experience, the embolization of the posterior cerebral territory has been the safest intracranial embolization procedure to follow.

Few investigators have reported the embolization of the posterior cerebral territory with small balloons and intravascular adhesive. The experi-

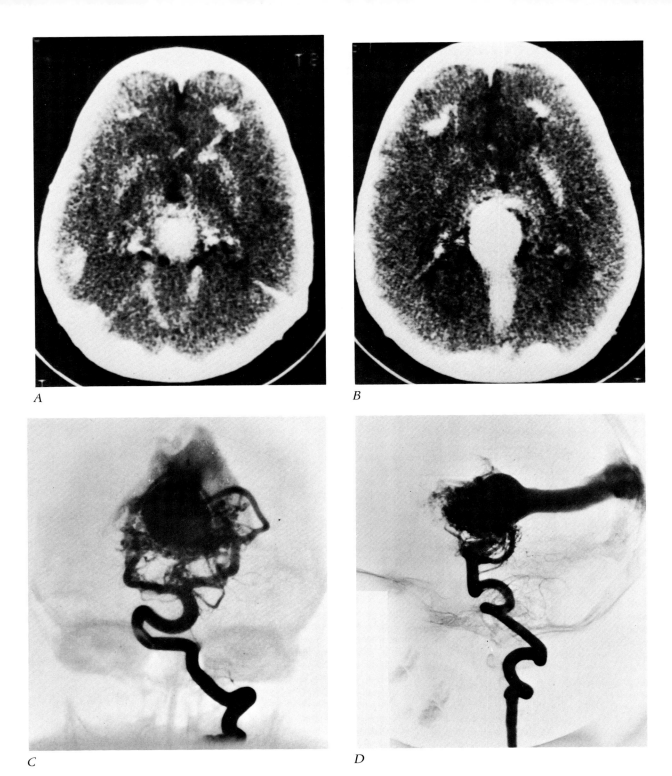

A

B

C

D

Figure 97-6. Aneurysm and vascular malformation of the vein of Galen. (A and B) A computed tomographic scan with contrast material demonstrates a large enhancing lesion in the region of the vein of Galen. The straight sinus is very large owing to the drainage of the malformation toward the torcula. (C and D) Preembolization vertebral angiogram at 2 seconds shows large and tortuous basilar and vertebral arteries. Branches of the posterior cerebral arteries supply a malformation of the midbrain and thalamus, which ultimately drains into the distal vein of Galen. (E and F)

After embolization of approximately 30 pellets (1.5-mm) into the vertebral artery, there is obliteration of a significant number of the small arterial feeders to the malformation. The frames shown were obtained at 3.5 seconds after the injection. The prolongation in the circulation time can be seen when the frames are compared with the preembolization frames obtained at 2 seconds (C and D). The patient made a remarkably good clinical recovery as a result of the reduction of the steal from the brain stem.

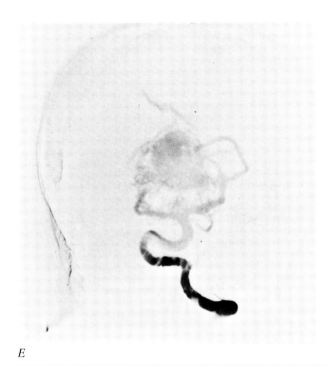

E

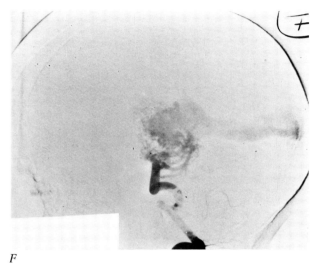

F

ence with these balloon catheters is still limited, and the work at this stage should be considered investigational. It is not clear whether the intravascular adhesive offers an advantage in the posterior cerebral artery territory over simple embolization by silicone spheres.

Most of the malformations supplied by the posterior cerebral artery are also supplied by the pericallosal branch of the anterior cerebral artery. Many of them are also supplied by the middle cerebral branches. The purpose of embolizing the posterior cerebral component is to facilitate the surgical removal. The embolization of the posterior cerebral artery may preclude the surgical exposure of this vessel and limit the operation to the clipping of the anterior cerebral or middle cerebral branches feeding the lesion. Such a case is illustrated in Figure 97-5. Vascular malformations associated with aneurysms of the great vein of Galen can, in most cases, be greatly reduced by embolizing the posterior cerebral circulation. The purpose of the procedure in these cases is to block the thalamoperforate arteries and the posterior choroidal arteries supplying the malformation. It was possible to decrease the size of the malformation remarkably, but the greatest benefit resulted from the improvement in the blood flow to the brain stem. Patients with long-standing lesions with a variety of motor function

disturbances and ataxia have shown a remarkable improvement as a result of the embolization alone. On one occasion, a child who had shown a decreased level of consciousness for several weeks because of a midbrain malformation associated with an aneurysm of the vein of Galen improved remarkably as a result of the embolization, to the point where he was able to carry on a useful conversation a few days after the embolization procedure (Fig. 97-6).

In most cases, the size of the aneurysm of the vein of Galen decreases only slightly. The most important effect, however, is the decrease in the size of the malformation, with the resultant improvement of the blood flow to the brain stem and significant obliteration of the neurologic symptoms. It should be pointed out that, since the aneurysm of the vein of Galen does not significantly decrease in size, the block to the cerebral spinal fluid circulation in the aqueduct and the posterior third ventricle is not diminished. The management of these patients may have to include, in addition to vascular embolization, the consideration of a ventricular shunt.

Infants with aneurysms of the great vein of Galen often present with cardiac failure. In these cases, embolization of the posterior circulation may be very helpful in controlling the cardiac decompensation until the child gets to an age where surgery is feasible. Also, as a result of growth, the amount of blood shunted through the malformation becomes a less significant fraction of the total cardiac output. Embolization of these infants may present technical difficulties. Often the vertebral artery leading to the malformation is larger than the descending aorta or is equal to it in size. In such a case, a catheter passed from the femoral artery to the vertebral artery has to be of such a large diameter that it is impossible to use the small femoral artery as the site of the arterial entry. Two approaches are possible. One approach consists of surgically introducing a large catheter into the vertebral artery near its origin from the subclavian artery. This approach requires a skillful surgical team, because the patient's condition is generally poor. Embolization carried out through the large catheter with Silastic spheres is easily controlled in regard to the number and size of the injected pellets. The other approach is the selective catheterization of the vertebral artery with a small catheter introduced via the femoral approach. The embolization material must be an expandable sponge (e.g., Ivalon or silicone sponge) that can be compressed in the catheter and delivered in the larger artery. Extreme care must be used since there is the danger that the expandable embolic material will be trapped in the basilar artery.

VASCULAR MALFORMATIONS OF THE ANTERIOR CEREBRAL ARTERY

Embolization of the anterior cerebral artery territory is very difficult to achieve with nonguided emboli. An embolic particulate substance released in the internal carotid artery tends in almost all cases to enter the middle cerebral artery rather than the anterior cerebral artery, primarily because of the geometry of branching of the internal carotid artery. As a rule, vascular malformations in the territory of the anterior cerebral artery are better managed surgically. It is possible, however, to use percutaneous techniques that involve a guided balloon catheter in the anterior cerebral artery with the injection of liquid embolic material. This approach, however, carries a risk of an insufficiently selective catheterization, leading to the obliteration of vessels supplying part of the motor cortex or resulting in a loss of sphincter control. Another approach to the embolization of the anterior cerebral artery that has been tried with partial success is the temporary occlusion of the middle cerebral ar-

tery with the balloon catheter and the injection of particulate emboli into the internal carotid artery.

DURAL VASCULAR MALFORMATIONS

Dural vascular malformations are supplied mostly by branches of the external carotid artery or by meningeal branches of the internal carotid and vertebral arteries. A smaller contribution may come from the cerebral leptomeningeal vessels. Embolization is only possible with the meningeal branches of the external carotid artery. The meningeal branches of the internal carotid and vertebral arteries are not readily accessible for selective embolization.

A dural malformation may present clinically as an audible bruit, a subarachnoid hemorrhage, or increased intracranial venous pressure resulting in papilledema and proptosis. It is not uncommon for the lesion to be associated also with venous thrombosis, causing a further increase in the intracranial venous pressure. Large dilated scalp veins and periorbital veins are sometimes encountered in children with dural vascular malformations.

In regard to their management, dural malformations can be classified in four groups: (1) posterior dural malformations, supplied primarily by the occipital artery; (2) middle cranial fossa and tentorial malformations, supplied primarily by the posterior division of the middle meningeal artery; (3) anterior dural malformations, supplied primarily by the anterior division of the middle meningeal artery; (4) pericavernous malformations, supplied by middle meningeal and internal maxillary branches.

Dural malformations supplied primarily by the occipital artery are present in the occipital region and the tentorium. Selective catheterization of the occipital artery is usually easily achieved with a small balloon catheter that can be threaded distal to the origin of the posterior auricular artery. This latter branch may supply the seventh nerve, and its inadvertent obliteration may cause facial palsy. The case illustrated in Figure 97-7 is an example of such a selective embolization with silicone rubber that filled retrogradely the middle meningeal branch feeding the malformation.

Dural malformations supplied by the posterior division of the middle meningeal artery may involve the tentorium and the floor of the middle cranial fossa and extend in the posterior fossa. Embolization of this region may result in facial palsy since the seventh nerve may get a part of its

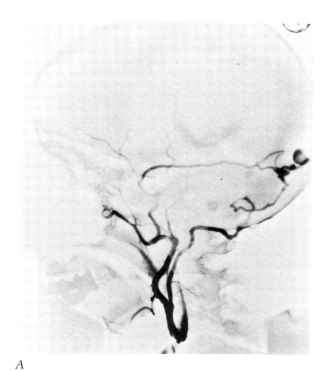

A

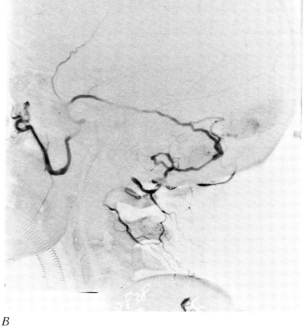

B

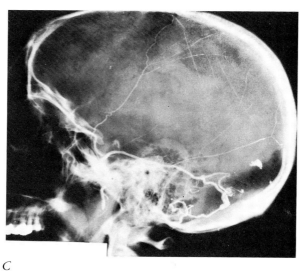

C

Figure 97-7. Dural vascular malformation. (A) Common carotid injection shows an AVM supplied by the occipital artery and the posterior division of the middle meningeal artery arising from the external carotid artery. The nidus of the AVM is close to the torcula. (B) Superselective injection of the occipital artery shows the nidus of the AVM around the posterior part of the lateral sinus and retrograde filling of the middle meningeal artery. (C) After embolization with silicone rubber, the vulcanized material fills both suppliers to the AVM and the AVM, resulting in its complete occlusion. The material was injected in the occipital artery and filled the middle meningeal artery retrogradely.

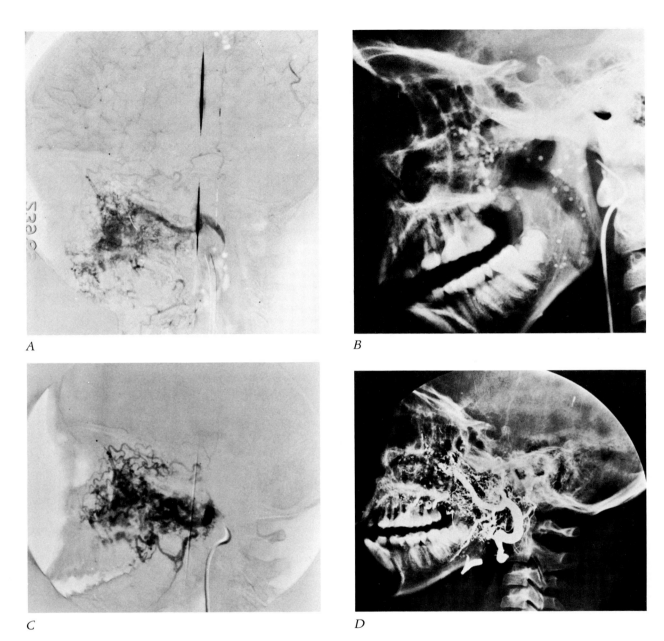

Figure 97-8. Embolization of a facial AVM. (A) Superselective external carotid angiography shows a large AVM supplied by the internal maxillary and lingual arteries. Small vessels are seen to reach the skin of the face, a phenomenon that incurs the risk of embolizing the skin, with ensuing necrosis. (B) Multiple Silastic spheres have been injected into the external carotid artery and are seen lodged in the AVM. The spheres block the small arteries and protect the capillary bed of the skin from the liquid silicone. (C) A repeat angiogram shows a reduction in the size of the AVM but no filling of the facial vessels. Ascertaining lack of filling of the facial vessels is essential before the injection of the silicone rubber. (D) The vulcanized silicone fluid is seen as a cast of the internal maxillary artery. Note the absence of the radiopaque silicone material from the skin of the face. Some of the silicone rubber reached the socket of the last two molar teeth, where there was bleeding. (E) A common carotid arteriogram shows complete obstruction of the flow to the AVM through the external carotid artery and a small supply from the internal carotid artery. This small feeder remained. No further bleeding occurred after prolonged follow-up.

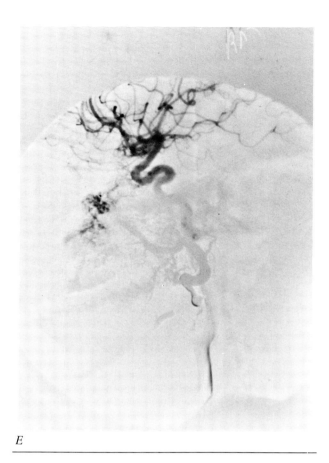

E

blood supply from the posterior branch of the middle meningeal artery. If possible, small particulate emboli should be used in preference to liquid silicone rubber.

Dural malformations supplied by the anterior division of the middle meningeal artery are usually in the dura covering the cerebral convexity. These lesions are relatively easy to embolize, particularly if one is careful to thread the embolization catheter through the foramen spinosum within the intracranial cavity. Care should be taken that the liquid embolic material does not reach the posterior meningeal division and so does not affect the blood supply of the seventh nerve.

Dural malformations in the region of the cavernous sinus usually have a dual blood supply—from both the internal carotid artery and the external carotid artery. Only the meningeal branches from the external carotid artery are accessible for embolization. Pericavernous dural malformations are usually low-flow lesions that tend to thrombose spontaneously. They also respond well to partial embolization of the internal maxillary artery branches. The procedure used in these cases tends to accelerate the natural tendency of these

lesions to thrombose. In our experience, a very partial obliteration of a few branches leading to the lesion has been sufficient to result in a complete thrombosis within a week or two. The trauma of the diagnostic angiogram, in a few cases, was sufficient to initiate the process of spontaneous thrombosis and cure.

VASCULAR MENINGEAL TUMORS

The preoperative embolization of meningiomas should be considered with great conservatism. As a rule, there is no point in embolizing a meningioma whose blood supply can be easily controlled at surgery. Examples of such lesions are convexity meningiomas supplied by branches of the middle meningeal artery. During the surgical dissection of these lesions, the feeding vessels are reached before the meningioma itself. It is easy, therefore, to ligate the meningeal branches supplying the lesion; they are usually ligated early during the surgery, at the time the craniotomy flap is being made (and before the tumor is reached). In such a case, there is little to be gained from preoperative obliteration of the meningeal vessels. In other lesions (e.g., a medial sphenoid wing meningioma or some tentorial meningiomas supplied by the middle meningeal arteries or branches of the internal maxillary artery), the surgeon may not reach the feeding artery before he reaches the lesion. The embolization of such meningiomas has the obvious advantage that it permits the surgeon to start the dissection of the neoplasm with reduced vascularity and, often, partial infarction.

EXTRACRANIAL VASCULAR MALFORMATIONS

Extracranial vascular malformations involving the maxilla, face, nasal cavity, orbit, tongue, and mandible can be greatly helped by percutaneous embolization for the purpose of achieving two goals: (1) the reduction of vascularity either as a definitive procedure or preoperatively to facilitate surgical resection and (2) the management of otherwise uncontrollable hemorrhage from the nose or the mouth. In this instance, the procedure can be lifesaving.

Embolization of vascular malformations of the facial structures carries certain risks, and its pitfalls should be understood. The following paragraphs discuss the potential hazards of such embolization.

(1) *Reflux of embolization material into the internal carotid artery.* Patients with vascular malformations of the extracranial structures usually have normal cerebral vessels and cannot tolerate the reflux of even the smallest amount of embolic material into the cerebral circulation. These patients are to be clearly distinguished from those with cerebral vascular malformations, who can well tolerate a few stray emboli because of the unusually high vascularity of the brain, which provides very ample collateral circulation. Utmost care must be taken to prevent the reflux of embolic material into the internal carotid artery during the therapeutic embolization of the external carotid circulation. The use of balloon catheters in the external carotid artery while the emboli are being delivered distally is an important precaution, and it should be taken whenever embolization of the extracranial structures is being performed. Wedging of a large outer catheter in the external carotid artery can achieve the same goal.

(2) *Discoloration and/or necrosis of the skin.* The potential embolization of the cutaneous vascular bed is an important problem in the treatment of vascular malformations of the facial structures. The risk is partially significant when one is using liquid emboli, which could reach the capillary bed and obliterate it completely. To avoid these complications, an initial embolization with particulate emboli of small (approximately 1 mm) diameter should be carried out prior to the injection of liquid emboli. These particles prevent the liquid embolic material from reaching the vascular capillary bed of the skin or the mucosa of the mouth. Particulate emboli will permit a sufficient collateral circulation through the anastomosis at the capillary level to maintain adequate vascular supply to the skin. The adequacy of embolization of the particles should be checked with selective angiography of the external carotid vessels and subtraction films to demonstrate the lack of vessels reaching the skin from the artery intended to be embolized with liquid materials. Optimally, one should not be able to obtain an angiogram of the vessels reaching the skin.

(3) *Superselective catheterization.* External carotid artery embolization should always be carried out in a superselective fashion as close as possible to the lesion. If, for example, a malformation is supplied by the distal branches of the internal maxillary artery, the catheter must be advanced into the branches of the internal maxillary artery as close as possible to the lesion. If the catheter is kept in the main external carotid artery or near the origin of the internal maxillary artery, the embolization of these large vessels can lead to serious complications, such as facial palsy and skin lesions due to indiscriminate obliteration of the arterial supply to the face or the facial nerve.

The plan for embolization should be studied carefully so that obliteration of the deep vessels supplying the lesions gets priority over obliteration of the other vessels. As a rule, deep vessels can be reached at the end of the surgical dissection of the lesion and thus contribute significantly to the bleeding during surgery. Negligible blood loss has been achieved during surgery on large vascular malformations. The surgeon was able to ligate the superficial feeders to a lesion at the beginning of surgery (the deep feeders had been blocked preoperatively by percutaneous embolization).

It is important to stress that embolization of arterial feeders resulting in their occlusion close to the malformation is much more effective in reducing the blood supply than is mere ligation of a major vascular trunk supplying the entire region of the malformation. Ligation of the main external carotid artery stem or even the main trunk of the internal maxillary artery has not significantly altered the blood flow in vascular malformations that affect the deep facial structures. Particulate emboli and liquid emboli occlude vessels close to the nidus of the malformation and often succeed in obliterating the angioarchitecture of the nidus itself, thus leading to an effective reduction in the blood flow through the lesion.

Percutaneous embolization of *superficial vascular malformations of the face* can be done as a preoperative procedure before skin grafting. In such a case, particulate emboli measuring 0.5–1.0 mm in diameter are usually used to block small arterial vessels close to the skin and, at the same time, to allow enough collateral circulation through the surface capillary bed to permit the success of a partial-thickness skin graft. But liquid emboli obliterate the very fine capillary bed so effectively that skin necrosis could result, with little chance of success for a subsequent skin graft operation.

The case illustrated in Figure 97-8 is that of a patient with a large vascular malformation involving the maxilla; he presented with uncontrollable bleeding from the gums. Initial embolization of silicone pellets was undertaken to protect the skin circulation; it was followed by silicone rubber injection that obliterated the internal maxillary artery distally and its major branches, leaving enough capillary circulation for the face. The silicone pellets prevented the silicone rubber from reaching the face. The bleeding stopped as a result of this lifesaving procedure.

Extracranial Vascular Tumors of the Head and Neck

Glomus jugulare tumors and juvenile angiofibromas are the two most commonly embolized vascular tumors of the head and neck [9, 15]. In the case of juvenile angiofibromas, the embolization is done preoperatively, to facilitate surgery. There is agreement among head and neck surgeons that preoperative embolization of glomus jugulare tumors is useful. Embolization is even used in certain cases as a definitive management without surgery. In the case of juvenile angiofibromas, however, many head and neck surgeons believe that adequate exposure of the neoplasm at the beginning of surgery permits the control of the entire vascular supply to the lesion and, therefore, preoperative embolization does not facilitate surgery as these surgeons perform it.

The most reliable and most effective technique of embolizing glomus jugulare tumors involves the selective injection of liquid silicone rubber into the ascending pharyngeal artery or branches of the internal maxillary or occipital arteries. The injection must be performed after careful superselective catheterization at a point as close as possible to the tumor. The silicone rubber mixture is prepared so that polymerization occurs in approximately 4 minutes. This delay in polymerization permits the filling of the fine tumor angioarchitecture. It has been possible on occasion to fill the entire glomus jugulare tumor by injecting the silicone rubber mixture into only the ascending pharyngeal artery using a small balloon catheter. The ascending pharyngeal artery provides the deep blood supply to the tumor and can be reached surgically, only toward the end of the dissection, which has to be carried out on a usually very friable and extremely vascular neoplasm. The injection of silicone rubber into the ascending pharyngeal artery or branches of the occipital artery has resulted in the filling of the intracranial component of these tumors, which may be supplied by branches of the vertebrobasilar artery system. In our series of more than 30 glomus jugulare tumors, we had no complications resulting from the escape of the silicone rubber material in the vertebrobasilar system by either antegrade or retrograde flow. (Recently one such case occurred with amblyopia caused by blockage of the terminal branches of the posterior cerebral artery. The patient eventually recovered.)

In the first few days after embolization of a vascular neoplasm, there is usually swelling of the tumor and mild-to-moderate pain at the site of the infarcted tumor. There may also be a transient worsening of the symptoms due to pressure on the cranial nerves arising close to the jugular foramen. These changes are, however, transient, and within a week most symptoms usually disappear. The end result uniformly has been an improvement over the preembolization symptoms.

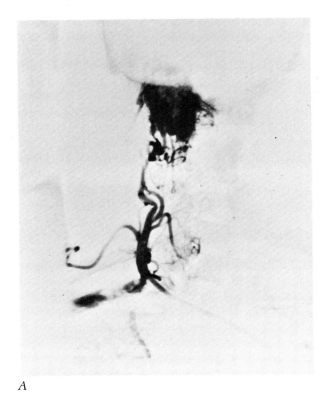

A

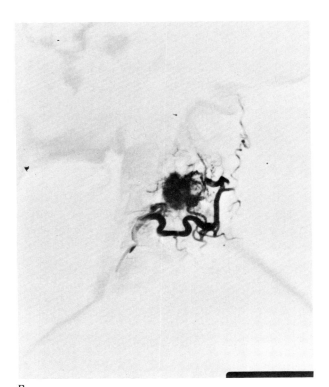

B

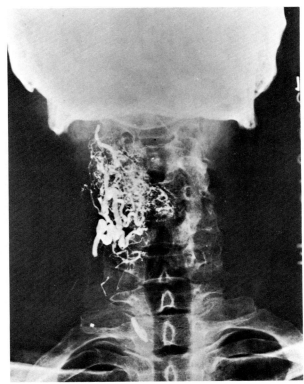

C

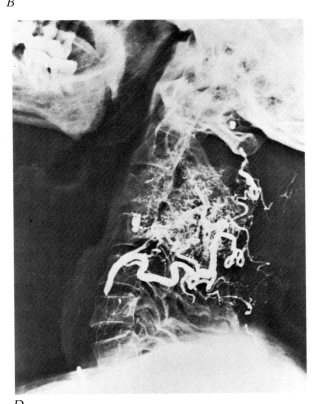

D

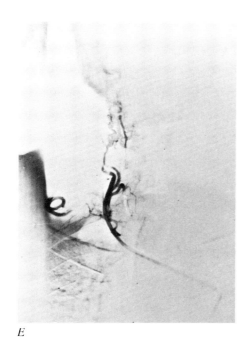

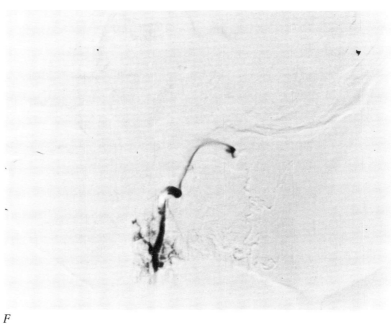

E *F*

Figure 97-9. Glomus vagale tumor. (A and B) Super-selective catheterization of the thyrocervical trunk. An enhancing soft tissue mass on the lateral side of the neck is demonstrated, representing a glomus vagale tumor. (C and D) Plain films of the neck obtained after selective catheterization and embolization with Silastic fluid and withdrawal of the catheter. The radiopaque vulcanized silicone rubber outlines the angioarchitecture of the tumor. (E and F) Repeat angiography in the same vessel after embolization shows complete disappearance of the stain owing to the complete filling of the mass by the embolization material.

Surgery on a neoplasm embolized with silicone rubber requires somewhat different techniques of dissection because the tumor is hard and rubbery. In our experience, even in the most complete embolization of glomus jugulare tumors, the postoperative histologic study shows areas of viable neoplasm surrounded by extensive regions of necrosis. Cell culture of tissue obtained from these tumors confirmed the presence of viable tumor cells. As a rule, embolization greatly facilitates surgery because it limits the bleeding and allows a more complete dissection of the neoplasm from the surrounding tissue. The boundary of the neoplasm is much more easily recognized after embolization because of the discoloration of the tumor by the tantalum powder.

Embolization of glomus jugulare tumors with silicone rubber has been a very effective method of filling the entire angioarchitecture, even in those parts of the tumor that are located in difficult areas, such as the jugular vein or the region of the cerebellopontine angle. The case illustrated in Figure 97-9 is that of a glomus vagale tumor of the neck that has been completely embolized with silicone rubber. The case in Figure 97-10 is that of a glomus jugulare tumor, in which an initial surgical approach failed. The embolization of silicone rubber shows the angioarchitecture of the tumor filled with the radiopaque rubber cast to correspond to the angiographic stain.

Figure 97-11 shows the base and lateral views of a glomus jugulare tumor after embolization with silicone rubber. The silicone rubber outlines the entire angioarchitecture of the lesion that underwent necrosis and was easily removed later by surgery.

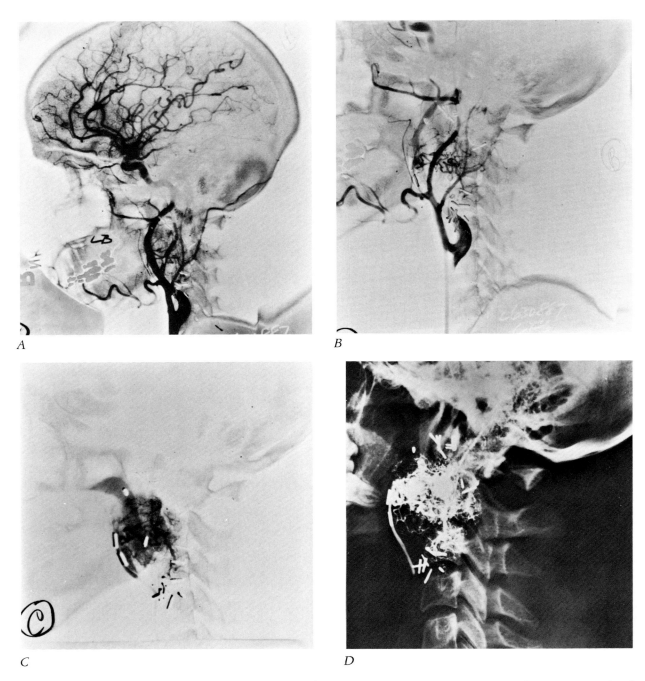

A

B

C

D

Figure 97-10. Glomus jugulare tumor. (A) Lateral view of a common carotid injection shows anterior displacement of the extracranial part of the internal carotid artery by a soft tissue mass, with a small stain arising from the external carotid artery. Several metallic clips are present from previously attempted unsuccessful surgery for this lesion. (B) A selective injection of the external carotid artery demonstrates abnormal tortuous neovascularity in a soft tissue mass in the neck displacing the external carotid artery distal to the takeoff of the facial and lingual arteries. (C) Selective catheterization of the ascending pharyngeal artery shows a large vascular stain at the base of the skull. (D) Silastic fluid injected through a superselective catheter is filling the glomus jugulare tumor. Good penetration of the angioarchitecture of the tumor is seen.

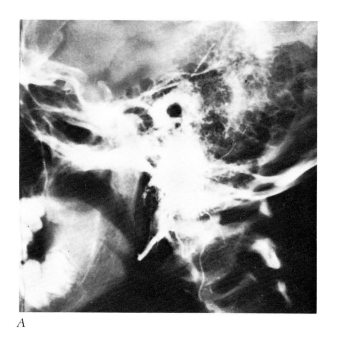

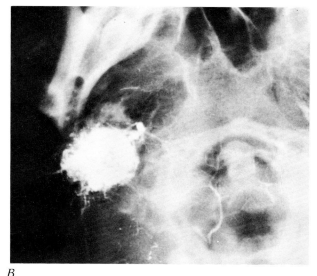

A

B

Figure 97-11. Embolized glomus jugulare tumor. (A and B) Base and lateral views obtained after the embolization of a glomus jugulare tumor with low-viscosity silicone rubber mixed with tantalum powder.

Only one arterial feeder was injected, using a catheter wedged in the superior branch of the ascending pharyngeal artery. The silicone rubber refluxed into the other arterial feeders after filling the tumor.

Treatment of Carotid-Cavernous Fistulas and Vertebral Arteriovenous Fistulas with Detachable Balloons

Detachable balloons have been very successfully used to block carotid-cavernous fistulas and vertebral venous fistulas. The technique described by Debrun is preferred because it permits the detachment of the balloon independently of the degree of its inflation. In some other detachable balloon systems, the balloon must be inflated to the point where it firmly rubs against the wall of the vessel or the fistula cavity before it can be detached. As explained earlier, one limitation of the detachable balloon is that it may shrink when it is filled with a water-soluble contrast medium. This shrinking usually occurs over a period of a few weeks. To avoid this undesirable result, the balloon may be inflated with low-viscosity silicone rubber mixed with tantalum powder for opacification. This approach assures a reasonable long-term stability of the balloon inflation. The case illustrated in Figure 97-12 is an example of a detachable balloon filled with silicone rubber and used to correct a carotid-cavernous fistula with complete restoration of the internal carotid artery.

A carotid puncture in the neck is preferred for the treatment of a carotid-cavernous fistula because it permits easier manipulation of the balloon into the fistula. In the case of an arteriovenous fistula involving the vertebral artery, a femoral catheterization is an easier approach. The manipulation of a long balloon catheter system from the femoral artery to the site of a vertebrovenous fistula requires patience and skill. One should always keep in mind that an inadvertent release of the balloon before complete inflation may result in the accidental lodging of the deflated balloon, or part of it, in the basilar artery.

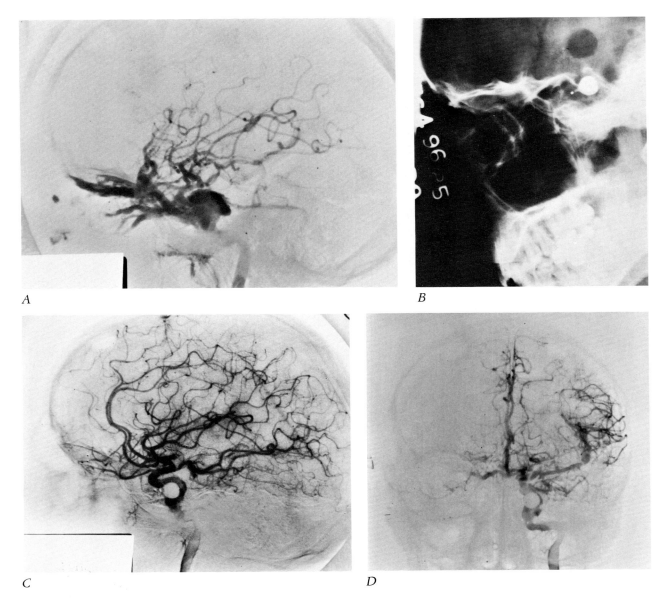

A

B

C

D

Figure 97-12. Carotid-cavernous fistula. (A) Injection of the internal carotid artery shows the presence of a communication between the internal carotid artery and the cavernous sinus, with shunting of the contrast medium into the superior and inferior ophthalmic veins. (B) A plain film of the skull shows a silicone-filled balloon after its detachment into the cavernous sinus. The balloon was introduced through a carotid puncture and manipulated through the fistula. (C and D) Internal carotid artery angiogram after the placement of the detachable balloon in the cavernous fistula. The shunt has been completely blocked and the carotid artery lumen completely restored.

Embolization of Vascular Malformations of the Spinal Cord

The vascular supply of the spinal cord can be divided essentially into the following two systems:

1. The *anterior spinal arterial system,* which consists primarily of a single longitudinal channel running along the ventral aspect of the spinal cord. The anterior spinal artery receives its blood supply from a limited number of anterior radiculomedullary arteries. The branches of the anterior spinal artery are end arteries supplying the anterior two-thirds of the spinal cord.

2. The *posterior spinal arterial system,* which consists primarily of two incomplete channels

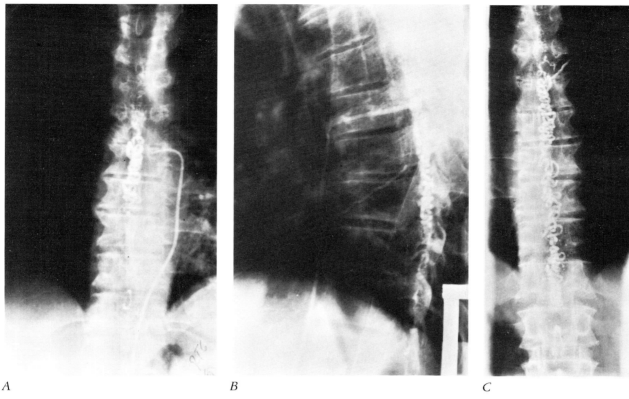

A   *B*   *C*

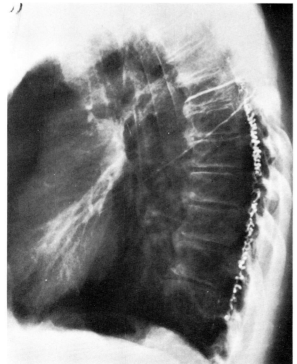

D

Figure 97-13. Spinal AVM. (A and B) With a catheter in place, the contrast material is injected into the right sixth intercostal artery, filling the AVM of the thoracic cord. (C and D) After embolization and withdrawal of the catheter, the vulcanized silicone rubber has produced a cast of the entire AVM from T6 to T12. The lateral film shows that the lesion is on the dorsal aspect of the cord. Embolization of a ventral malformation of the spinal cord carries a high risk of cord ischemia.

running dorsolaterally on the posterior aspect of the spinal cord. Since the posterior spinal arterial system receives posterior radicular arteries at almost every level of the spine and since it branches frequently, there is often a network of collateral vessels between the two posterolateral spinal arteries.

In embolizing vascular malformations, one should avoid embolizing the anterior spinal arterial system because it has inadequate collateral vessels and because all its branches are end arteries. The few attempts that were made at our institution to embolize the anterior spinal circulation resulted in worsening of the patient's condition in every case. It is therefore recommended that patients with demonstrated vascular malformations of the spinal cord be studied extensively with selective spinal angiography on both sides of the thoracic and lumbar segmental arteries. And when the malformation is in the upper dorsal spine or the cervical cord, the subclavian arteries and their branches potentially supplying the cervical spinal cord should also be studied in a selective fashion. The extensive angiographic exploration is done to determine all the radicular arterial feeders that supply the malformations.

The rationale for embolizing these lesions is that spinal vascular malformations supplied entirely by posterior radicular vessels can be easily embolized by the injection of silicone rubber in the proper intercostal or posterior radicular vessels. The vascular malformations supplied entirely by the anterior spinal system are better avoided at this stage of development of the technology. Vascular malformations supplied by both anterior and posterior spinal radicular feeders may be embolized through the posterior radicular vessels during the temporary occlusion of the anterior radicular arteries, with a small balloon catheter or a flow-guided catheter. This was done in a few cases in our institution, and resulted in the obliteration of the malformation without worsening the patient's condition. The only embolization material we now use for the management of malformations of the spinal cord is low-viscosity silicone rubber [11]. The injection of silicone pellets was tried in a dozen cases; it did not prove as satisfactory as the silicone rubber. Bucrylate has been used by other investigators for the management of these lesions; it does not seem to provide, in most cases, as complete an obliteration of the malformation as may be obtained from the silicone rubber. Recently 0.5-mm particles of polyvinyl alcohol sponge were used at other centers with satisfactory results.

Physiologic monitoring of the patient during the procedure is a new addition to the embolization of the spinal cord malformation. Somatosensory evoked responses are conducted during the procedure with a temporary occlusion of the artery to be embolized. Changes in the evoked responses are considered evidence of intolerance of the patient to the embolization.

The patient whose case is illustrated in Figure 97-13 had an extensive vascular malformation of the dorsal aspect of the spinal cord that was filled by the injection of silicone rubber into an intercostal vessel. It is interesting to note the completeness of the filling of the malformation on the dorsal aspect of the spinal cord on the lateral projections. The patient recovered from his paraplegia and actually walked out of the hospital. Favorable results such as this one occur in 60 to 70 percent of cases. In 25 percent of cases, the patient's condition is unchanged, and, in the remaining 5 percent, there may be worsening of the neurologic condition.

Conclusions

The percutaneous therapeutic embolization of particulate and liquid emboli and the use of detachable balloons have progressed remarkably in the last decade. To perform these procedures adequately, the radiologist must be familiar with all the available possibilities in catheters and embolization materials. The radiologists should work in conjunction with a neurosurgeon, in order to establish a plan for the embolization and for the occlusion of vessels that will facilitate any intended surgical procedure. Intraoperative evoked responses require collaboration with a neurologist. This work is a true interdisciplinary activity and should be performed by the neuroradiologist and the neurosurgeon and the neurologist functioning as a team. It is also important that in any one institution interventional procedures be performed by the same angiographers so that the skills may be maintained by concentrating the experience in a few hands. The patient's safety and continuing progress in the technology require that these techniques be done by a few skilled operators.

References

1. Berenstein, A., and Kricheff, I. Catheter and material selection for transarterial embolization. Technical considerations. *Radiology* 132:619, 1979.
2. Debrun, G., Lacour, P., Caron, J. P., Hurth, M., Comoy, J., and Keravel, Y. Inflatable and released balloon technique experimentation in dog—application in man. *Neuroradiology* 9:267, 1975.
3. Debrun, G., Lacour, P., Caron, J. P., Hurth, M., Comoy, J., Keravel, Y., and Laborit, G. Experimental approach to the treatment of carotid fistulas with an inflatable and isolated balloon. *Neuroradiology* 9:9, 1975.
4. Debrun, G., Lacour, P., Caron, J., Hurth, M., Comoy, J., and Keravel, Y. Detachable balloon

and calibrated-leak balloon techniques in the treatment of cerebral vascular lesions. *J. Neurosurg.* 49:635, 1978.

5. Debrun, G., Vinuda, F., and Fox, A. Latex Detachable Calibrated Leak Balloon. Experimental Work. Clinical Applications. Presented at the annual meeting of the American Society of Neuroradiology, Chicago, Ill., April 5–9, 1981.

6. Doppman, J. L., Zapol, W., and Pierce, J. Transcatheter embolization with a silicone rubber preparation: Experimental observations. *Invest. Radiol.* 6:304, 1971.

7. Dotter, C. T., Goldman, M. L., and Rösch, J. Instant selective arterial occlusion with isobutyl-2-cyanoacrylate. *Radiology* 114:227, 1975.

8. Dotter, C. T., Rösch, J., Lakin, P. C., Lakin, R. C., and Pegg, J. E. Injectable flow-guided coaxial catheters for selective angiography and controlled vascular occlusion. *Radiology* 104:421, 1972.

9. Hilal, S. K., Michelsen, W. J., Driller, J., and Leonard, E. Magnetically guided devices for vascular exploration and treatment. *Radiology* 113:529, 1974.

10. Hilal, S. K., and Michelsen, W. J. Therapeutic percutaneous embolization for extra-axial vascular lesions of the head, neck and spine. *J. Neurosurg.* 43:275, 1975.

11. Hilal, S. K., Sane, P., Michelsen, W. J., and Kosseim, A. The embolization of vascular malformations of the spinal cord with low-viscosity silicone rubber. *Neuroradiology* 16:430, 1978.

12. Kerber, C. W., Bank, W. O., and Manelfe, C. Control and placement of intracranial microcatheters. *Am. J. Neuroradiol.* 1:157, 1980.

13. Kricheff, I., Madayag, M., and Braunstein, P. Transfemoral catheter embolization of cerebral and posterior fossa arteriovenous malformations. *Radiology* 103:107, 1972.

14. Luessenhop, A. J., and Spence, W. T. Artificial embolization of cerebral arteries. Report of use in a case of arteriovenous malformation. *J.A.M.A.* 172:1153, 1960.

15. Michelsen, W. J., Hilal, S. K., Sane, P., and Janecka, I. Glomus Jugulare Tumors. In H. Silverstein and H. Norell (eds.), *Neurological Surgery of the Ear.* Birmingham: Aesculapius, 1979. Vol. 2, pp. 364–369.

16. Pevsner, P. H., and Doppman, J. L. Therapeutic embolization with a microballoon catheter system. *Am. J. Neuroradiol.* 1:171, 1980.

17. Serbinenko, F. A. Balloon catheterization and occlusion of major cerebral vessels. *J. Neurosurg.* 41:125, 1974.

18. White, R., Ursic, T. A., Kaufman, S. L., Barth, K. H., Kim, W., and Gross, G. S. Therapeutic embolization with detachable balloons. Physical factors influencing permanent occlusion. *Radiology* 126:521, 1978.

19. Wolpert, S. M., and Stein, B. M. Catheter embolization of intracranial arteriovenous malformations as an aid to surgical excision. *Neuroradiology* 10:73, 1975.

20. Wolpert, S. M., and Stein, B. M. Factors governing the course of emboli in the therapeutic embolization of cerebral arteriovenous malformations. *Radiology* 131:125, 1979.

Nonsurgical Closure of Patent Ductus Arteriosus (14 Years' Experience)

WERNER PORSTMANN
LECH WIERNY

Patent ductus arteriosus (PDA) is one of the commonest cardiovascular malformations, accounting for 12 to 17 percent of all congenital cardiac defects. Its first successful surgical treatment was achieved in 1939 by Gross [1], an accomplishment that marked the beginning of cardiac surgery.

A new technique employed by our team makes use of the catheter instead of the scalpel. The first nonsurgical closure of PDA was done by us in 1966, following several years of model and animal experiments [4–6]. The working principle is described in the text that follows (Fig. 98-1).

A closure plug of Ivalon is passed over a guidewire and forced from the aortic side into the open duct. The guidewire is removed, leaving the occluding plug permanently in place in the ductus. Although the basic approach remains valid, details have been modified with growing experience. The site of the catheter entry is at the femoral vessels. Originally, the femoral artery and vein were surgically exposed in all patients; that is now done only in small children or in patients with oversized ductus; that is, only when the ductal diameter exceeds the diameter of the femoral artery. To begin the procedure, special catheters are percutaneously introduced into the femoral artery and vein under local anesthesia.

The arterial catheter is passed via the aorta into the open duct. A guidewire is threaded through this catheter across the open duct and into the pulmonary artery, where the venous catheter with a protruding loop snare is waiting. The arterial guidewire is caught in that loop snare and is pulled out the venous side (Fig. 98-2).

The arterio-transductal-venous guidewire loop thus formed is essential to the entire closing procedure. A coaxial plug introducer is now inserted into the femoral artery over the arterial end of the guidewire loop. This introducer consists of thin-walled Teflon tubes that telescope into one another and provide for gradual dilatation of the artery. The inner tubes of the introducer assembly are removed when the outermost tube has reached the aortic bifurcation (Fig. 98-3). The closing plug, passed through a central hole onto the guidewire, is forced through the outermost tube into the aorta and from there is pushed and pulled into the duct by means of the catheter arrangement (Fig. 98-4). Plug introducers used with the percutaneous technique range from 12 to 22 French, depending on the size of the duct to be closed.

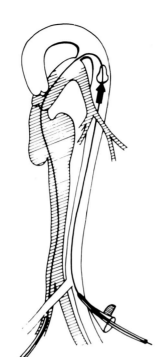

Figure 98-1. Diagrammatic representation of percutaneous closure of a patent ductus arteriosus. The plug is moved into position along a previously placed arterio-transductal-venous loop. Here, it is depicted in the aorta. (From Porstmann et al. [6]. Reproduced with permission from *Radiol. Clin. North Am.*)

Figure 98-2. Capture of the arterially introduced guidewire in the superior vena cava aids in establishing the necessary arterio-transductal-venous guidewire loop. This can also be done in the pulmonary artery or the aorta. The dotted catheter is arterial; the hatched catheter lies on the venous side. (From Porstmann et al. [6]. Reproduced with permission from *Radiol. Clin. North Am.*)

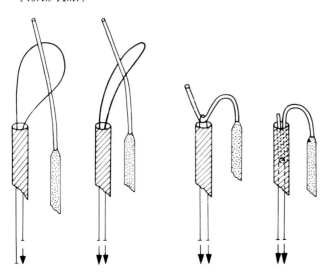

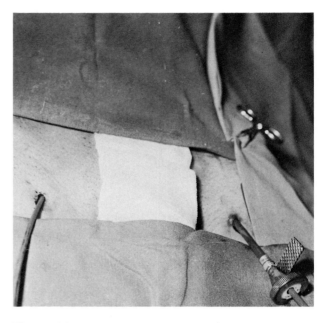

Figure 98-3. Catheter in the right femoral vein. The applicator for plug transportation is in the left femoral artery.

Closure plug shape is also dependent on ductal size and shape, as shown by preliminary lateral aortography (Fig. 98-5A, B).

The closure plug is conical and is made of precompressed Ivalon foam (polyvinyl alcohol foam; Unipoint Industries) (Fig. 98-6). Once forced into the duct, it is "self-retained." Its reinforcement, necessary for transport through the introducer and fixation within the PDA, is achieved by a frame of stainless wire. Plug radiopacity is based either on the wire frame alone or on the concomitant use of radiopaque polyvinyl alcohol foam.

Thus far, we have used this technique in closing ducts in 180 patients without mortality and with a high success rate. The method has been adopted by others in Japan, Taiwan, and Poland [2, 8, 9]. By the end of 1979, more than 500 patients had been treated.

The average mortality in surgical PDA closure is about 1 or 2 percent; it increases with age. However, in over 500 catheter-treated patients in a Japanese group, only one death occurred, giving a collective mortality of less than 0.2 percent.

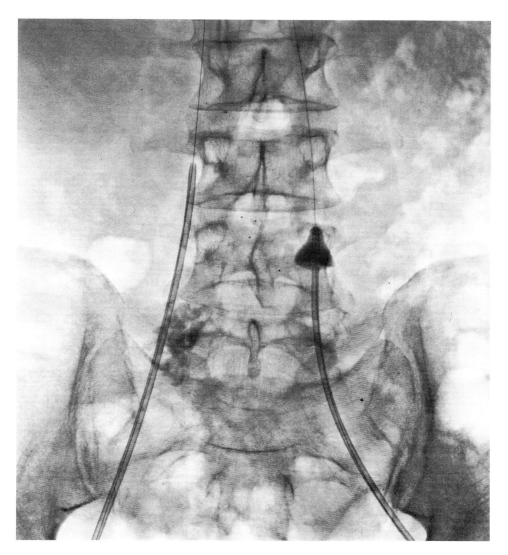

Figure 98-4. Radiopaque plug traveling on the arterial-transductal-venous guidewire on its way to the patent ductus arteriosus.

In general, cardiac surgeons and pediatric cardiologists have not accepted catheter closure, because, as they say, PDA can be treated surgically in infants whereas transfemoral closure is not yet possible in the first 3 or 4 years of life (depending on body size, PDA width, and the width of the femoral vessels).

That view is not consistent with reality. Patent ductus is often first discovered in older children and adults, who are candidates for transfemoral, nonoperative closure. We agree with the surgical dictum that every isolated patent ductus with left-to-right shunting should be closed. Three conditions must be met before we undertake nonsurgical closure:

1. The duct must be smaller than the femoral artery.
2. The duct must be conical or cylindrical.
3. The transductal shunt must be left to right.

The presence of these conditions can be established by heart catheterization and arteriography. They were present in 173 of our 180 patients. In the other seven patients, although shunting was left to right, the ducts were unusually large. A modified catheter technique was used on these high-risk patients [3]. More details are given below.

Pulmonary artery pressures were normal to moderately increased in most of our patients.

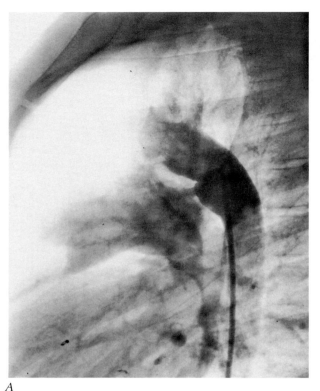

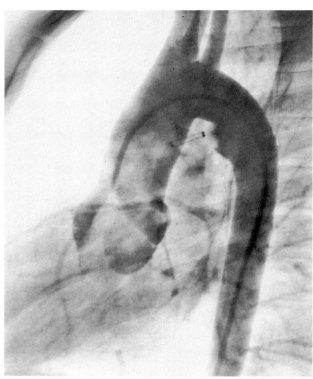

A   *B*

Figure 98-5. Aortography in the lateral projection before (A) and after (B) closure of the patent ductus arteriosus.

Figure 98-6. Schematic drawing of closure plug with its inner steel wire frame.

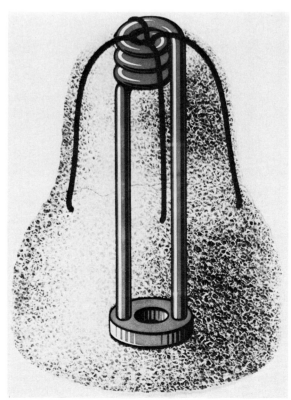

Pressures as high as 60 to 100 mm Hg were encountered in only 10 patients.

Left-to-right shunting, as determined by dye dilution, ranged from 20 to 80 percent of pulmonary blood flow. The patients were from 5 to 57 years old.

Japanese workers have treated a larger number of children than we have. Their youngest patient was 3 years old at the time of treatment [2]. We believe that with our current technique, uncomplicated patent ductus can be closed in most patients, even those of preschool age. In other words, a widespread pediatric demand can be met without the need for a thoracotomy. Surgical treatment continues to be necessary when PDA in infants leads to cardiac failure. Rashkind [7] has developed a modification of transluminal ductal closure that has been used with success on infants and small children. Following femoral arteriotomy, ductal closure was effected from the aortic side without a transductal guidewire/security loop, using an umbrella-like device fixed in place by wire hooks. Thus, in one form or another, transvascular ductal closure appears to be applicable to all age groups.

Most patients with PDA are female; in our series the ratio of females to males was 4 to 1. Thus the transfemoral technique has avoided thoracotomy scars in 112 young girls and women below 35. The cosmetic effect of a thoracotomy scar and its psychologic impact on the girl or woman is rarely discussed by the cardiac surgeon.

Failures and Complications

Transfemoral closure of PDA using a precompressed, self-retaining plug, proved impossible in 10 of 173 patients (the failure rate was 5.8%). The ducts of these 10 patients were subsequently ligated surgically.

In rare instances early in our experience, efforts had to be discontinued because plugs that were too small slipped through the duct. Such plugs were pushed along the guidewire into the femoral vein and removed by venotomy. Experience has taught us that in such (rare) circumstances, a second attempt with a larger plug will lead to success in the same session. In four cases, following removal of the safety guidewire, the closure plug embolized to the aortic bifurcation and had to be removed by arteriotomy. This complication can be avoided by checking the plug fixation before the guidewire is withdrawn. This is done by attempting to push the plug into the aorta using the transvenous catheter.

Following the procedure, close attention was

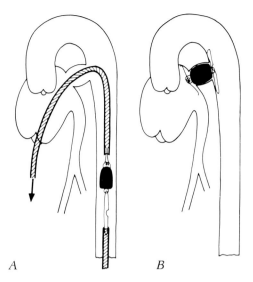

Figure 98-8. Principle of plug anchorage in a patent ductus arteriosus with a diameter larger than that of the femoral artery. (A) A transarterially introduced plug with springs at both ends fitted between the two catheters prepared for transportation through the pelvic arteries and the aorta. (B) The plug in position fixed by latches at both the aortic and the pulmonary ends. (From Porstmann et al. [3]. Reproduced with permission from *Circulation*.)

given to leg blood flow. Follow-up checks disclosed femoral bruits in several patients and the absence of a femoral pulse in 13 patients. Corrective vascular surgery was done in seven patients. This complication was attributed to the early design of the plug introducer, which has since been improved. That it was unrelated to the percutaneous technique itself may be seen from Figure 98-7, in which complications are summarized over three periods of time, in relation to modes of entry into the vascular system. In our 180-case series, the complication rate has continued to decline, no doubt because of improved instruments and accumulated experience (Fig. 98-7).

Surgery, too, has complications; among our successfully treated patients, there were five with postsurgical patency.

The standard technique was not applicable to seven patients with excessively large ducts, large left-to-right shunts, and hypervolemic pulmonary hypertension. Ductal diameters in these cases exceeded femoral artery diameters. Therefore, an attempt was made to modify the closure technique. An almost uncompressed plug was introduced percutaneously through the femoral artery. A special anchoring device was provided to

Figure 98-7. Mode of entrance into the femoral artery (percutaneous or surgical exposure) during three periods of time in relation to arterial complications (shown below the graph) at the entry side.

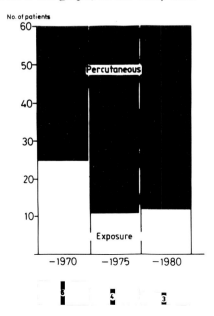

fix it in the aorta and pulmonary artery (Fig. 98-8). Most of the seven cases in which this modified approach was tried had been rejected by cardiac surgeons. Two of our attempts failed, incomplete closure was achieved in another two, and complete closure was achieved in the remaining three.

Conclusions

Although the modified technique could be further improved, we have put our developmental efforts elsewhere because the technique is rarely needed. Nevertheless, the switch from precompressed self-retaining closure plugs to uncompressed closing material, anchored in the duct by other means, offers further improvement, not only by facilitating closure of excessively large ducts but also by allowing percutaneous closure in smaller children, as in Rashkind's modification [7].

Percutaneous transfemoral closure of PDA takes about 30 minutes. Less than 10 minutes is required for fluoroscopy. Blood loss is usually less than 50 cc. The patient stays in bed 3 days, and then leaves the hospital after another 2 days.

PDA was the first congenital cardiovascular defect to be treated surgically. It is also the first such defect to be cured without surgery, as is shown by our results and confirmed by others during the last 14 years.

References

1. Gross, G. W., and Hubbard, J. P. Surgical ligation of a patent ductus arteriosus. *J. Am. Med. Assoc.* 112:729, 1939.
2. Kitamura, S., Sato, K., Naito, Y., Shimizu, Y., Fujino, M., Oyama, C., Nakano, S., and Kawashima, Y. Plug closure of patent ductus arteriosus by transfemoral catheter method: Cooperative study with surgery and a new technical modification. *Chest* 70:631, 1976.
3. Porstmann, W., Hieronymi, K., Wierny, L., and Warnke, H. Nonsurgical closure of oversized PDA with pulmonary hypertension. *Circulation* 50:376, 1974.
4. Porstmann, W., Wierny, L., and Warnke, H. Der Verschluss des Ductus arteriosus persistens ohne Thorakotomie: I. Mitteilung. *Thoraxchirurgie* 15:199, 1967.
5. Porstmann, W., Wierny, L., and Warnke, H. Der Verschluss des Ductus arteriosus persistens ohne Thorakotomie: II. Mitteilung *ROEFO* 109:133, 1968.
6. Porstmann, W., Wierny, L., Warnke, H., Gerstberger, G., and Romaniuk, P. A. Catheter closure of patent ductus arteriosus. *Radiol. Clin. North Am.* 9:203, 1971.
7. Rashkind, W. J., and Cuaso, Ch. C. Transcatheter closure of patent ductus arteriosus. *Pediatr. Cardiol.* 1:3, 1979.
8. Sato, K., Fujino, M., Kozuka, T., Naito, Y., Kitamura, S., Nakano, S., Ohyama, C., and Kawashima, Y. Transfemoral plug closure of patent ductus arteriosus. *Circulation* 51:337, 1975.
9. Takamiya, M., Tadokoro, M., and Okada, Y. Nonsurgical closure of PDA: Report of 23 cases. *Nippon Kyobu Geka Gakkai Zasshi* 21:196, 1973.

Therapeutic Renal Angiography

JOSEF RÖSCH
FREDERICK S. KELLER
CHARLES T. DOTTER

The kidney is one of the parenchymal organs best suited for therapeutic angiography. In the majority of people (about 70%), it is supplied by a single, large, well-localized renal artery that is easy to catheterize. Usually a catheter can also be advanced into segmental and, occasionally, interlobar renal branches, thus enabling selective therapy of peripheral lesions. Specific characteristics of the rich renal arterial vascular bed also contribute to the suitability of the kidney for angiographic treatment. For instance, its high vasoactive sensitivity makes it amenable to selective pharmacoangiotherapy, and its terminal type of branching, without the presence of significant parenchymal communications, makes the kidney ideal for selective transcatheter occlusive therapy of focal lesions located in segmental or subsegmental portions of the renal parenchyma. Absence of arterial collateral vessels between renal segments also prevents the development of hypertension after arterial occlusion since total infarction rather than ischemia of the corresponding renal tissue results and, therefore, the renin-angiotensin mechanism is not activated.

A relatively high index of safety is another positive factor in therapeutic renal angiography. Even though the kidney is one of the most richly perfused parenchymal organs, receiving 20 to 25 percent of the cardiac output, it has a relatively low sensitivity to ischemia. At body temperature, renal tissue can tolerate up to 20 minutes of ischemia with rapid and complete recovery of function. Longer ischemic periods of up to 60 minutes lead to an initial loss of function and a delayed recovery in 1 to 2 weeks [32, 65]. Organ bilaterality makes the kidney amenable to one-sided renal ablation; and, in addition, renal dialysis or renal transplantation makes even bilateral renal ablation possible when life-threatening pathologic renal function is present.

The kidney has, therefore, been one of the organs most often exposed to therapeutic angiography, and a wide range of procedures has been used for a variety of indications in the management of pathologic renal processes. Angiography has occasionally been used to protect the kidney from insults, such as radiation and surgical ischemia, or for the treatment of medical diseases, such as hepatorenal failure and acute transplant rejection. Most often, however, therapeutic angiography has been used for surgical indications, as an adjunct to surgery or even an alternative to surgery. Therapeutic angiography can replace surgery in controlling renal hemorrhage of various origin, in obliterating major nonbleeding arteriovenous connections, in treating varicocele or acute thromboembolism of the renal artery, and, occasionally, for therapy of renovascular hypertension. In selected cases, catheter therapy can be used instead of surgery, even for nephrectomy or for palliation of renal tumors. Preoperative angiographic embolotherapy is a useful adjunct to nephrectomy, particularly for large tumors, since it substantially simplifies the operative procedure. Furthermore, angiographic therapeutic techniques can also be applied successfully to the urinary tract, with percutaneous nephrostomy as an attractive alternative to surgery for decompression of an obstructed urinary tract.

General Considerations

Successful and safe angiographic treatment requires a detailed diagnostic angiographic study, as well as considerable knowledge, experience, technical skill, and responsibility on the part of the angiographer.

Accurate and detailed anatomic delineation of the lesion(s) with evaluation of regional vascular anatomy is a prerequisite for making decisions concerning therapeutic angiography. The extent of the lesion and the number and location of the feeding arteries and draining veins should be demonstrated. Careful attention must always be directed to the presence and size of direct arteriovenous communications. Diagnostic angiography should, if possible, be separated from the therapeutic procedure, thus giving additional time to gather necessary information about the patient, to select the optimal therapeutic approach, and to prepare both the patient and the necessary angiographic equipment for a successful and safe therapeutic procedure. Often, however, emergency conditions exist, and the angiographer has to be ready to combine the diagnostic and therapeutic procedures. This combination, particularly if performed on patients in unstable condition, has limitations and must be executed carefully because it not only increases the risk of therapeutic angiography but also may limit the angiographer's method of treatment.

Furthermore, therapeutic angiography requires additional responsibility from the angiographer. The decision for angiographic treatment must be made on the basis of knowledge of the natural course of the specific disease process and familiarity with the available therapeutic alternatives. Decisions about therapy are then made only after the benefits of angiographic therapy are carefully weighed against the risks. Selection of the appropriate angiographic therapeutic technique (which can vary widely, depending on the type of lesion and on the therapeutic goals) requires basic experience with a variety of methods and occlusive means. The angiographer's technical skill, knowledge of his own limitations, awareness of complications, and ability to avoid or manage them are important factors affecting the safety of angiographic treatment.

Therapeutic angiography also has certain technical requirements; it should be performed with an excellent fluoroscopic image-intensifying system and television monitor. A videodisk recorder with replay capability and, particularly, with superimposition of past- and real-time images can aid the work of the therapeutic angiographer.

Technical Notes

In preparing the patient for occlusive procedures resulting in renal infarction, a moderate dose of narcotics is recommended. For other types of procedures, only mild sedation similar to that used in diagnostic studies is usually employed.

The *femoral approach* is used in the majority of cases, and either side is suitable for catheterization of the renal arteries. In transplant patients with anastomosis of the renal artery to a hypogastric artery, the contralateral femoral approach gives good catheter access to the transplant. With anastomosis of the transplant renal artery to the external iliac artery, the ipsilateral femoral approach is preferred. The left axillary approach may occasionally be useful for superselective catheterization in patients with caudally oriented renal arteries. If multiple catheter exchanges or the use of nontapered catheters is anticipated, a thin-wall sheath should be used for catheter introduction and exchanges.

Catheters for angiographic treatment are mostly the same as those used for diagnosis—preshaped and with high torque control. They are sufficiently large to allow passage of occlusive materials and devices. For application of larger obstructive devices, nontapered catheters are often necessary.

Selective and superselective *catheterization* is often possible with traditional diagnostic, single-curve catheters used in conjunction with guidewires or external deflector systems. Double-curve catheters, preshaped according to the vascular anatomy, or coaxial catheters may sometimes be necessary to achieve the desired superselective position. With high-flow lesions, flow-guided balloon catheters are useful for superselective catheterization. Conventional balloon catheters are usually used as an ancillary means to prevent reflux of embolic material; fixed balloons are used for temporary vascular occlusion, and detachable balloons are used for permanent vascular occlusion.

The *selection of materials or devices* (described in detail in previous chapters) for renal vascular occlusion depends on several factors, particularly on the type of lesion to be occluded and the character of its vessels, the desired duration of occlusion, the catheter accessibility, the availability of suitable occlusive materials or devices, and the angiographer's preference and familiarity with their use. There is no one occlusive material or device that is appropriate under all circumstances for all lesions. Therapeutic angiographers must, therefore, be familiar with a variety of materials and devices in order to choose from them as indicated by case-specific needs. Fortunately, several occlusive means are capable of achieving equally good results, and, therefore, experience with a few suitable methods usually suffices to achieve the ultimate goal of the therapeutic angiographer—a safe and effective vascular occlusion.

Generally, balloon catheters of various sizes offer an effective and safe means for temporary, immediately reversible occlusion, even of the large arteries, particularly in cases of massive bleeding. For short-term occlusion (hours to a few days), autologous clot or its modification with Amicar may be a useful occlusive material. For medium-term occlusion (days to weeks), such materials as absorbable gelatin sponge (Gelfoam) and microcrystalline collagen (Avitene) can be used in the form of either particles or powder. Permanent vascular occlusion is usually achieved by the application of microparticles of polyvinyl alcohol sponge (Ivalon), liquid polymers, such as cyanoacrylate tissue adhesive (bucrylate) or silicone rubber mixtures, or by the installation of mechanical devices, particularly Gianturco coil spring occluders or detachable balloons. Simple and effective permanent occlusion of the desired amount of vasculature is often also achieved by a combination of peripheral Gelfoam emboli and central placement of a coil spring occluder.

Kidney Protection

Therapeutic angiography has been used relatively rarely to protect the kidney. Promising original reports that documented good results of angiographic techniques in the prevention of radiation nephritis, the management of hepatorenal failure and acute transplant rejection, and the prevention of renal damage during surgery have not been widely accepted. The theoretic potential of therapeutic angiography for these indications thus remains to be further substantiated by greater clinical use.

PREVENTION OF RADIATION NEPHRITIS

Decreased radiosensitivity of hypoxic tissue is the rationale for preventing or reducing radiation nephritis. Of several techniques for inducing hypoxia, a selective infusion of epinephrine that produces a marked but rapidly reversible vasoconstriction has been used to achieve temporary renal ischemia. After successful exploration in animals, this technique has been used clinically in patients receiving radiotherapy for advanced retroperitoneal or diffuse abdominal malignancies [52, 90, 91]. An indwelling renal arterial catheter was left in place for the duration of the course of radiotherapy, lasting from 12 to 23 days. Several minutes prior to and during periods of actual radiation treatment, small doses of epinephrine (4–8 μg/min) were infused into the renal artery. The mean time of the vasoconstrictive period was about 10 minutes. Between treatments, the catheter was kept open by a microinfusion of heparinized saline. This technique has helped preserve renal function and prevent radiation nephritis without any undue side effects despite high doses of radiation.

HEPATORENAL SYNDROME

Therapeutic angiography with a selective infusion of dopamine has been used in attempts to alter the renal component of the hepatorenal syndrome. Renal failure in decompensated cirrhosis is accompanied by significant vasoconstriction of the cortical arteries leading to cortical ischemia and redistribution of renal flow [1, 28]. Dopamine hydrochloride infused selectively into the renal artery in subpressor doses (2–6 μg/kg/min) can reverse most of these renal hemodynamic changes and, particularly, can relieve cortical vasospasm and improve the cortical blood flow [10]. Infusions lasting 1 hour have resulted in some temporary improvement of the renal component of the hepatorenal syndrome. The effects of long-term infusions on the prognosis of this grave disease complex remain to be explored.

ACUTE TRANSPLANT REJECTION

Acute allograft rejection with secondary oliguric renal failure also has a high component of cortical vasoconstriction [1, 51]. The effects of selective infusions of vasodilators on cortical vasospasm have not yet been clinically studied; however, preliminary experience has shown that an acute episode of rejection can be treated successfully by a continuous selective infusion of methylprednisolone into the transplanted renal artery [35].

SURGICAL RENAL DAMAGE

Percutaneous balloon occlusion of the renal artery combined with intermittent hypothermic perfusion of the kidney has been used successfully to facilitate kidney surgery and to prevent or diminish operative renal damage, particularly during an extensive nephrolithotomy [62, 63]. The inflated balloon of a double-lumen balloon catheter can cause renal ischemia as effectively as clamp occlusion. Intermittent perfusion of the kidney with Ringer's lactate solution cooled to 4 to 6°C via the other catheter lumen can keep the temperature of the kidney between 18 and 25°C. This degree of hypothermia prevents renal damage due to the ischemia necessary for detailed dissection, exploration, and reconstructive work. With this technique, complicated surgery with ischemia times of up to 1 hour can be performed without significant deterioration of function, even on kidneys that are already impaired [62, 63].

Renal Hemorrhage

Renal bleeding is the most frequent indication for therapeutic renal angiography. "Catheter hemostasis" in this setting is a safe, simple, and effective alternative to surgical arterial ligation. It can be the definitive mode of treatment of hemorrhage from a medical disease of the kidney or from traumatic or nontumorous vascular renal lesions. In these settings, angiographic treatment

enables renal tissue and function to be preserved; partial or total nephrectomy would be the only alternative. In hemorrhage from benign and, particularly, malignant tumors, angiographic control of bleeding helps to avoid emergency surgery and permits the definitive surgical procedure to be performed on an elective basis and on a stable patient. Catheter hemostasis can be used in every type of renal hemorrhage, regardless of its etiology. Expeditiously applied techniques are efficient in controlling renal bleeding, whether it is unifocal, multifocal, or diffuse, localized inside the renal parenchyma or extending into the subcapsular, perirenal, or retroperitoneal spaces. The etiology of successfully controlled renal hemorrhage includes various types of traumas—among them, iatrogenic injury after renal biopsy or complicated renal surgery—vascular malformation, and tumors. Gross hematuria is the most common clinical manifestation of renal bleeding for which angiography therapy is used.

The method chosen to control bleeding—vasoconstrictive infusion or vascular occlusion—and, when vascular occlusion is chosen, the selection of the appropriate technique of occlusion depend on several factors. The type, location, extent, and etiology of bleeding, the size of the bleeding vessels, and the nature of the underlying lesion is most important in making decisions about therapy. Success in selective catheterization of the vessels supplying the bleeding lesions also has to be considered. After evaluating these variables, the angiographer can decide whether to attempt only to control bleeding or whether to attempt also to treat definitively the underlying renal lesion by angiographic therapy.

VASOCONSTRICTIVE INFUSIONS

Vasoconstrictive infusions have been used only rarely for the control of renal hemorrhage; however, they should always be considered since they have the lowest risks and are the least invasive. For good indications, vasoconstrictive infusions can be an effective therapeutic modality [50].

Epinephrine, which affects both the peripheral arteries and the major renal arteries, has been the vasoconstrictive drug used most frequently. A 10-minute infusion of epinephrine at 10 μg per minute may be sufficient to control bleeding. We have usually performed two or three 10-minute infusions with interruptions of 10 minutes between them to avoid potential renal damage from prolonged ischemia. No significant side effects or complications have been encountered from infusions of these minimal doses of epinephrine. The dosage, however, should not be increased because prolonged infusions of high doses of epinephrine may induce acute renal failure [56]. Furthermore, caution is necessary in patients with cardiac disease.

Vasoconstrictive infusions are particularly effective in controlling bleeding from small vessels and multifocal hemorrhages (Fig. 99-1). We have also used these infusions successfully to control hemorrhage from a transplanted kidney after biopsy. Infusion may be the primary therapeutic angiographic treatment in cases in which satisfactory catheterization of the bleeding artery cannot be achieved and in which vasoocclusive techniques therefore carry a high risk of unnecessary infarction of normal renal tissue.

Vasoconstrictive infusions cannot be expected to give good results in bleeding from tumors because malignant neoplastic vessels do not respond to vasoactive substances. Epinephrine infusions, however, may be useful in combination

Figure 99-1. Hemorrhage in a renal transplant following open biopsy; the hemorrhage was successfully controlled by selective vasoconstriction. The bleeding was mostly from small vessels (*arrowheads*) and was clinically manifested by gross hematuria. After two 10-minute infusions of 10 μg per minute of epinephrine into the main renal artery, with a 10-minute interval between them, the hematuria ceased and did not recur.

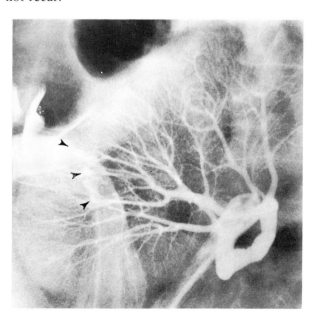

with embolization in treating tumors when vessels supplying the tumor lesion cannot be selectively catheterized. A preliminary epinephrine infusion constricts normal arteries and directs the occlusive material to the nonconstricted tumor vessels.

VASOOCCLUSIVE TECHNIQUES

Vascular occlusive techniques are the most commonly used techniques of angiographic therapy for the control of renal bleeding. Selection of the appropriate occlusive material and/or device depends on the success of selective catheterization and on the nature and degree of bleeding; that is, whether it is a massive hemorrhage, focal traumatic bleeding without an underlying lesion, or a hemorrhage from an underlying pathologic renal process.

Massive Bleeding
Massive bleeding of any type, particularly when the bleeding vessel itself cannot be selectively catheterized, is best controlled by temporary balloon catheter occlusion [82, 102]. This simple technique can be a lifesaver. Placed in the main renal artery and sufficiently inflated, the balloon completely blocks flow. However, the potential for renal damage due to ischemia must be carefully considered and weighed against the risk of recurrent bleeding on deflation of the balloon. A reasonable approach in these situations is the use of a double-lumen catheter for occlusion of the renal artery for 15 to 20 minutes interrupted by periods of balloon deflation ranging from 5 to 10 minutes (Fig. 99-2). During balloon inflation, the kidney could be perfused via the second catheter lumen with cooled Ringer's solution in order to promote some protective renal hypothermia. The deflation periods can be used for follow-up studies.

Focal Traumatic Bleeding Without Underlying Pathologic Processes
Such bleeding is usually treated by vascular occlusion with short- or medium-term occlusive material [54, 59]. Autologous clot or its modification and Gelfoam have been the materials most frequently used for control of this type of bleeding irrespective of whether the hemorrhage presented angiographically by intrarenal, subcapsular, or perinephric extravasation, by pseudoaneurysm, or by traumatic arteriovenous or arteriopelvic fistula of minor dimensions [53,

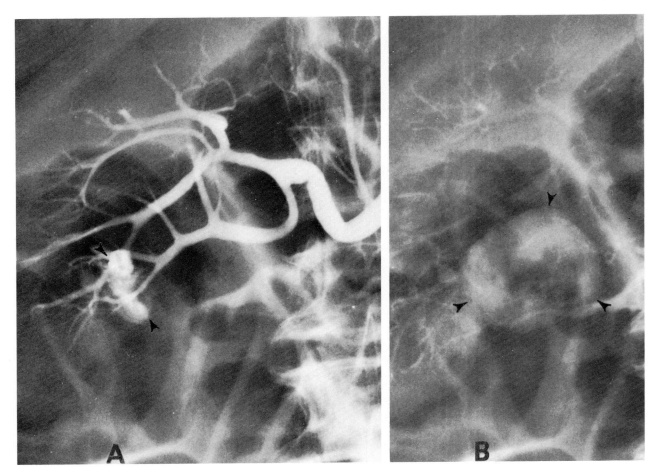

Figure 99-2. Massive renal hemorrhage after percutaneous biopsy controlled by temporary balloon occlusion. The bleeding was clinically manifested by gross hematuria and a rapid fall in the hematocrit. (A) The initial and (B) the late arterial phases of the right renal angiogram demonstrate extravasation of the contrast medium from the lower pole renal artery and a large pseudoaneurysm (*arrowheads*). The hematuria ceased and did not recur after three 15-minute periods of balloon occlusion of the main renal artery separated by 5-minute periods of deflation.

54, 83, 84, 98]. For larger traumatic arteriovenous connections, permanent occlusive devices are recommended [64, 99, 101].

Selective occlusion of the bleeding vessel as close as possible to the bleeding site is the therapeutic objective in focal hemorrhage. It allows maximum conservation of the renal tissue while minimizing the size of renal infarction. Therefore, in these cases, superselective catheterization is of primary importance, as is careful injection of embolic material under fluoroscopic control to avoid reflux and embolization of normal parenchyma. Occlusion therapy resulting in minor renal infarction usually causes only minor transient flank pain.

The use of *autologous clot*, a readily available and usually easily prepared embolic material, is often a satisfactory treatment of this type of bleeding [15, 22, 23, 54, 68, 80, 83, 84]. It is relatively safe and should be used especially when a satisfactory selective catheter position cannot be achieved. Animal research and clinical experience have shown that clot lysis in damaged, bleeding vessels is retarded and that the embolized artery remains occluded for several days. Lysis of clots in the nontraumatized vessels, on the other hand, occurs rapidly, usually within a matter of hours. Therefore, with the use of autologous clot, unintentionally embolized normal renal tissue sustains only minor damage. Like other particulate materials, autologous clot is to be injected in small increments and followed with contrast medium to achieve optimal results.

Gelfoam should be used only when safe selec-

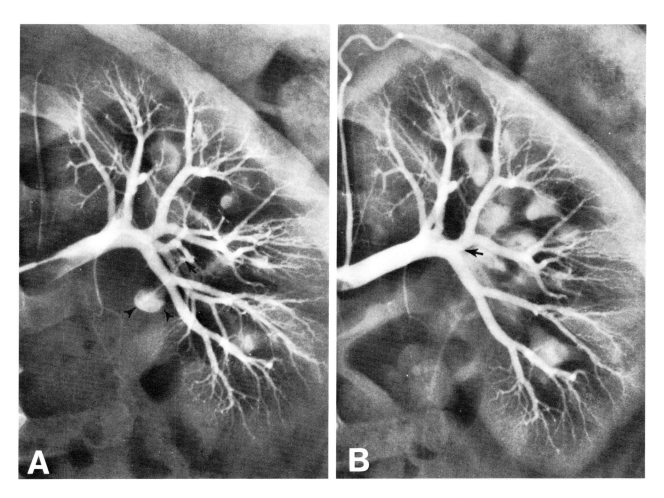

Figure 99-3. Posttraumatic renal hemorrhage successfully controlled by selective Gelfoam vasoocclusion. (A) A control selective renal angiogram demonstrates a traumatic pseudoaneurysm (*arrowheads*) supplied by a small branch of the dorsal segmental artery (*arrow*). (B) A follow-up angiogram immediately after the selective placement of two Gelfoam particles into the segmental artery supplying the pseudoaneurysm demonstrates its occlusion (*arrow*). Avascularity of the corresponding renal parenchyma is present.

tive catheterization of the target vessels can be achieved [21, 37, 78] (Fig. 99-3). The particles of Gelfoam should be large enough not to pass through arteriovenous communications. The particles are tailored to the size of vessel to be occluded and usually are partially opacified by soaking in contrast medium; occasionally they are marked by an attached silver slip. Like autologous clot, their delivery is monitored by injections of contrast medium after each small aliquot of Gelfoam emboli.

Detachable balloons or spring coil occluders—*permanent occlusive devices*—are indicated for the treatment of traumatic fistulas with large arteriovenous communications [99, 101]. Small embolic particles would pass through these fistulas, with resultant pulmonary embolism. A spring coil occluder should be used only when the catheter can be positioned in the involved artery or (optimally) directly into the origin of the fistula. Detachable balloons have an advantage in these cases since they do not require such high selectivity. Because a detachable balloon is flow directed, it can be injected at a considerable distance from the fistula; the high blood flow usually carries it into the fistula's origin. The possibility of testing its position prior to detachment is another advantage.

Bleeding from Underlying Nontraumatic Renal Processes

These processes include aneurysms, congenital vascular malformations, and benign hypervascular tumors; however, nontraumatic hematuria is usu-

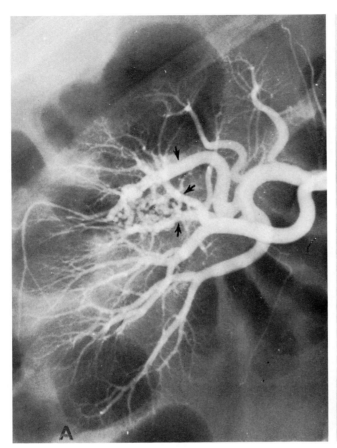
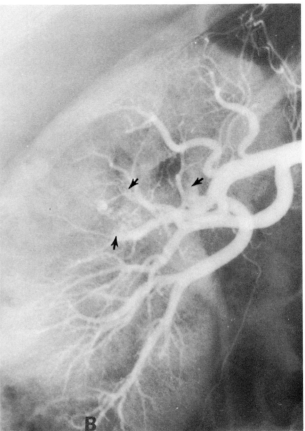

Figure 99-4. Congenital vascular malformation of the right kidney presenting clinically with recurrent gross hematuria. The malformation was treated by selective Gelfoam vasoocclusion without recurrence of the hematuria. (A) A control selective renal angiogram demonstrates a nidus of small vessels and lakes in the midportion of the right kidney supplied mainly by three renal branches (one segmental and two interlobar branches) (*arrows*). (B) A follow-up angiogram immediately after embolization of the nidus and placement of Gelfoam particles into the three supplying branches reveals their occlusion (*arrows*) and only minimal residual filling of the nidus.

ally due to a primary or a metastatic renal malignancy. In such a case, therapeutic angiography is directed not only to controlling the hemorrhage but also to treating the underlying lesion. Permanent vasoocclusive means are usually employed.

Aneurysms are often localized centrally, particularly aneurysms due to atherosclerosis or fibromuscular dysplasia. Their origin from major vessels often permits superselective catheterization and occlusion, avoiding the loss of any renal parenchyma. Expandable devices, mainly the spring coil occluder, are ideal occlusive devices for this type of problem, and their use results in rapid occlusion of the aneurysm. The size and/or eventually the number of coil springs necessary for transcatheter occlusion depends on the size of aneurysm. The use of rapidly polymerizing bu-crylate tissue adhesive is another method of occluding renal aneurysms.

Congenital renal arteriovenous malformations are somewhat more difficult than renal aneurysms to treat angiographically. In contrast to traumatic fistulas, which for the most part are fed by one artery and represent a direct arteriovenous communication, congenital malformations are formed by a nidus of small vessels and lakes usually supplied by several segmental branches (Fig. 99-4). They often occur in peripheral portions of the kidney, which may make their selective occlusion without secondary renal infarction difficult. Skillful catheterization, however, permits occlusive therapy with only minimal infarction of the renal tissue [12, 13, 15, 21, 31, 47, 55, 99].

Congenital malformations are best treated by

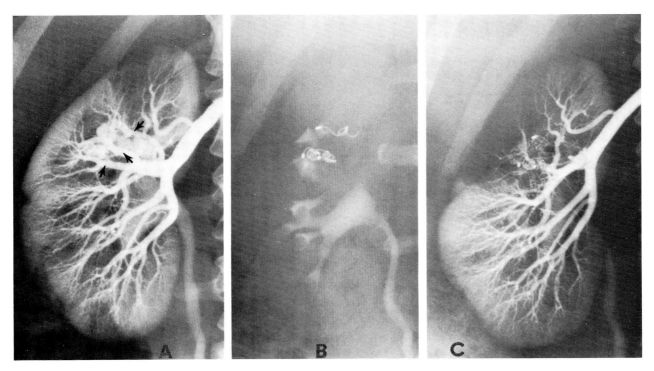

Figure 99-5. A congenital vascular malformation of the right kidney clinically manifested by recurrent gross hematuria. The malformation was treated by a combination of selective Gelfoam embolization and selective placement of small (3-mm) spring coil occluders. (A) A control selective renal angiogram reveals a nidus of small vessels and lakes in the upper half of the right kidney, with early venous filling. Three of the supplying branches (*arrows*) were occluded. (B and C) Follow-up studies 3 months later, after vasoocclusive therapy. An intravenous pyelogram (B) shows good renal function and 3 spring coil occluders. An angiogram (C) reveals continuous occlusion of the three branches, with infarction of the corresponding renal parenchyma and no filling of the malformation.

occlusion of their nidus by the use of a temporary or permanent occlusive material followed by a permanent material or device to occlude the feeding arteries. In the past, when temporary occlusive materials were used mostly for embolization, some malformations recurred. For occlusion of a nidus, small particles of Gelfoam or Ivalon are generally used only in minute quantities, since the nidus of renal malformations is relatively small. An occlusion device, a spring coil occluder or a detachable balloon, is then placed into the feeding vessel, ideally just at the fistula [101] (Fig. 99-5). Small (2–3 mm) spring coil occluders are usually sufficient because of the small vessel size. When tissue adhesive is used, mixing it with Pantopaque enables "timed" polymerization and "cast" occlusion of both the nidus and the feeding vessel [25].

If selective catheterization of all feeding vessels is not possible, it is better to leave one or two small arteries open rather than risk major renal infarction by the occlusion of larger vessels. The nidus of congenital renal malformations has a relatively low tendency for growth. Cases have been reported in which occlusion of the nidus and only one supplying vessel prevented further bleeding. Even if bleeding recurs, occlusive therapy can be repeated with favorable prospects since a residual vessel or vessels may have enlarged after the first vasoocclusion.

Hemorrhage from *benign renal tumors* is a relatively rare indication for angiographic therapy. The benefits of controlling hemorrhage with maximal preservation of renal tissue, however, should not be forgotten for those patients who are not good surgical candidates or for whom radical operations, such as partial or total nephrectomy, are not suitable. This concept is particularly important in patients with angiomyolipoma involving a solitary kidney and in patients having multifocal tumor involvement of both kidneys [17, 71]. Control of bleeding by infarction of the entire tumor or as much tumor as possible is the therapeutic objective in such cases. Successful positioning of the catheter close to or directly in the tumor can often be achieved because the supplying vessels are usually enlarged. Gelfoam or Ivalon is frequently used for embolization of the tumor vasculature. Feeding vessels are then occluded, with a permanent occluding device when necessary. Acrylic tissue adhesive is also very useful in this situation. Even when a tumor cannot be completely occluded because of the inability to catheterize all the supplying arteries, particularly the smaller ones, the infarcted and later necrotic portion of the tumor shrinks and the rest of the tumor often does not rebleed. Infarction of large tumor masses is usually accompanied by side effects, mainly pain requiring narcotics and/or fever for a few days.

Most *malignant tumors* referred for angiographic control of their bleeding are in their late stages. The therapeutic objectives and occlusive techniques are the same as those for the general treatment of renal malignancies, which are discussed in the section that follows.

Malignant Tumors

Selective chemotherapeutic infusions, selective intraarterial irradiation, and, particularly, therapeutic infarction by vasoocclusion are the available techniques of angiographic treatment of primary and metastatic kidney malignancies.

SELECTIVE INTRAARTERIAL CHEMOTHERAPY

Selective intraarterial administration of cytostatic agents was suggested prior to the advent of therapeutic tumor infarction for the palliation of unresectable renal malignancies [57]. Its use has not been explored further clinically. This technique, however, remains a possibility when other therapeutic modes cannot be employed. In combination with selective application of epinephrine during short-term infusions to divert most of the toxic drug from normal renal parenchyma to the tumor, it would be possible to deliver high doses of cytostatic agents. Selective chemotherapy, however, would not be indicated in tumors with multiple large arteriovenous connections, which would permit rapid passage of the drug through the tumor.

SELECTIVE INTRAARTERIAL IRRADIATION

Implantation of radioactive pellets via an angiographic catheter directly inside the tumor mass has been successfully used clinically for therapy of renal cell carcinoma but has not had wide application following the introduction of tumor infarction with nonradioactive occlusive means [57, 58, 85]. Pellets containing isotopes of gold, radon, or yttrium were injected through catheters positioned deep in the renal branches supplying the tumor or, preferably, directly in the tumor and, in the case of extrarenal tumor extension, into the perirenal vessels. Infusion of epinephrine prior to injection of the pellets helps to channel them into the tumor if a satisfactory superselective catheter position cannot be achieved. Isotope seeds must be large enough to lodge deep inside the tumor and not pass through arteriovenous shunts into the venous circulation. To avoid tumor hypoxia with concomitant radioresistance, arterial feeders to the tumor are not occluded.

This method has enabled selective high-dose therapeutic tumor irradiation without damage to normal renal tissue or the small intestine. It has usually resulted in a substantial decrease in tumor size and has been used for palliation or (preoperatively) to facilitate tumor resection [58]. Tumors once considered inoperable were later found to be amenable to resection after selective irradiation. The radioisotopes employed have a relatively short half-life, ranging from 2 to 4 days. Therefore, the radioactivity was only minimal when nephrectomy was performed about 3 weeks after isotope implantation, and safe handling of the specimen was possible.

VASOOCCLUSION

Therapeutic infarction of the entire tumor is an objective of the vasoocclusive-embolization therapy of renal malignancies. Occasionally, when the tumor is fairly localized, it can be selectively embolized with only segmental infarction of surrounding renal parenchyma and preservation of the rest of the renal tissue. Most malignancies referred for vasoocclusive therapy, however, are large, involve major parts of the kidney, and sometimes extend into the extrarenal tissues so that infarction of the whole kidney is usually done. Vasoocclusive treatment of renal malignancies is performed either as a preoperative step to facilitate nephrectomy or for tumor palliation.

The value of *preoperative tumor infarction* has been widely debated by surgeons; most agree that it should not be done routinely but consider it a valuable ancillary procedure in the treatment of large, hypervascular tumors. Preoperative renal vascular occlusion facilitates surgery in these tumors by decreasing the operative time and blood loss [3–5, 16, 18, 30, 38, 44, 46, 49, 60, 61, 76, 81, 86, 93] (Fig. 99-6). Preoperative renal infarction substantially reduces or completely eliminates the blood flow to the tumor and kidney, allowing initial ligation of the renal vein without tumor engorgement [49, 86, 93]. Furthermore, preoperative renal infarction results in a reduction in the tumor size. Even large tumors invading the renal veins are easier to re-

sect [38]. Preoperative infarction also induces perirenal edema, which makes tissue planes more distinct, thereby aiding the dissection of the kidney during nephrectomy [3–5]. A hypothetical reason for preoperative renal infarction is that it decreases the chance of embolization of tumor cells into the venous circulation during surgical manipulation [44, 59, 60]. Opinions concerning the timing of preoperative vasoocclusion have widely differed. Some surgeons prefer that it be done immediately before the operation, to avoid the early side effects of embolization, whereas others have delayed surgery 1 to 2 weeks after infarction to maximize the immunologic response [16, 17, 39, 70]. In most cases, however, surgery has been done about 48 hours after embolization.

Vasoocclusive treatment for *tumor palliation* is performed in patients who cannot sustain ne-

Figure 99-6. Preoperative vasoocclusion of a large renal cell carcinoma of the right kidney by Gelfoam. (A) A control selective renal angiogram reveals a large renal cell carcinoma involving a major portion of the

right kidney. (B) A follow-up angiogram immediately after Gelfoam embolization shows obliteration of the entire tumor vasculature and most of the kidney vasculature.

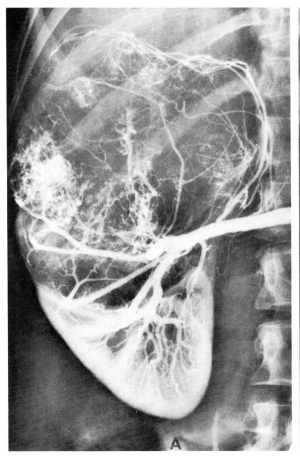
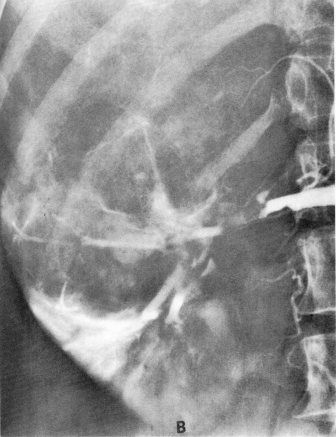

phrectomy and in patients with unresectable tumors, particularly for control of local symptoms, such as bleeding and pain. Embolization is effective for both these symptoms [24, 26, 30, 34, 38, 43, 45, 79, 94, 95, 100]. There has been some evidence that embolization also decreases tumor progression and that it both prolongs and improves survival [4, 38, 70, 92]. In several cases, reduction in size or complete disappearance of the tumor metastases has been documented. These responses are possibly due to stimulation of immunologic activity; that is, tumor necrosis following embolization and infarction may enhance the organism's autoimmune response to tumor cells and tissue [26, 70]. The unpredict-

able natural course of renal cell carcinoma, however, makes it difficult to evaluate therapeutic successes.

The technique of *preoperative vasoocclusion* of renal malignancies may be simple, particularly when surgery follows immediately. Inflation of a balloon catheter in the main renal artery or placement of a spring coil occluder is sometimes all that is necessary [60, 63]. Often, however, tumor embolization is done with Gelfoam particles [49]. Some angiographers follow tumor embolization by spring coil occlusion of the main renal artery. The spring coil should be placed in the distal portion of the main renal artery, because if it is inserted close to the renal artery ori-

Figure 99-7. Therapeutic infarction of a large renal cell carcinoma of the right kidney by a combination of Gelfoam embolization and spring coil occluders for tumor palliation. (A) A control selective renal angiogram shows a huge hypervascular renal cell carcinoma of the right kidney extending into the surrounding tis-

sues. (B) A follow-up angiogram after Gelfoam tumor embolization and placement of six spring coil occluders (*arrows*) in vessels supplying the tumor (five occluders are in the renal branches and one occluder is in the adrenal artery) shows almost complete obliteration of the tumor vasculature.

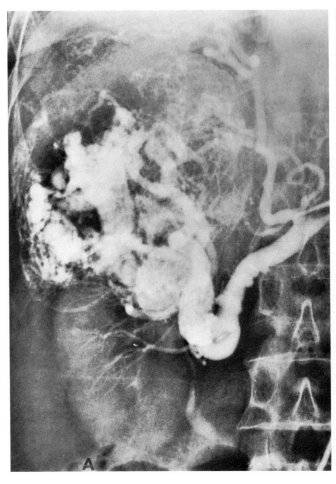
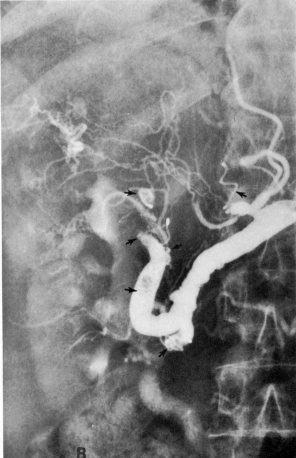

gin, it could be dislodged into the aorta during the surgical manipulation, particularly during ligature of the renal artery [104].

The aim of *palliative treatment* is embolization of the entire tumor vasculature, from its main feeders to its peripheral branches (Fig. 99-7). Without occlusion of the peripheral vessels, collateral vessels could form from capsular branches, and the peripheral portions of the tumor could revascularize [14, 26, 30, 70, 81]. Permanent occlusive material, such as Ivalon or isobutyl 2-cyanoacrylate tissue adhesive, bucrylate, is preferable for embolization (Fig. 99-8). If Gelfoam is used for peripheral embolization, the central renal branches and/or the main renal artery should be occluded by an obstructive device to prevent recanalization. A spring coil occluder

is ideal for this. Depending on the size and the vascularity of the tumor, several spring coil occluders may be placed in major vessels to ensure permanent occlusion (see Fig. 99-7). The size of occlusive particles or the timing of polymerization of bucrylate is selected to obstruct peripheral vessels but not to pass through tumorous arteriovenous shunts. In the presence of large, high-flow tumor shunts, a balloon catheter obstructing the renal artery and renal vein may help to slow down the renal flow and allow the safe delivery of the occlusive material. Usually the whole kidney is embolized, and no renal parenchyma on the involved side is preserved (Fig. 99-9). With tumor extension outside the kidney, all the additional supply arteries (i.e., the adrenal, phrenic, and lumbar arteries) are also

Figure 99-8. Therapeutic infarction of a hypervascular renal cell carcinoma of the left kidney by bucrylate mixed with tantalum for palliative tumor therapy. (A) A control selective renal angiogram reveals a hypervascular tumor involving mostly the medial portion of the kidney without major arteriovenous communications. (B) A follow-up open film after bucrylate embolization shows an opaque "cast" in the entire tumor vasculature, in most of the kidney, and within the main renal artery.

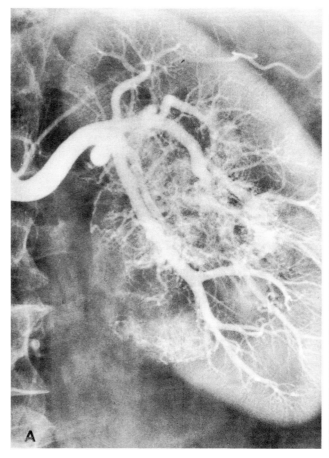

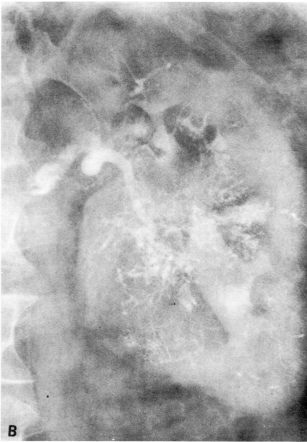

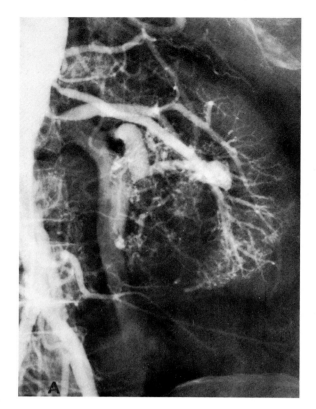

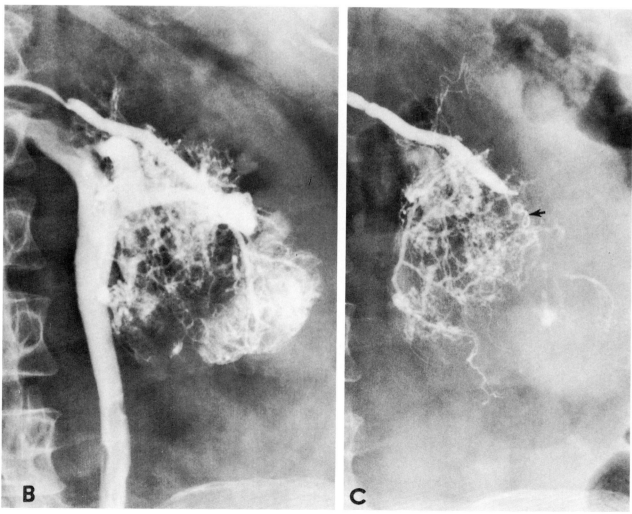

2276

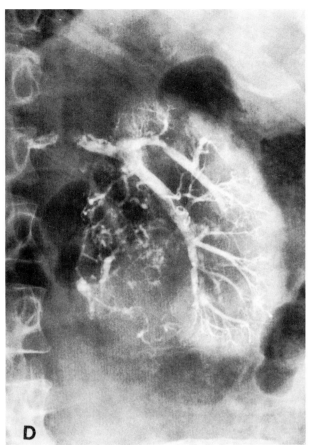

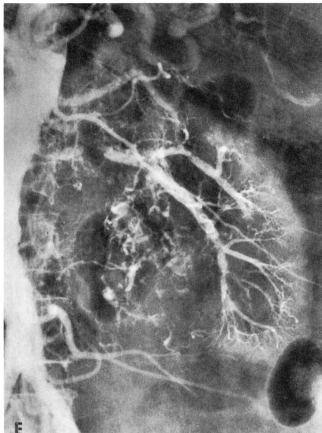

Figure 99-9. Palliative infarction of a hypervascular renal cell carcinoma containing a large, direct, arteriovenous communication. A combination of bucrylate tissue adhesive and a spring coil occluder was employed for infarction. (A) A control abdominal aortogram shows a hypervascular tumor in the left kidney supplied by two stenotic renal arteries and containing a large arteriovenous fistula. (B) A control selective angiogram of the upper renal artery demonstrates both the extent of the tumor vasculature and the size of the arteriovenous fistula. The left renal vein is obstructed centrally, and an enlarged testicular vein is filled. (C) A selective angiogram of the upper renal artery after embolization of the tumor vasculature in the lower pole of the kidney distal to the fistula with tissue adhesive (using a coaxial catheter) and by placement of a spring coil occluder (*arrow*) in the fistula. The fistula was occluded in this manner to prevent pulmonary embolism during embolization of the residual tumor vasculature. (D) A follow-up open film after embolization of both renal arteries supplying the tumor reveals an opaque "cast" of the entire vasculature of the kidney and tumor. (E) A follow-up abdominal aortogram demonstrates occlusion of both left renal arteries and only minimal supply to the tumor via the adrenal artery, its capsular branch, and the lumbar artery. These arteries were embolized in the second therapeutic session.

occluded (see Fig. 99-7). Depending on the extent of the procedure, the number of vessels to be occluded, the volume of contrast medium used, and the condition of the patient, vasoocclusive therapy of major tumors is sometimes done in two sessions, with a few days between them.

Vasoocclusive treatment of major tumors has *side effects*, and usually a typical "postembolization" syndrome develops: flank pain, increased temperature, moderate gastrointestinal symptoms, and occasional transient blood pressure elevation [66, 92]. Localized flank pain in the area of the infarcted kidney starts just after embolization, lasts 2 to 4 days, and usually requires narcotics for relief. Lidocaine injected during embolization into the renal artery may delay the onset of this pain for several hours [49]. A febrile response, sometimes with temperatures up to 39°C, occurs in almost all patients the first day after embolization. The fever lasts a few days but its course does not necessarily parallel that of the flank pain. The initial gastrointestinal symptoms may include nausea and vomiting, and often a moderate localized paralytic ileus develops later. Laboratory studies indicate leukocytosis and increased lactic dehydrogenase levels secondary to tumor necrosis.

Tubular necrosis of the nonembolized kidney and acute renal failure as a complication of vasoocclusive therapy have been reported but can and should be avoided. They occur in debilitated patients who have been "overtreated," particularly those who have received an enormous amount of contrast medium during diagnostic angiography and cavography performed at the same time as vasoocclusion. Sufficient hydration of the patient before, during, and after the procedure, the use of a small amount of contrast medium, and the performance of the diagnostic and therapeutic procedures in two or even three sessions help prevent this complication.

Miscellaneous Conditions

RENAL ABLATION

The ablation of renal functions is a medical alternative to nephrectomy. It is accomplished by renal infarction intended to eliminate pathologic renal function in critically ill patients whose precarious condition precludes safe surgical nephrectomy. Therapeutic renal ablation can be indicated in severe nephrotic syndrome, renal amyloidosis, or postdialysis cachexia to eliminate proteinuria with excessive protein losses [48, 67, 97, 105] (Fig. 99-10). It can also be requested to control severe, otherwise uncontrollable malignant hypertension [2, 7, 27, 36, 97]. End-stage renal disease with chronic renal failure requiring nephrectomy prior to transplantation is another potential indication for this angiographic procedure [31]. Occasionally, renal ablation alone or in combination with transcatheter ureteral obliteration is performed to treat ureterocutaneous or ureterovaginal fistulas, which usually are caused by an incurable pelvic malignancy [42, 103]. Properly performed, renal ablation immediately destroys renal function, with the patient becoming anuric. In patients in whom hypertension is the indication for renal ablation, high blood pressure becomes controllable medically.

Technically, renal ablation is performed by embolization of the kidneys with some permanent occlusive material or with a combination of Gelfoam and spring coil occluders. The entire renal vasculature, from the central vessels to the small peripheral branches, should be occluded; if it is not, preexisting capsular collateral vessels may enlarge and supply peripheral renal vessels. If this occurs, uncontrollable hypertension persists because peripheral renal tissue continues to be ischemic and, therefore, produces large amounts of renin [2, 97]. In these patients with advanced renal disease and a marked decrease in renal blood flow, a reflux of embolic material during embolization can easily occur [11, 33]. Use of a balloon catheter, together with a slow, very careful injection of emboli, should be done to prevent this complication.

Complete infarction of the diseased kidneys usually produces only short-term pain and fever, lasting 2 to 3 days. The kidney undergoes severe atrophy, and histologic studies done several months later show complete infarction in various stages of healing, with fibrosis and sclerosis.

CLOSURE OF LARGE ARTERIOVENOUS FISTULAS

Large arteriovenous fistulas occasionally develop after nephrectomy, particularly when the artery and the vein were ligated together without detailed dissection. These arteriovenous fistulas usually have a pseudoaneurysm and/or irregular, occasionally tortuous channel interposed between the stumps of the artery and the vein [20, 29, 74]. A large arteriovenous fistula can cause high-output cardiac failure and even cardiac decompensation. Therapeutic angiography is an effective and safe method of closure of these lesions. Large mechanical devices that will not pass through the fistula are the occlusive agents of choice. The aim is to occlude the pseudoaneurysm or channel and the distal portion of the arterial stump. A large occlusive balloon left in the pseudoaneurysm cavity for several days may result in thrombosis of the fistula [74]. Immediate occlusion, however, is preferable, using a large detachable balloon or spring coil occluder [20, 101]. A modified large coil occluder (10–15 mm in helix diameter) may be first introduced and embedded in the pseudoaneurysm to form a baffle (Fig. 99-11). Several smaller wire occluders can then be safely placed to complete the closure of the fistula.

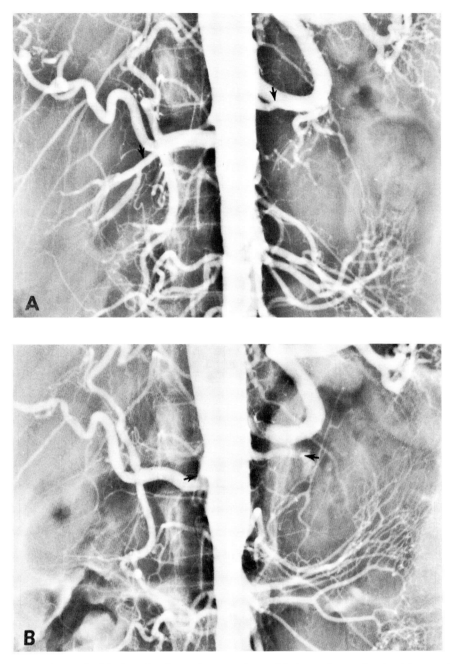

Figure 99-10. Bilateral renal ablation by bucrylate embolization to eliminate proteinuria in a patient with severe nephrotic syndrome. (A) A control abdominal aortogram reveals small renal arteries (*arrows*), atrophy of both kidneys, and a slow renal blood flow. (B) A follow-up abdominal aortogram after renal emboliza- tion with bucrylate mixed with tantalum shows occlu- sion of the right renal artery at its origin (*arrow, left*) and the left renal artery prior to its bifurcation (*arrow, right*). The renal blood flow to both kidneys is com- pletely interrupted.

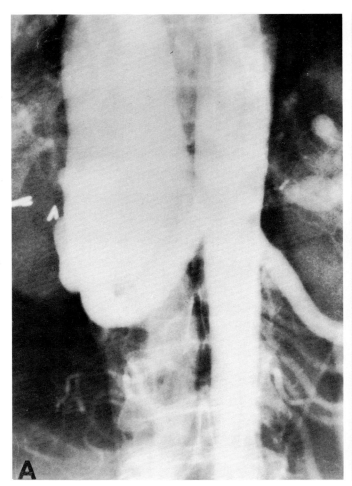

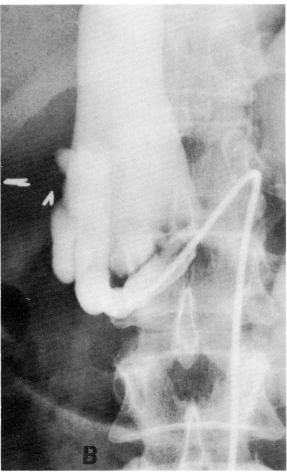

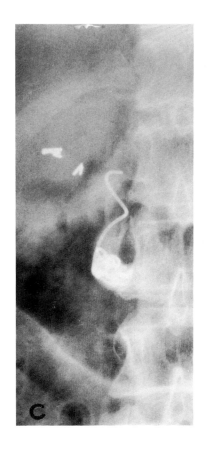

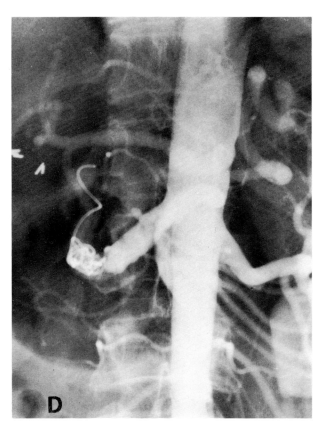

THROMBOEMBOLECTOMY

Transcatheter thromboembolectomy of an acute renal artery occlusion is an alternative to direct arterial surgery in restoring renal flow and function. It has been used mainly in poor-risk patients with acute or recent renal thrombosis either as a definitive procedure or in preparation for a subsequent surgical correction of an accompanying renal artery stenosis [69]. Acute renal artery embolism, in patients with mitral valve disease or developing as a complication of angiography, can also be successfully treated [18, 69]. Removal of the thrombus or embolus can be accomplished by suction of the clot through a large-diameter catheter [18, 19]. Use of a Fogarty balloon catheter introduced through the angiographic catheter is another possibility [69]. The balloon catheter is passed through the clot and inflated, and the clot is then pulled out into the aorta. Several passages are usually necessary to remove enough clot to restore adequate renal arterial flow. The dislodged clot is embolized into the distal aorta, but, in the reported cases, these emboli have not had untoward effects [69]. If distal embolism compromises the circulation to a lower extremity, a simple percutaneous or surgical Fogarty embolectomy can be performed.

RENAL ANGIOPLASTY

Renal angioplasty, an alternative to aorticorenal bypass graft surgery for the treatment of renovascular hypertension caused by stenosis of the main renal artery or its branches, is discussed in Chapter 90.

VARICOCELE

The angiographic treatment of varicocele consists of occlusion of the spermatic vein with interruption of the retrograde blood flow to the plexus pampiniformis. Appropriate occlusive therapy

◀ **Figure 99-11.** Closure of a large postnephrectomy renal artery–renal vein fistula by spring coil occluders. (A) A control abdominal aortogram and (B) a selective renal angiogram demonstrate a large, high-flow arteriovenous fistula with immediate dense filling of the dilated inferior vena cava. (C) An open film after the placement of a large (15-mm) spring coil occluder in the fistula and three 8-mm occluders in the distal portion of the renal artery stump. (D) A follow-up abdominal aortogram demonstrates occlusion of the fistula.

eliminates the possibility of recurrence and thus has been reported to be superior to surgical ligation [96, 106]. Performed on an outpatient basis, gonadal vein occlusion not only treats the varicocele but also improves spermatogenesis and fertility by decreasing scrotal congestion and temperature [106].

A diagnostic selective venogram is performed first, to visualize the spermatic vein anatomy, particularly the size of the vein and the location of its branching. Selective catheterization on the left side, where most varicoceles are located, is usually easy; catheterization of the right spermatic vein, which is involved in about 10 percent of cases of varicocele, is more difficult because of the variable origin of the vein on this side. For occlusion, sclerotic agents may be used, preferably with a balloon catheter blocking the superior portion of the spermatic vein, to prevent reflux of the sclerosing material into the renal vein [106]. Obstructive devices, such as spring coil occluders or detachable balloons (Fig. 99-12), are, however, superior and give an immediate and definitive occlusion without damage to the testicular veins [96, 101, 106]. The size of the obstructive device is selected according to the diameter of the spermatic vein, and often devices 10 mm in size or larger are necessary. The obstructive device should be placed in the spermatic vein superior to the origin of its branches in order to prevent recurrence of the varicocele. With double spermatic veins, both channels have to be occluded.

Occlusion of the spermatic vein is usually asymptomatic or causes only minimal flank tension. Mild transient scrotal tenderness may develop, with secondary thrombosis of the varicocele, which occurs more often with the use of sclerosing agents than with the use of obstructive devices.

PERCUTANEOUS NEPHROSTOMY

Although not a vascular procedure, percutaneous nephrostomy is often performed by vascular radiologists. Their expertise with catheterization, together with the support of an experienced team, ensures high efficiency and safety in the performance of this therapeutic radiologic intervention. The relief of acute or chronic, simple or complicated, supravesical urinary tract obstruction is the primary aim of percutaneous nephrostomy [9, 40, 73, 89]. It is often used as a temporary measure to allow the kidney to re-

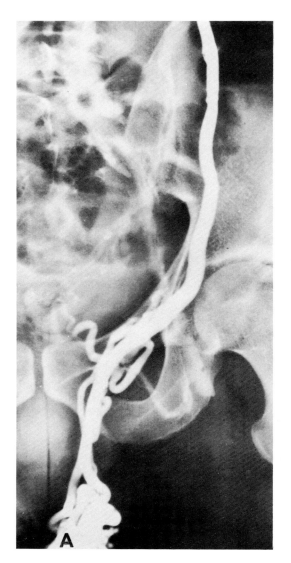

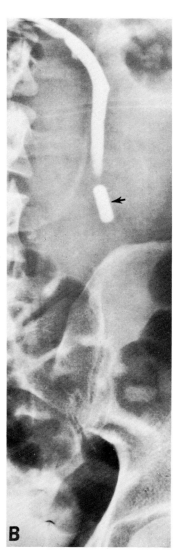

Figure 99-12. Occlusion of the spermatic vein with a detachable balloon for the treatment of varicocele. (A) A control left spermatic venogram demonstrates a large varicocele. (B) A follow-up venogram after the placement of a detachable balloon (*arrow*) shows occlusion of the spermatic vein, with complete interruption of the flow to the varicocele. (Courtesy of R. I. White, Jr., M.D.)

cover from obstruction prior to final corrective surgery; occasionally it is performed for long-term or permanent diversion of the upper urinary tract. Percutaneous nephrostomy is also a route for the performance of additional interventional, nonsurgical procedures, such as dilatation of stenoses, dissolution or removal of renal or ureteral stones, direct installation of antibiotics or chemotherapeutic drugs, stent catheter placement, and permanent occlusion of the ureter or its fistulas [9, 73, 87–89]. Patients of all ages, even infants, can benefit from percutaneous nephrostomy and associated therapeutic techniques, which can be performed on one kidney, both kidneys, or even a renal transplant [6, 8, 40, 41, 89].

Percutaneous nephrostomy may be performed under fluoroscopic guidance after intravenous contrast-medium opacification of the pelvicaliceal system. Ultrasonography also provides good control of puncture, particularly in the non-visualized collecting system [6, 72, 73]. A prone or a slight oblique position is used for puncture, which may be done with vertical or oblique di-

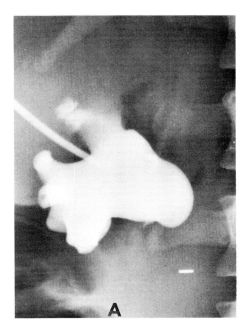
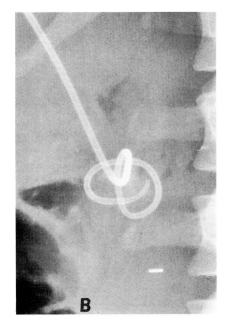

Figure 99-13. Percutaneous nephrostomy of the right kidney for an obstruction of the ureteropelvic junction. (A) A catheter placed in the enlarged pelvis visualized by antegrade pyelography. (B) After drainage, the distal catheter tip is well coiled in the pelvis.

rection. The oblique direction is preferable for long-term nephrostomy. In the nonvisualized kidney, a fine needle is usually inserted into the pelvis first and antegrade pyelography is done. With pelvic visualization, a larger (18-gauge) thin-wall needle, frequently one with an overlying sheath, is used. After entry into the pelvis, the usual angiographic techniques of catheter introduction are employed: use of the guidewire (preferably a safety J guidewire), satisfactory dilatation of the puncture tract, and, finally, insertion of the catheter. Usually, polyethylene catheters having multiple side holes and a pigtail tip are used. The size of the catheter depends on the patient's age and weight; usually a 6 to 8 French catheter is placed at the first sitting. When it is possible to introduce only a small catheter, that catheter should be exchanged a few days later for a larger one. In patients with ureteropelvic junction obstruction, the tip of the catheter is coiled in the enlarged pelvis (Fig. 99-13). With a more distal obstruction and an enlarged ureter, the catheter may be placed distally so that its tip is located well in the ureter (Fig. 99-14). All the side holes of the catheter should be in the collecting system. The catheter is fixed to the skin by sutures and tape adhesive. Irrigation of the catheter prevents its occlusion by blood clot during the initial 24 hours, when traumatic hematuria secondary to the procedure often occurs. Subsequent irrigations minimize the deposition of crystals within the catheter. If long-term drainage is contemplated, the catheter can be exchanged for a larger one; and once a permanent tract is established, a 20 to 24 French Foley-type balloon catheter can be inserted.

A number of procedures may be performed in association with percutaneous nephrostomy. Dilatation of ureteral strictures can be done using an angioplasty balloon catheter. Renal or ureteral stones may be dissolved with direct infusions of alkalizing solutions or, depending on their composition, organic acids [87, 88]. Stones can also be extracted with a stone basket retriever or a steerable catheter used for the removal of biliary calculi [73, 87]. The placement of a stent-splint catheter permits internal drainage of the ureteral obstruction. It is usually placed after the dilatation of the ureteral stricture. The stent catheter is placed over a guidewire introduced from the nephrostomy site and snared distally in the bladder, or, in the case of a urinary tract diversion, in the ileal or colon conduit via a cystoscope. With short or long stent catheters, internal drainage or internal drainage combined with external drainage is available [73].

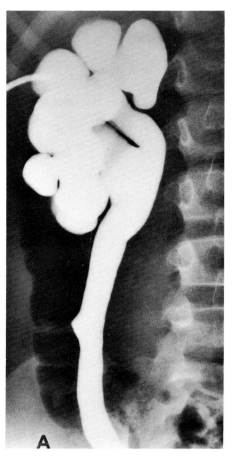 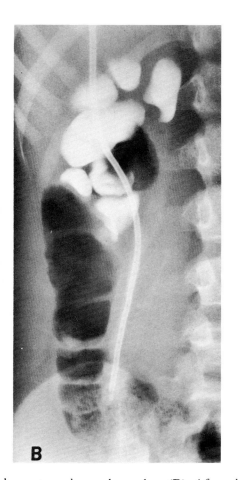

Figure 99-14. A percutaneous nephrostomy in a child with a distal ureteral obstruction. (A) A catheter placed in the enlarged ureteropelvic system visualized by antegrade pyelography. (B) After drainage, the catheter tip is seen in the distal ureter.

References

1. Abrams, H. L.   Quantitative derivates of renal radiologic studies: An overview. *Invest. Radiol.* 7:240, 1972.
2. Adler, J., Einhorn, R., McCarthy, J., Goodman, A., Solangi, K., Varanasi, U., and Thelmo, W.   Gelfoam embolization of the kidneys for treatment of malignant hypertension. *Radiology* 128:45, 1978.
3. Almgård, L. E., Fernström, I., Haverling, M., and Ljungqvist, A.   Treatment of renal adenocarcinoma by embolic occlusion of the renal circulation. *Br. J. Urol.* 45:474, 1973.
4. Almgård, L. E., and Slezak, P.   Treatment of renal adenocarcinoma by embolization: A follow-up of 38 cases. *Eur. Urol.* 3:279, 1977.
5. Arkell, D. G., Cotter, K. P., Fitz-Patrick, J. D., and Shaw, R. E.   Pre-operative arterial embo-lisation in renal carcinoma. *Br. J. Urol.* 50:469, 1978.
6. Babcock, J. R., Jr., Shkolnik, A., and Cook, W. A.   Ultrasound-guided percutaneous neph-rostomy in the pediatric patient. *J. Urol.* 121: 327, 1979.
7. Bachman, D. M., Casarella, W. J., Spiegel, R., and Bregman, D.   Selective renal artery em-bolization: Treatment of acute renovascular hypertension. *J.A.M.A.* 238:1534, 1977.
8. Barbaric, Z. L., and Thomson, K. R.   Per-cutaneous nephropyelostomy in the manage-ment of obstructed renal transplants. *Radiology* 126:639, 1978.
9. Barbaric, Z. L., and Wood, B. P.   Emergency percutaneous nephropyelostomy: Experience with 34 patients and review of the literature. *AJR* 128:453, 1977.
10. Bennett, W. M., Keefe, E., Melnyk, C., Mahler, D., Rösch, J., and Porter, G. A.   Response to

dopamine hydrochloride in the hepatorenal syndrome. *Arch. Intern. Med.* 135:964, 1975.

11. Bergreen, P. W., and Woodside, J. R. Treatment of uncontrolled hypertension by therapeutic renal infarction. *Urology* 8:593, 1976.

12. Bischoff, W., and Goerttler, U. Aktuelle Aspekte der renalen Gefässembolisation. *Dtsch. Med. Wochenschr.* 102:901, 1977.

13. Bischoff, W., Pohle, W., and Goerttler, U. Treatment of arteriovenous angiomas of the kidney: Surgical intervention and intra-arterial embolization. *J. Urol.* 122:825, 1979.

14. Bischoff, W., Thomas, C., Elsässer, E., and Schnitzer, A. Wachstumsbeeinflussung experimenteller Nephroblastome durch Nierenarterienokklusion. *Radiologe* 17:503, 1977.

15. Bookstein, J. J., and Goldstein, H. M. Successful management of postbiopsy arteriovenous fistula with selective arterial embolization. *Radiology* 109:535, 1973.

16. Bracken, R. B., Johnson, D. E., Goldstein, H. M., Wallace, S., and Ayala, A. G. Percutaneous transfemoral renal artery occlusion in patients with renal carcinoma: Preliminary report. *Urology* 6:6, 1975.

17. Bücheler, E. E., Wiessbach, L., Müller, R., and Thelen, M. Katheterembolisation eines blutenden Nierenhamartoms. Zugleich ein Beitrag zur angiographischen Diagnostik. *ROEFO* 122:107, 1975.

18. Bücheler, E., Hupe, W., Hertel, E. U. and Klosterhalfen, H. Katheterembolisation von Nierentumoren. *ROEFO* 124:134, 1975.

19. Buxton, D. R., Jr., and Mueller, C. F. Removal of iatrogenic clot by transcatheter embolectomy. *Radiology* 111:39, 1974.

20. Castaneda-Zuniga, W. R., Tadavarthy, S. M., Murphy, W., Beranek, I., and Amplatz, K. Nonsurgical closure of large arteriovenous fistulas. *J.A.M.A.* 236:2649, 1976.

21. Cho, K. J., and Stanley, J. C. Non-neoplastic congenital and acquired renal arteriovenous malformations and fistulas. *Radiology* 129:333, 1978.

22. Chuang, V. P., Reuter, S. R., and Schmidt, R. W. Control of experimental traumatic renal hemorrhage by embolization with autogenous blood clot. *Radiology* 117:55, 1975.

23. Chuang, V. P., Reuter, S. R., Walter, J., Foley, W. D., and Bookstein, J. J. Control of renal hemorrhage by selective arterial embolization. *AJR* 125:300, 1975.

24. Chuang, V. P., Wallace, S., Swanson, D., Zornoza, J., Handel, S. F., Schwarten, D. E., and Murray, J. Arterial occlusion in the management of pain from metastatic renal carcinoma. *Radiology* 133:611, 1979.

25. Cromwell, L. D., and Kerber, C. W. Modification of cyanoacrylate for therapeutic emboliza-

tion: Preliminary experience. *AJR* 132:799, 1979.

26. Ekelund, L., Månsson, W., Olsson, A. M., and Stigsson, L. Palliative embolization of arterial renal tumor supply: Results in 10 cases. *Acta Radiol.* [*Diagn.*] (Stockh.) 20:323, 1979.

27. Eliscu, E. H., Haire, H. M., Tew, F. T., and Newton, L. W. Control of malignant renovascular hypertension by percutaneous transluminal angioplasty and therapeutic renal embolization. *AJR* 134:815, 1980.

28. Epstein, M., Berk, D. P., Hollenberg, N. K., Adams, D. F., Chalmers, T. C., Abrams, H. L., and Merrill, J. P. Renal failure in the patient with cirrhosis: The role of active vasoconstriction. *Am. J. Med.* 49:175, 1970.

29. Formanek, A., Probst, P., Tadavarthy, S., Castaneda-Zuniga, W. R., and Amplatz, K. Transcatheter embolization (interventive radiology) in the pediatric age group and adolescent. *Ann. Radiol.* (Paris) 22:150, 1979.

30. Frasson, F., Fugazzola, C., Bianchi, G., Franzolin, N., Caresano, A., Del Favero, C., and Comelli, S. Selective arterial embolization in renal tumors. *Radiol. Clin.* 47:239, 1978.

31. Freeny, P. C., Bush, W. H., Jr., and Kidd, R. Transcatheter occlusive therapy of genitourinary abnormalities using isobutyl 2-cyanoacrylate (bucrylate). *AJR* 133:647, 1979.

32. Friedman, S. M., Johnson, R. L., and Friedman, C. L. The pattern of recovery of renal function following renal artery occlusion in the dog. *Circ. Res.* 2:231, 1954.

33. Gang, D. L., Dole, K. B., and Adelman, L. S. Spinal cord infarction following therapeutic renal artery embolization. *J.A.M.A.* 237:2841, 1977.

34. Giuliani, L., Garmignani, G., Belgrano, E., and Puppo, P. Transcatheter arterial embolization in urological tumors: The use of isobutyl-2-cyanoacrylate. *J. Urol.* 121:630, 1979.

35. Gold, R. E., Stiller, C. R., Ulan, R. A., Blair, D. C., and Quadir, H. Intra-arterial therapy of acute rejection of renal transplants. Presented at the 23rd Annual Meeting of the Association of University Radiologists in San Diego, California, April 30–May 2, 1975.

36. Goldin, A. R., Naude, J. H., and Thatcher, G. N. Therapeutic percutaneous renal infarction. *Br. J. Urol.* 46:133, 1974.

37. Goldman, M. L., Fellner, S. K., and Parrott, T. S. Transcatheter embolization of renal arteriovenous fistula. *Urology* 6:386, 1975.

38. Goldstein, H. M., Medellin, H., Beydoun, M. T., Wallace, S., Ben-Menachem, Y., Bracken, R. B., and Johnson, D. E. Transcatheter embolization of renal cell carcinoma. *AJR* 123:557, 1975.

39. Goldstein, H. M., Wallace, S., Anderson, J. H.,

Bree, R. L., and Gianturco, C. Transcatheter occlusion of abdominal tumors. *Radiology* 120:539, 1976.

40. Günther, R., and Alken, L. P. Perkutane Nephropyelostomie bei Kindern. *ROEFO* 130:586, 1979.

41. Günther, R., Alken, P., and Altwein, J. E. Percutaneous nephropyelostomy using a fine-needle puncture set. *Radiology* 132:228, 1979.

42. Günther, R., Marberger, M., and Klose, K. Transrenal ureteral embolization. *Radiology* 132:317, 1979.

43. Günther, R., Schubert, U., Bohl, J., Georgi, M., and Marberger, M. Transcatheter embolization of the kidney with butyl-2-cyanoacrylate: Experimental and clinical results. *Cardiovasc. Radiol.* 1:101, 1978.

44. Habighorst, L. V., Kreutz, W., Eilers, H., Sparwasser, H. H., and Klug, B. Katheterembolisation der Nierenarterie, eine Alternative zur präoperativen Radiotherapie bei Nierentumoren? *Radiologe* 17:509, 1977.

45. Haertel, M., Zaunbauer, W., and Zingg, E. Die Katheterembolisation maligner urologischer Tumoren. *Schweiz. Med. Wochenschr.* 107:584, 1977.

46. Harrison, M. R., de Lorimier, A. A., and Boswell, W. O. Preoperative angiographic embolization for large hemorrhagic Wilms' tumor. *J. Pediatr. Surg.* 13:757, 1978.

47. Hawkins, I. F., and Garin, E. H. Therapeutic renal embolization in children. *J. Pediatr.* 94:415, 1979.

48. Henrich, W. L., Goldman, M., Dotter, C. T., Rösch, J., and Bennett, W. M. Therapeutic renal arterial occlusion for elimination of proteinuria. *Arch. Intern. Med.* 136:840, 1976.

49. Hlava, A., Steinhart, L., and Navratil, P. Intraluminal obliteration of the renal arteries in kidney tumors. *Radiology* 121:323, 1976.

50. Hoffman, R. B., and Zucker, M. O. A new technique in the treatment of renal bleeding: Epinephrine infusion in a patient with sickle cell trait. *Calif. Med.* 118:49, 1973.

51. Hollenberg, N. K., Retik, A. B., Rosen, S. M., Murray, J. E., and Merrill, J. P. The role of vasoconstriction in the ischemia of renal allograft rejection. *Transplantation* 6:59, 1968.

52. Johnson, R. E., Doppman, J. L., Harbert, J. C., Steckel, R. J., and MacLowry, J. D. Prevention of radiation nephritis with renal artery infusion of vasoconstrictors: Experimental and preliminary clinical studies. *Radiology* 91:103, 1968.

53. Jorest, R., Monneins, F., Olier, C., Steg, A., and Harry, G. Hémorragie cataclysmique après néphrolithotomie traitée avec succès par embolisation artérielle rénale hypersélective. *Ann. Urol.* 12:177, 1978.

54. Kalish, M., Greenbaum, L., Silber, S., and

Goldstein, H. Traumatic renal hemorrhage treatment by arterial embolization. *J. Urol.* 112:138, 1974.

55. Kerber, C. W., Freeny, P. C., Cromwell, L., Margolis, M. T., and Correa, R. J., Jr. Cyanoacrylate occlusion of a renal arteriovenous fistula. *AJR* 128:663, 1977.

56. Knapp, R., Hollenberg, N. K., Busch, G. J., and Abrams, H. L. Prolonged unilateral acute renal failure induced by intraarterial norepinephrine infusion in the dog. *Invest. Radiol.* 7:164, 1972.

57. Lang, E. K. Superselective arterial catheterization of tumors of the urogenital tract: A modality used for perfusion with chemotherapeutic agents and infarction with radioactive pellets. *J. Urol.* 104:16, 1970.

58. Lang, E. K. Superselective arterial catheterization as a vehicle for delivering radioactive infarct particles to tumors. *Radiology* 98:391, 1971.

59. Lemaitre, G., Merland, J. J., and Berger, P. Embolisation and its application to urogenital pathology. *J. Belge. Radiol.* 61:127, 1978.

60. Lopatkin, N. A., Mazo, E. B., and Nabiev, Y. N. Nephrectomy with prior intraluminal balloon occlusion of the renal artery in kidney cancer. *Eur. Urol.* 5:255, 1979.

61. MacErlean, D. P., Owens, A. P., and Bryan, P. J. Hypernephroma embolisation: Is it worthwhile? *Clin. Radiol.* 31:297, 1980.

62. Marberger, M., Georgi, M., Guenther, R., and Hohenfellner, R. Simultaneous balloon occlusion of the renal artery and hypothermic perfusion in in situ surgery of the kidney. *J. Urol.* 119:463, 1978.

63. Marberger, M., Georgi, M., Günther, R., Schäfer, R., and Hohenfellner, R. Die intraluminale Ballonokklusion der Nierenarterie. Klinische Anwendungsmöglichkeiten und Erfahrungen. *Urologe* 16:146, 1977.

64. Marshall, F. F., White, R. I., Jr., Kaufman, S. L., and Barth, K. H. Treatment of traumatic renal arteriovenous fistulas by detachable silicone balloon embolization. *J. Urol.* 122:237, 1979.

65. Marshall, V. Renal Preservation. In P. J. Morris (ed.), *Kidney Transplantation: Principles and Practice.* London: Academic Press; New York: Grune & Stratton, 1979. P. 89.

66. Marx, F. J., Eisenberger, F., and Bassermann, R. Komplikationen nach transfemoraler Nierentumorembolisation. *Urologe* 17:79, 1978.

67. McCarron, D. A., Rubin, R. J., Barnes, B. A., Harrington, J. T., and Millan, V. G. Therapeutic bilateral renal infarction in end-stage renal disease. *N. Engl. J. Med.* 294:652, 1976.

68. Meaney, T. F., and Chicatelli, P. D. Obliteration of renal arteriovenous fistula by transcatheter clot embolization. *Cleve. Clin. Q.* 41:33, 1974.

69. Millan, V. G., Sher, M. H., Deterling, R. A., Packard, A., Morton, J. R., and Harrington, J. T. Transcatheter thromboembolectomy of acute renal artery occlusion. *Arch. Surg.* 113:1086, 1978.

70. Mohr, S. J., and Whitesel, J. A. Spontaneous regression of renal cell carcinoma metastases after preoperative embolization of primary tumor and subsequent nephrectomy. *Urology* 14:5, 1979.

71. Moorhead, D. J., Fritzsche, P., and Hadley, H. L. Management of hemorrhage secondary to renal angiomyolipoma with selective arterial embolization. *J. Urol.* 117:122, 1977.

72. Pedersen, J. F., Cowan, D. F., Kuist, J., Kristensen, J. K., Holm, H. H., Hancke, S., and Jensen, F. Ultrasonically-guided percutaneous nephrostomy: Report of 24 cases. *Radiology* 119:429, 1976.

73. Pfister, R. C., and Newhouse, J. H. Interventional percutaneous pyeloureteral techniques: Percutaneous nephrostomy and other procedures. *Radiol. Clin. North Am.* 17:351, 1979.

74. Pingoud, E. G., Glickman, M. G., and Pais, S. O. Balloon-induced thrombosis of renal arteriovenous fistula. *AJR* 135:605, 1980.

75. Pontes, J. E., Parekh, N., McGuckin, J. T., Banks, M. D., and Pierce, J. M. Percutaneous transfemoral embolization of arterio-infundibular-venous fistula. *J. Urol.* 116:98, 1976.

76. Porstmann, W., Münster, W., Futh, M., Krebs, W., and Schwozer, A. Die präoperative Embolisation der Arteria renalis bei Nierentumoren. *Z. Urol.* 70:165, 1977.

77. Reuter, S. R., Pomeroy, P. R., Chuang, V. P., and Cho, K. J. Embolic control of hypertension caused by segmental renal artery stenosis. *AJR* 127:389, 1976.

78. Richman, S. D., Green, W. M., Kroll, R., and Casarella, W. J. Superselective transcatheter embolization of traumatic renal hemorrhage. *AJR* 128:843, 1977.

79. Riedl, P., and Flamm, J. Kontrollangiographische Befunde nach palliativer Nierenarterienokklusion mit der GAW- (Gianturco, Anderson-Wallace-) Spirale. *ROEFO* 130:398, 1979.

80. Rosen, R. J., Feldman, L., and Wilson, A. R. Embolization for postbiopsy renal arteriovenous fistula: Effective occlusion using homologous clot. *AJR* 131:1072, 1978.

81. Schulman, C. C., Struyven, J., Giannakopoulos, X., and Mathieu, J. Preoperative embolization of renal tumors: Comparison of different methods. *Eur. Urol.* 6:154, 1980.

82. Selman, S. H., Zelch, J. V., and Kursh, E. D. Successful treatment of a renal arteriovenous fistula with a Fogarty catheter. *J. Urol.* 122:387, 1979.

83. Silber, S. Renal trauma: Treatment by angiographic injection of autologous clot. *Arch. Surg.* 110:206, 1975.

84. Silber, S. J., Collins, E., and Clark, R. Treatment of hemorrhage from renal trauma by angiographic injection of clot. *J. Urol.* 116:15, 1976.

85. Simon, N., Silverstone, S. M., Roach, L. C., Warner, R. R. P., Baron, M. G., and Rudavsky, A. Z. Intra-arterial irradiation of tumors, a safe procedure. *AJR* 112:732, 1971.

86. Singsaas, M. W., Chopp, R. T., and Mendez, R. Preoperative renal embolization as adjunct to radical nephrectomy. *Urology* 14:1, 1979.

87. Smith, A. D., Reinke, D. B., Miller, R. P., and Lange, P. H. Percutaneous nephrostomy in the management of ureteral and renal calculi. *Radiology* 133:49, 1979.

88. Spataro, R. F., Linke, C. A., and Barbaric, Z. L. The use of percutaneous nephrostomy and urinary alkalinization in the dissolution of obstructing uric acid stones. *Radiology* 129:629, 1978.

89. Stables, D. P., Ginsberg, N. J., and Johnson, J. L. Percutaneous nephrostomy: A series and review of the literature. *AJR* 130:75, 1978.

90. Steckel, R. J., Tobin, P., Ross, G., Stein, J. J., and Stevens, G. H. Radiation protection of vital organs, using a selective arterial catheter: Experimental and clinical aspects. *AJR* 106:841, 1969.

91. Steckel, B. J., Tobin, P. L., Stein, J. J., and Bennett, R. L. Intra-arterial epinephrine protection against radiation nephritis: A progress report. *Radiology* 92:1341, 1969.

92. Steckenmesser, R., Bayindir, S., Rothauge, C. F., Nöske, K., and Weidner, W. Embolisation maligner Nierentumoren. *ROEFO* 125:251, 1976.

93. Struyven, J., Mathieu, J., Brion, J. P., Potvliege, R., and Schulman, C. Transcatheter embolization in renal pathology. *J. Belge. Radiol.* 60:289, 1977.

94. Thelen, M., Brühl, P., Bücheler, E., Hupe, H., and Gerlach, F. Erfahrungen mit der arteriellen Katheterembolisation in der Urologie. *Urologe* 17:160, 1978.

95. Thelen, M., Brühl, P., Gerlach, F., and Biersack, H. J. Katheterembolisation von metastasierten Nierenkarzinomen mit Butyl-2-Cyanoacrylat. *ROEFO* 124:232, 1976.

96. Thelen, M., Weissbach, L., and Franken, T. Die Behandlung der idiopathischen Varikozele durch transfemorale Spiralokklusion der Vena testicularis sinistra. *ROEFO* 131:24, 1979.

97. Thiebot, J., Merland, J. J., Duboust, A., Rottembourg, J., and Bories, J. Néphrectomie bilatérale par embolisation der artères rénales: A propos de cinq cas. *Ann. Radiol.* (Paris). 22:502, 1979.

98. Thomas, M. L., and Lamb, G. H. R. Selective arterial embolization in the management of post operative renal haemorrhage. *Acta Radiol.* [*Diagn.*] (Stockh.) 18:49, 1977.

99. Wallace, S., Schwarten, D. E., Smith, D. C., Gerson, P. L., and Davis, L. J. Intrarenal arteriovenous fistulas: Transcatheter steel coil occlusion. *J. Urol.* 120:282, 1978.

100. Walther, P. J., Marks, L. S., Stern, D., and Smith, R. B. Renal metastasis of adenocarcinoma of the lung: Massive hematuria managed by therapeutic embolization. *J. Urol.* 122:398, 1979.

101. White, R. I., Barth, K. H., Kaufman, S. L., DeCaprio, V., and Strandberg, J. D. Therapeutic embolization with detachable balloons. *Cardiovasc. Intervent. Radiol.* 3:299, 1980.

102. Wholey, M. H. The technology of balloon catheters in interventional angiography. *Radiology* 125:671, 1977.

103. Williams, J. D., Maddison, F. E., Imray, T. J., and Lawson, R. K. Transcatheter renal artery embolization in treatment of ureterocutaneous fistula. *Urology* 13:188, 1979.

104. Wirthlin, L. S., Gross, W. S., James, T. P., and Sadiq, S. Renal artery occlusion from migration of stainless steel coils. *J.A.M.A.* 243:2064, 1980.

105. Wu, M. J., Moorthy, A. V., Beirne, G. G., and Crummy, A. B. Renal infarction with Gianturco wool coils: Use in the management of massive proteinuria. *J.A.M.A.* 243:2425, 1980.

106. Zeitler, E., Jeckt, E., Richter, E. I., and Seyferth, W. Perkutane Behandlung männlicher Infertilität im Rahmen der selektiven Spermatikaphlebographie mit Katheter: Technik, Indikation, Komplikationen, Ergebnisse. *ROEFO* 132:294, 1980.

Hepatic Artery Infusion Therapy of Liver Metastases

SACHIO KURIBAYASHI
DAVID C. LEVIN

Among all patients with carcinoma, 30 to 50 percent show liver metastases at autopsy [54]. Carcinomas in the portal area (gastrointestinal tract, pancreas, and gallbladder) are especially likely to metastasize to the liver. The prognosis of patients with metastatic liver disease is poor. According to Jaffe et al. [32], the overall median survival in the absence of therapy was 75 days from the date of diagnosis of liver metastases, and only 6.6 percent of these patients survived for more than 1 year. In addition, hepatic metastases had a dominant influence on survival despite the presence of metastatic lesions in other sites. The results of efforts at treatment have not been encouraging.

The indications for surgical resection of metastatic liver tumors are limited because the metastases may involve both lobes of the liver or may be associated with impairment of liver function. Fairly good survival after resection has been reported for patients with colorectal carcinoma when the metastasis is single [23, 71] or localized to one lobe [25]. However, the fairly high mortality, which varies with the extent of resection [25], cannot be ignored.

Surgical ligation of the hepatic artery has been attempted as a method of treating liver metastases by devascularizing the tumors [2, 59]. Although transient relief of symptoms has been obtained with this method, there has been no definitive evidence of increased survival. Autopsies in a small number of patients who have had hepatic artery ligation have generally shown necrosis within the central portion of the tumor but viable tumor cells at the margins of the lesions. One reason for the relative lack of effectiveness of this form of therapy is the very rapid development of collateral circulation following hepatic artery ligation [37, 46, 55]. Experience with transcatheter hepatic artery embolization for metastatic liver tumor is limited [1, 21, 29, 56, 67], and there are no conclusive data regarding response and survival.

Systemic 5-fluorouracil (5-FU) has been widely employed in patients with metastatic liver disease, utilizing a variety of dose schedules and routes of administration [3, 8, 17, 30, 31, 35, 39, 41]. The data from these clinical studies can be summarized by stating that the overall response rate is approximately 20 percent without associated prolongation of survival [51, 57, 74].

A number of reports have indicated that direct hepatic arterial infusion of chemotherapeutic agents has achieved significant increases in both

2289

the response rate and the survival time [4, 53, 60, 70]. Furthermore, in patients in whom systemic chemotherapy has failed, hepatic arterial infusion chemotherapy can still be effective in controlling progressive liver metastases [4, 6, 65].

The following discussion deals with hepatic arterial infusion chemotherapy, especially that involving the percutaneous transbrachial approach, and emphasizes the important role of the vascular radiologist in the joint management of patients with cancer metastatic to the liver.

Rationale for Hepatic Arterial Infusion Chemotherapy

There is substantial experimental evidence in vivo and in vitro to indicate that most antitumor agents have a steep dose-response curve [26]. That is, the higher the dose and/or concentration, the greater the antitumor effects.

The normal liver derives 20 to 25 percent of its blood supply from the hepatic artery and 75 to 80 percent of its blood supply from the portal vein [58], whereas primary and metastatic tumors of the liver receive 80 to 100 percent of their blood supply from the hepatic artery [12, 27]. Therefore, when chemotherapeutic agents are infused directly into the hepatic artery, there is selective concentration of the drug within the tumor, as compared with uninvolved parenchyma. Another advantage that hepatic arterial infusion provides over systemic intravenous infusion is that a number of chemotherapeutic drugs are biotransformed to less active products in the liver; hence the systemic side effects are diminished.

According to Ensminger et al. [22], 94 to 99 percent of 5-fluoro-2'-deoxyuridine (FUDR) and 19 to 51 percent of 5-FU are extracted in one pass through the liver when these drugs are infused directly into the hepatic artery. This results in a drug concentration in the tumor capillary bed that is 4 times as high for FUDR infusion and 1.5 times as high for 5-FU infusion as can be achieved by intravenous infusion. Systemic FUDR levels with hepatic arterial infusion are about 25 percent of corresponding levels obtained after peripheral venous infusion, and systemic levels of 5-FU with hepatic arterial infusion are 60 percent of the levels achieved following peripheral venous infusion. Thus, from the pharmacologic standpoint, when chemotherapeutic agents are infused directly into the hepatic artery, the tumor in the liver is exposed to higher concentrations of the drug while the systemic levels and resultant side effects are significantly diminished.

Catheterization Technique

Catheters can be placed in the hepatic artery by (1) the percutaneous left brachial approach or the femoral approach [18, 45, 72, 73] or (2) a surgical procedure [69]. In the surgical approach, the hepatic and gastroduodenal arteries are exposed and a Teflon catheter is introduced through the gastroduodenal artery and advanced into the hepatic artery. The gastroduodenal artery is then ligated around the catheter. The mortality of laparotomy for catheter placement in patients with extensive hepatic metastases ranges up to 30 percent, depending on the patient selection [70]. Because the percutaneous approach permits the selective catheterization of the hepatic artery to be performed simply and routinely, with relatively low morbidity and almost no mortality, this approach has come to be preferred [18, 45, 72]. The percutaneous approach has an additional advantage in that it permits the patient to be ambulatory, with little restriction of activity.

In the percutaneous approach, a preshaped 100-cm catheter (5 French) with a gentle J curve at the tip is inserted into the high left brachial artery using the Seldinger technique under local anesthesia. The catheter is passed into the thoracic aorta with a J guidewire, and the hepatic artery is then catheterized with or without the aid of the guidewire or a deflector apparatus. A high axillary puncture should be avoided, since it can cause problems if bleeding occurs at the puncture site. Also, sterility of the catheter entry site is very difficult to maintain in the axillary area. The right-arm approach should be avoided if possible because of the risk of stroke caused by embolization from the catheter surface into the right carotid artery. The femoral approach can be used if needed, but the brachial artery approach is preferred because it permits the patient to be ambulatory and is less likely to result in displacement of the catheter from the desired position.

The superior mesenteric artery should be checked fluoroscopically to ascertain the absence of important variations of hepatic artery branching. A replaced or accessory right hepatic artery is noted in 22 percent of cases, and a replaced common hepatic artery is noted in 4.5 percent of cases [48]. In 22 percent of cases, the left hepatic artery is derived from the left gastric artery.

If the catheter tip cannot be satisfactorily positioned distal to the origin of the gastroduodenal artery, the angiographer must determine whether the flow in this vessel is antegrade or retrograde. Often the flow is retrograde in patients with metastatic liver disease, due to hypervascularity and lowered vascular resistance within the liver. The direction of the flow in the gastroduodenal artery is determined by a low-flow-rate contrast injection (1–3 cc/sec) into the hepatic artery proximal to the gastroduodenal origin. If the gastroduodenal artery does not fill with contrast material, it can be assumed that the flow in the vessel is retrograde and that drugs infused into the hepatic artery will therefore not reach the stomach or duodenum. A high-flow-rate hepatic arteriogram may be misleading in that it artificially raises pressure in the gastroduodenal artery

and produces transient antegrade flow [42]. A low-flow-rate injection is necessary to determine the true direction of the hepatic artery blood flow. We have also used radionuclide flow studies to assess the flow pattern in the hepatic circulation. In patients who do not have reversal of flow in the gastroduodenal artery, embolization of this artery should be considered to prevent chemotherapeutic drugs injected into the hepatic artery from reaching the stomach or duodenum and producing gastrointestinal toxicity.

After catheterization of the hepatic artery, hepatic artery anatomy and angiographic changes in the liver are studied by injecting 25 to 40 cc of contrast medium at flow rates of 6 to 7 cc per second and obtaining serial films at a rate of 2 films per second for 8 seconds (Fig. 100-1). Once the catheter is in a satisfactory position, it is sutured and taped in place and connected to a portable infusion pump for drug infusion.

Complications

The most common complication of transbrachial hepatic artery catheterization is thrombosis or dissection of the hepatic artery (Fig. 100-2). The incidence, including complete and partial thrombosis, is 15 to 40 percent [18, 28, 44]. Thrombosis or dissection of the hepatic artery generally does not cause serious problems, because it occurs gradually and collateral vessels develop fairly rapidly (Fig. 100-3) from the gastroduodenal, pancreaticoduodenal, and phrenic arteries, as well as via intrahepatic arterial anastomoses [37, 47, 49, 50, 55]. The development of hepatic artery thrombosis or dissection is usually heralded clinically by abdominal or back pain accompanying drug infusion through the catheter.

Displacement of the catheter tip from the hepatic artery occurs in 15 to 40 percent of cases [13, 18]. It is more likely to occur if the catheter is not far enough into the hepatic artery or if the patient engages in excessive physical activity. Usually the catheter can be repositioned satisfactorily.

The incidence of clinically demonstrated ischemia of the hand secondary to brachial artery thrombosis has been reported to be low [7, 13, 18, 28, 72]. However, the actual incidence of brachial artery occlusion without symptoms is not well known. Brachial artery thrombosis cannot be prevented by heparinization of the catheter or

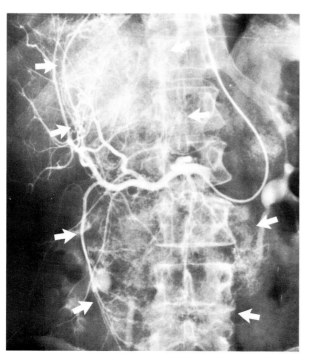

Figure 100-1. Selective hepatic arteriogram after catheter placement reveals multiple large liver metastases in the right hepatic lobe (arrows) in a patient with carcinoma of the colon. The tip of the catheter is in a good position for infusion chemotherapy.

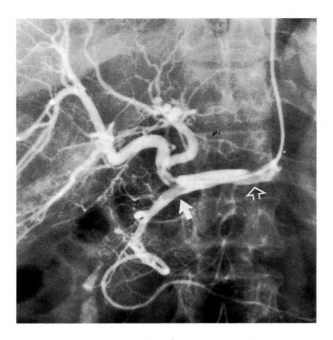

Figure 100-2. Thrombus formation in the common hepatic artery around the indwelling catheter (*open arrow*) and at the bifurcation of the common hepatic artery (*closed arrow*).

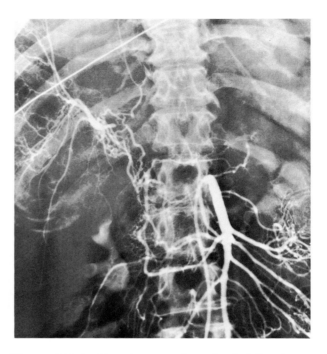

Figure 100-3. Hepatic artery thrombosis following an initial course of intraarterial infusion chemotherapy. Superior mesenteric arteriography reveals good collateral flow to the liver from the pancreaticoduodenal arteries.

systemic heparinization [28, 66]. Therefore, it is important to use catheters of the smallest possible caliber (generally 5 French) and to manipulate the catheter smoothly and gently during the angiographic procedure.

Aneurysm formation of the common hepatic artery, attributed to a direct toxic effect of 5-FU on the arterial wall, was reported by Forsberg et al. [24]. In our experience, this complication is quite rare.

Other complications, such as bleeding at the puncture site, infection at the puncture site, peripheral septic embolization, stroke, peptic ulcer, and gastrointestinal hemorrhage, have been reported in small percentages of patients [7, 18, 28, 44, 45, 72].

Radionuclide Flow Studies

The angiographer must be sure the catheter tip is properly positioned for optimal delivery of the drug to the tumor-bearing areas. This is particularly important because much of the effect of

chemotherapy depends on drug extraction during the first pass through the liver.

As mentioned earlier, high-flow-rate contrast arteriography is not an ideal method of determining this [42] because the flow rate and the pressure in the artery are increased during selective injection [43]. This increase results in a different distribution of flow than that which occurs during a very slow infusion with an infusion pump.

The best way to assess the distribution pattern of chemotherapeutic agents is a radionuclide flow study that uses ^{99m}Tc macroaggregated albumin (MAA) as a radiotracer [33, 34] infused slowly through the catheter. The MAA particles are distributed throughout the liver by the hepatic artery blood flow and trapped by capillary blockade on the first pass. A subsequent gamma camera scan indicates precisely what portions of the liver or other organs will receive drugs similarly infused through the catheter.

In the method in use in our institution, a baseline ^{99m}Tc sulfur colloid (SC) liver-spleen scan is obtained before chemotherapy is started. The MAA flow study is then performed within

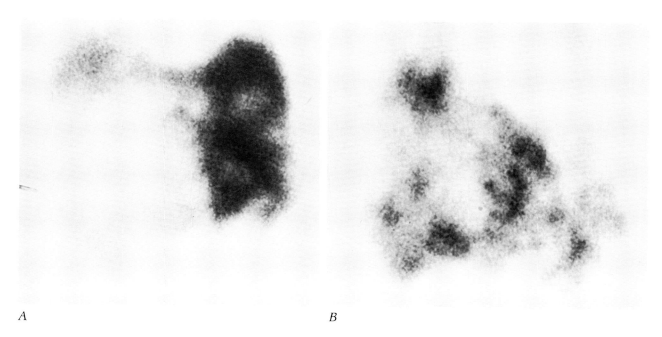

A   B

Figure 100-4. (A) A ^{99m}Tc sulfur colloid liver scan demonstrates large filling defects in the liver due to metastatic colon carcinoma. (B) A ^{99m}Tc macroaggre- gated albumin (MAA) flow study reveals a good ac- cumulation of radioaggregates in the tumor-bearing areas noted in (A).

Figure 100-5. Sequential flow studies 5 days apart. (A) The initial flow study after the catheter placement shows good perfusion of tumor-bearing areas in both lobes of the liver. (B) However, a follow-up study performed 5 days later reveals perfusion of only the spleen and stomach, suggesting either a change of catheter position or occlusion of the hepatic artery. A contrast injection under fluoroscopic control demon- strated displacement of the catheter tip into the splenic artery.

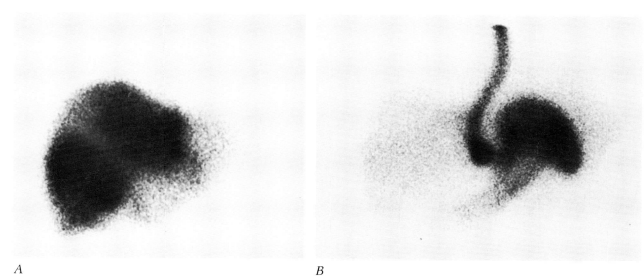

A   B

24 hours after hepatic artery catheter placement. For this flow study, we use approximately 4 mCi of ^{99m}Tc MAA in a volume of less than 0.2 cc introduced through the catheter into the hepatic artery by the pump at a flow rate of 10 to 21 cc per hour, which is the actual flow rate used for chemotherapy infusions. Sequential images are obtained with a gamma camera at a rate of 2 frames per second for a total of 80 frames. Immediately after the completion of the pump infusion, the catheter is cleared with a rapid hand flush (approximately 1 cc/sec) of 10 cc saline, and scans are again obtained to determine whether additional areas of the liver are covered when this more rapid flow pattern is used. Figure 100-4 shows good perfusion to tumor-bearing areas. In Figure 100-4A, a standard ^{99m}Tc SC scan shows filling defects in the liver due to metastatic carcinoma of the colon. Figure 100-4B shows a static image of the flow study that uses ^{99m}Tc MAA infused through the hepatic artery catheter. An accumulation of MAA is shown in the tumor-bearing areas noted on Figure 100-4A. This technique is useful not only for placing the catheter in the optimal position but also for subsequent follow-up and monitoring of the distribution pattern and catheter position. Figure 100-5 shows a case of carcinoma of the colon with liver metastases. The initial flow study (Fig. 100-5A) shows good perfusion to the tumor-bearing areas of both lobes of the liver. However, a follow-up study 5 days later (Fig. 100-5B) showed perfusion of only the spleen and stomach, suggesting either a change in the catheter position or occlusion of the hepatic artery. A contrast injection under fluoroscopic control demonstrated that the catheter tip had slipped back into the splenic artery.

The technique is also useful for determining the optimal flow rate to use in delivering the drug to the tumor-bearing areas. If rapid flushing of the catheter with 10 cc of saline results in a better flow pattern to the tumor than occurs with the slower infusion, the patient should be treated by intermittent, relatively rapid, bolus injections of chemotherapy several times a day, rather than by the continuous low-flow-rate infusion.

Finally, this technique is helpful in differentiating between nonresponse due to inadequate drug perfusion and nonresponse due to a failure of the drug effect. It may prove possible to predict the response of patients to hepatic arterial infusion chemotherapy from the distribution patterns seen on flow studies [34].

Therapeutic Effects of Hepatic Arterial Infusion Chemotherapy

Chemotherapeutic agents were first delivered directly into the arterial blood supply of tumors in 1950 by Bierman et al. [9, 10] and Klopp et al. [36]. The technique was repopularized by Sullivan et al. in 1959 [61], who first reported hepatic arterial infusion of chemotherapeutic agents for metastatic liver cancer in 1964 [62]. Since that time, numerous reports of hepatic arterial infusion chemotherapy using 5-FU or FUDR have appeared describing variations of drug dosage schedules and different durations of therapy.

In 1965, Sullivan and Zurek [64] reported response rates of 60 percent with metastatic liver cancer. These rates were confirmed by Cady and Oberfield [14], who reported clinical response rates of 67 percent, with a median survival of 15 months in responders as opposed to 4.5 months in nonresponders. Following these reports, several additional studies were done in the Lahey Clinic [15, 53, 69, 70]; in each study, objective response rates were on the order of 60 percent, with up to threefold prolongation of survival.

Labelle [38] reported an 82 percent objective response rate, which was defined as a decrease in the liver size by more than 50 percent and a return to normal or nearly normal liver function tests. This rate, however, dropped to 47 percent if only the responses that lasted longer than 3 months were considered.

Cady and Oberfield [15] described 51 patients with hepatic metastases from colon carcinoma treated with intraarterial FUDR infusion. In these patients, Cady and Oberfield attempted to evaluate the response by various objective parameters. They observed a decrease in the liver size of over 2 cm on palpation in 57 percent, an improved liver scan in 61 percent, improved liver function tests in 59 percent, and "improved" angiograms in 39 percent. Subjective improvement (defined as return to a normal or nearly normal life-style with marked symptomatic improvement) was noted in 71 percent.

Ansfield and Ramirez [4] treated 528 patients with hepatic arterial infusion 5-FU chemotherapy followed by systemic 5-FU chemotherapy, and achieved a 55 percent response rate. A response meant that all the following criteria had been present for at least a 2-month period: (1) a reduction of at least 5 cm in liver size; (2) a reduction of at least 50 percent in at least two of three major liver enzymes, such as alkaline phosphatase, serum glutamic-oxaloacetic transaminase, and lactic dehydrogenase; and (3) the elimination of jaundice, if present, and a return to normal levels of total bilirubin. The median survival of responders was 7.5 months, compared with 2.4 months for nonresponders.

It is difficult to compare these numerous data accurately, but in general it can be said that most studies have revealed the superiority of hepatic arterial infusion chemotherapy over systemic chemotherapy for hepatic metastases [4, 20, 53, 60, 65, 70]. The data from these arterial infusion studies suggest that response rates of 35 to 85 percent can be achieved if adequate doses are administered and that the median survival times are 8.5 to 15 months in responders, compared with only 2.5 to 4.5 months in nonresponders [60]. Thus, a two- or threefold prolongation of survival has been reported. In addition, responses were noted in patients refractory to intravenous 5-FU therapy.

In conclusion, patients with cancer metastatic to the liver have a very poor prognosis in the absence of therapy. Various types of treatment have been attempted in an effort to control these metastases. Among them, hepatic arterial infusion chemotherapy seems to be the most effective method, in that it produces a clinical response and an increased survival in a significant percentage of patients. It will undoubtedly continue to be used until a more effective mode of therapy becomes available. Hepatic artery catheters can be placed either percutaneously, using angiographic techniques, or surgically. The surgical approach has not been discussed in this chapter, but it also is fraught with pitfalls and complications, mainly related to difficulty in finding the proper vessels to catheterize and in properly positioning the catheter tip. The percutaneous approach seems preferable in that better control of catheter tip placement is achieved and the procedure does not require laparotomy with prolonged hospitalization in this group of patients, whose life span is already greatly shortened. In most instances, patients can become fully ambulatory within a few hours after completion of the procedure, and continued therapy can be administered on an outpatient basis. The vascular radiologist will undoubtedly continue to play an important role in the proper management of patients with liver metastases, along with his colleagues in the fields of oncology, surgery, and nuclear medicine.

References

1. Allison, D. J., Modlin, I. M., and Jenkins, W. J. Treatment of carcinoid liver metastases by hepatic artery embolization. *Lancet* 2:1323, 1977.
2. Almersjö, O., Bengmark, S., Hafström, L., and Leissner, K. H. Results of liver dearterialization combined with regional infusion of 5-fluorouracil for liver cancer. *Acta Chir. Scand.* 142:131, 1976.
3. Ansfield, F. J., and Curreri, A. R. Further clinical studies with 5-fluorouracil. *J. Natl. Cancer Inst.* 22:497, 1959.
4. Ansfield, F. J., and Ramirez, G. The clinical results of 5-fluorouracil intrahepatic arterial infusion in 528 patients with metastatic cancer to the liver. *Prog. Clin. Cancer* 7:201, 1978.
5. Ansfield, F. J., Ramirez, G., Davis, H. L., Wirtanen, G. W., Johnson, R. O., Bryan, G. T., Manalo, F. B., Borden, E. C., Davis, T. E., and Esmaili, M. Further clinical studies with intrahepatic arterial infusion with 5-fluorouracil. *Cancer* 36:2413, 1975.
6. Ansfield, F. J., Ramirez, G., Skibba, J. L., Bryan, G. T., Davis, H. L., and Wirtanen, G. W. Intrahepatic arterial infusion with 5-fluorouracil. *Cancer* 28:1147, 1971.
7. Antonovic, R., Rösch, J., and Dotter, C. T. Complications of percutaneous transaxillary catheterization for arteriography and selective chemotherapy. *AJR* 126:386, 1976.
8. Bateman, J., Irwin, L., Pugh, R., Cassidy, F., and Weiner, J. Comparison of intravenous and oral administration of 5-fluorouracil for colorectal carcinoma. *Proc. Am. Assoc. Cancer Res.* 16:242, 1975.
9. Bierman, H. R., Byron, R. L., and Kelly, K. H. Therapy of inoperable visceral and regional metastases by intra-arterial catheterization. *Cancer Res.* 11:236, 1951.
10. Bierman, H. R., Byron, R. L., Miller, E. R., and Shimkin, M. B. Effects of intra-arterial administration of nitrogen mustard. *Am. J. Med.* 8:535, 1950.
11. Breedis, C., and Young, G. Blood supply of neoplasms in the liver. *Fed. Proc.* 8:351, 1949.
12. Breedis, C., and Young, G. The blood supply of neoplasms in the liver. *Am. J. Pathol.* 30:969, 1954.
13. Burrows, J. H., Talley, R. W., Drake, E. L., San Diego, F. I., and Tucker, W. G. Infusion of fluorinated pyrimidines into hepatic artery for treatment of metastatic carcinoma of the liver. *Cancer* 20:1886, 1967.
14. Cady, B., and Oberfield, R. A. Infusion chemotherapy of liver metastases from large bowel cancer. *Lahey Clin. Found. Bull.* 21:89, 1972.
15. Cady, B., and Oberfield, R. A. Regional infusion chemotherapy of hepatic metastases from

carcinoma of the colon. *Am. J. Surg.* 127:220, 1974.

16. Cady, B., and Oberfield, R. A.   Arterial infusion chemotherapy of hepatoma. *Surg. Gynecol. Obstet.* 138:381, 1974.

17. Carter, S. K.   Large bowel cancer—the current status of treatment. *J. Natl. Cancer Inst.* 56:3, 1976.

18. Clouse, M. E., Ahmed, R., Ryan, R. B., Oberfield, R. A., and McCaffrey, J. A.   Complications of long term transbrachial hepatic arterial infusion chemotherapy. *AJR* 129:799, 1977.

19. Curry, J. L., and Howland, W. J.   Guided percutaneous arterial infusion chemotherapy. *AJR* 102:562, 1968.

20. Donegan, W. L., Harris, H. S., and Spratt, J. S., Jr.   Prolonged continuous hepatic infusion. Results with fluorouracil for primary and metastatic cancer of the liver. *Arch. Surg.* 99:149, 1969.

21. Doppman, J. L., Girton, M., and Kahn, E. R.   Proximal versus peripheral hepatic artery embolization: Experimental study in monkeys. *Radiology* 128:577, 1978.

22. Ensminger, W. D., Rosowsky, A., Raso, V., Levin, D. C., Glode, M., Come, S., Steele, G., and Frei, E., III.   A clinical-pharmacological evaluation of hepatic arterial infusion of 5-fluoro-2'-deoxyuridine and 5-fluorouracil. *Cancer Res.* 38:3784, 1978.

23. Flanagan, L., Jr., and Foster, J. H.   Hepatic resection for metastatic cancer. *Am. J. Surg.* 113:551, 1967.

24. Forsberg, L., Hafström, L., Lunderquist, A., and Sundqvist, K.   Arterial changes during treatment with intrahepatic arterial infusion of 5-fluorouracil. *Radiology* 126:49, 1978.

25. Foster, J. H., and Berman, M. M.   Resection of Metastatic Tumors. In P. A. Ebert (ed.), *Solid Liver Tumors: Major Problems in Clinical Surgery*. Philadelphia: Saunders, 1977. Vol. 22, pp. 209–234.

26. Frei, E., III.   Effect of Dose and Schedule on Response. In J. F. Holland and E. Frei III (eds.), *Cancer Medicine*. Philadelphia: Lea & Febiger, 1973. Pp. 717–730.

27. Gelin, L. E., Lewis, D. H., and Nilsson, L.   Liver blood flow in man during abdominal surgery: II. The effect of hepatic artery occlusion on the blood flow through metastatic tumor nodules. *Acta Hepatogastroenterol.* (Stuttg.) 15:21, 1968.

28. Goldman, M. L., Bilbao, M. K., Rösch, J., and Dotter, C. T.   Complications of indwelling chemotherapy catheters. *Cancer* 36:1983, 1975.

29. Goldstein, H. M., Wallace, S., Anderson, J. H., Bree, R. L., and Gianturco, C.   Transcatheter occlusion of abdominal tumors. *Radiology* 120:539, 1976.

30. Hahn, R. G., Moertel, C. G., Schutt, A. J., and Bruckner, H. W.   A double-blind comparison of intensive course 5-fluorouracil by oral vs intravenous route in the treatment of colorectal carcinoma. *Cancer* 35:1031, 1975.

31. Jacobs, E. M., Reeves, W. J., Jr., Wood, D. A., Pugh, R., Braunwald, J., and Bateman, J. R.   Treatment of cancer with weekly intravenous 5-fluorouracil. *Cancer* 27:1302, 1971.

32. Jaffe, B. M., Donegan, W. L., Watson, F., and Spratt, J. S., Jr.   Factors influencing survival in patients with untreated hepatic metastases. *Surg. Gynecol. Obstet.* 127:1, 1968.

33. Kaplan, W. D., D'Orsi, C. J., Ensminger, W. D., Smith, E. H., and Levin, D. C.   Intra-arterial radionuclide infusion: A new technique to assess chemotherapy perfusion patterns. *Cancer Treat. Rep.* 62:699, 1978.

34. Kaplan, W. D., Ensminger, W. D., Come, S. E., Smith, E. H., D'Orsi, C. J., Levin, D. C., Takvorian, R. W., and Steele, G. D.   Radionuclide angiography to predict patient response to hepatic artery chemotherapy. *Cancer Treat. Rep.* 64:1217, 1980.

35. Khung, C. L., Hall, T. C., Piro, A. J., and Dederick, M. M.   A clinical trial of oral 5-fluorouracil. *Clin. Pharmacol. Ther.* 7:527, 1966.

36. Klopp, C. T., Bateman, J., Berry, N., Alford, C., and Winship, T.   Fractionated regional cancer chemotherapy. *Cancer Res.* 10:229, 1950.

37. Koehler, R. E., Korobkin, M., and Lewis, F.   Arteriographic demonstration of collateral arterial supply to the liver after hepatic artery ligation. *Radiology* 117:49, 1975.

38. Labelle, J. J., Lucas, R. J., Eisenstein, B., Reed, M. D., Vaitkevicius, V. K., and Wilson, G. S.   Hepatic artery catheterization for chemotherapy. *Arch. Surg.* 96:683, 1968.

39. Lahili, S. R., Boileau, G., and Hall, T. C.   Treatment for colorectal carcinoma with 5-fluorouracil by mouth. *Cancer* 28:902, 1971.

40. Lee, Y. N.   Nonsystemic treatment of metastatic tumors of the liver—a review. *Med. Pediatr. Oncol.* 4:185, 1978.

41. Leone, L. A.   The chemotherapy of colorectal cancer. *Cancer* 34:972, 1974.

42. Levin, D. C.   Augmented arterial flow and pressure resulting from selective injections through catheters: Clinical implications. *Radiology* 127:103, 1978.

43. Levin, D. C., Phillips, D. A., Lee-Son, S., and Maroko, P. R.   Hemodynamic changes distal to selective arterial injections. *Invest. Radiol.* 12:116, 1977.

44. Lucas, R. J., Tumacder, O., and Wilson, G. S.   Hepatic artery occlusion following hepatic artery catheterization. *Ann. Surg.* 173:238, 1971.

45. Massay, W. H., Fletcher, W. S., Judkins, M. P., and Dennis, D. L.   Hepatic artery infusion for metastatic malignancy using percutaneously placed catheters. *Am. J. Surg.* 121:160, 1971.

46. Mays, E. T., and Wheeler, C. S. Demonstration of collateral arterial flow after interruption of hepatic arteries in man. *N. Engl. J. Med.* 290:993, 1974.

47. Michels, N. A. Collateral arterial pathways to the liver after ligation of the hepatic artery and removal of the celiac axis. *Cancer* 6:708, 1953.

48. Michels, N. A. *Blood Supply and Anatomy of the Upper Abdominal Organs.* Philadelphia: Lippincott, 1955. Pp. 152–154, 372–375.

49. Michels, N. A. Newer anatomy of the liver: Variant blood supply and collateral circulation. *J.A.M.A.* 172:125, 1960.

50. Michels, N. A. Newer anatomy of the liver and its variant blood supply and collateral circulation. *Am. J. Surg.* 112:337, 1966.

51. Moertel, C. G. Clinical management of advanced gastrointestinal cancer. *Cancer* 36:675, 1975.

52. Moertel, C. G., Reitemeier, R. J., and Hahn, R. G. Therapy with the Fluorinated Pyrimidines. In C. G. Moertel and R. J. Reitemeier (eds.), *Advanced Gastrointestinal Cancer.* New York: Hoeber Div., Harper & Row, 1969. Pp. 86–107.

53. Oberfield R. A. Current status of regional arterial infusion chemotherapy. *Med. Clin. North Am.* 59:411, 1975.

54. Pack, G. T., and Miller, T. R. The treatment of hepatic tumors. *N.Y. State J. Med.* 53:2205, 1953.

55. Plengvanit, U., Vhearanai, O., Sindhvananda, K., Damrongsak, D., Tuchinda, S., and Viranuvatti, V. Collateral arterial blood supply of the liver after hepatic artery ligation: Angiographic study of twenty patients. *Ann. Surg.* 175:105, 1972.

56. Pueyo, I., Jiménez, J. R., Hernández, J., Brugarolas, A., Garcia-Moran, M., Garcia-Muñiz, J. L., and Arroyo, F. Carcinoid syndrome treated with hepatic embolization. *AJR* 131:511, 1978.

57. Rapoport, A.H., and Burleson, R. L. Survival of patients treated with systemic fluorouracil for hepatic metastases. *Surg. Gynecol. Obstet.* 130:773, 1970.

58. Reuter, S. R., and Redman, H. C. *Gastrointestinal Angiography.* Philadelphia: Saunders, 1977. P. 308.

59. Sparks, F. C., Mosher, M. B., Hallauer, W. C., Silverstein, M. J., Rangel, D., Passaro, E., Jr., and Morton, D. L. Hepatic artery ligation and postoperative chemotherapy for hepatic metastases: Clinical and pathophysiological results. *Cancer* 35:1074, 1975.

60. Sullivan, R. D. Systemic and arterial infusion chemotherapy for metastatic liver cancer. *Int. J. Radiat. Oncol. Biol. Phys.* 1:973, 1976.

61. Sullivan, R. D., Miller, E., and Sikes, M. P. Antimetabolite-metabolite combination cancer chemotherapy. *Cancer* 12:1248, 1959.

62. Sullivan, R. D., Norcross, J. W., and Watkins, E., Jr. Chemotherapy of metastatic liver cancer by prolonged hepatic artery infusion. *N. Engl. J. Med.* 270:321, 1964.

63. Sullivan, R. D., Young, C. W., Miller, E., Glatstein, N., Clarkson, B., and Burchenal, J. H. The clinical effects of the continuous administration of fluorinated pyrimidines (5-fluorouracil and 5-fluoro-2'-deoxyuridine). *Cancer Chemother. Rep.* 8:77, 1960.

64. Sullivan, R. D., and Zurek, W. Z. Chemotherapy of liver cancer by protracted ambulatory infusion. *J.A.M.A.* 194:481, 1965.

65. Tandon, R. N., Bunnell, I. L., and Cooper, R. G. The treatment of metastatic carcinoma of the liver by the percutaneous infusion of 5-fluorouracil. *Surgery* 73:118, 1973.

66. Tylén, U., Forsberg, L., and Owman, T. Heparinized catheters for long-term intraarterial infusion of 5-fluorouracil in liver metastases. *Cardiovasc. Radiol.* 2:111, 1979.

67. Wallace, S., Gianturco, C., Anderson, J. H., Goldstein, H. M., Davis, L. J., and Bree, R. L. Therapeutic vascular occlusion utilizing steel coil technique: Clinical applications. *AJR* 127:381, 1976.

68. Watkins, E., Jr. Chronometric infusor: An apparatus for protracted ambulatory infusion therapy. *N. Engl. J. Med.* 269:850, 1963.

69. Watkins, E., Jr., Khazei, A. M., and Nahra, K. S. Surgical basis for arterial infusion chemotherapy of disseminated carcinoma of the liver. *Surg. Gynecol. Obstet.* 130:581, 1970.

70. Watkins, E., Jr., Oberfield, R. A., Cady, B., and Clouse, M. E. Arterial infusion chemotherapy of diffuse hepatic malignancies. *Prog. Clin. Cancer* 7:235, 1978.

71. Wilson, S. M., and Adson, M. A. Surgical treatment of hepatic metastases from colorectal cancers. *Arch. Surg.* 111:330, 1976.

72. Wirtanen, G. W. Percutaneous transbrachial artery infusion catheter techniques. *AJR* 117:696, 1973.

73. Wirtanen, G. W., Bernhardt, L. C., Mackman, S., Ramirez, G., Curreri, A. R., and Ansfield, F. J. Hepatic artery and celiac axis infusion for the treatment of upper abdominal malignant lesions. *Ann. Surg.* 168:137, 1968.

74. Wooley, P. V., III, Macdonald, J. S., and Schein, P. S. Chemotherapy of colorectal carcinoma. *Semin. Oncol.* 3:415, 1976.

3. Biopsy

Transthoracic Lung Biopsy

PETER G. HERMAN

Leyden [13], in 1883, and subsequently Menetrier [15], in 1886, were the first to perform direct percutaneous lung biopsy in order to diagnose pneumonia and lung cancer. Although transthoracic lung biopsy has been known for almost 100 years, the technique became more widely used only during the past 20 years. The introduction of image-amplified television fluoroscopy, which allows the precise localization of the lesion, and the development of modern cytopathologic techniques and smaller and better biopsy instruments have markedly improved the success rate of the transthoracic approach. The technique is relatively simple, and the equipment required is available in most hospitals. A successful biopsy program, however, requires close cooperation among the radiologist, the cytopathologist, the microbiologist, and the thoracic surgeon.

Definitions

Transthoracic needle biopsy is the sampling of the thoracic contents by a needle introduced through the chest wall in order to obtain cytologic, microbiologic, and histopathologic specimens. The needle biopsy may also be considered as either an aspiration biopsy or a tissue core biopsy. *Aspiration biopsy* yields only tissue fluids and therefore is limited to cytologic and/or microbiologic assessment, whereas *tissue core biopsy* provides, in addition, tissue fragments that are suitable for histopathologic examination.

Indications

In general, transthoracic biopsy may give useful information in the presence of any radiographically visible pulmonary abnormality of unknown etiology, either focal or disseminated. This is particularly true when an unexpected pulmonary abnormality cannot be related to any past or current illness. In practice, an a priori judgment as to the most likely cause based on the clinical presentation, the history, the occupational and epidemiologic data, and the x-ray findings will influence the indications for biopsy. The following are the more commonly encountered specific indications.

For patients with solitary pulmonary mass or nodule who are poor operative risks, transthoracic

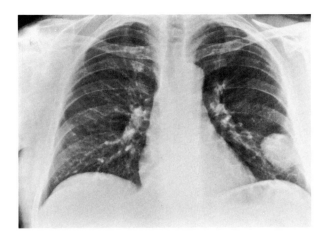

Figure 101-1. A 49-year-old man who was a heavy smoker. A chest x-ray taken 3 months earlier showed a large mass in the left lower lobe. In the 3-month interval, there had been no change in the mass.

needle biopsy is indicated, provided that it will have an impact on patient management. The role of needle biopsy in patients with solitary pulmonary nodules who are good surgical candidates is not clearly defined. In these patients, the risks of surgery have to be weighed against the risks of needle biopsy, which include the possibility of a false diagnosis. For patients with a high clinical suspicion of cancer, either aspiration biopsy or core biopsy is often diagnostic. If the purpose of the biopsy is to establish a specific benign diagnosis, tissue core biopsy allowing histopathologic

examination is usually required. If surgery will inevitably be carried out, needle biopsy should not be done.

Multiple pulmonary nodules or masses may be diagnosed with cytologic techniques; however, a core biopsy will permit a more specific classification of the abnormality.

Cavitary processes will frequently yield both cytologic and microbiologic material using the aspiration technique.

Focal or disseminated confluent opacities are often biopsied at the time of bronchoscopy using the transbronchial technique. It is well documented, however, that aspiration biopsy and core biopsy [4, 9] yield the correct diagnosis in both neoplastic and inflammatory diseases.

Disseminated interstitial processes are usually best biopsied either by the transbronchial route or by open lung biopsy; however, needle biopsy may be diagnostic [18, 19].

Mediastinal abnormalities have recently been successfully biopsied with small-gauge aspiration needles with a high diagnostic accuracy and low morbidity [1, 11]. The technique is not yet widely used.

ASPIRATION BIOPSY VERSUS CORE BIOPSY

In a nationwide survey in the United States that compared diagnostic yields and complications, no significant differences were found between tissue

Figure 101-2. (A) Biopsy specimen, low power (× 10). Diagnostic for hamartoma. The vacuoles in the center represent the presumed areas of fat dissolved in

processing. (B) Hyaline cartilage (×70). (Courtesy of Fredrick P. Stitik, M.D.)

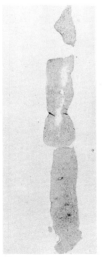
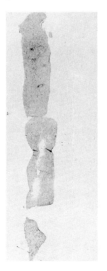
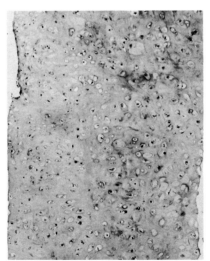
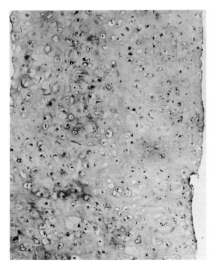

A   *B*

core biopsy and aspiration needle biopsy [9]. It is our impression, however, that small needles (18–23 gauge) are associated with lower morbidity. As a practical compromise, we are currently using a 22-gauge modified Chiba needle [8] that is sharpened around its entire circumference and that yields both aspirate and tissue fragments.

In general, to confirm the malignant nature of a pulmonary abnormality, cytologic study usually is sufficient. On the other hand, to establish the definitely benign nature of a lesion, core biopsy is desirable for obtaining a specific histologic diagnosis (Figs. 101-1, 101-2A, B).

Contraindications

Specific contraindications include patients who are unable to tolerate a unilateral pneumothorax, uncooperative patients, patients with bleeding diathesis, patients on anticoagulation therapy, and patients with suspected vascular lesions or severe pulmonary hypertension [23]. The relative indications and contraindications, however, have to be weighed for each patient individually.

Informed Consent

The patient should be informed about the indication for the procedure and its relevance to his management. The potential complications, such as pneumothorax, occasional hemorrhage, and the possible need for a chest tube, should be explained. It is useful to describe in advance the steps of the procedure and the probabilities of making the needed diagnosis. Since a successful biopsy also depends on the patient's cooperation, making sure that the patient is well informed not only fulfills the legal requirements but also makes it easier to carry out the procedure.

Prebiopsy Evaluation and Orders

In addition to the routine laboratory tests, we require a recent platelet count of more than 100,000 per cubic millimeter and a prothrombin time that is within 3 seconds of normal. The patient is instructed not to eat or drink for 4 hours before the biopsy. Sedation is usually not required, but a mild tranquilizer or phenobarbital may be given to the apprehensive patient. The patient's chart and his radiographic studies should be available in the biopsy room.

Biopsy Procedure

NEEDLE SELECTION

Needles of various sizes and shapes have been successfully used in the past [1, 5, 6, 9, 10, 12, 14, 20, 21, 23, 25]. As was mentioned earlier, the most commonly used needle in our institution at the present time is a 22-gauge modified Chiba needle, which is not only suitable for aspiration biopsy but which frequently yields diagnostic tissue fragments [8] (the modified Chiba needle was designed by R. Greene for Cook Inc.). The needle is usually advanced through a 19-gauge disposable Chiba needle placed in the proximity of the lesion. The use of the introducer needle allows numerous passes to be made through a single puncture of the chest wall and the pleura (Figs. 101-3, 101-4).

For tissue core biopsy in the lung periphery, we occasionally use an 18-gauge Turner needle (see Fig. 101-3) [25], which will also yield both aspirate and tissue fragments.

For aspiration biopsy, we use a 19- or a 22-gauge Chiba needle. For mediastinal biopsies, however, we use only the modified or the standard 22-gauge Chiba needle.

The sizes and shapes of the various biopsy needles are shown in Figure 101-3.

Figure 101-3. Transthoracic lung biopsy instruments and their outer diameters (left to right): Vim Tru-Cut needle; Nordenström screw needle; 16-gauge Turner needle (0.0645–0.0655); 18-gauge Turner needle (0.0495–0.0505); 19-gauge Chiba needle (0.0415–0.0425); 22-gauge modified Chiba needle (0.0280–0.0285).

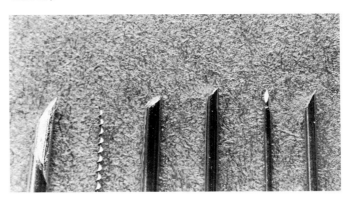

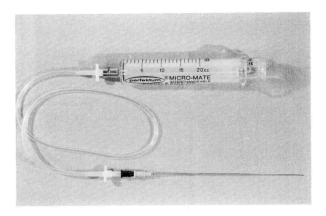

Figure 101-4. Biopsy assembly: 19-gauge introducer needle, 22-gauge biopsy needle, 12-inch connecting tubing, 20-cc suction syringe.

RADIOLOGIC LOCALIZATION OF THE ABNORMALITY

The patient's radiographs, including his computed tomographic scans, are reviewed and those images that best illustrate and localize the abnormality are displayed on a view box in the biopsy room. Based on the depth from the skin and the proximity of sensitive structures, a decision is made as to the best entry point. If the prebiopsy localization seems to be particularly difficult, additional radiographs, tomograms, or computed tomograms are obtained. With computed tomography, we often mark the most appropriate entry point on the skin and confirm it with a repeat cut. We have found computed tomography to be particularly useful in the lung apex and the paravertebral areas.

In the biopsy suite, the patient is placed on the fluoroscopic couch in the recumbent position. The fluoroscopic unit should have either a biplane arrangement or a C arm that allows for the

Figure 101-5. Biopsy tray contains syringes, needles, culture tubes, glass slides, scalpel, hemostats, etc.

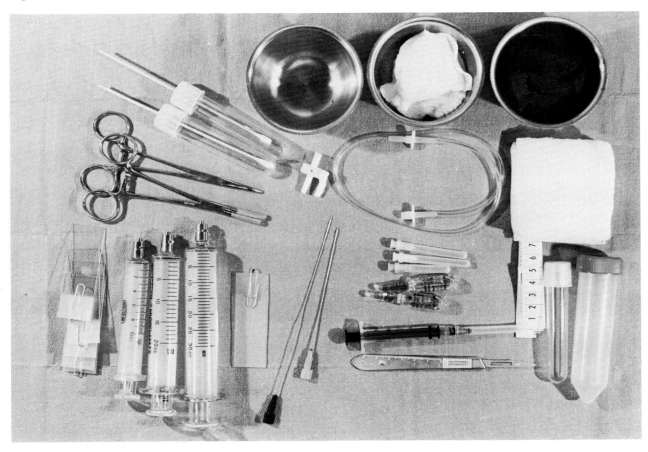

control of the direction of the needle and the confirmation of the target in two planes. Although biplane fluoroscopy is preferred, single plane fluoroscopy may be used. The depth of the lesion from the entry point has to be determined from the radiographs.

After the entry point has been decided, a metallic marker (BB) is placed on the patient's skin. The position of the metallic marker is reconfirmed by fluoroscopy and the skin is then marked with ink. The skin surrounding the site of entry is prepared with alcohol and iodine and is draped with sterile towels (Fig. 101-5). The subcutaneous tissues reaching the parietal pleura are anesthetized with 1 percent lidocaine. The biopsy site is again verified fluoroscopically by placing a small-gauge needle at the planned site of entry. A tiny incision is then made in the skin and subcutaneous tissue with a #11 scalpel blade to facilitate the passage of the needle through the skin. The biopsy (or introducer) needle is then inserted over the superior border of the lower rib to avoid the intercostal vessels that are situated at the inferior margin of the upper rib. The needle is always advanced parallel with the central ray of the fluoroscopy tube. During the puncture of the pleura, the patient is instructed to hold his breath and then to maintain shallow, quiet respiration. The needle is advanced in 1-to-2-cm increments, with frequent observation under fluoroscopy. The operator's hand is outside the fluoroscopic field. A long, sterile clamp may be used for the advancement of the needle. When the 19-gauge needle has reached the proximity of the abnormality, the needle mandrin is removed and the 22-gauge modified Chiba needle is passed through the introducer needle. When the 22-gauge biopsy needle has reached the periphery of the abnormality, the stylet is removed and a 20-millimeter glass syringe is attached to the needle with a 12-inch flexible plastic connecting tube filled with sterile Hank's solution. Under fluoroscopic guidance, several short thrusts are made with the needle by the operator while an assistant applies suction with the 20-cc syringe. During the biopsy, the needle is both advanced and rotated. At the completion of the biopsy, the suction is released, and the needle, the connecting tube, and the syringe are removed. The mandrin is replaced into the introducer needle. At this point, the operator concentrates his attention on the proper handling of the specimen while an assistant observes and fluoroscopes the patient to evaluate him for pneumothorax or hemothorax.

Specimen Handling

It is essential to decide before the biopsy whether an inflammatory or a noninflammatory process is more likely to be present. If sufficient material is available, it should be routinely submitted for cytologic, histopathologic, and microbiologic study. All specimen handling is done with sterile technique.

The biopsy needle, the connecting tube, and the suction syringe are removed as a unit (see Fig. 101-4). The biopsy needle is then detached from the connecting tube, and, with a 10-cc wetted syringe, the contents of the needle are expressed and smeared on sterile glass slides. If a tumor is suspected, the glass slides are immediately dropped in 96 percent alcohol for cytologic study. If an inflammatory process is considered, the glass slides are air dried. If tissue fragments are recovered from the needle tube, they are immediately placed in 10 percent formalin for histologic study.

The contents of the connecting tube and the suction syringe are then injected into a 25-cc sterile, clear-plastic jar. The syringe and the connecting tube are flushed repeatedly with sterile Hank's solution into the same jar.

Larger tissue fragments settling to the bottom of the container are removed and put in formalin for histologic study. The remaining contents of the jar are gently shaken, and small aliquots are sent for microbiologic study. We routinely submit cultures to be studied for aerobic and anaerobic organisms, acid-fast bacilli, and fungi.

The alcohol-fixed smears and the plastic jar are sent for cytologic study. The smears are stained with a Papanicolaou stain, and the contents of the jar are passed through a Millipore filter and stained. If larger tissue fragments are still present, they are submitted for histologic study.

The air-dried slides are routinely stained with Gram's and acid-fast stain and with Gomori methenamine silver stain (for microorganisms).

It should be emphasized that the success of the biopsy depends to a large extent on proper planning of the specimen handling and making collaborative arrangements with the cytology, pathology, and microbiology laboratories.

Postbiopsy Care

If the patient is asymptomatic and if no evidence of pneumothorax or hemothorax is seen fluoroscopically, an upright posteroanterior chest film is obtained during expiration to rule out pneumothorax. If there is no evidence of pneumothorax, a follow-up chest radiograph is obtained 5 hours later. In the event of a small pneumothorax that does not require a chest tube, the patient must remain in the hospital for follow-up x-rays at appropriate intervals until the pneumothorax subsides or becomes stable. If a significant pneumothorax occurs, a thoracic surgeon is consulted for chest tube placement. The patient immediately receives oxygen through a face mask. If necessary, a large-bore Intracath can be inserted into the pleural cavity and the pleural air removed with suction using a 50-mm syringe.

Following an uncomplicated lung biopsy, the patient has little discomfort. Nevertheless, we recommend 2 hours of bed rest. The patient may resume a normal diet.

Diagnostic Yield

MALIGNANT TUMORS

It is somewhat difficult to compare the results of the various reported series (Table 101-1) since there are differences in patient population,

biopsy technique, and specimen handling. There is general agreement, however (provided that the biopsy needle has not missed the lesion), that the diagnostic accuracy using cytologic study will be 80 percent or higher [5, 6, 8, 9, 12, 20–24]. False-positive results will not exceed 1 to 2 percent, while false-negative results (in which a malignant tumor that is indeed present is not detected by the biopsy) will be 4 to 25 percent. The accuracy varies somewhat with the experience of the operator, the handling of the specimen, and the number of passes made. A second pass increases the diagnostic accuracy [20].

The diagnostic accuracy of the tissue core histologic study is similar to that of the cytologic study [8]. However, the former permits more specific classification of the lesion. Since a biopsy may be in error in 4 to 25 percent of the cases, these limitations have to be considered in the management of the patient.

BENIGN TUMORS

Successful diagnosis of benign tumors using cytologic study alone has been reported, but definitive diagnosis of these lesions requires histologic confirmation [23]. In our institution we

Table 101-1. Diagnostic Accuracy and Complications of Transthoracic Lung Biopsy in Various Types of Abnormalities

Abnormality	Number of Patients	Overall Accuracy (%)	Number of Deaths	Pneumothorax (%)	Chest Tube (%)	Comments
Mostly malignancy						
Sinner (1961–1975) [21, 22]	2,726	90.7	0	27.2	2.6	0.9-, 1.0-, and 1.1-mm needles
Sagel (1978) [20]	896	96	0	24	14	Turner 18-gauge needle
Herman & Hessel (1977) [8]	1,940	83	2	15	5	Various needles
Lalli et al. (1978) [12]	1,223	86.4	1	24.2	4.4	18-gauge needle
Stitik (1980) [24]	225	93	0	25	4	Turner needle
Inflammatory process						
Castellino (1979) [4]	82	73	0	26	13	18-gauge spinal needle
Herman & Hessel (1977) [8]	112	73	0	—	—	Various needles
Mediastinal abnormality						
Jereb & Us-Drasovec (1976) [10]	50	72	0	13.8	3.4	22-gauge needle
Adler & Rosenberger (1979) [1]	38	76	0	16	2	22-gauge needle

accept a report that a mass is benign only if a specific diagnosis (e.g., of a hamartoma) can be made histologically (see Figs. 101-1, 101-2A, B).

Inflammatory Processes

The diagnostic accuracy for inflammatory processes is more difficult to evaluate because of the variety and extent of these processes and the problems inherent in confirming the causative organisms. We estimate that approximately 60 to 70 percent of the correct microbiological diagnoses can be made from smears or cultures [4, 7, 8, 18]. Very often, primarily in protozoal and fungal processes, histologic study will be diagnostic (Table 101-1).

Complications

Small pneumothorax is present in 8 to 50 percent of patients, and the chest tube is required in 4 to 50 percent of patients [6, 8, 12, 14, 20, 22–24]. With the use of small needles (18 gauge and smaller), hemoptysis occurs in 3 to 5 percent of patients; significant hemoptysis (30 mm or more) is very rare. Major hemothorax or air embolization has been reported occasionally, but it also is considered a very rare complication [16, 17, 26].

The mortality in aspiration biopsy is approximately 0.1 percent; in core biopsy it is 0.3 percent [8]. Dissemination of malignancy along the needle track is a potential complication [3], but it is exceedingly rare (3 of 5,000 biopsies) [23]. Dissemination of inflammation is even more unusual.

The complication rate varies, depending on the patient selection, the needle type, the number of passes, and the experience of the operator.

General Comments

It is mandatory that accurate records be kept, including records of the type of needle used, the number of passes made, and the certainty that the needle has entered the lesion. The records should also note the type of specimen submitted and the results. The occurrence and the severity of complications must be carefully noted.

The success of transthoracic needle biopsy has to be judged on the diagnostic yield and the complication rate. To confirm a suspected malignancy, the diagnostic yield should exceed 80 percent, with negligible false-positive results.

In general, the smallest, least traumatic needle should be used, and the minimal number of passes should be made. Each patient has to be evaluated individually, and the specimen-handling strategy tailored accordingly. Collaboration among the departments of cytology, pathology, and thoracic surgery is essential. The prebiopsy and postbiopsy care should be standardized. Small-needle transthoracic biopsy is a very useful, relatively simple diagnostic technique that yields accurate diagnosis and has a low complication rate.

References

1. Adler, O., and Rosenberger, A. Invasive radiology in the diagnosis of mediastinal masses: Use of fine needle for aspiration biopsy. *Radiologe* 19:169, 1979.
2. Ballard, G. L., and Boyd, W. R. A specially designed cutting aspiration needle for lung biopsy. *AJR* 130:899, 1978.
3. Berger, R. L., Dargan, E. L., and Huang, B. L. Dissemination of cancer cells by needle biopsy of the lung. *J. Thorac. Cardiovasc. Surg.* 63:430, 1972.
4. Castellino, R. A., and Blank, N. Etiologic diagnosis of focal pulmonary infection in immunocompromised patients by fluoroscopically guided percutaneous needle aspiration. *Radiology* 132:563, 1979.
5. Chin, W. S., and Sng Tsun Kee, I. Percutaneous aspiration biopsy of malignant lung lesions using the Chiba needle: An initial experience. *Clin. Radiol.* 29:617, 1978.
6. Dahlgren, S., and Nordenström, B. *Transthoracic Needle Biopsy.* Chicago: Year Book, 1966. P. 59.
7. Giglia, A. R., Morgan, P. N., and Bates, J. H. Rapid definitive diagnosis of Legionnaire's disease. *Chest* 76:98, 1979.
8. Herman, P. G., and Hessel, S. J. The diagnostic accuracy and complications of closed lung biopsies. *Radiology* 125:11, 1977.
9. Hutton, L. Percutaneous pulmonary aspiration biopsy using the Chiba needle. *J. Can. Assoc. Radiol.* 30:148, 1979.
10. Jereb, M., and Us-Drasovec, M. Transthoracic needle biopsy of mediastinal and hilar lesions. *Cancer* 40:1354, 1977.

11. Koss, L. G. Thin needle aspiration biopsy (editorial). *Acta Cytol.* 24:1, 1980.

12. Lalli, A. F., McCormack, L. J., Zelch, M., Reich, N. E., and Belovich, D. Aspiration biopsies of chest lesions. *Radiology* 127:35, 1978.

13. Leyden, H. Verhandlungen des Vereins für innere Medizin. *Dtsch. Med. Wochenschr.* 9:52, 1883.

14. McCartney, R., Tait, D., Stilson, M., and Seidel, G. F. A technique for the prevention of pneumothorax in pulmonary aspiration biopsy. *AJR* 120:872, 1974.

15. Menetrier, P. Cancer primitif du poumon. *Bull. Soc. Anat. Paris* 4:643, 1886.

16. Meyer, J. E., Ferrucci, J. T., and Janowner, M. C. Fatal complications of percutaneous lung biopsy: Review of the literature and report of a case. *Radiology* 96:47, 1970.

17. Milner, L. B., Ryan, K., and Gullo, J. Fatal intrathoracic hemorrhage after percutaneous aspiration lung biopsy. *AJR* 132:280, 1979.

18. Ramzy, I., Geraghty, R., Lefcoe, M. S., and Lefcoe, N. M. Chronic eosinophilic pneumonia: Diagnosis by fine needle aspiration. *Acta Cytol.* 22:366, 1978.

19. Roub, L. W., Dekker, A., Wagenblast, H. W., and Reece, G. J. Pulmonary silicatosis: A case diagnosed by needle-aspiration biopsy and energy-dispersive x-ray analysis. *Am. J. Clin. Pathol.* 72:871, 1979.

20. Sagel, S. S., Ferguson, T. B., Forrest, J. V., Roger, C. L., Weldon, C. S., and Clark, R. E. Percutaneous transthoracic aspiration needle biopsy. *Ann. Thorac. Surg.* 26:399, 1978.

21. Sinner, W. N. Transthoracic needle biopsy of small peripheral malignant lung lesions. *Invest. Radiol.* 8:305, 1973.

22. Sinner, W. N. Pulmonary neoplasms diagnosed with transthoracic needle biopsy. *Cancer* 43:1533, 1979.

23. Stitik, F. P. Percutaneous Lung Biopsy. In S. S. Siegelman and W. R. Summer (eds.), *Multiple Imaging Procedures. Vol. 1: Pulmonary System: Practical Approaches to Pulmonary Diagnoses.* New York: Grune & Stratton, 1972. P. 181.

24. Stitik, F. P. Personal communication, 1980.

25. Turner, F. T., and Sargent, E. N. Percutaneous pulmonary needle biopsy: An improved needle for a simple direct method of diagnosis. *AJR* 104:846, 1968.

26. Westcott, J. L. Air embolism complicating percutaneous needle biopsy of the lung. *Chest* 63:108, 1973.

Percutaneous Biopsy of the Pancreas, Retroperitoneum, and Liver

EDWARD H. SMITH

Percutaneous biopsy of organs or masses for diagnostic purposes is by no means a new technique, and considerable experience has been obtained and much information has been accumulated as to its accuracy, safety, and utility.

Percutaneous biopsy provides direct confirmation of the nature of the lesion under question, often in the safest, shortest, and least expensive way, obviating the need for more complex invasive procedures. Previously, the limitation of percutaneous biopsy has been the inability to place the needle accurately within the lesion. Several new techniques have been developed to overcome this limitation, enabling percutaneous biopsy to become one of the major diagnostic tools available. These techniques, as well as the older methods, are described in this chapter. Ultrasound guidance, using the specially developed biopsy transducer, is emphasized, and the application of this technique to and its effects on lesions of the pancreas, retroperitoneum, and liver are discussed.

Techniques

Although the term *percutaneous biopsy* appears to be self-explanatory and to need no further definition, the type (and size) of the needle used and the method of needle guidance employed are critical in determining the accuracy, safety, and, indeed, the place of the technique in the modern diagnostic array of methods.

BLIND BIOPSY

Until recently, percutaneous biopsy was limited to situations in which "blind" biopsy was indicated; e.g., liver biopsy in which the needle is placed blindly within the organ from which only a representative sample of tissue is desired or in which the disease process is thought to be so diffuse that biopsy of any site will yield a diagnosis. In other situations, a mass is palpated and the needle placement guided by the palpating fingers.

Certainly in the latter circumstance, blind biopsy would be acceptable. However, that circumstance is not very common, and even then, one may be deceived as to the size of the mass by physical examination. In addition, biopsy of a certain portion of the mass may be more likely to yield a diagnosis (Fig. 102-1).

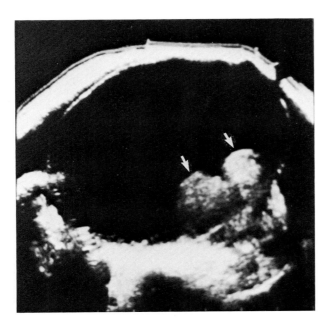

Figure 102-1. A nubbin of solid tissue (*arrows*) in a scan of a patient with ascites. It is unlikely that a blind biopsy would fortuitously strike the solid elements.

Even if blind biopsy is perhaps satisfactory, it stands to reason that if the lesion to be biopsied can be visualized and the needle placement guided, the yield will be higher and, possibly, a finer-gauge needle can be used, reducing the risk of the procedure.

GUIDED BIOPSY

Radiologic-Assisted Techniques
The usual methods of needle guidance have been radiologic ones, with identification of a mass on plain films or, more commonly, by fluoroscopy. If the target is seen on the radiograph, the needle can be introduced, either in steps guided by further films or by a mark made on the skin, with subsequent introduction of the needle and completion of the biopsy in one step.

Fluoroscopy alone remains the method of choice when the lesion can be clearly identified by this means (usually a lesion in the lung or in bone); fluoroscopy has very little application in the abdomen. Extensive experience in the needle aspiration of pulmonary lesions has been gained over the years, and aspiration and cytologic techniques have been adapted for use in other areas of the body [3].

Obviously, both radiographic and fluoroscopic methods can be performed in conjunction with

contrast enhancement to improve further visualization of the lesion to be biopsied. Thus opacification of the upper gastrointestinal tract with barium may outline a mass in the head of the pancreas and allow successful needle aspiration of the lesion during fluoroscopy or with plain-film guidance. Opacification of the ureters during excretory urography may enable indirect visualization of a retroperitoneal mass, facilitating more accurate needle placement. However, these methods allow visualization of only relatively large or opportunely located masses and will not provide any information concerning the internal architecture of the lesion. Thus the optimal site within the mass may not be chosen, or a vascular lesion, such as an aortic aneurysm, may be inadvertently biopsied.

Any one of a number of more complex fluoroscopic procedures can be carried out as a guide to needle placement [24]. Contrast material may be injected via a percutaneously placed vascular catheter with subsequent identification of an area of tumor "blush," tumor vasculature, or encasement. Then, with the aid of hand injections of small amounts of contrast material via the catheter, the area of abnormality produced by the tumor can be visualized fluoroscopically while the needle is guided to this area [22]. If the appropriate equipment is available, fluoroscopy can be done simultaneously in two planes so that the depth of the lesion can be determined as well.

Similarly, biopsy can be performed in conjunction with such procedures as percutaneous transhepatic cholangiography, endoscopic retrograde pancreatography [14], and lymphangiography [10], with fluoroscopic visualization of the area of abnormality and guidance of the needle to this area.

All these methods are complex, invasive, time consuming, and involve irradiation; also, they are expensive, usually requiring hospitalization of the patient. However, if any of these procedures is the only one by which the lesion can be visualized, it becomes the method of choice.

Radionuclide Techniques
Radionuclide techniques may similarly be used to identify an area of abnormality with demarcation of the biopsy site on the skin overlying the lesion and subsequent introduction of a biopsy needle [18]. This study can be done either with a static scan or in conjunction with a computer-assisted dynamic flow study that provides information regarding the vascularity of the lesion to be biop-

sied. Multiple projections of the lesion can be obtained so that its depth can be determined.

Computed Tomography

Computed tomography (CT) as a guide for needle placement is becoming increasingly popular [6, 11, 12]. With this technique, the lesion is localized on the CT scan, the skin overlying the lesion is marked, and a needle is percutaneously introduced into the subcutaneous tissues. The patient is then moved back into the CT scanner, and the study is repeated, with further introduction of the needle toward the lesion; or, if the needle appears to be off course, it is removed and redirected or a second needle is introduced alongside the first one. The process is continued until the lesion is successfully negotiated. This technique is most convenient when the needle pathway can be perpendicular to the skin surface. When the lesion is small, or if it is deep and the needle pathway has to be severely angulated, the procedure may be quite difficult and time consuming. The advantage of this method is that the needle tip most often can be identified and confirmed to be within the lesion and the depth of the target can be readily determined. In addition, smaller lesions are more easily visualized than with ultrasonography, and bowel gas does not present a problem.

ULTRASONICALLY GUIDED PUNCTURE

Ultrasonography can be used as an aid to percutaneous biopsy in several ways. Most simply, a scan is performed, the lesion is identified in two planes, it is characterized as cystic or solid and its depth from the surface is measured, and the skin overlying the lesion is marked. The needle can then be inserted and the biopsy done. This is a satisfactory approach, but it is of great advantage to visualize the target during the procedure. For this purpose, a specially constructed B-scan biopsy transducer has been developed [17]. The transducer has a central channel through which the needle is introduced (Fig. 102-2). The transducer connector to the scanning arm is displaced off-axis to allow sufficient room for needle manipulation. The canal should be wide enough to permit the introduction of a cutting-biopsy needle; adapters can be inserted for smaller caliber needles. Once the lesion is discovered, the optimal plane and direction of the puncture is determined. The skin overlying the lesion is marked, and the conventional transducer is exchanged for

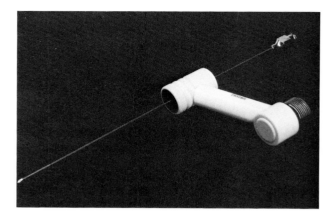

Figure 102-2. B-scan biopsy transducer containing a central channel through which the needle is introduced.

a sterile biopsy transducer. The skin overlying the region is sterilized, and the area is rescanned, using the biopsy transducer. The lesion is again visualized, and the transducer is positioned so that when the depth-marker button is pressed, an array of dots is electronically flashed across the monitor such that the dots pass directly through the center of the lesion. These dots pass through the central axis of the transducer, exactly demarcating the needle pathway. The depth of the part of the lesion to be biopsied is then measured. This distance is added to the length of the biopsy transducer, and a needle stop is placed at this distance along the needle shaft. After local anesthesia is administered, the needle is inserted through the puncture transducer up to the needle stop, and the biopsy is performed. All the while, the needle direction is monitored with the depth-marker array of dots, to ensure that the desired angulation of the needle is maintained (Fig. 102-3). With cystic lesions and with certain homogeneous solid lesions, the tip of the needle may be seen on the A-mode display and occasionally on the B-scan as well.

When it is determined that the needle is within the area in question, a 10-cc syringe is attached, full suction is applied, and the needle tip is moved vertically three or four times to ensure that an adequate sample is obtained. The suction is released and the needle withdrawn. The syringe is detached and filled with air; the aspirate is expelled from the needle onto glass slides, which are then placed immediately in 95 percent alcohol and stained by the Papanicolaou technique. (The staining procedure varies with the cytologist, and he must be consulted prior to the

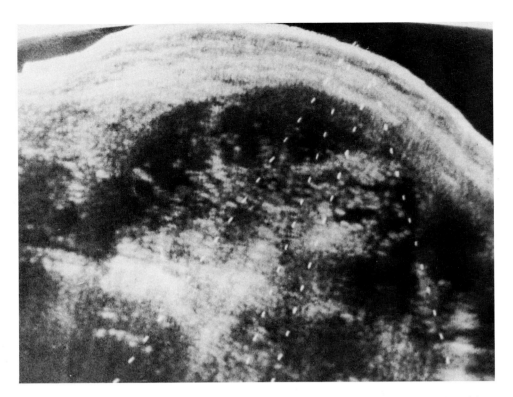

Figure 102-3. Large abdominal mass. An array of centimeter depth-marker dots that pass through the central axis of the biopsy transducer is flashed on the monitor until the desired pathway is obtained. The needle introduced through the biopsy transducer channel follows this path. These dots are flashed onto the monitor continuously as the needle is introduced to ensure that the desired angulation is maintained.

procedure.) Three or four aspirates are usually obtained, if possible, from different parts of the mass.

The method just described has a number of advantages over the others previously described. The imaging is rapid, the lesion is visualized in at least two planes, its depth is accurately determined, its internal architecture is demonstrated, and the surrounding organs are identified. Most important, the target is visualized during the needle insertion, which is extremely helpful when small, deeply situated structures are biopsied. Ultrasound equipment is relatively inexpensive and commonly available in most hospitals, and it does not involve the use of radiation.

Certain objections to the technique have been raised. It has been claimed that the use of a biopsy transducer makes the system too rigid, increasing the risk of laceration [6, 20]. However, if the scanner is set up parallel to the long axis of the patient and the connector arm of the biopsy transducer is set up perpendicular to the plane of the scanning arm, the biopsy transducer (and

needle) will be free to move with the patient's respiratory excursions (Fig. 102-4). For a distortion-free image, the biopsy transducer must always be attached so that the connector arm is at all times perpendicular to the plane of the scanning arm, not parallel to it (Fig. 102-5) [28].

Variations of the technique, using dynamic scanning or an A-mode biopsy transducer, can be employed. In certain circumstances they are quite satisfactory. The introduction of a real-time aspiration biopsy transducer promises to simplify the technique even further, and this will in all likelihood become the method of choice [8].

In general, if moderate-to-large amounts of fluid are to be removed, a 19-gauge needle is used. If it must be decided whether a solid lesion is malignant, a fine (22-gauge) needle is employed and several aspirations from different parts of the mass are taken in the same session. This technique yields a cytologic aspirate, not a tissue sample. If a tissue sample is required, special cutting-biopsy needles are used. When fine-needle biopsy is carried out, the procedure is

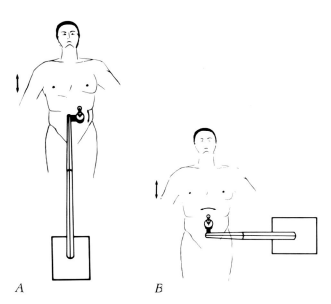

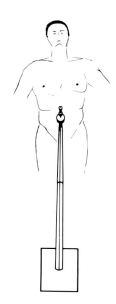

Figure 102-4. (A) Correct attachment of the biopsy transducer to the scanning arm. The scanning arm is set up *parallel* to the long axis of the patient. The connector arm of the biopsy transducer is *perpendicular* to this plane. The motion of the biopsy transducer (*curved arrow*) is in the same direction as the patient's respiratory motion (*straight arrow*). This scheme allows free movement of the needle, and it does not create a rigid system. (B) Incorrect orientation of the scanning arm *perpendicular* to the long axis of the patient. Transducer motion, and hence needle motion, is *perpendicular* to the patient's respiratory excusions and creates a rigid system that increases the risk of needle laceration.

Figure 102-5. Incorrect attachment of the biopsy transducer to the scanning arm. The biopsy transducer should be *perpendicular* to the plane of the scanning arm to ensure a distortion-free image. (Adapted from Yeh et al. [28].)

quite safe and can be performed on an outpatient basis, provided the patient is observed for a suitable period of time following the procedure.

Applications and Results

PANCREATIC BIOPSY

Despite the many advances in diagnostic techniques, pancreatic malignancy is difficult to diagnose, and exploratory surgery is often resorted to as the definitive diagnostic step. Unfortunately, by the time the disease becomes clinically manifest, it is most often surgically unresectable. In situations in which a solid mass in the pancreas is detected by ultrasonography and is seen to be unresectable (by evidence of metastases or by extrapancreatic vascular encasement), percutaneous fine-needle biopsy under ultrasound guidance

should be undertaken if a tissue diagnosis is required. Arnesjö et al. and others have shown that cytodiagnosis by means of needle aspiration during laparotomy compares favorably with the histologic diagnosis of surgical specimens [1, 19]. When a fine (22- or 23-gauge) needle is used, essentially none of the morbidity associated with the cutting-biopsy technique during laparotomy has occurred.

Technique
The technique for pancreatic biopsy is essentially that just described (Fig. 102-6). The procedure can be performed on an inpatient or an outpatient basis. A routine hematologic workup is done to exclude an occult bleeding dyscrasia, and the patient is kept fasting the morning of the procedure. The shortest, most direct needle pathway is selected; puncture through the liver is avoided, but the gastrointestinal tract is routinely traversed without untoward sequelae. (It must be kept in mind that a 22-gauge needle creates a hole smaller than does the surgeon's suture.)

Results
Pancreatic biopsy is now being done successfully in a number of institutions [4, 6, 9, 27]. The largest series reported to date has been that of

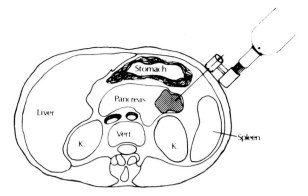

Figure 102-6. Diagrammatic representation of a biopsy of the tail of the pancreas. The needle is seen to pass through the channel of the biopsy transducer directly into the pancreatic mass (*shaded portion*). It is not always possible to avoid passing the needle through the stomach or the small intestine, but this can be done without any apparent risk. *Vert* = vertebral body.

Holm et al. [16] at the University of Copenhagen Hospital, at Herlev, with Holm pioneering the technique. Of 90 patients referred for biopsy with suspected carcinoma of the pancreas, 53 were subsequently proved to have carcinoma. Of the 53, 43 had cytologic aspirates conclusive for malignancy, while in 10, no malignant cells were recovered despite an adequate aspirate. No malignant cells were aspirated in 35 of 37 benign lesions, while in 2 cases the aspirate was inadequate (Table 102-1). No false-positive results occurred. The success rate of 81 percent compares favorably to that of open surgical biopsy and may be explained by the frequently scirrhous nature of pancreatic tumors, which may be surrounded by relatively large areas of inflammatory tissue, preventing the surgeon from palpating a focal mass [1, 19]. In addition, the surgeon is more hestitant in obtaining a biopsy from deep within the pancreas and may miss the tumor [2]. Our own more limited experience has shown similar results with no false-positive results and an ap-

proximate 80 percent success rate. It goes without saying that before this procedure is undertaken, the presence of a skilled and interested cytologist is required.

In Holm's series, no significant complications occurred, including hemorrhage, infection, or fistula formation [16]. In contrast, in an older series of 159 patients, in which pancreatic biopsy was carried out intraoperatively, either by wedge resection or the use of a large-bore (Vim-Silverman) cutting-biopsy needle, there was a complication rate of 9.5 percent, a mortality of 3.8 percent, and an accuracy rate of only 65 percent [26].

To date, only one instance of needle tract seeding in a patient undergoing percutaneous fine-needle biopsy of the pancreas has been reported [5].

The reasons for aspirating a pancreatic cystic lesion include verification of the diagnosis of pseudocyst and exclusion of a pancreatic abscess or cystic malignancy. The procedure may be therapeutic in that the fluid may not reaccumulate and surgery may be avoided entirely; or, in cases of threatened rupture, decompression by aspiration (several aspirations if necessary) may allow time for "maturation" of the cyst wall, making subsequent elective surgery safer and easier to carry out.

The technique for cyst aspiration differs from the previously described technique only in the use of a larger needle, frequently a 19-gauge needle.

The Danish experience consists of 40 patients who underwent ultrasonically guided pancreatic cyst puncture. The diameters of the cysts ranged from 3 to 20 cm. Nine patients had 2 cysts, all of which were punctured. Nine patients had repunctures, with 1 patient undergoing a total of 5 aspirations. All the punctures were successful. Twenty-one patients had recurrences within several months; 3 were without recurrence after 12 months. In 4 patients, a pancreatic abscess was

Table 102-1. Results of Pancreatic Aspiration Biopsy

Final Diagnosis	Total	Cytologic Findings		
		Malignant Cells	No Malignant Cells	Insufficient Material
Malignant	53	43	10	0
Benign	37	0	35	2
Total	90	43	45	2

From Holm et al. [16].

found and appropriate therapy was instituted [13].

RETROPERITONEAL BIOPSY

The experience with percutaneous fine-needle biopsy of retroperitoneal masses has, in general, been less rewarding than that with most other lesions within the abdomen. This is especially true when the material examined includes a large number of lymphomas. When a primary adrenal tumor is to be aspirated, it is important to exclude the presence of a pheochromocytoma by chemical studies before proceeding with the biopsy, in order to avoid provoking a hypertensive crisis. In fact, if the history is at all suggestive, it would be wise to exclude that diagnosis with any retroperitoneal mass (especially when partially cystic) since a pheochromocytoma can occur in an extraadrenal, retroperitoneal site (Fig. 102-7).

Technique

Again, the technique is the same as for a biopsy of any abdominal mass. If the lesion is large enough to be visualized with ultrasonography, it should be able to be successfully biopsied (Fig.

102-8). Very often, however, the suspected lesion is discovered by lymphangiography and is quite small, below the threshold for ultrasound detection. In such a case, it is obvious that fluoroscopically guided biopsy of the opacified lymph nodes is the method of choice; indeed, it is the only method. The lower abdomen and the upper pelvis are frequently obscured by bowel gas, and when they are, they cannot be optimally imaged by ultrasonography. In such a case, CT-guided biopsy may be the preferred method if the masses are large enough to be seen.

Results

In one series of ultrasonically guided biopsy of retroperitoneal masses, of 18 cases of malignant tumors, 14 were successfully diagnosed by fine-needle aspiration. In 1 case, no malignant cells were obtained and subsequent histologic examination revealed the tumor to be completely necrotic, with no identifiable tumor cells. In the 3 remaining cases, the aspirated material was insufficient for diagnosis. It is of interest that the series included only 2 lymphomas and 16 carcinomas (15 of them metastatic) [7]. Comparable results were obtained in a study of similar material [21], but one in which biopsy was guided

Figure 102-7. Large cystic pheochromocytoma of the right adrenal gland. Sagittal scan through the right kidney, the liver, and a cystic lesion of the adrenal. The echo-free white area above the upper pole of the right kidney represents a cystic component of the lesion surrounded by an echogenic rim. On other sections, the tumor was seen to extend into the liver and to involve the retroperitoneum as well. With any cystic retroperitoneal or adrenal lesion the possibility of a pheochromocytoma should be considered.

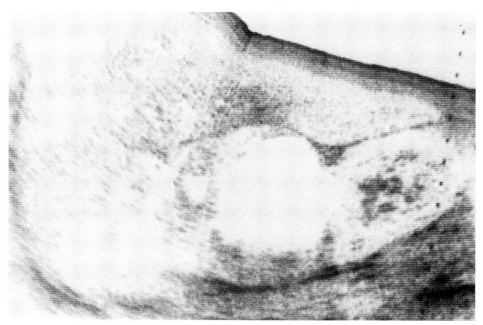

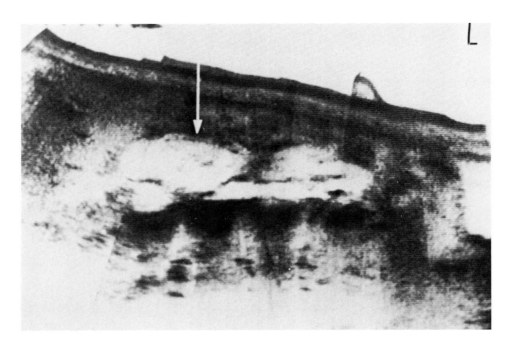

Figure 102-8. Retroperitoneal adenopathy in a patient with lymphoma. Sagittal scan revealing extensive lymphadenopathy (*arrow*) surrounding and indenting the inferior vena cava. This is an example of a lymphoma that can be easily biopsied under ultrasound guidance.

by fluoroscopy following lymphangiography. In a report from the M. D. Anderson Hospital in Houston, of 14 patients with lymphoma undergoing lymph node biopsy under fluoroscopic guidance following lymphangiography, there were 5 false-negative results (6 were true positive and 3 were true negative). This is in contrast to 58 patients (in the same study) with carcinomatous lymph node metastases among whom there were only 8 false-negative results (37 were true positive, 13 were true negative) [30]. No significant complications occurred in 109 patients. With lymphomas, the aspirated material is usually scanty, and correct diagnosis is difficult, especially the determination of histologic type.

LIVER BIOPSY

The liver is probably the abdominal organ most frequently biopsied. Biopsy is often the only way to sort out which of the various diseases affecting the liver is present; also, the liver is very frequently the site of metastatic disease and it is often the most convenient and accessible area from which to obtain a tissue diagnosis of malignancy before surgery is excluded and chemotherapy or some other type of therapy is embarked on.

Technique

Traditionally, the procedure is performed blindly (i.e., without any guidance), and a core of tissue is obtained with a large-bore cutting-biopsy needle. In the presence of diffuse liver disease, this approach is usually quite appropriate. However, in an obese patient who has a small or unusually shaped liver or an enlarged gallbladder or who has ascites, tissue may not be obtainable or another organ may be inadvertently punctured. In these situations, and probably in most cases, the biopsy should be preceded by an ultrasound scan of the liver so that a safe pathway can be chosen. Use of a biopsy transducer or other means of guidance is usually unnecessary.

In the presence of focal liver disease when proof of metastases is required, the situation is entirely different. Blind biopsy, with a large cutting-biopsy needle providing a tissue core, is successful in 20 to 91 percent of cases [23, 25]; it has a complication rate of about 10 percent, including a definite (but low) mortality [29]. But ultrasonically guided biopsy with a 22-gauge needle and a biopsy transducer carries essentially no risk, allows visualization of the lesion to be biopsied throughout the procedure, and is more accurate. If more than verification of the presence of malignant cells in a cytologic aspirate is required (i.e., a detailed histologic analysis to

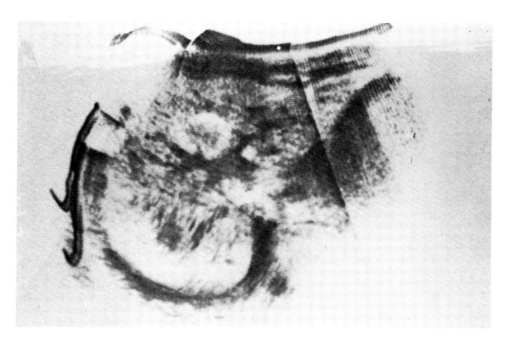

Figure 102-9. Solitary liver metastasis. Echo-poor focal lesion with an echogenic center. A blind biopsy would have a very poor chance of success. Ultrasonically guided biopsy was readily carried out.

define, for example, the site of origin of an unknown primary tumor), a core of tissue is usually needed. The cutting-biopsy needle can then be introduced via the biopsy transducer and the procedure carried out under ultrasound guidance. Unless the liver is diffusely invaded with confluent metastases, it appears to make no sense to do the procedure blindly (Fig. 102-9).

Aspiration of hepatic abscesses, amebic or pyogenic, may be carried out using the basic technique outlined previously, for both diagnostic and therapeutic purposes. The presence of hydatid disease of the liver is probably a contraindication to aspiration, because aspiration may result in peritoneal dissemination or even anaphylaxis, either of which may end in death.

Results

A study comparing the accuracy of ultrasonically guided fine-needle biopsy of focal liver lesions with ultrasonically guided core biopsy in the same patients was recently completed in Holm's laboratory [15]. Where possible, a fine-needle biopsy was followed by a core biopsy of the same lesion using a Vim Tru-Cut needle. In each case, the biopsy transducer was used, and in most cases, both biopsies were done by the same person.

Table 102-2. Comparison of Ultrasonically Guided Fine-Needle Biopsy of Focal Liver Lesions with Ultrasonically Guided Core Biopsy in the Same Patients

	50 Fine-Needle Biopsies of Liver Lesions		
	Malignant Cells	No Malignant Cells	Insufficient Material
36 Malignant lesions	33	2	1
14 Benign lesions	0	14	0
	26 Vim Tru-Cut Needle Biopsies of Liver Lesions		
	Malignant Tissue	No Malignant Tissue	Insufficient Material
22 Malignant lesions	16	3	3
4 Benign lesions	0	4	0

From Holm [15].

The results are shown in Table 102-2. The fine-needle technique was successful in detecting malignant cells in 33 of 36 metastatic liver lesions; the core biopsy was successful in 16 of 22 metastatic lesions.

From the results of this study and others [31] and the obviously greater risk involved in performing a core biopsy, it makes no sense to perform a core biopsy when only a cytologic diagnosis of a malignancy is required. When a histologic examination is required, core biopsy under ultrasound guidance seems indicated.

Summary

Ultrasonically guided fine-needle percutaneous biopsy, a very valuable and underutilized technique, is a safe, rapid, inexpensive, and relatively painless way to provide a definitive cytologic diagnosis, often obviating the need for more hazardous and expensive studies, including exploratory surgery. When the lesion to be biopsied cannot be visualized by ultrasound examination, many other methods of needle guidance are available, the choice depending on what study allows optimal visualization of the target and accuracy of needle placement.

References

1. Arnesjö, B., Stormby, N., and Åkerman, M. Cytodiagnosis of pancreatic lesions by means of fine-needle biopsy during operation. *Acta Chir. Scand.* 138:363, 1972.
2. Bowden, L. The fallibility of pancreatic biopsy. *Ann. Surg.* 139:403, 1954.
3. Dahlgren, S., and Nordenström, B. *Transthoracic Needle Biopsy.* Chicago: Year Book, 1966.
4. Evander, A., Ihse, I., Lunderquist, A., Tylén, U., and Åkerman, M. Percutaneous cytodiagnosis of carcinoma of the pancreas and bile duct. *Ann. Surg.* 188:90, 1978.
5. Ferrucci, J. T., Jr., Wittenberg, J., Margolies, M. N., and Carey, R. W. Malignant seeding of the tract after thin-needle aspiration biopsy. *Radiology* 130:345, 1979.
6. Ferrucci, J. T., Jr., Wittenberg, J., Mueller, P. R., Simeone, J. F., Harbin, W. P., Kirkpatrick, R. H., and Taft, P. D. Diagnosis of abdominal malignancy by radiologic fine-needle aspiration biopsy. *AJR* 134:323, 1980.
7. Gammelgaard, J., Pedersen, P. H., and Henriksen, O. B. Puncture of Retroperitoneal, Gastrointestinal and Gynecological Mass Lesions. In H. H. Holm and J. K. Kristensen (eds.), *Ultrasonically Guided Puncture Technique.* Copenhagen: Munksgaard, 1980.
8. Goldberg, B. B., Pollack, H. M., Cole-Beuglet, C., Kurtz, A. B., and Rubin, D. O. Real-time aspiration-biopsy transducer. *J. Clin. Ultrasound* 8:107, 1980.
9. Goldstein, H. M., Zornoza, J., Wallace, S., Anderson, J. H., Bree, R. L., Samuels, B. I., and Lukeman, J. Percutaneous fine needle aspiration biopsy of pancreatic and other abdominal masses. *Radiology* 123:319, 1977.
10. Göthlin, J. Percutaneous transperitoneal fluoroscopy-guided fine-needle biopsy of lymph nodes. *Acta Radiol. [Diagn.]* (Stockh.) 20:660, 1979.
11. Haaga, J. R. New techniques for CT-guided biopsies. *AJR* 133:633, 1979.
12. Haaga, J. R., and Alfidi, R. J. Precise biopsy localization by computed tomography. *Radiology* 118:603, 1976.
13. Hancke, S., and Jacobsen, G. W. Puncture of Pancreatic Mass Lesions. In H. H. Holm and J. K. Kristensen (eds.), *Ultrasonically Guided Puncture Technique.* Copenhagen: Munksgaard, 1980.
14. Ho, C. S., McLoughlin, M. J., McHattie, J. D., and Tao, L. C. Percutaneous fine needle aspiration biopsy of the pancreas following endoscopic retrograde cholangiopancreatography. *Radiology* 125:351, 1977.
15. Holm, H. H. Personal communication, 1979.
16. Holm, H. H., Als, O., and Gammelgaard, J. Percutaneous Aspiration and Biopsy Procedures Under Ultrasound Visualization. In K. J. W. Taylor (ed.), *Clinics in Diagnostic Ultrasound. Diagnostic Ultrasound in Gastrointestinal Disease* (vol. 1). New York, Edinburgh, London, Melbourne: Churchill Livingstone, 1979.
17. Holm, H. H., Kristensen, J. K., Rasmussen, S. N., Northeved, A., and Barlebo, H. Ultrasound as a guide in percutaneous puncture technique. *Ultrasonics* 10:83, 1972.
18. Johansen, P., and Svendsen, K. N. Scan-guided fine needle aspiration biopsy in malignant hepatic disease. *Acta Cytol.* 22:292, 1978.
19. Kline, T. S., and Neal, H. S. Needle aspiration biopsy. A safe diagnostic procedure for lesions of the pancreas. *Am. J. Clin. Pathol.* 63:16, 1975.
20. Lang, E. K. Renal cyst puncture and aspiration: A survey of complications. *AJR* 128:723, 1977.
21. Macintosh, P. K., Thomson, K. R., and Barbaric, Z. L. Percutaneous transperitoneal lymph-node biopsy as a means of improving lymphographic diagnosis. *Radiology* 131:647, 1979.
22. Oscarson, J., Stormby, N., and Sundgren, R. Selective angiography in fine-needle aspiration cytodiagnosis of gastric and pancreatic

tumours. *Acta Radiol. [Diagn.]* (Stockh.) 12:737, 1972.

23. Øvlisen, B., and Baden, H. Liver biopsy by the method of Menghini. *Nord. Med.* 83:297, 1970.

24. Pereiras, R. V., Meiers, W., Kunhardt, B., Troner, M., Hutson, D., Barkin, J. S., and Viamonte, M. Fluoroscopically guided thin needle aspiration biopsy of the abdomen and retroperitoneum. *AJR* 131:197, 1978.

25. Rasmussen, S. N., Holm, H. H., Kristensen, J. K., and Barlebo, H. Preliminary communications: Ultrasonically-guided liver biopsy. *Br. Med. J.* 2:500, 1972.

26. Schultz, N. J., and Sanders, R. J. Evaluation of pancreatic biopsy. *Ann. Surg.* 158:1053, 1963.

27. Smith, E. H., Bartrum, R. J., Chang, Y. C., D'Orsi, C. J., Lokich, J., Abbruzzese, A., and Dantono, J. Percutaneous aspiration biopsy of the pancreas under ultrasonic guidance. *N. Engl. J. Med.* 292:825, 1975.

28. Yeh, E. L., Kronenwetter, C., Meade, R. C., and Ruetz, P. P. Technical considerations in B-mode scanning with an aspiration transducer. *Radiology* 129:527, 1978.

29. Zamcheck, N., and Klausenstock, O. Liver biopsy (concluded): II. The risk of needle biopsy. *N. Engl. J. Med.* 249:1062, 1953.

30. Zornoza, J., Jonsson, K., Wallace, S., and Lukeman, J. M. Fine needle aspiration biopsy of retroperitoneal lymph nodes and abdominal masses: An updated report. *Radiology* 125:87, 1977.

31. Zornoza, J., Wallace, S., Ordonez, N., and Lukeman, J. Fine-needle aspiration biopsy of the liver. *AJR* 134:331, 1980.

Percutaneous Renal Biopsy in the Assessment of Renal Parenchymal Disease

RICHARD D. SWARTZ
KYUNG J. CHO
DOUGLASS F. ADAMS

Renal biopsy via the surgical, or "open," route dates back more than 50 years [27]. Recognition of the clinical utility of biopsy was delayed some 20 to 30 years, however, until a reliable method for nonsurgical percutaneous biopsy was developed [25]. In general, newer radiologic techniques for localization and guidance have simplified the procedure, reduced the morbidity, and improved the tissue yield of percutaneous renal biopsy. Furthermore, the development of newer histopathologic techniques, particularly immunofluorescent and electron microscopy, has enhanced the diagnostic value of renal biopsy. Experience with biopsy techniques and familiarity with the wider spectrum of findings have expanded the use of percutaneous renal biopsy, and this technique now has an accepted role in the evaluation, treatment, and understanding of primary and secondary disease affecting the kidney. This chapter outlines the indications, the technical aspects including the radiologic localization of the kidney, the histopathologic findings, and the relationship of angiography and percutaneous renal biopsy.

Indications

Renal biopsy has its greatest use in the early diagnosis of renal disease marked by proteinuria, hematuria, or loss of renal function. The following paragraphs discuss the major clinical situations in which renal biopsy is indicated.

(1) *Proteinuria* is a marker for renal parenchymal disease, and the amount of proteinuria indicates the likelihood of glomerular disease versus tubular-interstitial disease. Heavy proteinuria—more than 3.5 gm per day—strongly suggests glomerular proteinuria and the nephrotic syndrome and indicates the need for renal biopsy along with clinical and serologic evaluations for accompanying systemic immunologic disease. Moderate proteinuria—2 gm or less per day—is consistent with glomerular and/or tubular-interstitial disease of the kidney, and, unless accompanied by hematuria or red blood cell casts in the urinary sediment, should prompt evaluation for historical data or radiologic evidence of chronic interstitial nephritis before percutaneous renal biopsy is undertaken.

(2) *Hematuria* strongly suggests renal or genitourinary tract pathology and may indicate

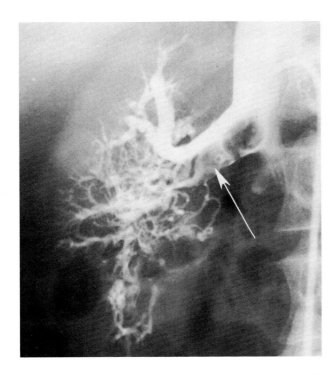

Figure 103-1. Right renal venogram in a 61-year-old man with chronic glomerulonephritis and nephrotic syndrome that demonstrates thrombosis in intrarenal and main renal veins (*arrow*).

the need for renal biopsy. In the presence of proteinuria, renal insufficiency, or evidence of systemic immune disease, renal biopsy is indicated for the renal as well as for the systemic diagnosis. In the absence of these ancillary findings, however, hematuria should prompt anatomic evaluation with pyelography, cystoscopy, and, occasionally, angiography before percutaneous renal biopsy is considered. On occasion, clinical suspicion of renal vein thrombosis in a patient with hematuria, proteinuria, and renal insufficiency may warrant renal venography. However, even in the presence of positive venography (Fig. 103-1), renal biopsy may still be indicated because renal vein thrombosis usually accompanies glomerular disease and nephrotic syndrome in the adult patient [35, 42, 48].

(3) *Acute renal failure* of unknown etiology may necessitate renal biopsy to determine the underlying cause. In the presence of proteinuria or hematuria, immune glomerular disease is likely and biopsy is needed to make the diagnosis. If there is suspicion of deposition or infiltration with histologically demonstrable material, such as oxalate crystals, leukemic infiltrates, or atheromatous emboli, then renal biopsy is also war-

ranted to attempt to explain renal failure. On the other hand, renal injury may occur in several clinically obvious situations: exposure to nephrotoxic drugs (e.g., aminoglycoside antibiotics or contrast agents), acute hemodynamic events (e.g., shock or myocardial infarction), or metabolic derangements (e.g., severe hyperuricemia or hypercalcemia). A strong history of such injury may well explain acute renal failure and so obviate renal biopsy or other radiologic intervention.

(4) Finally, renal biopsy may be indicated in determining the progression of known renal disease primary to the kidney or secondary to systemic immunologic processes and may indicate the proper therapeutic program. Systemic lupus erythematosus is a good example of such a disease, in which renal histopathology in each of the various forms of lupus nephritis appears to indicate the aggressiveness with which steroid and immunosuppressive treatment should be applied [2, 3, 23, 24].

Technical Considerations

LOCALIZATION

Figure 103-2 shows the normal location of the kidney as seen at intravenous pyelography or fluoroscopy. The normal kidney measures 11 to 15 cm and spans 3 to 3.5 lumbar vertebral bodies and interspaces. The hilus of the left kidney is ordinarily located opposite the second lumbar vertebra, and the right hilus is lower by about one-half the span of a lumbar vertebra. The sagittal plane of the kidney is usually 7 to 9 cm from the midline, and the normal kidney may move as much as 3 cm with respiration. The lower pole of the kidney is accessible posteriorly through a relatively thin layer of subcutaneous fat and muscle [40].

Several radiologic techniques can be used to localize the kidney for percutaneous biopsy and to guide the biopsy needle into a safe area in the lower pole away from the hilus. First, the "normal" position of the kidney can be confirmed using a recent intravenous pyelogram, and the "blind" biopsy can be performed at the patient's bedside. With the advent of accurate methods of localization, this approach is used less often.

Second, the biopsy can be performed at the time of intravenous pyelography, with fluoroscopic guidance of renal localization and needle

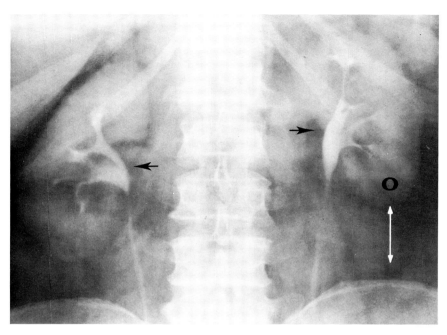

Figure 103-2. Pyelogram demonstrating normal renal position and excursion during respiration. The left hilus is at the level of L2, and the right hilus is lower by one-half the span of the lumbar vertebra (*arrows*). The respiratory excursion of the kidney is marked by the two-headed arrow, and the site of the renal biopsy is marked by the circle.

placement [31]. This method is widely used because it allows direct guidance as well as the possibility of rechecking needle placement during the procedure. The image intensifier is necessary in utilizing fluoroscopy for biopsy guidance. The fluoroscopic method has the potential complications of contrast-agent administration and radiation exposure to the patient and the personnel.

Third, ultrasonic localization for percutaneous renal biopsy is becoming an accepted technique. This method has several advantages [4]. As illustrated in Figure 103-3, ultrasonography can map the lower pole of the kidney, determining the depth, thickness, and proper angle for penetration of the capsule into the renal cortex. Furthermore, some centers now have a B-scan ultrasonic transducer through which a biopsy needle can be passed to allow direct ultrasonic guidance during needle placement. Although ultrasonic guidance avoids contrast-agent and radiation exposure, assurance of intact bilateral function is desirable in some circumstances, and this may require concomitant intravenous pyelography or radioisotope scanning of the kidneys before biopsy. Radioisotope scanning has not been widely employed as a primary localizing technique because of poor resolution of the exact margins and detail of the kidney. Computed to-

Figure 103-3. Renal ultrasonography showing a sagittal section for biopsy localization, with the needle track perpendicular to the surface of the lower pole (*arrow*). The depth for the biopsy, shown by the scale marker, is 5 cm.

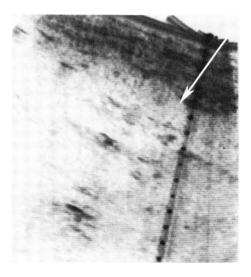

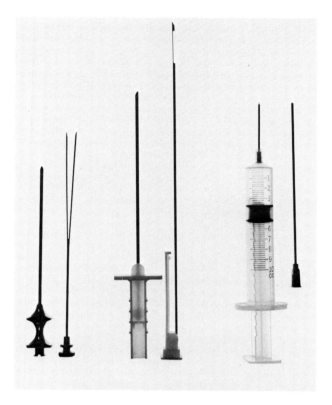

Figure 103-4. Three different types of renal biopsy needles: the Vim-Silverman type, with the Franklin modification (*left*); the slotted disposable biopsy needle (*center*); and the aspiration biopsy needle of the Jamshidi type (*right*).

mography may prove useful as a localizing procedure for percutaneous biopsy because it can precisely determine size, depth, thickness, and position without the risk involved in contrast-agent administration.

BIOPSY NEEDLES AND TECHNIQUES

Three major types of biopsy needles are currently in wide use; they are shown in Figure 103-4. First, the hollow cutting needle of the Vim-Silverman type has been modified so that the tissue core is cut off by the tip of the needle, which is filled in (Franklin modification) [33, 41]. Second, a disposable cutting needle is available (Tru-Cut; Baxter-Travenol Laboratories) that avoids the need for resterilization and resharpening [29]. The disposable needle employs a 20-mm slot for the biopsy core and a hollow sleeve that slides over the slot and cuts off the tissue core. Third, there is now available a hollow aspiration biopsy needle of the Jamshidi type, which some nephrologists feel is easier to use [8].

The relative merits and problems of each type of needle have not been scrutinized in a controlled manner, and the needle choice is an individual decision of the physician performing the biopsy.

At the time of biopsy, the patient may be premedicated to alleviate anxiety and pain. The patient is placed prone on the biopsy table or bed, with a prop or sponge under the xiphoid process to assure posterior localization of the kidneys during the procedure. After sterile preparation of the skin with iodine and local anesthesia, a small (5-mm) incision is made to prevent binding of the skin when the biopsy needle is advanced or twisted. The kidney may be probed with a thin (22–25-gauge) spinal needle before introduction of the actual biopsy needle, allowing additional deep local anesthesia once the cortical surface is identified. The location of the spinal needle or the biopsy needle can be sensed by the resistance felt on the capsular surface, by the respiratory and cardiac-pulsatile motion of the needle placed on the cortical surface, and by ultrasonic depth guidance or fluoroscopic visualization of respiratory motion. In all cases, the needle must be advanced only during suspended respiration since advancement during respiratory motion of the kidney may result in laceration of the cortical surface or malplacement of the needle away from the lower pole. It is most comfortable for the patient if breathing is suspended in midrespiration. After completion of the biopsy and removal of the needle, the patient should remain at bed rest with frequent monitoring of his vital signs and visual observations for gross hematuria during the first 24 hours. Thereafter the patient may be discharged from the hospital with a warning to watch for any signs of late complications.

BIOPSY OF THE RENAL TRANSPLANT

The renal transplant allograft is usually implanted superficially in the lower quadrant of the abdomen, outside the peritoneum. Therefore, the transplant can be readily palpated and is easily accessible for percutaneous needle biopsy. In addition, there is no respiratory movement of the transplant kidney, and the biopsy procedure is considerably easier to perform using a shorter needle of the same type as that used for biopsy of the in situ kidney. Radiographic localization is usually not needed for biopsy of the transplant, although prebiopsy ultrasonography is advisable to identify abnormalities that might be contraindications to the procedure.

Complications and Management

The complication rate following percutaneous renal biopsy is in the range of 5 to 10 percent overall, with serious morbidity confined to less than 1 percent and mortality to less than 0.1 percent [7, 13, 14, 40, 46] (Table 103-1). The most common complications are gross hematuria or perinephric hematoma, which usually are self limited and require no therapeutic intervention. Computed tomography after percutaneous biopsy has revealed that as many as 85 percent of patients have at least a small perinephric hematoma and an accompanying hematocrit decrease of 1 to 4 vol% [38]. Transfusion is required in perhaps 10 to 20 percent of such episodes [40]. In the past, refractory bleeding occasionally required surgical intervention to ligate the bleeding site, to evacuate the hematoma, or to remove the kidney if complications could not be

Table 103-1. Complications of Renal Biopsy

Early complications
  Bleeding
    Gross hematuria
    Perinephric hematoma
  Ureteral obstruction (clot)
  Perforation or injury of internal organs (pancreas, spleen, liver, bowel, peritoneum)
  Vasomotor changes, changes in blood pressure
  Septicemia
  Pain
Late complications
  Abscess in perinephric hematoma
  Delayed bleeding
  Arteriovenous fistula

Figure 103-5. (A) Left renal angiogram showing a small pseudoaneurysm and arteriovenous fistula (*arrow*) in the lower pole following a renal biopsy. (B) Transplant renal angiogram demonstrating a pseudoaneurysm associated with an arteriovenous communication (*arrow*) in the lower pole of the transplant. Note the distal interlobar arterial irregularity and the nonvisualization of the interlobular arteries, indicating chronic transplant rejection.

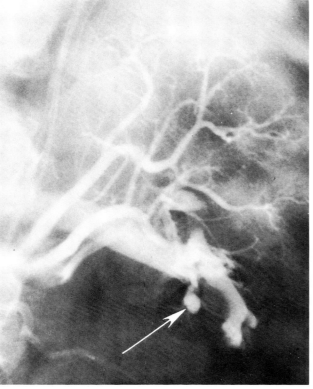

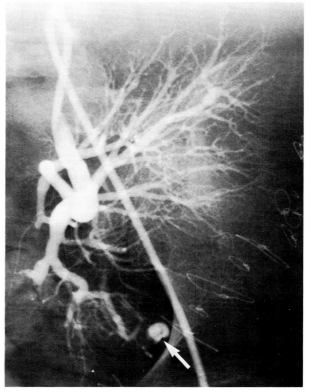

A   *B*

otherwise managed. However, selective angiographic techniques now allow precise localization of bleeding sites as well as therapeutic control of hemorrhage using autologous clot or some other embolic agent [44].

Other early complications, which occur in approximately 1 percent of cases, are often self limited, but they can be serious and can require intervention on occasion. Ureteral obstruction due to blood clots during gross bleeding [13] is usually managed by attention to the bleeding itself and is most often self limited. Perforation of visceral structures or injury to nearby organs, such as the pancreas, liver, or spleen, is avoidable with radiologic guidance during biopsy but must be ruled out in patients with severe pain or clinical signs after biopsy. Vasomotor changes following biopsy may result in hemodynamic instability with increased or decreased blood pressure [13]; however, such vasomotor changes usually regress spontaneously and require no treatment. Septicemia may develop if the skin is not prepared properly or if the needle perforates an unsuspected septic focus in or around the kidney. However, septicemia should be avoidable with strict aseptic techniques and with prior pyelographic or ultrasonic studies. Mild-to-moderate pain following biopsy is usually managed with analgesic medication; however, persistent and severe pain may indicate the development of perinephric hematoma.

Less than 1 percent of patients develop late complications [13, 40]. Abscess formation may complicate previous perinephric hematoma and require surgical drainage. Delayed bleeding, which has been reported as long as 10 to 37 days after biopsy [21], should be managed in the same manner as acute hemorrhage. Aspirinlike analgesics should be avoided in the period after biopsy to obviate any late bleeding due to platelet dysfunction. Finally, arteriovenous fistulas (Fig. 103-5A, B) may form at the biopsy site, representing the most common biopsy complication next to early bleeding and pain [17]. Severe hypertension, parenchymal renal disease, and vasculitis appear to predispose the patient to the formation of fistulas [16]. The reported incidence among severely hypertensive patients is as high as 36 percent; however, the incidence of fistula formation overall is probably much lower. Fistulas usually close spontaneously or remain asymptomatic, detectable only by a persistent bruit. Rarely, hypertension or hemorrhage is associated with such fistulas and necessitates intervention. Recent experience indicates that symptomatic small arteriovenous fistulas can be managed angiographically by using embolic techniques or electrocoagulation [6, 32, 37].

Contraindications

Because the array of complications of renal biopsy is well known, the contraindications can be reasonably defined (Table 103-2). Biopsy via the percutaneous route is contraindicated absolutely in the presence of a bleeding diathesis. Therefore, abnormalities in coagulation factors and platelet function must be ruled out. The recent use of an aspirinlike analgesic should prompt the assessment of platelet function via measurement of the bleeding time or in vitro platelet testing. Platelet dysfunction in the patient with uremia can be readily corrected by dialysis before biopsy. Sustained severe hypertension may predispose the patient to bleeding and should be controlled medically before a biopsy is undertaken. A cyst, tumor, or vascular malformation, such as that shown in Figure 103-6, may also be the source of postbiopsy hemorrhage and should be excluded before biopsy by the radiologic study used to guide needle placement. Malposition or malformation of the kidney may make the proper area of the kidney inaccessible and so predispose the patient to hilar injury and complication; therefore, such abnormalities are contraindications to percutaneous renal biopsy. Percutaneous biopsy in the uncooperative patient can be performed by the open, surgical route or by the percutaneous route with general anesthesia and mechanical control of ventilation during the procedure. Finally, the danger of deep biopsy and hemorrhage is increased when the kidneys are small and atrophic;

Table 103-2. Contraindications to Percutaneous Renal Biopsy

Coagulation abnormality
  Circulating coagulation factors
  Platelet dysfunction (aspirinlike drugs, uremia)
Severe hypertension
Cyst, tumor, or vascular malformation of kidney
Malposition or malformation of kidney
Comatose or uncooperative patient
Small, atrophic kidneys
Solitary kidney

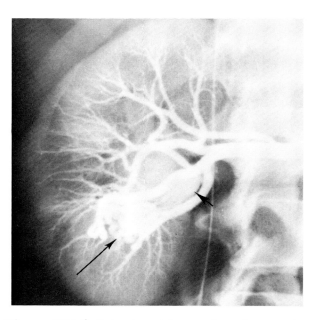

Figure 103-6. Selective right renal angiogram that demonstrates an arteriovenous malformation adjacent to the anticipated site of a renal biopsy (*long arrow*) and dense opacification of the renal vein, indicating an arteriovenous communication (*short arrow*).

therefore, percutaneous biopsy of small, atrophic kidneys should not be undertaken. In such circumstances, the diagnostic yield of a treatable, reversible cause of renal failure is generally low.

The patient with only one kidney presents a special dilemma, since this patient is subject to the same maladies that indicate the need for renal biopsy as is the patient with two functioning kidneys. The solitary kidney should not be jeopardized unless it is absolutely necessary to establish the diagnosis and treatment of the renal disease by biopsy. If necessary, such a biopsy is probably best performed via the open, surgical route. This situation underscores an important consideration in evaluating all patients before percutaneous renal biopsy: before a percutaneous or a surgical renal biopsy is performed, it must be ascertained that the patient has two functioning kidneys. All patients should have an evaluation before biopsy that ensures that there is bilateral perfusion if not bilateral function.

In cases in which the biopsy is deemed absolutely necessary but the risk is high, open surgical biopsy (i.e., sampling of the renal cortex with direct vision through a flank incision under general anesthesia) can obviate some of the complications of percutaneous renal biopsy. Examples of such situations include many of those listed as con-

traindications in Table 103-2. The advantages of open biopsy are the avoidance of injury to the renal hilus and to nonrenal structures and the availability of direct hemostasis. The complications of open biopsy are similar to those of percutaneous biopsy, with a significant incidence of hemorrhage and incisional flank pain, and there are the dangers of general anesthesia [5, 34]. Also, there is occasional ureteral injury with obstruction or urinary leaking. In situations in which percutaneous biopsy is definitely contraindicated, even open surgical biopsy should be undertaken only after careful consideration.

Tissue Processing

Once a percutaneous biopsy sample has been obtained, the tissue core must be prepared for each of three different microscopic examinations, namely, light microscopy, immunofluorescent microscopy, and electron microscopy. In the light of our present level of knowledge and technology, all renal biopsy samples should be examined by these modalities if the quantity of tissue suffices.

At the time of biopsy, fixative materials for each preparation should be available at the bedside in order that the tissue can be fixed without delay before delivery to the pathology laboratory for further processing. If available, a dissecting microscope or a hand lens can be used to examine the tissue core to confirm the presence of renal cortex with glomeruli, using the distinctive vascular corticomedullary junction or the vascular pattern of glomeruli as markers. The tissue sample usually consists of a cylinder measuring 1 to 2 mm in diameter and 10 to 25 mm in length. The sample can be sectioned in many ways, but a reasonable method involves division of the sample into three sections. The middle section should be the largest and should be kept intact, with fixation in buffered formalin or Bowen's solution for paraffin imbedding and sectioning for light microscopy. One-half of each of the other two sections should be fixed in glutaraldehyde for plastic imbedding and ultramicrotome sectioning for electron microscopy. The other half of each fragment should be immediately frozen or placed in iced saline for prompt frozen sectioning and incubation with fluorescein-labeled antisera for ultraviolet immunofluorescent microscopy. Such a method assures the more likely availability of cortex with glomeruli for each microscopic modality and thus a higher yield of suitable tissue for diagnosis. Needless to say, cooperation among the nephrologist performing the biopsy, the radiologist helping with the biopsy guidance, and the pathologist processing the biopsy sample is crucial to the ultimate success of the procedure.

Histopathology of Renal Biopsy

The development of several modalities for examining the renal biopsy sample has had a major impact on the ability to distinguish among the various forms of renal disease and to define better the pathogenetic processes causing these diseases (Table 103-3). The following discussion gives a brief overview of the basic data obtained from renal biopsy, showing what data are contributed by each microscopic modality employed in processing the biopsy sample.

Table 103-3. Histopathologic
Findings on Renal Biopsy

Light microscopy
    Structure involved (glomeruli, tubules, interstitium, blood
        vessels)
    Glomerular changes
      Cell type (epithelium, endothelium, mesangium)
      Patterns (proliferation, membranous change, sclerosis,
        necrosis, crescent formation, lobulation)
      Extent, uniformity (focal, diffuse)
      Specific patterns (diabetes mellitus, amyloidosis,
        "myeloma kidney," vasculitis)
    Nonglomerular changes (interstitial nephritis,
        nephrosclerosis)
Immunofluorescent microscopy
    Specific materials deposited (immunoglobulins,
        complement components, fibrin)
    Location of deposits (capillary loop, mesangium, tubular
        wall, blood vessel wall)
    Pattern of deposition (linear; fine, granular, coarse; and
        irregular)
Electron microscopy
    Location of immune deposits (subepithelial,
        subendothelial, mesangial, intramembranous)
    Ultrastructural basement membrane changes (thickening,
        splitting, thinning)
    Other ultrastructural changes (podocyte fusion,
        microtubular bodies, endothelial vacuolization)

LIGHT MICROSCOPY

Light microscopy provides the best definition of the basic type and extent of renal disease, that is, a descriptive pathologic diagnosis. This diagnosis is based on a number of elements:

1. The actual structures affected (glomeruli, tubules, interstitium, or blood vessels)
2. The type of glomerular cell affected (epithelium, mesangium, or endothelium)
3. The patterns of glomerular involvement (e.g., proliferation, membranous change, sclerosis, necrosis, crescent formation, or lobulation)
4. The extent and uniformity of involvement (focal or diffuse)
5. The specific diagnostic patterns (e.g., diabetic glomerular change, amyloid deposition, "myeloma kidney," or vasculitis)
6. The nonglomerular changes (e.g., interstitial inflammation or nephrosclerosis)

Light microscopic diagnoses are given in descriptive terms, such as *diffuse proliferative glomerulonephritis* (Fig. 103-7B), *membranous nephropathy,* and *focal glomerulosclerosis.* Refinements of these descriptive diagnoses are provided by the immunofluorescent and electron microscopic findings, which better define the ultrastructural and immune processes causing the observed changes in light microscopy.

IMMUNOFLUORESCENT MICROSCOPY

Incubation of frozen sections with fluorescein-labeled antibody that is directed against specific immunoglobulins (e.g., IgG, IgM, or IgA), against individual complement component (e.g., C3, C4, or properdin), and against other circulating mediators (e.g., fibrin) determines the presence and general location of such substances within the kidney. These data refine the light microscopic diagnosis and suggest pathogenetic mechanisms for some lesions. For example, the *rapidly progressive (crescentic) glomerulonephritis* seen in Goodpasture's syndrome of pulmonary hemorrhage and renal failure is characterized by a fine, homogeneous, linear deposition of IgG and C3 along the capillary basement membrane (Fig. 103-8). This pattern suggests deposition of a specific nephrotoxic IgG directed against basement membrane, and we now measure anti-glomerular–basement-membrane antibody in the serum of patients suspected of having this lesion

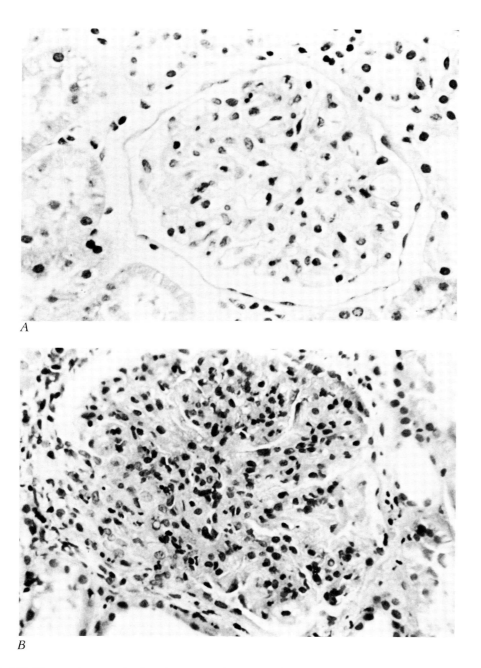

Figure 103-7. (A) Photomicrograph showing normal histology on light microscopy. (H&E, ×400.) (B) Photomicrograph showing diffuse proliferative glo-merulonephritis in a patient with poststreptococcal disease. (H&E, ×400.)

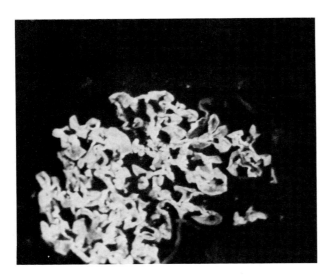

Figure 103-8. Photomicrograph under ultraviolet light showing diffuse linear deposition of IgG in a patient with Goodpasture's syndrome. (×400.)

[49]. Another example, *membranous nephropathy*, is characterized on light microscopy by a fine, granular capillary loop deposition of IgG and C3 on immunofluorescent sections, suggesting immune complex deposition. In further work with immunofluorescent microscopy, it may be possible to detect the presence of specific antigens, such as hepatitis B surface antigen or carcinoembryonic antigen, which may be pathogenetic for immune complex renal diseases. In fact, there are reports of several cases in which such antigen has been detected in the kidney [10, 11]. Finally, other data have shown that in certain light microscopic lesions the inflammatory process may involve alternate rather than classic complement activation. Immunofluorescent microscopy in such cases shows C3 and properdin but no C4 [39].

ELECTRON MICROSCOPY

Ultrastructural examination of the kidney can aid in specifying the disease process that eventuates in the light microscopic picture seen on biopsy. In immune complex diseases, such as systemic lupus erythematosus or poststreptococcal glomerulonephritis, electron-dense material can be detected by electron microscopy in various locations within the glomeruli, tubules, or blood vessel walls. This electron-dense material is analogous to the immune complex deposits seen on immunofluorescent microscopy, but the exact location with reference to the basement membrane can be defined only by electron microscopy. The exact location of the deposit is characteristic of certain underlying diseases and aids in the differential diagnosis. For example, the diffuse proliferative glomerulonephritis in postinfectious states, such as that after streptococcal infection or during subacute bacterial endocarditis, is characterized by electron-dense deposits between the glomerular basement membrane and epithelial cell, termed *subepithelial* [28], and illustrated by the electron micrograph shown in Figure 103-9B. On the other hand, the diffuse proliferative glomerulonephritis in systemic lupus erythematosus is characterized by electron-dense deposits located between the glomerular basement membrane and endothelial cell, termed *subendothelial* [2, 3, 23, 24]. Other locations within the glomerulus or outside the glomerulus are characteristic of other disease processes. Precise localization of the deposits has helped refine the diagnostic accuracy of renal biopsy.

Electron microscopy also defines other ultrastructural changes in the basement membrane itself that signal specific renal diagnoses. Some examples are diabetes mellitus, with a two- to threefold uniform thickening of the basement membrane early in the disease process [12], hereditary nephritis (Alport's syndrome), characterized by well-defined splitting of the basement membrane with areas of decreased density between layers [43], and the syndrome benign familial hematuria, characterized by numerous areas of extremely thin basement membrane [36].

Finally, specific changes in other elements of the glomerular ultrastructure can be detected only by electron microscopy. The following are examples in which such findings add to the diagnostic specificity of the biopsy: fusion of the epithelial cell projections, or podocytes, that abut the glomerular capillary basement membrane is characteristic of the nephrotic syndrome and may be the only detectable biopsy change in children with *lipoid nephrosis* [9, 19]; microtubular bodies, often referred to as *myxoviruslike bodies*, are seen in the endothelial cells of some biopsy samples but are most characteristic of lupus nephritis [20]; and endothelial vacuolization is the major finding in patients with severe eclampsia [47]. Again, these examples demonstrate the additional diagnostic utility of electron microscopy in further refining the specific diagnosis available from biopsy samples.

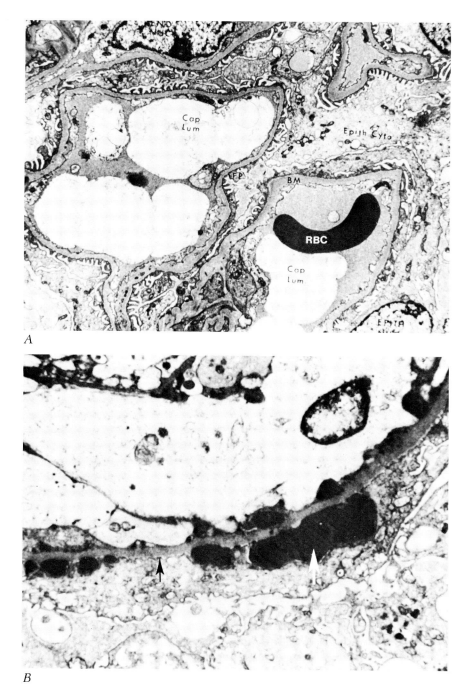

Figure 103-9. (A) Electron micrograph showing normal glomerular ultrastructure, including the capillary lumen (*Cap Lum*), the epithelial cytoplasm (*Epith Cyto*) and foot process (*FP*), and the basement membrane (*BM*). *RBC* = red blood cell. (B) Electron micrograph showing large subepithelial electron-dense deposits (*white arrow*) along the basement membrane (*black arrow*) in a case of poststreptococcal glomerulonephritis.

Clinical Correlations of Angiography with Renal Biopsy

Angiography and renal biopsy may complement each other as diagnostic tools in the evaluation of renal disease seen by the clinician. The evaluation of hematuria or acute renal failure may be best pursued by one or the other of these interventions, depending on the clinical circumstances encountered. For example, if tumor or vascular malformation is suspected, then angiography should precede renal biopsy. On the other hand, when proteinuria exists and clinical or serologic testing indicates possible glomerulonephritis, renal biopsy is the procedure of choice. In some cases, both procedures may be necessary. Renal allograft transplant rejection and polyarteritis nodosa are two excellent examples of disease processes in which the results of angiography and biopsy complement each other. In acute transplant rejection, renal biopsy reveals interstitial inflammatory cells and a striking hyaline sclerosis of small arterioles in the renal cortex [18, 30]. This vascular pathology leads to hypoperfusion of the renal cortex with the characteristic clinical sequelae of decreased glomerular filtration rate, sodium retention, and hypertension. Angiography may clearly show this decrease in cortical perfusion and is marked by "pruning" of the small interlobar arteries and lack of visualization of the interlobular arteries (see Fig. 103-5B) [1, 22, 26]. In the failing renal transplant, angiography may also show major arterial stenosis amenable to surgical correction in situations in which the biopsy shows no specific lesion. Angiographic findings in classic polyarteritis nodosa are characterized by multiple small arterial aneurysms in the kidney as well as other visceral organs, as shown in Figure 103-10 [15]. Renal biopsy in polyarteritis nodosa may show only a focal glomerulonephritis and usually misses arteries large enough to show typical vasculitis. Therefore, angiography may be needed to make this diagnosis, even if renal biopsy is performed.

Angiography and renal biopsy occasionally may complement each other in radiologic localization for percutaneous biopsy. In acute renal failure with nonvisualization via routine intravenous pyelography, angiography to rule out vascular occlusion can be used as the procedure to map the area for biopsy. The angiography in this situation will also define the renal size and

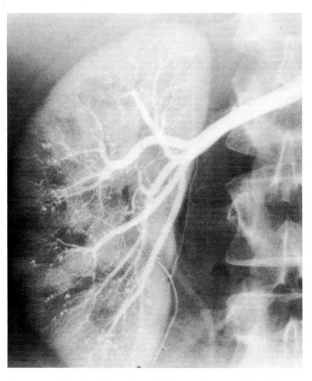

Figure 103-10. Selective right renal magnification angiogram demonstrates numerous microaneurysms in medium and small renal arteries in a 31-year-old woman with polyarteritis nodosa.

parenchymal thickness, data that may have prognostic significance as to the outcome of acute renal failure. However, now that ultrasound techniques are widely available, angiography is seldom used as a primary localizing technique for renal biopsy. In most circumstances, combined renal scanning to assure bilateral renal perfusion and mapping for biopsy with ultrasonography have replaced angiography and have obviated the potential morbidity of arteriotomy and contrast-agent administration.

The most important area in which angiography complements renal biopsy is in the management of postbiopsy complications. Angiography is the best method to detect the site of arterial bleeding or arteriovenous fistula in the patient with gross hematuria or perinephric hematoma. As noted previously, angiography may also serve as a nonsurgical means of treating such bleeding lesions.

In general, advances in nephrology, radiology, and histopathology have made percutaneous renal biopsy an accepted and reliable procedure in clinical medicine. The development of new serologic and biochemical tests to determine systemic immunologic disease, the development of reliable radiographic methods for both imaging the kidney and managing biopsy complications, and the development of sophisticated histopathologic methods of processing biopsy material have all made percutaneous renal biopsy a safer, more reliable, and more accurate diagnostic tool.

References

1. Alfidi, R. J., Meaney, T. F., Buonocore, E., and Nakamoto, S. Evaluation of renal homotransplant by selective angiography. *Radiology* 87:1099, 1966.
2. Appel, G. B., Silva, F. G., Pirani, C. L., Meltzer, J. I., and Estes, D. Renal involvement in systemic lupus erythematosus. *Medicine* 57:371, 1978.
3. Baldwin, D. S., Lowenstein, J., Rothfield, N. F., Gallo, G., and McCluskey, R. T. The clinical course of proliferative and membranous forms of lupus nephritis. *Ann. Intern. Med.* 73:929, 1970.
4. Bolton, W. K., Tully, R. J., Lewis, E. J., and Ranniger, K. Localization of the kidney for percutaneous biopsy. *Ann. Intern. Med.* 81:159, 1974.
5. Bolton, W. K., and Vaughan, E. D. A comparative study of open surgical and percutaneous renal biopsies (abstract). American Society of Nephrology, Washington, D.C., November, 1975.
6. Bookstein, J. J., and Goldstein, H. M. Successful management of post-biopsy arteriovenous fistula with selective arterial embolization. *Radiology* 109:535, 1973.
7. Carvajal, H. F., Travis, L. B., Srivastava, R. N., DeBeukelaer, M. M., Dodge, W. F., and Dupree, E. Percutaneous renal biopsy in children—an analysis of complications in 890 consecutive biopsies. *Tex. Rep. Biol. Med.* 29:253, 1971.
8. Charytan, C. A new aspiration needle-syringe for percutaneous renal biopsy (abstract). American Society of Nephrology, Washington, D.C., November, 1976.
9. Churg, J., Grishman, E., Goldstein, M. H., Yunis, S. L., and Porush, J. G. Idiopathic nephrotic syndrome in adults: A study and classification based on renal biopsies. *N. Engl. J. Med.* 272:165, 1965.
10. Costanza, M. E., Pinn, V., Schwartz, R. S., and Nathanson, L. Carcinoembryonic antigen-antibody complexes in a patient with colonic carcinoma and nephrotic syndrome. *N. Engl. J. Med.* 289:520, 1973.
11. Couser, W. G., Wagonfeld, J. B., Spargo, B. H., and Lewis, E. J. Glomerular deposition of tumor antigen in membranous nephropathy associated with colonic carcinoma. *Am. J. Med.* 57:962, 1974.
12. Dachs, S., Churg, J., Mautner, W., and Grishman, E. Diabetic nephropathy. *Am. J. Pathol.* 44:155, 1964.
13. Diaz-Buxo, J. A., and Donadio, J. V. Complications of percutaneous renal biopsy: An analysis of 1000 consecutive biopsies. *Clin. Nephrol.* 4:223, 1975.
14. Dodge, W. F., Daeschner, C. W., Brennan, J. C., Rosenberg, H. S., Travis, L. B., and Hopps, H. C. Percutaneous renal biopsy in children. *Pediatrics* 30:287, 1962.
15. Dornfeld, L., Lecky, J. W., and Peter, J. B. Polyarteritis and intrarenal renal artery aneurysms. *J.A.M.A.* 215:1950, 1971.
16. Ekelund, L., Göthlin, J., Lindholm, T., Lindstedt, E., and Mattsson, K. Arteriovenous fistulae following renal biopsy with hypertension and hemodynamic changes: Report of a case studied by dye-dilution technique. *J. Urol.* 108:373, 1972.
17. Ekelund, L., and Lindholm, T. Arteriovenous fistulae following percutaneous renal biopsy. *Acta Radiol. [Diagn.]* (Stockh.) 11:38, 1971.
18. Finkelstein, F. O., Siegel, N. J., Bastl, C., Forrest, J. N., and Kashgarian, M. Kidney transplant biopsy in the diagnosis and management of acute rejection episodes. *Kidney Int.* 10:171, 1976.
19. Folli, G., Pollak, V. E., Reid, R. T., Pirani, C. L., and Kark, R. M. Electron microscopic studies of reversible glomerular lesions in the adult nephrotic syndrome. *Ann. Intern. Med.* 49:775, 1958.
20. Gyorkey, F., Min, K.-W., Syncovics, J. G., and Györkey, P. Systemic lupus erythematosus and myxovirus. *N. Engl. J. Med.* 280:333, 1969.
21. Hampers, C. L., and Prager, D. Massive bleeding ten days after renal biopsy. *J.A.M.A.* 114:782, 1964.
22. Hamway, S., Novicks, A., Braun, W. E., Levin, H., Banowsky, L., Alfidi, R., and Magnusson, M. Impaired renal allograft function: A comparative study with angiography and histopathology. *J. Urol.* 122:292, 1979.
23. Hecht, B., Siegel, N., Adler, M., Kashgarian, M., and Hayslett, J. Prognostic indices in lupus nephritis. *Medicine* 5:163, 1976.
24. Hill, G. S., Hinglais, N., Tron, F., and Bach, J.-F. Systemic lupus erythematosus: Morphologic correlations with immunologic and clinical data at the time of biopsy. *Am. J. Med.* 64:61, 1978.
25. Iverson, P., and Brun, C. Aspiration biopsy of the kidney. *Am. J. Med.* 11:324, 1951.
26. Jones, B. J., Palmer, F. J., Charlesworth, J. A., Shirley, D. V., MacDonald, G. J., Williams, R. M., and Robertson, M. R. Angiography in the

diagnosis of renal allograft dysfunction. *J. Urol.* 119:461, 1978.

27. Jungmann, E. Über chronische Streptokokkeninfektionen. *Dtsch. Med. Wochenschr.* 50:71, 1924.

28. Kimmelstiel, P. The hump—a lesion of acute glomerulonephritis. *Bull. Pathol.* 6:187, 1965.

29. Lavastida, M. T., Musil, G., and Hulet, W. H. A disposable needle for percutaneous renal biopsy. *Clin. Pediatr.* 7:170, 1968.

30. Lindquist, R. R., Gutmann, R. D., Merrill, J. P., and Dammin, G. J. Human renal allografts: Interpretations of morphological and immunohistological observations. *Am. J. Pathol.* 53:851, 1968.

31. Lusted, L. B., Mortimore, G. E., and Hopper, J., Jr. Needle renal biopsy under image amplifier control. *AJR* 75:953, 1956.

32. McAlister, D. S., Johnsrude, I., Miller, M. M., Clapp, J., and Thompson, W. M. Occlusion of acquired renal arteriovenous fistulae with transcatheter electrocoagulation. *AJR* 132:998, 1979.

33. Muehrcke, R. C., Kark, R. M., and Pirani, C. L. Technique of percutaneous renal biopsy in prone position. *J. Urol.* 74:267, 1955.

34. Patel, J., Bailey, G. L., and Mahoney, E. F. Open renal biopsy in uremic patients. *Urology.* 3:293, 1974.

35. Pollak, V. E., Kark, R. M., Pirani, C. L., Shafter, H. A., and Muehrcke, R. C. Renal vein thrombosis and the nephrotic syndrome. *Am. J. Med.* 21:496, 1956.

36. Rogers, P. W., Kurtzman, N. A., Bunn, S. M., and White, M. G. Familial benign essential hematuria. *Arch. Intern. Med.* 131:257, 1973.

37. Rosen, R. J., Feldman, L., and Wilson, A. R. Embolization for post biopsy renal arteriovenous fistula: Effective occlusion using homologous clot. *AJR* 131:1072, 1978.

38. Rosenbaum, R., Hoffsten, P. E., Stanley, R. J., and Klahr, S. Use of computerized tomography

to diagnose complications of percutaneous renal biopsy. *Kidney Int.* 14:87, 1978.

39. Rothfield, N., Ross, H. A., Minta, J. O., and Lepow, I. H. Glomerular and dermal deposition of properdin in systemic lupus erythematosus. *N. Engl. J. Med.* 287:681, 1972.

40. Schreiner, G. Renal Biopsy. In M. B. Strauss and L. G. Welt (eds.), *Diseases of the Kidney.* Boston: Little, Brown, 1971. Pp. 197–209.

41. Schreiner, G. E., and Berman, L. B. Experience with 150 consecutive renal biopsies. *South. Med. J.* 50:733, 1957.

42. Schwartz, M. M., and Lewis, E. J. Immunopathology of the nephrotic syndrome associated with renal vein thrombosis. *Am. J. Med.* 54:528, 1973.

43. Sherman, R. L., Churg, J., and Yudis, M. Hereditary nephritis with a characteristic renal lesion. *Am. J. Med.* 56:44, 1974.

44. Silber, S. J., and Clark, R. E. Treatment of massive hemorrhage after renal biopsy with angiographic injection of clot. *N. Engl. J. Med.* 292:1387, 1975.

45. Silverberg, D. S., Dossetor, J. B., Eid, T. C., Mant, M. J., and Miller, J. D. R. Arteriovenous fistulae and prolonged hematuria after renal biopsy. *Can. Med. Assoc. J.* 110:671, 1974.

46. Slotkin, E. A., and Madsen, P. O. Complications of renal biopsy: Incidence in 5000 reported cases. *J. Urol.* 87:13, 1962.

47. Spargo, B., McCartney, C. P., and Winemiller, R. Glomerular capillary endotheliosis in toxemia of pregnancy. *Arch. Pathol.* 68:593, 1959.

48. Trew, P. A., Biava, C. G., Jacobs, R. P., and Hopper, J. Renal vein thrombosis in membranous glomerulonephropathy: Incidence and association. *Medicine* 57:69, 1978.

49. Wilson, C. B., and Dixon, F. J. Anti-glomerular basement membrane antibody induced glomerulonephritis. *Kidney Int.* 3:74, 1973.

4. Drainage Techniques and Intravascular Foreign Body Removal

Catheter Drainage of Abscesses

STEPHEN G. GERZOF

Until recently, the radiologic diagnosis of intraabdominal abscess was based on subtle and indirect plain-film findings. Restricted to a one-dimensional image, conventional radiographs could not localize abscesses in relation to surrounding structures. Guidance for needle aspiration was incomplete and fraught with the danger of perforating surrounding structures and disseminating sepsis. Prior to antibiotics, the results of this complication were often disastrous. As a result, needle aspiration of abscesses was felt by most surgeons to be contraindicated as "useless, irrational, and distinctly dangerous" [26].

Early nuclear medicine techniques were similarly limited to indirect demonstration of abscesses as photon-deficient masses on liver or liver-lung scans. Recently, the use of gallium for direct abscess imaging has improved isotopic diagnosis [14]. However, radionuclide studies remain nonspecific and provide little or no guidance for needle aspiration.

Angiography has been successful in demonstrating hepatic and renal abscesses. Based on fluoroscopy and rapid-sequence films, however, angiography suffers from the same limitations as conventional radiographs and isotopic scans. It is unable to image the abscess directly while simultaneously demonstrating its relationship to surrounding structures. These two factors are basic requirements for safe drainage route planning and guidance.

It is only with the advent of sectional imaging by computed tomography (CT) and ultrasonography that abscesses have become directly visible. These modalities display both the abscess and its surrounding structures in two dimensions so that percutaneous aspiration can be performed safely.

Basic Principles of Abscess Drainage

Traditionally, abscesses have been treated surgically, with wide incision and drainage as the cardinal principles of operative management. Surgical exposure was necessary to view the abscess directly, confirm the diagnosis, break down any internal loculation, exclude the presence of other abscesses, and place large drains intraoperatively to provide continuous drainage.

In percutaneous drainage, sectional imaging by CT and ultrasonography replaces operative exposure for diagnosis and localization. Instead of large surgically placed drains, catheters of relatively small bore are placed percutaneously, guided by CT or ultrasonography. Despite their small size, they remain patent and provide continuous and definitive drainage.

There are four basic steps in percutaneous abscess drainage: (1) CT or ultrasonography is performed to identify the abscess with respect to its surrounding structures; (2) based on the images, a safe percutaneous route that avoids the surrounding structures is planned; (3) using this route, a diagnostic needle aspiration is performed to confirm both the diagnosis and the route; and (4) following confirmation by needle aspiration, a drainage catheter is inserted, the abscess is evacuated, and the catheter is sutured in place.

Signs of Abscess

Because abscesses are fluid collections of water density, they blend with the surrounding tissues and are not well seen on conventional radiographs. Plain film signs of abscess include (1) a soft tissue mass, (2) a collection or a pattern of extraluminal gas, (3) viscus displacement, (4) loss of normally visualized structures or fascial planes, and (5) fixation of a normally mobile organ [22].

Arteriography of parenchymal abscesses shows displacement of arteries and veins, with a hypervascular rim of compressed inflammatory tissue contiguous to the abscess. There may be tissue staining, with an indistinct interface between the abscess and the adjacent tissues [13]. Irregular inflammatory vessels may be seen, but tumor vessels are absent. The hypervascular rim, described angiographically as a "blush," has been termed the *rind sign* when demonstrated by contrast-enhanced CT [7, 9].

There are five CT signs of abscess (Figs. 104-1A, 104-2B, 104-3A) [7–9, 12, 18]:

1. A soft tissue mass of low attenuation (0–25 Hounsfield units). It may have either irregular contours or sharply defined walls, depending on its age and organization.
2. The rind sign, a rim of peripheral enhancement that appears after the infusion of intravenous contrast material, circumscribes the abscess and clearly demarcates it from the surrounding structures. In this regard, the CT and angiographic signs of abscess are similar.
3. Inappropriate gas, presenting as small bubbles or air-fluid levels.
4. Edema of the contiguous tissue planes.
5. Displacement of surrounding structures. It is by this displacement that the majority of intraabdominal abscesses actually provide themselves with safe percutaneous drainage routes.

Figure 104-1. (A) Prone computed tomographic scan shows an oval perinephric abscess (*arrowheads*) posterior to the right kidney (*RK*). Note the convex borders and the ill-defined tissue planes compared to the left kidney (*LK*). Percutaneous drainage was performed and is shown in Figure 104-7. The high attenuation coefficient of this abscess was due to hemorrhage. *L* = liver; *Sp* = spleen. (B) Prone transverse sonogram corresponding to the scan shown in (A). The abscess (*A*) is echo free and has irregular walls. Sonographic markers (*arrows*) indicate planned entry site, route, and depth. *K* = kidney.

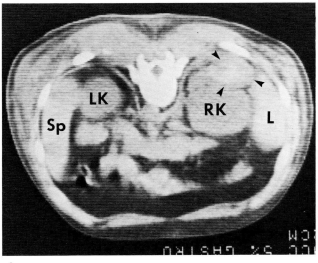

A

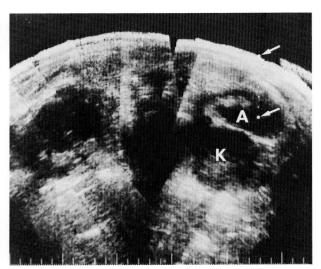

B

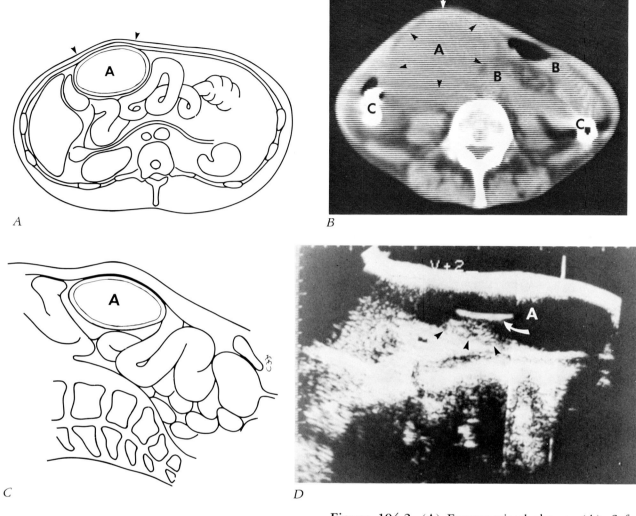

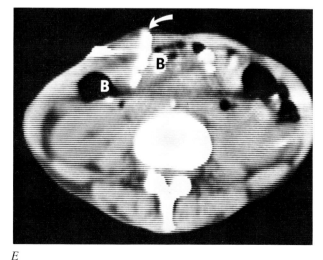

Figure 104-2. (A) Enteroparietal abscess (*A*). Safe percutaneous access for drainage is found in the area of peritoneal contact (*arrowheads*). (B) Computed tomographic scan of an enteroparietal abscess (*arrowheads*) documents the absence of bowel interposed between the abscess and the peritoneum. *Arrow* = entry site; *C* = barium in colon; *B* = small bowel. (C) Sagittal diagram of an enteroparietal abscess (*A*) shows displaced loops of bowel. Both axial and sagittal scans are used to confirm the absence of interposed bowel and to provide localization and guidance in two planes. (D) Sagittal sonogram of the enteroparietal abscess (*A*) shown in (B) demonstrates its full 16-cm cephalocaudad extent. There is dependent layering debris (*arrowheads*) in the otherwise echo-free abscess. The linear echo within the abscess (*arrow*) represents a percutaneously placed catheter scanned after insertion but before aspiration of the abscess contents. (E) Postdrainage computed tomographic scan shows the catheter (*arrow*) in the former abscess cavity seen in (B). Note how the bowel loops (*B*) have returned to a normal position, which would rule out a safe repeat aspiration.

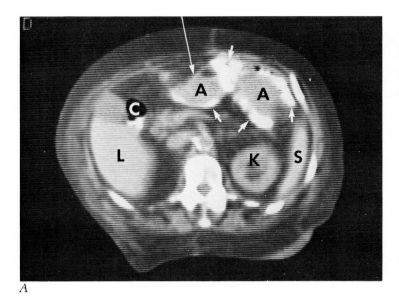

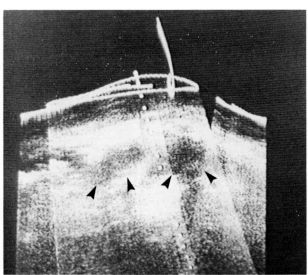

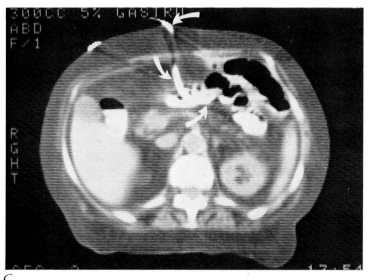

Figure 104-3. (A) Computed tomographic (CT) scan of a bilobate interloop abscess (*A*) surrounded by contrast-filled loops of small bowel (*short arrows*). *L* = liver; *C* = colon; *K* = left kidney; *S* = spleen. The long arrow indicates proposed CT-guided drainage route. (B) Transverse sonogram corresponding to the scan shown in (A) shows two ill-defined areas of lower echogenicity (*arrowheads*) that were unrecognized as abscesses by ultrasonography prior to the CT scan. The relationship of the abscess to bowel loops cannot be determined by this sonogram. (C) CT scan after drainage under CT guidance shows a pigtail catheter (*arrows*) draining both portions of the abscess cavity.

With the use of these signs, CT has proved to be the most accurate and effective method for diagnosis of abdominal abscesses and is the current diagnostic standard against which other modalities must be compared [8, 18, 24].

The sonographic signs of abscesses vary with the homogeneity of the abscess contents and with the scan techniques used [6]. Most abscesses present as echo-free masses with good through transmission of sound because of their fluid nature (see Figs. 104-1B, 104-2D) [4, 5, 21]. Occasionally, fluid-fluid levels are seen within the abscess when internal debris layers dependently [6]. Gas bubbles within the abscess may produce

an echogenic pattern indistinguishable from surrounding structures [19]. When frank air-fluid levels are present, the gas may shield the deeper portions from sonographic view. The abscess may then be inapparent or mistaken for bowel gas and overlooked [6, 19].

Guidance and Route Planning

The physical properties of contact scanning ultrasonography inherently limit its reliability for the initial diagnosis of abscess. Computed tomography is far more dependable in providing a

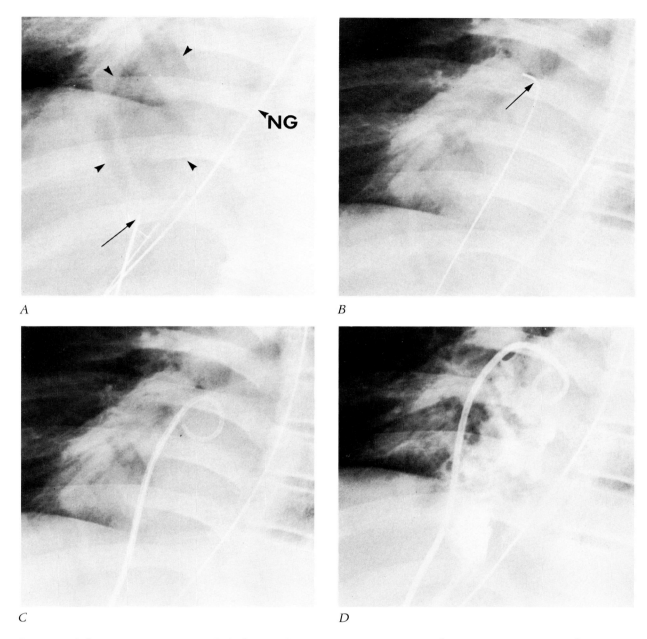

A

B

C

D

Figure 104-4. Fluoroscopically guided abscess drainage. (A) Fluoroscopic spot film of a gas-containing abscess (*arrowheads*). Its posterior extrapleural location had earlier been determined by a computed tomographic scan. The long arrow indicates the needle tip placed on the skin under fluoroscopic control to localize the site for percutaneous entry. *NG* = nasogastric tube. (B) After the abscess is entered ex- trapleurally, a guidewire (*arrow*) is inserted. (C) Pigtail catheter is inserted over the guidewire. Note how the pigtail tip immediately regains its coil after extending beyond the guidewire tip. (D) As the catheter is advanced, the pigtail ensures coiling of the body of the catheter within the abscess and prevents perforation of the far wall. An injection of contrast material defines the entirety of the abscess cavity.

rapid, accurate, and complete diagnosis, particularly postoperatively, when extensive bowel gas, open wounds, drain sites, suture lines, and bandages severely curtail sonographic examination [8, 18, 24].

Ultrasonography alone can be used for guidance and route planning in retroperitoneal, renal, and hepatic abscesses when there is no danger of encountering interposed bowel [7, 8]. It is also sufficient in large enteroparietal abscesses [23]. These are abscesses that by virtue of their size have expanded and displaced bowel loops such that the abscess wall lies in contact with the parietal peritoneum. This point of contact becomes the "window" for sonic imaging, diagnostic aspiration, and insertion of drainage catheters (see Fig. 104-2A–D).

In general, CT is the best modality for route planning and exclusion of synchronous disease. It is the only modality that directly and simultaneously images the bowel and the abscess, as well as their spatial relationship. This is most important for route planning in intraperitoneal and interloop abscesses when bowel must be identified in order to be avoided [7, 8] (Fig. 104-3A–C).

The combination of CT for diagnosis and route planning followed by ultrasonography for three-dimensional guidance is often the best sequence for integrating the strengths of these two modalities. With the use of CT for route planning, an inability to define a safe percutaneous access route is unusual and should occur in less than 10 percent of cases.

Guidance by fluoroscopy is usually limited to those cases in which the access route lies parallel to the x-ray beam and the central ray can be placed perpendicularly above the abscess (Fig. 104-4A–D). Fluoroscopy alone can be used for route planning and guidance for enteroparietal abscesses when the bowel is opacified and is displaced by the abscess. Renal abscesses discovered at angiography can be aspirated in this fashion when the patient is rotated into an appropriate position. However, percutaneous abscess drainage is a septic procedure and is best performed elsewhere than in an angiography suite, where sterility should prevail.

There are four factors to consider when planning a projected drainage route: (1) the cutaneous entry site, (2) the angle of entry, (3) the depth, and (4) the surgical anatomy [3, 7, 8]. The first three factors are derived from the CT and sonographic scans and are carefully defined prior to needling. As an integral part of route planning,

the projected route should be correlated with the surgical anatomy and the established operative approaches for that location [3].

After the proposed entry site is marked on the skin, its localization is confirmed with a repeat scan. From that point, the angle of entry to the abscess is measured from the scan with a gonionmeter. The distance from the entry site to the near wall of the abscess is the depth. To prevent perforation of the far wall, this distance should be transposed to the aspiration needle with a needle stop.

The peritoneum is not a barrier to percutaneous drainage. Transperitoneal routes have been used routinely without peritonitis or dissemination of sepsis [8]. However, in accordance with general surgical principles, extraperitoneal routes may be preferred to transperitoneal routes when possible [25].

Techniques of Catheter Drainage

DIAGNOSTIC ASPIRATION

For diagnostic aspiration, a 20-gauge, 10- to 12-inch Teflon-sleeve needle is used. It is preferred to the 22-gauge needle, whose lumen may be too small to allow aspiration of viscous purulent material. However, when the diagnosis or the route is uncertain, a 22-gauge needle may be used initially.

The skin at the entry site is prepared and draped as for an arteriogram. After infiltration with local anesthesia, a #11 blade is used to make a 4-mm incision, which is widened by blunt dissection with a curved hemostat. A rubber-shod Kelly clamp is recommended for use as the needle stop and is placed on the Teflon-sleeve needle at the premeasured depth. The needle is then inserted over the projected route in a single pass. After the clamp and the stylet are removed, a small (5-cc) sample is aspirated for Gram's staining and culturing [7, 8, 10, 15, 28].

If the aspirated material is purulent, drainage should proceed immediately by either the modified Seldinger technique or the trochar catheter technique. At this point, the patient should not be moved, since any change in position may alter the anatomic relationships and compromise the selected drainage route. If the aspirate is sterile, the remainder of the fluid should be totally aspirated and the Teflon sleeve removed.

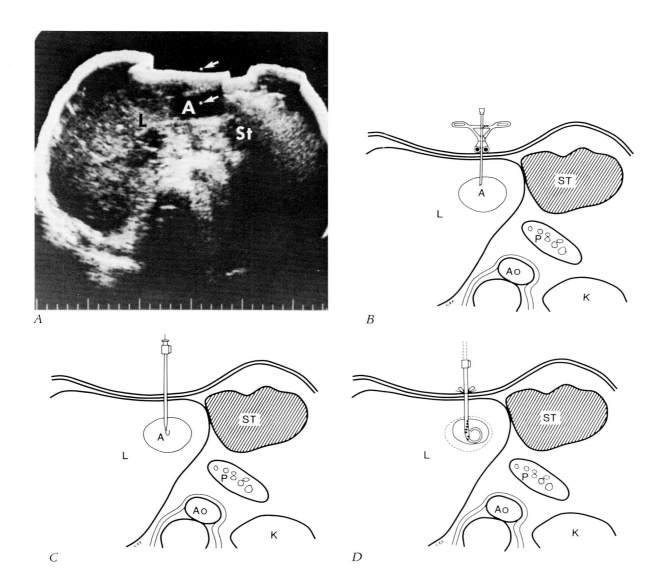

A

B

C

D

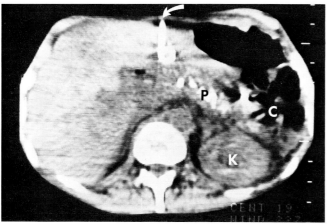

E

Figure 104-5. (A) Transverse sonogram shows a 4-×-6-cm echo-free abscess (*A*) in the left lobe of the liver (*L*), with good sound transmission and irregular walls. The white sonographic cursor marks (*arrows*) indicate the cutaneous entry site, angle, and depth. Note how stomach gas (*St*) obscures the left upper quadrant. (B) A 20-gauge Teflon-sleeve needle with a needle stop is inserted over the planned route shown in (A). (C) After the insertion of a J guidewire, an 8 French dilator is passed over the guidewire. (D) An 8 French pigtail catheter is inserted over the guidewire and advanced until it engages the far wall. The abscess is evacuated by manual syringe suction; the catheter is sutured securely to skin and connected to closed biliary drainage system, as is shown in Figure 104-8. (E) Follow-up computed tomographic scan 7 days following drainage shows the pigtail catheter (*arrow*) in place with no residuum. Such confirmation of complete resolution prevents too early catheter removal and possible recurrence. As compared with the sonogram shown in (A), this computed tomographic scan clearly demonstrates the colon (*C*), pancreas with calcification (*P*), and left kidney (*K*), with detail that allows the exclusion of synchronous disease. *Ao* = Aorta. (B to E from Gerzof et al. [10]. Reproduced by permission from *Semin. Roentgenol.*)

2341

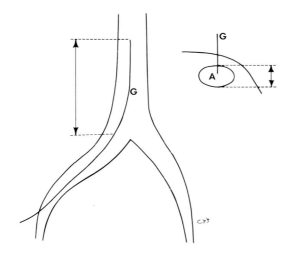

Figure 104-6. Diagram shows wide latitude (*arrows*) in the positioning of the guidewire (*G*) during catheter exchange at angiography. However, the narrow anteroposterior diameter of this perinephric abscess (*A*) requires meticulous care in maintaining the tip of the guidewire in the abscess.

Some aspirates are indeterminate, and it may be unclear whether the aspirate is sterile or infected. One must then await the results of the immediate Gram's stain to decide whether to insert a drainage catheter or simply to aspirate the remainder of the fluid. This is an important decision. Catheters cannot be reinserted after a fluid collection has been evacuated since displaced viscera return to their normal positions and so prevent further percutaneous access (see Figs. 104-2E, 104-3C).

All aspirates should be routinely cultured for anaerobic as well as aerobic organisms [1]. Special transport vials or capped syringes should be used for anaerobic specimens.

MODIFIED SELDINGER ANGIOCATHETER TECHNIQUE

A 0.035-inch 80-cm floppy-tip Amplatz or J-tip angiographic guidewire is inserted into the abscess through the Teflon sleeve [7, 8, 11] (Fig.

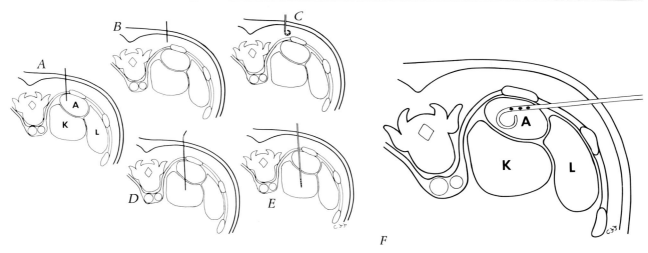

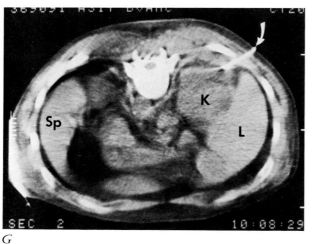

Figure 104-7. Perinephric abscess shown in Figure 104-1. (A) The guidewire in the proper position. (B and C) Result of inadvertent withdrawal of the guidewire from the abscess cavity: the pigtail catheter coils in subcutaneous tissues. (D and E) Results of inadvertent advancement of the guidewire through the far wall of the abscess into the kidney, with the catheter tip following into renal parenchyma. *A* = abscess; *K* = kidney; *L* = liver. (F) Diagram shows lateral approach to the abscess (*A*) to take advantage of the wider transverse diameter after attempts at a posterior approach were unsuccessful. (G) Postdrainage computed tomographic scan shows a lateral approach of the pigtail catheter (*arrow*) in a perinephric abscess. The pigtail tip is out of the scan plane. Note the resolution of the abscess compared to that shown in Figure 104-1A. *Sp* = spleen.

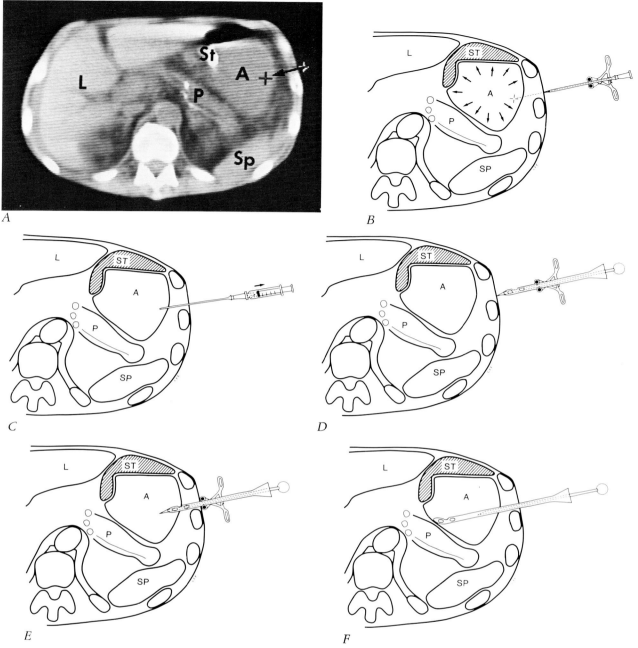

Figure 104-8. (A) Computed tomographic scan shows a lesser sac abscess (*A*) displacing the stomach (*St*) ventrad. The splenic flexure is displaced caudad and therefore is not seen on this scan. Thus the abscess has provided itself with a safe percutaneous drainage route (*arrow and electronic cursor marks*) from a point just below the left costal margin. To avoid the diaphragm, this route enters from below upward. *P* = pancreas; *Sp* = spleen; *L* = liver. (B) Aspiration needle in position. The depth to the near side of the abscess has been transposed to the aspiration needle with a rubber-shod clamp. (C) After the aspiration needle is inserted in a single pass over the planned route, a small sample of material is aspirated for an immediate Gram's stain. (D) Trocar catheter in position. Note that the trocar catheter is being inserted with cephalad angulation to avoid the diaphragm. The direct intercostal approach may traverse the pleura, causing pyopneumothorax.

(E) Trocar catheter is advanced in a single motion into the abscess over the preselected route. (F) After removal of the clamp, a central stylet is held fixed in position while the outer catheter is gently advanced over the stylet. The catheter should slide easily until a slight resistance indicates that it has engaged the far wall. During this maneuver, the central stylet functions like a guidewire. Note that care must be taken not to advance the cutting edge of the stylet as the leading point beyond the near wall of the abscess. Doing so may perforate the far wall. (G) The stylet is removed, and the abscess is manually evacuated by syringe suction. The catheter is sutured securely to the skin with two 1-0 silk sutures and then connected to closed biliary bag drainage. With the decrease in mass effect (*arrows*), the surrounding structures return to a normal position and close the percutaneous access window. The catheter must now be protected against **2343**

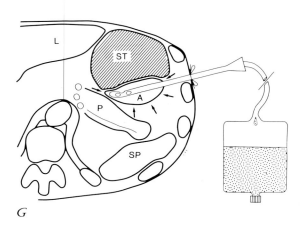

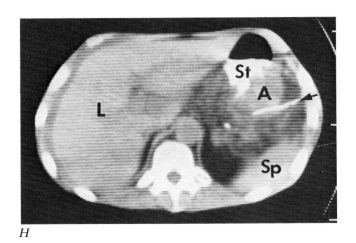

G

H

inadvertently falling out since reinsertion may be impossible. (H) A follow-up computed tomographic scan shows the catheter (*arrow*) with a small residuum (*A*). The outermost portion of the catheter is not seen since it lies below the scan plane and was inserted from below upward. The catheter remained in place for several days until complete resolution and then was removed. (B to H from Gerzof et al. [10]. Reproduced by permission from *Semin. Roentgenol.*)

104-5A–E). With care taken not to withdraw or advance the tip of the guidewire inside the abscess cavity, the Teflon sleeve is removed. This is somewhat at variance with the commonly employed Seldinger technique. In aortography, there is often wide latitude for advancement or withdrawal of the guidewire without danger of inadvertently perforating or pulling out of the arterial tree (Fig. 104-6). However, in small abscesses or in abscesses with narrow diameters, one must beware of advancing the guidewire beyond the far wall or withdrawing it from the near wall during this maneuver (Fig. 104-7A–G; see also Fig. 104-5A–E).

As in the Seldinger technique, the track is slightly widened by passage of an 8 French angiographic dilator over the wire. An 8.2 French pigtail catheter with 12 side holes (Cook) is introduced over the guidewire into the abscess cavity. The pigtail tip immediately resumes its tight coil within the abscess, preventing perforation of the far wall and promoting coiling of the catheter within the abscess cavity, a further safety factor. The abscess is then manually evacuated by syringe suction, and the catheter is sutured in position and connected to a closed biliary bag drainage system (see Management, p. 2345).

TROCAR CATHETER TECHNIQUE

Localization, route planning, and diagnostic aspiration are the same as in the angiocatheter technique. However, this technique employs a 12 French or 16 French Argyle trocar catheter (Sherwood) [16, 17] (Fig. 104-8A–H), a Silastic catheter with multiple side holes that has a self-contained central stylet. It is inserted over the same route confirmed by diagnostic aspiration. The central stylet provides rigidity to the catheter, while its cutting edge permits its insertion through subcutaneous tissue. However, considerable force may be required to advance the trocar catheter across deeper tissue planes and a sturdy rubber-shod Kelly clamp must be used as a needle stop to prevent insertion beyond the desired depth [8]. Once in the abscess, the central stylet is held in a fixed position, like an angiographic guidewire, while the outer catheter is gently advanced. Slight resistance is felt when the catheter tip has engaged the far wall of the abscess. At this point, the stylet is removed, and the abscess is evacuated by syringe suction. The catheter is then sutured in position and connected to a closed biliary bag system (see Management, p. 2345).

In both techniques, the aspirated volume is compared with the estimated volume and repeat imaging studies are performed to exclude undrained residuum. Small volumes may remain after initial drainage and will usually drain out over the next 24 to 48 hours. A large residuum may require manipulation of the catheter—or placement of a second catheter if the residuum persists.

Choice of Drainage Technique

The location and accessibility of the abscess determine which catheter technique to use. In turn, these factors are determined by the size and depth of the abscess and its proximity to surrounding structures. It is recommended that the less traumatic 8 French pigtail catheter be used for smaller, deeper abscesses, for abscesses in parenchymal organs, and for abscesses in close proximity to the bowel or other vital structures. The trocar catheter may be used for larger, more superficial, enteroparietal abscesses to which there is safe, easy percutaneous access and for retroperitoneal abscesses in which there is no concern for interposed bowel [7, 8, 10].

While the 8 French pigtail catheter can be used in any location, its insertion is more involved than that of the trocar catheter and its use may be difficult in uncooperative patients. The trocar catheter can be inserted rapidly, and, because of its larger bore, it provides faster drainage for the larger collections. There is no significant difference in the complication rates of the two catheter systems. Experience with over 70 cases suggests that the side holes in both systems, small as they are, provide equal and adequate drainage. When there is a doubt, the angiocatheter system is suggested because it requires only one initial needle pass as opposed to two with the trocar catheter system.

Indications and Contraindications

Percutaneous abscess drainage should be performed when the following criteria are met: (1) a well-defined abscess cavity without internal loculation, (2) a safe percutaneous access route, (3) concurring surgical opinion, and (4) capability for immediate operative intervention in case of failure or complication.

Contraindications include the absence of any of the above criteria or the presence of a bleeding diathesis [8]. In addition, like any angiographic procedure, percutaneous abscess drainage has relative contraindications, such as severe coagulopathy. Internal loculation of an abscess is only a relative contraindication since it occurs rarely and since loculated abscesses may be treated by placement of separate catheters to drain each loculation.

Infected hematomas and septic pancreatic phlegmona may be diagnosed by needle aspiration, but the presence of solid clot or necrotic, partially digested tissue requires surgical evacuation. In such cases, when the patient is a poor operative risk, percutaneous catheter drainage may be used as a temporizing measure to provide decompression until the patient can better tolerate surgery [8, 10].

Management

Immediately after aspiration is completed, a follow-up scan is performed to document complete evacuation of the abscess. The catheters are then carefully sutured to the skin at their entry site with two 1-0 silk sutures covered with dry sterile dressings. In both drainage techniques, a closed biliary bag collection system is attached to the catheters by a short length of connecting tubing. The outer portion of the catheter is securely taped to the skin to avoid traction by the collection bag. Anteroposterior and lateral radiographs are then obtained to document the position of the radiopaque catheters.

In general, percutaneously placed catheters are managed like surgically placed drains. Irrigation is usually unnecessary since purulent abscess contents do not clot. Daily drainage volumes are measured and recorded to assess progress. The system is left to gravity drainage only, since active suction may erode the abscess wall and surrounding vessels and viscera.

The decision to remove a drainage catheter is based on the clinical response of the patient. When the patient's temperature and white blood cell count return to normal, when there is cessation of drainage (less than 5–10 cc/day), and when follow-up scans exclude undrained residuum, the catheter can be removed, usually by 14 days [8].

Sinograms should be performed when a persistent residuum is demonstrated by follow-up scan, there is significant drainage that lasts beyond 5 to 7 days, or an enteric fistula is suspected. Sinograms should be performed with low pressure by hand injection under close fluoroscopic control by one who is familiar with the case.

Comparison of Percutaneous Drainage and Surgical Drainage

At first glance, percutaneous abscess drainage appears to be a radical departure from the traditional methods of surgical treatment, which are based on wide incision and open drainage. However, percutaneous drainage does adhere to basic surgical principles. Surgical exposure provides decompression and evacuation, and surgically placed drainage catheters provide continuous drainage. These same mechanical processes are performed by percutaneously placed drainage tubes without damage to surrounding tissues. In fact, percutaneously inserted catheters appear to function better than surgically placed drains since there are no clotting factors present to block the catheter. As a result, smaller bore catheters placed percutaneously function better than larger bore catheters placed surgically.

Furthermore, percutaneous drainage routes closely parallel surgical approaches to abscesses in comparable locations. This often requires a combination of CT and ultrasonography for guidance, particularly when cephalad angulation is necessary to approach a subphrenic abscess situated high under the diaphragm (Fig. 104-9A, B). In this case, the subcostal approach of Ochsner is the route of choice [27]. Renal and perinephric abscesses are approached posterolaterally extraperitoneally, as in the usual lumbodorsal surgical approach to this area [20]. Enteroparietal abscesses are approached through their point of contact with the parietal peritoneum [23, 25]. Hepatic abscesses are variously approached anteriorly, laterally, or posteriorly, depending on their intrahepatic location and their proximity to the abdominal wall. In all cases, knowledge of surgical anatomy is necessary for safe percutaneous access.

Percutaneous abscess drainage has many advantages over operative drainage [8]. The most basic advantage is the total avoidance of general anesthesia and surgery as well as their related perioperative complications. Performed under local anesthesia only, percutaneous abscess drainage is better accepted by the patient. Morbidity, mortality, and recurrence of percutaneously drained abscesses are lower than for operatively drained abscesses [8]. This may be due in part to the fact that sectional imaging usually provides earlier diagnosis and permits earlier treatment.

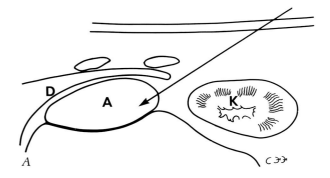

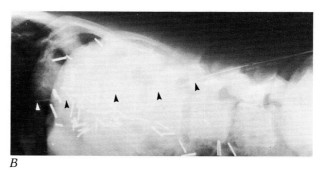

B

Figure 104-9. (A) A prone sagittal diagram of the recommended percutaneous access route to the posterior subphrenic space. It is an extraperitoneal subcostal approach from below upward. The route passes cephalad and dorsad to the kidney and caudad and ventrad to the diaphragm. Ultrasonography is ideal for guidance when this degree of cephalocaudad angulation is required. *A* = abscess; *D* = diaphragm; *K* = kidney; *arrow* = drainage route. (B) A lateral radiograph shows a trocar catheter (*arrowheads*) draining a subphrenic abscess from the subcostal approach.

Sectional imaging displays the entirety of the abscess and identifies internal septation, which may not be apparent by operative exposure alone. It can exclude synchronous disease, which may be missed by limited operative exposure. Nursing care is simpler since emptying the closed collection system replaces the frequent changes of absorbent bandages necessary for wide incisions with multiple drains.

Discussion

As with any interventional radiologic procedure, thorough correlation with clinical data and all pertinent radiographic studies is essential before diagnostic aspiration or therapeutic drainage can be considered. Only after such a thorough review should aspiration be performed for confirmation. It should be reemphasized that the CT and sonographic findings of abscess are nonspecific. The simple presence of an abnormal postoperative fluid collection in a febrile patient is not an indication for surgery. Unnecessary surgery may be avoided by a sterile diagnostic aspirate.

Although angiocatheter exchange techniques are used for percutaneous placement of pigtail drains, the procedure is best performed by those experienced in sectional imaging, route planning, and needle aspirations guided by sectional imaging. Angiography and fluoroscopy can occasionally be used for guidance, but the majority of abscesses are best drained under CT or ultrasonography guidance.

From personal experience with over 70 cases, the following conclusions can be drawn:

1. The majority of intraabdominal and retroperitoneal abscesses have safe percutaneous drainage routes.
2. Percutaneous accessibility is determined by the size and location of the abscess.
3. The use of CT for diagnosis and route planning, followed by ultrasonography to provide guidance in three planes, is the most efficient and perhaps the safest approach.
4. When CT provides the necessary anatomic detail for avoidance of bowel loops or when enteroparietal abscesses displace bowel loops, transperitoneal drainage routes can be used safely.
5. The vast majority of intraabdominal abscesses are unilocular and are amenable to percutaneous drainage.
6. Most radiology departments with sectional imaging can perform percutaneous abscess drainage because the materials are readily available and the technique itself is relatively simple.

Summary

Percutaneous abscess drainage is a new procedure in the array of resources of the interventional radiologist [2]. Seemingly radically invasive for a radiologic procedure, it is rather conservative compared to surgery, the ultimate invasion. When a unilocular abscess cavity with a safe percutaneous route is demonstrated by sectional imaging, a trial of percutaneous drainage should be offered as a primary method of definitive treatment. Surgery should be performed only if this method fails.

References

1. Anderson, C. B., Marr, J. J., and Ballinger, W. F. Anaerobic infections in surgery: Clinical review. *Surgery* 79:313, 1976.
2. Athanasoulis, C. A. Therapeutic applications of angiography. *N. Engl. J. Med.* 302:1174, 1980.
3. Callender, C. L. *Surgical Anatomy.* Philadelphia: Saunders, 1941. Pp. 317, 345–349.
4. Doust, B. D., Quiroz, F., and Stewart, J. M. Ultrasonic distinction of abscesses from other intraabdominal fluid collections. *Radiology* 125:213, 1977.
5. Doust, B. D., and Thompson, R. Ultrasonography of abdominal fluid collections. *Gastrointest. Radiol.* 3:273, 1978.
6. Gerzof, S. G. The Role of Ultrasound in the Search for Intra-abdominal and Retroperitoneal abscesses. In K. J. W. Taylor and G. N. Viscomi (eds.), *Ultrasound in Emergency Medicine* (vol. 7). New York, Edinburgh, London, Melbourne: Churchill Livingstone, 1981.
7. Gerzof, S. G., Robbins, A. H., and Birkett, D. H. Computed tomography in the diagnosis and management of abdominal abscesses. *Gastrointest. Radiol.* 3:287, 1978.
8. Gerzof, S. G., Robbins, A. H., Birkett, D. H., Johnson, W. C., Pugatch, R. D., and Vincent, M. E. Percutaneous catheter drainage of abdominal abscesses guided by ultrasound and computed tomography. *AJR* 133:1, 1979.
9. Gerzof, S. G., Robbins, A. H., Pugatch, R. D., and Gerson, E. J. New applications of old radiographic techniques applied to computed tomography. *Comput. Tomogr.* 1:331, 1977.
10. Gerzof, S. G., Spira, R., and Robbins, A. H. Percutaneous abscess drainage. *Semin. Roentgenol.* 16:62, 1981.
11. Grønvall, J., Grønvall, S., and Hegedus, V. Ultrasound guided drainage of fluid-containing masses using angiographic catheterization techniques. *AJR* 129:997, 1977.
12. Haaga, J. R., Alfidi, R. J., Havrilla, T. R., Cooperman, A. M., Seidelmann, F. E., Reich, N. E., Weinstein, A. J., and Meaney, T. F. CT detection and aspiration of abdominal abscesses. *AJR* 128:465, 1977.
13. Halpern, M. Arteriography of the Alimentary Tract. In A. K. Margulis and J. S. Burhenne (eds.), *Alimentary Tract Roentgenology* (2nd ed.). St. Louis: Mosby, 1973. Pp. 1401–1405.

14. Hoffer, P. Gallium and infection. *J. Nucl. Med.* 21:484, 1980.

15. Holm, H. H., Rasmussen, S. N., and Kristensen, J. K. Ultrasonically guided percutaneous puncture technique. *J. Clin. Ultrasound* 1:27, 1973.

16. Ingram, J. M. Suprapubic cystotomy by trocar catheter: A preliminary report. *Am. J. Obstet. Gynecol.* 113:1108, 1972.

17. Ingram, J. M. Further experience with suprapubic drainage by trocar catheter. *Am. J. Obstet. Gynecol.* 121:885, 1975.

18. Koehler, P. R., and Moss, A. A. Diagnosis of intra-abdominal and pelvic abscesses by computerized tomography. *J.A.M.A.* 244:49, 1980.

19. Kressel, H. Y., and Filly, R. A. Ultrasonographic appearance of gas-containing abscesses in the abdomen. *AJR* 130:71, 1978.

20. Lutzeyer, W. Lumbodorsal Exploration. In J. F. Glenn (ed.), *Urologic Surgery* (2nd ed.). Hagerstown, Md.: Harper & Row, 1975. Pp. 127–133.

21. Maklad, N. F., Doust, B. D., and Baum, J. K. Ultrasonic diagnosis of postoperative intraabdominal abscess. *Radiology* 113:417, 1974.

22. Meyers, M. A., and Whalen, J. P. Radiologic Aspects of Intra-abdominal Abscesses. In I. M. Ariel and K. K. Kazarian (eds.), *Diagnosis and Treatment of Abdominal Abscesses.* Baltimore: Williams & Wilkins, 1971. Pp. 87–127.

23. Nagler, S. M., and Poticha, S. M. Intraabdominal abscess in regional enteritis. *Am. J. Surg.* 137:350, 1979.

24. Norton, L., Eule, J., and Burdick, D. Accuracy of techniques to detect intraperitoneal abscesses. *Surgery* 84:370, 1978.

25. Ochsner, A. Reminiscence: The development of the retroperitoneal operation of subphrenic abscess. *Rev. Surg.* 21:153, 1964.

26. Ochsner, A., and DeBakey, M. Subphrenic abscess: A collective review and an analysis of 3608 collected and personal cases. *Int. Abstr. Surg.* 66:426, 1938.

27. Ochsner, A., and Graves, A. M. Subphrenic abscess: An analysis of 3372 collected and personal cases. *Ann. Surg.* 98:961, 1933.

28. Pedersen, J. F., Hancke, S., and Kristensen, J. K. Renal carbuncle: Antibiotic therapy governed by ultrasonically guided aspirations. *J. Urol.* 109:777, 1973.

Interventional Biliary Radiology

ERNEST J. RING
JUAN A. OLEAGA
DAVID B. FREIMAN
GORDON K. McLEAN

Interventional radiology includes a diverse group of procedures that combine three basic elements:

1. Safe access for introduction of catheters and other devices into areas of internal pathology.
2. Fluoroscopically guided manipulations within the involved organ system.
3. Specialized catheter systems that have been modified to effect a beneficial change in a pathologic condition.

During the past 10 years, advances in all three of these areas have dramatically broadened the impact of interventional radiology on clinical medicine. Interventional radiologic techniques are especially applicable to the management of patients with biliary tract pathology. Percutaneous access into the bile ducts can be achieved either through surgically created drainage tracts or directly through percutaneous approaches. Fluoroscopy provides an excellent overview of the morbid anatomy, despite such complicating factors as obesity, tumor encasement, or scarring from previous surgery. Angiographic catheters can be readily manipulated throughout the intrahepatic and extrahepatic biliary tree. Interventional biliary procedures are performed without general anesthesia and many of the risks of surgery, and they can provide nonoperative solutions to a variety of clinical problems. Even when surgery is performed, preliminary instrumentation by the radiologist can, in many cases, facilitate the operative procedure. In this chapter, we review the interventional radiologic procedures currently being used in the management of patients with biliary tract pathology.

Interventions Through Surgically Created Drainage Tracts

REMOVAL OF RETAINED STONES

It has been estimated that stones are left in the biliary tree after 1 to 3 percent of cholecystectomies [1]. Since 500,000 patients have their gallbladders removed each year in the United States, retained stones is a relatively common clinical problem. Nonoperative techniques of extracting retained biliary calculi through T-tube tracts have proved to be so successful that reoperation for stone removal is now necessary in less than 10 percent of cases [2, 3]. Pancreatitis and sepsis have been reported as complications of the procedure, but they are exceedingly rare [4]. Mazzariello [4] has had impressive success removing stones with an extraction forceps placed directly through the fistulous tract, but the more common approach is to trap and remove the stone with a basket introduced through a modified angiographic catheter [3, 5].

The commonly used Dormia basket is constructed of four thin, stainless steel wires fused proximally and distally and arranged in a helical configuration. The wires fold together when the basket is introduced into a sheath catheter and return to their original configuration as the basket exits from the sheath. The basket is attached to one end of a long, rigid guidewire, and a handle is attached to the other end. When the handle is rotated, torque is transmitted to the basket, causing it to spin. It is the spinning motion that traps the stone within the helices of the basket.

Technique of Stone Removal

Stone retrieval (Fig. 105-1) is usually attempted 4 to 5 weeks after cholecystectomy and identification of a residual calculus. During this time, the

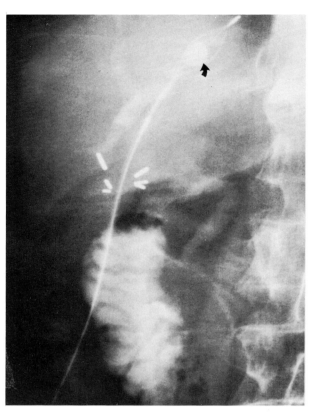

Figure 105-2. A retained common duct stone is demonstrated in the left hepatic duct (*arrow*). The stone has been trapped by a Dormia basket and was removed without difficulty.

Figure 105-1. Techniques of stone removal with a Dormia basket. (A) After a catheter is positioned adjacent to a stone, the basket is introduced. The wires of the helical basket fold together when the basket is passing through the sheath. (B) The basket opens as it exits from the sheath. Rotating the external handle causes the basket to spin. (C) The stone is trapped within the basket's wires. (D) The basket is closed by advancing the sheath toward the stone (*arrows*).

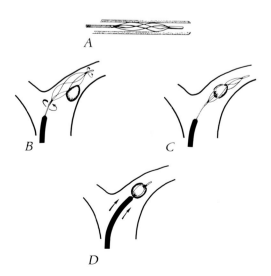

tract around the T tube matures so that catheters can be freely passed through the fistulous tract into the common duct. Before an extraction procedure is begun, the patient is placed on prophylactic, broad-spectrum antibiotic therapy. The skin around the tube entry site is cleansed with an antiseptic solution and isolated with sterile drapes. The T tube is removed with gentle traction on its external limb.

Burhenne advocates a steerable catheter system for manipulations through the fistulous tract and bile ducts [5]. This catheter has four wires in its wall that control motion at the tip. A channel is provided in the catheter through which the basket and its sheath can be passed. There is a second portal for injections of contrast material. Once the catheter has been maneuvered up to a stone, the basket and sheath are passed through the catheter. The basket is opened adjacent to the stone and rotated until the stone is seen fluoroscopically to project within its wires (Fig. 105-2). The basket is then closed by holding it in

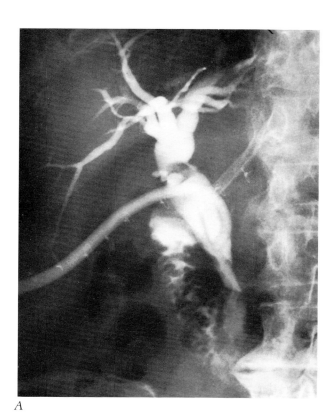

A

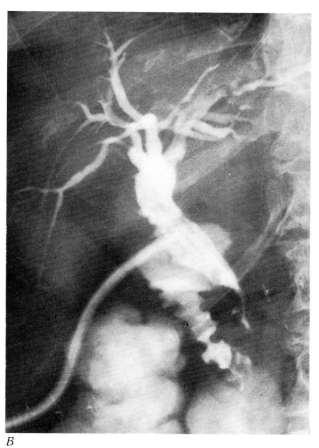

B

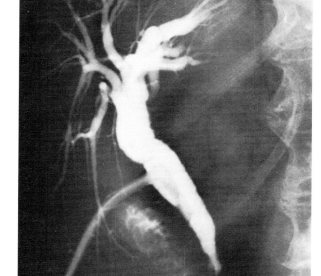

C

Figure 105-3. Debris in the common bile duct after the crushing of a stone in a basket. (A) A T-tube cholangiogram demonstrates a large retained stone in the upper part of the common bile duct. (B) The T tube was removed and a Dormia basket was introduced into the common bile duct. The stone was trapped in the basket and was crushed into multiple small fragments. A T tube was reintroduced through the tract. A cholangiogram shows considerable debris in the common bile duct. (C) A T-tube cholangiogram performed after 3 days of drainage shows that the residual material has cleared through the new T tube.

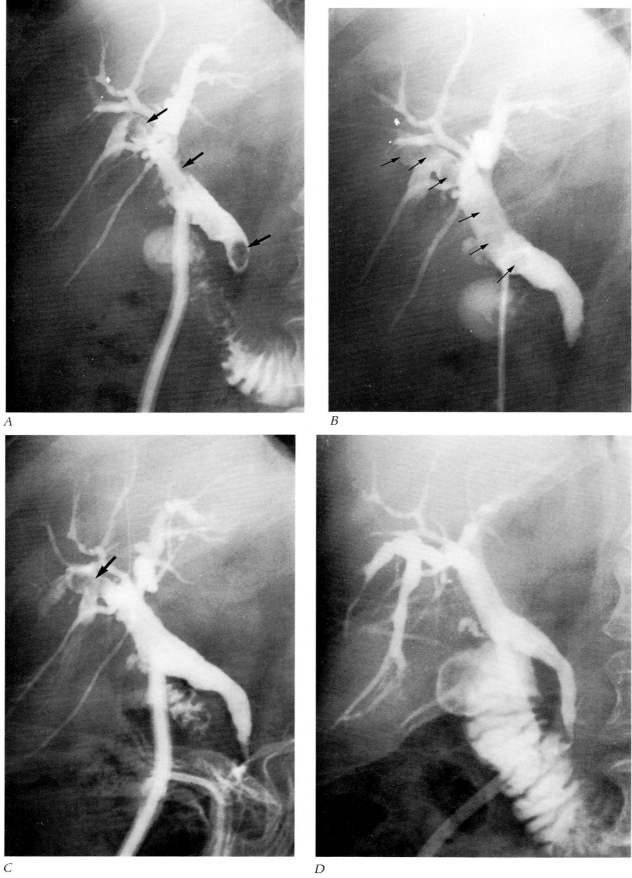

A

B

C

D

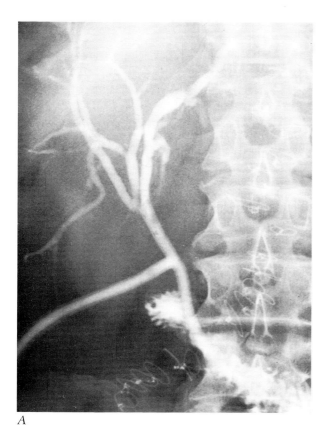

A

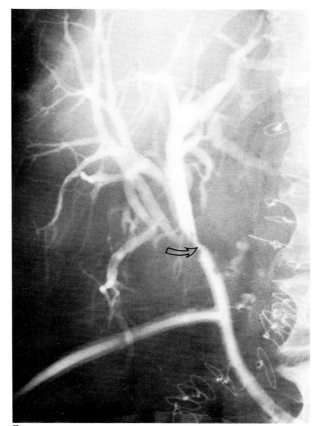

B

Figure 105-5. Overgrowth of tumor above a stenting
T tube. A T tube had been left in a 67-year-old man
after a choledochoenterostomy. (A) A T-tube cholangiogram demonstrates free flow into the intrahepatic
ducts and the duodenum. (B) After approximately 18
months, the signs and symptoms of obstructive jaundice developed. A T-tube cholangiogram demonstrates irregular stenosis of the duct just above the
proximal limb of the T tube consistent with recurrent
tumor (*arrow*). (C) The stenting tube was removed and
replaced by a longer T tube (*dots*) with multiple side
holes attached to the lesion. Free drainage was then
reestablished.

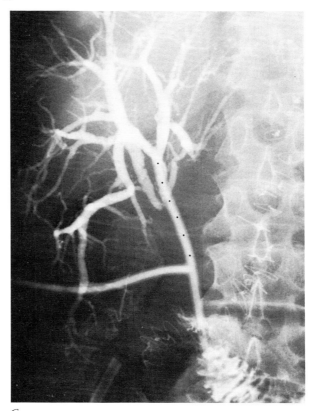

C

◀ **Figure 105-4.** Stage removal of retained common bile
duct stones. (A) A T-tube cholangiogram demonstrates multiple retained stones in the common bile
duct as well as the right hepatic duct (*arrows*). (B) The
T tube was removed and a Dormia basket was introduced through the common bile duct. Several stones
were removed (*arrows*). (C) Since a single stone in the
right hepatic duct could not be removed at that time,
the T tube was reintroduced. A T-tube cholangiogram
demonstrates the persistent stone (*arrow*). (D) Two
weeks later, the stone had moved into the common
bile duct, where it was easily trapped in the basket and
removed.

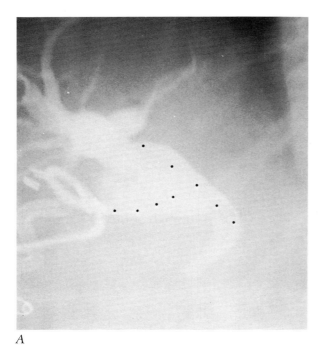

A

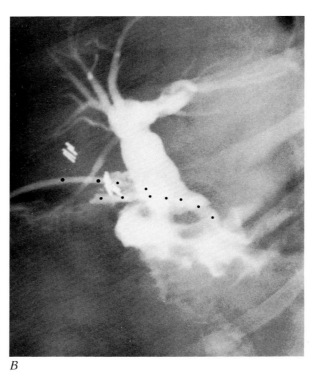

B

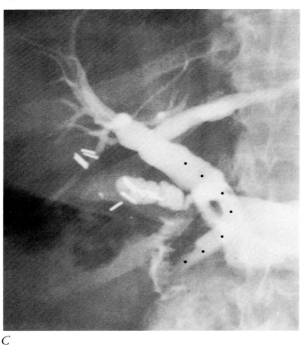

C

Figure 105-6. Malpositioning of a T tube. (A) This 52-year-old woman had a retained common bile duct stone after a cholecystectomy and a common bile duct exploration. An initial T-tube (*dots*) cholangiogram showed the stone obstructing the distal common bile duct. (B) Three weeks later, the woman became febrile, and a thick mucinous material came from the tube. A T-tube cholangiogram showed that the tube (*dots*) had rotated in such a way that the distal end had perforated the duct to create a fistulous communication with the duodenum cap. (C) The T tube was removed and the stone retrieved using a Dormia basket. A new T tube was introduced through the tract. The longer distal limb of the tube bypassed the fistulous communication (*dots*). This arrangement allowed the fistula to heal.

position and advancing the sheath. After the stone has been trapped, the basket and sheath are forcefully withdrawn through the tract. Stones of almost any size can be successfully removed in this fashion. To facilitate passage of an unusually large stone, the tract may be dilated prior to stone removal [6]. Either coaxial or balloon catheter dilatation techniques can be used.

After a stone has been removed, a catheter is reintroduced through the tract and any additional stones or fragments are removed in the same manner. Interpreting a cholangiogram performed immediately following stone extraction may be difficult because of residual air bubbles or clots in the biliary tree (Fig. 105-3). A rubber tube is usually left through the tract and a final cholangiogram performed at a later date. The tube is not removed completely until cholangiography demonstrates a normal-appearing biliary tree with no residual fragments. It is not uncommon in patients with multiple stones for the extraction procedure to be performed in several stages, with a few stones removed each time (Fig. 105-4).

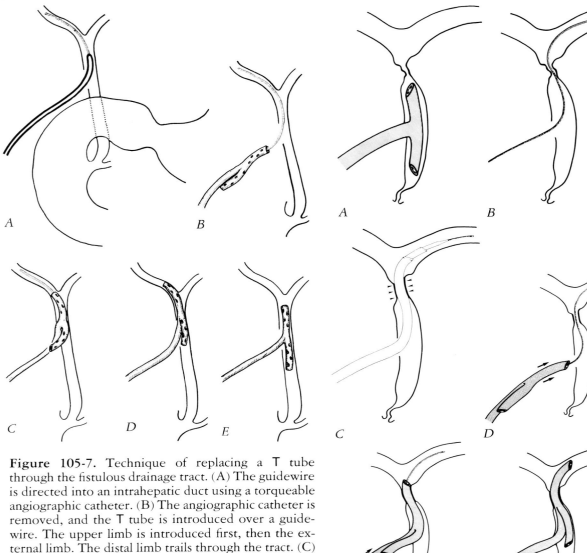

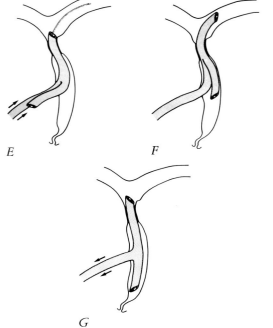

Figure 105-7. Technique of replacing a T tube through the fistulous drainage tract. (A) The guidewire is directed into an intrahepatic duct using a torqueable angiographic catheter. (B) The angiographic catheter is removed, and the T tube is introduced over a guidewire. The upper limb is introduced first, then the external limb. The distal limb trails through the tract. (C) Both the proximal and the distal limbs are advanced through the choledochotomy site and into the upper part of the common bile duct. (D) Once the lower limb has passed through the choledochotomy site, it springs freely into the lumen of the common bile duct. (E) Slight external pressure will then cause the lower limb to descend into the lower common bile duct.

Figure 105-8. Dilating a stricture prior to introducing a stenting T tube. (A, B, and C) The initial T tube is removed and a guidewire is passed through the tract and directed across the stricture. The narrowed area is dilated with a coaxial Teflon catheter of up to 24 French. (D to G) The T tube is introduced in the usual manner. The leading limb of the T tube is always directed at the narrowed area so that the free limb can spring into the normal segment of the common duct.

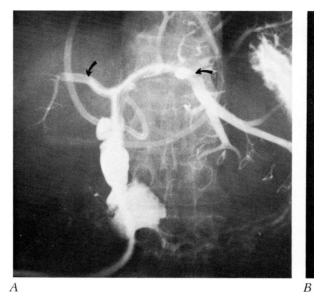

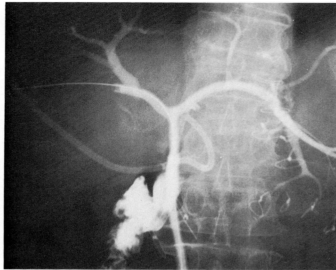

A   B

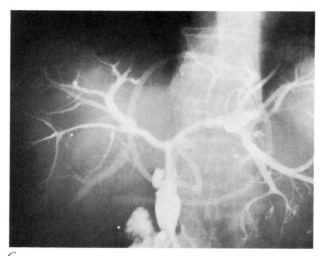

C

Figure 105-9. A 63-year-old man with a cholangiocarcinoma stented by a Y tube. The patient developed cholangitis when the tube became obstructed by sludge. (A) A T-tube cholangiogram demonstrated partial obstruction of the left limb and complete obstruction of the right limb of the tube (*arrows*). (B) Catheters and guidewires were used to break up the sludge. (C) A repeat cholangiogram after disimpaction of the tube showed free flow into both limbs. A cholangiogram was done every 3 months during the remaining 2 years of the patient's life.

Technique of T-Tube Replacement

After the original tube has been removed, a catheter is advanced through the tract into the common bile duct. To avoid false passage, a soft rubber tube should be used to catheterize the empty tract. A rigid guidewire with a floppy tip is then passed through the tube into either the proximal or the distal duct, and the new tube is fashioned. The rubber tube is removed and the new T tube is introduced over the guidewire (Fig. 105-7). The leading vertical limb of the T tube is placed on the guidewire first, followed by the long external limb. The other vertical limb trails freely through the tract. Because T tubes are made of rubber, which has a high coefficient of friction, a sterile lubricating jelly is applied. The T tube is advanced over the guidewire into the common duct. Passage through the tract is often difficult but can usually be accomplished by advancing the tube and guidewire as a unit for a few centimeters and then withdrawing the guidewire to its original position. The process is repeated until both limbs of the T tube have completely passed into the common bile duct. Once both of the vertical

T-TUBE REPLACEMENT

Indwelling tubes are frequently employed to palliate malignant biliary obstructions and to stent complicated strictures. However, a stenting tube will eventually stop functioning if it deteriorates or migrates (Fig. 105-5) or if the duct above or below the tube becomes obstructed by continued growth of tumor (Fig. 105-6). When a T tube stops functioning, it can almost always be replaced without surgery through the original drainage tract [7]. The new tube can be positioned under fluoroscopic guidance so that both vertical limbs are anchored in the common duct [8]. The limbs can be fashioned to match the original tube or lengthened to extend through new areas of obstruction.

limbs are through the choledochotomy, the free limb of the rubber T tube springs into the lumen of the duct. The guidewire is then removed. The vertical limbs are secured by slightly withdrawing the external limb. This causes the free vertical limb to catch on the lip of the choledochotomy and slide into position.

When tubes are being replaced to provide a longer limb through an obstruction, preliminary dilatation of the narrowed area with coaxial catheters facilitates introduction. In such a case, the leading limb of the new T tube is always directed toward the obstruction so that the free limb can spring into a normal segment of duct (Fig. 105-8).

Y TUBES

Primary cholangiocarcinoma that obstructs the common hepatic duct and extends into the right and left ducts commonly is palliated surgically by placing a Y tube [9]. Each of the proximal limbs of the tube extends into an intrahepatic duct, and the distal limb is positioned in the common bile duct. An external limb is also provided for drainage or irrigation. When a Y tube deteriorates, there is no technique that permits its replacement without surgery. Two T tubes may be placed fluoroscopically, each with an upper limb in a separate intrahepatic duct, or a single T tube can be placed through the tract to drain one lobe of the liver and a transhepatic catheter positioned to drain the other. When a Y tube ceases to function because it is obstructed with sludge, it can be disimpacted using a simple catheter technique (Fig. 105-9). Tube disimpaction is performed by passing an angiographic catheter through the lumen of the Y tube and directing it into each of its limbs. A guidewire passed through the angiographic catheter is used to fragment the obstructing material, which is cleared with suction and saline irrigation. Tube disimpaction is a totally painless procedure that can be performed on an outpatient basis. Broad-spectrum antibiotics are administered for 3 or 4 days following completion of the procedure.

Interventions Through a Direct Transhepatic Approach

Percutaneous catheterization of the bile ducts has been used for many years to establish temporary biliary drainage prior to surgery [10]. Recent technical improvements have made it possible to manipulate transhepatic catheters consistently through various types of obstructions into the distal duct and duodenum [11–13]. Special catheters with side holes positioned above and below the obstruction can be introduced to direct the flow of bile antegrade through the obstruction into the duodenum [14]. In addition to lowering serum bilirubin levels, antegrade drainage helps to improve the patient's nutritional status and avoids the electrolyte loss associated with external drainage. Because the drainage tube acts as a conduit for bile flow into the duodenum, it not only can be used for preoperative decompression but may also provide long-term palliation for patients who are not considered surgical candidates [15].

TECHNIQUE OF PERCUTANEOUS TRANSHEPATIC BILIARY DRAINAGE

The patient is placed supine on a fluoroscopic table, with his right arm extended. The skin around the upper lateral abdomen is prepared with an antiseptic solution and isolated by sterile drapes. The drainage procedure is performed in two stages (Fig. 105-10). Transhepatic cholangiography is performed first, with the 22-gauge Chiba needle, to confirm the presence of an obstruction and portray the nature and location of the obstructing lesion. This information is used to decide whether further catheterization and drainage are indicated. In addition, in the presence of an obstruction, the ducts remain filled with contrast material after the thin-needle cholangiogram, and this facilitates the subsequent introduction of the larger needle and catheter.

If it is decided that transcatheter drainage is indicated, an 18-gauge stylet within a thin-wall polyethylene sheath is introduced through the liver. The needle is directed under fluoroscopic guidance toward a duct that appears to have a straight course into the common bile duct. Once the needle/sheath has been observed fluoroscopically to cross the desired duct, the needle is removed and a syringe is attached to the sheath. The sheath is slowly withdrawn until a free flow of bile into the syringe indicates an intraluminal position. If the sheath passes without entering the desired duct, it is withdrawn to a point within the margin of the liver, and the stylet is reintroduced. The needle/sheath is then redirected with a slightly more dorsal or ventral angulation. Since complete removal of the sheath from

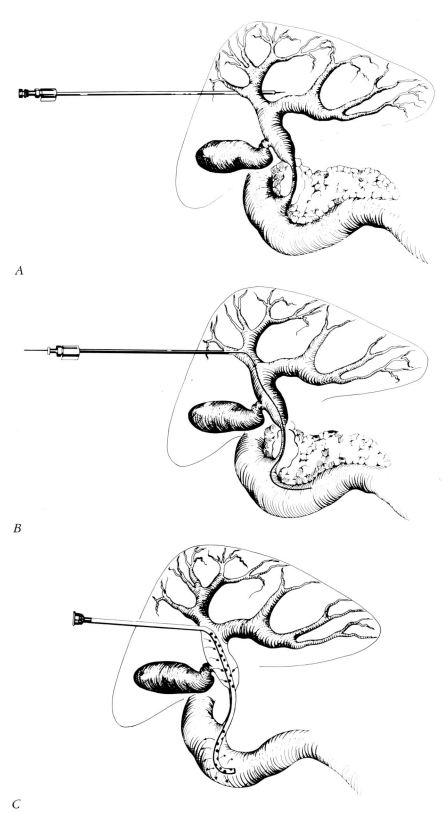

A

B

C

Figure 105-10. Technique of percutaneous transhepatic biliary drainage. (A) After the bile ducts have been opacified using a 22-gauge thin needle, an 18-gauge needle within a thin-wall polyethylene sheath is introduced into the liver and directed under fluoroscopic control toward the right hepatic duct. (B) The stylet is removed and the sheath is slowly withdrawn until a free flow of bile indicates an intraluminal position. A guidewire is then advanced through the sheath and directed through the distal common bile duct into the duodenum. (C) The sheath is replaced with a larger catheter, using the modified Seldinger technique. Multiple side holes in the catheter above and below the obstruction lesion allow antegrade drainage of bile through the catheter into the duodenum (*arrows*).

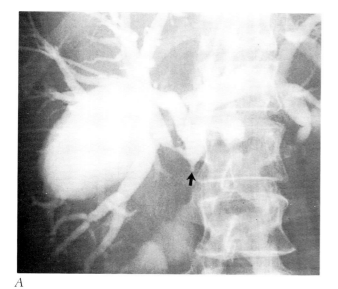

A

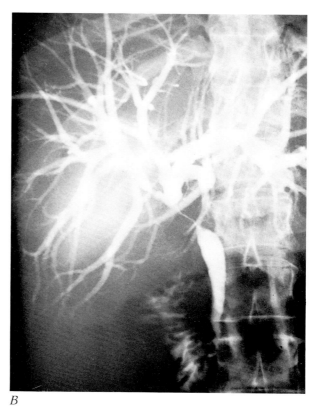

B

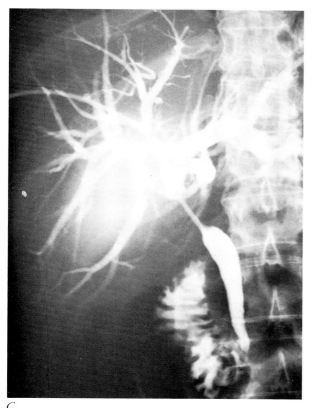

C

Figure 105-11. Staged catheterization across a complete obstruction of the common hepatic duct. (A) A transhepatic cholangiogram performed on a 51-year-old woman with obstructive jaundice caused by carcinoma of the gallbladder that had invaded the porta hepatis. The transhepatic catheter could be advanced only to the point of obstruction (*arrow*). (B) After 48 hours of external biliary drainage, the cholangiogram was repeated. A thin tract was then evident through the tumor. (C) The transhepatic catheter could then be advanced through the tract into the distal common bile duct and duodenum. Antegrade drainage was established, and the total bilirubin level fell from 22 to 3 mg per 100 cc.

the liver is not necessary, only a single capsular puncture is required.

Once the sheath is confirmed to be intraductal, a guidewire is directed through it toward the common bile duct. A special guidewire is used, one that can be curved with a small right-angle bend near its tip. The curved tip of this guidewire can be rotated by applying circular torque exter-

nally and can usually be directed into the entrance of a tract through an obstructing lesion. If the guidewire cannot be advanced past the obstruction, the catheter should be left in place in an intrahepatic duct and external drainage should be established. After 48 hours of external drainage, it is usually possible to advance the guidewire through the obstruction (Fig. 105-11).

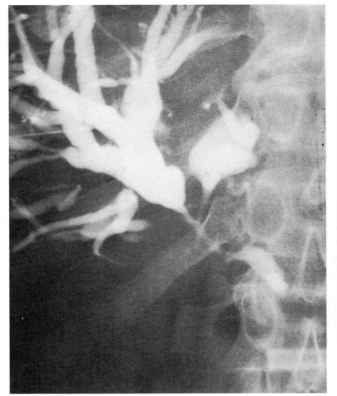

A

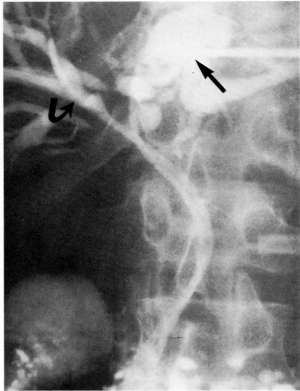

B

Figure 105-12. Obstruction at the porta hepatis by cholangiocarcinoma. (A) A thin-needle cholangiogram demonstrates obstruction of the upper common hepatic duct as well as separate obstructions involving the right and left hepatic ducts. (B) A catheter was introduced percutaneously through the right duct across the obstruction into the duodenum (*curved arrow*). A second catheter (*straight arrow*) was introduced from the anterior approach into the left duct and then through the obstruction into the duodenum. This provided total decompression of the intrahepatic biliary tree.

Figure 105-13. Obstruction of the common hepatic duct by a metastatic malignancy. (A) The transhepatic cholangiogram demonstrates an obstruction of the common hepatic duct (*arrow*) in a patient with a history of carcinoma of the colon. (B) Percutaneous transhepatic catheterization was performed, and the catheter was advanced through the obstruction into the duodenum. Over the next 6 weeks, the serum bilirubin level fell from 46 to 2 mg per 100 cc.

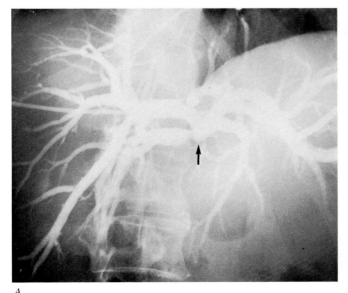

A

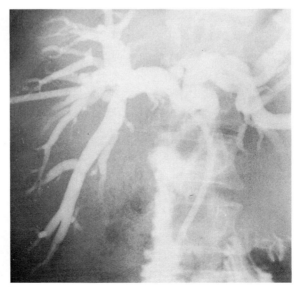

B

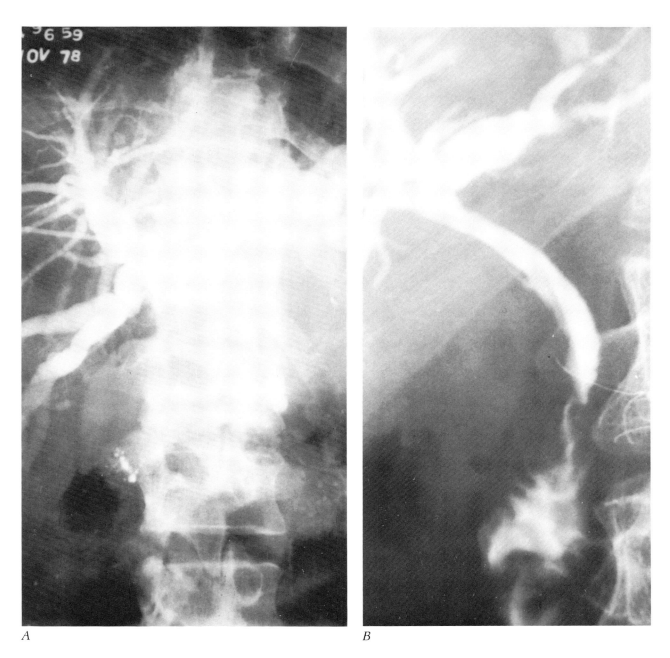

A   *B*

Figure 105-14. Obstruction of the common bile duct by metastatic gastric carcinoma. (A) A transhepatic cholangiogram shows obstruction of the proximal common hepatic duct. A percutaneous catheter was introduced and antegrade drainage was established. There was sufficient clinical improvement over the next several weeks that antineoplastic chemotherapy could be instituted. (B) Six months later, the patient had improved dramatically. The jaundice had disap-peared, and there was a 20-lb weight gain. A repeat cholangiogram through the transhepatic catheter demonstrates that the obstructing mass has responded to the chemotherapy. There is free flow of contrast material through the region previously obstructed. Three months later, the patient continued to improve and the catheter was removed. The patient was without jaundice 15 months later.

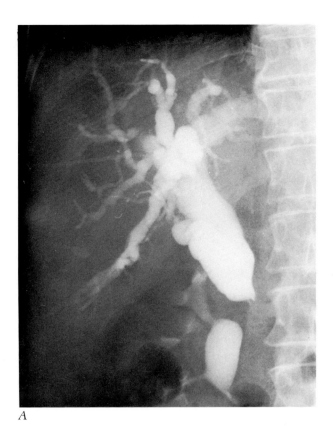
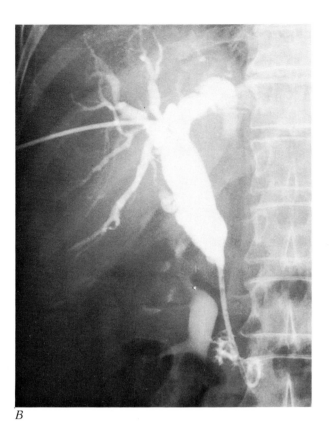

A   *B*

Figure 105-15. Preoperative decompression for resectable pancreatic carcinoma. (A) A transhepatic cholangiogram in a 57-year-old man with obstructive jaundice secondary to pancreatic carcinoma. (B) A catheter was introduced and antegrade drainage was established. The serum bilirubin level fell from 24 to 4 mg per 100 cc over the next 12 days. At surgery, a small carcinoma of the head of the pancreas was found, and a pancreaticoduodenectomy was performed.

Once the sheath has been advanced into the duodenum, it is replaced over a guidewire with a multiple side-hole drainage catheter. A special heavy-duty guidewire is used for the exchange. It is constructed of solid stainless steel and has a short, floppy segment welded to its tip. Before the catheter is introduced, side holes are made so that they will be located above and below the obstructing lesion. Correct positioning of the side holes can be precisely determined in the following manner: When the sheath has been positioned in the duodenum, a guidewire is passed through its lumen up to the ampulla. A kink is made in the guidewire as it exits from the sheath's hub. The guidewire is then withdrawn until its tip is at the site of entry into the duct, and a second kink is made at the catheter hub. The distance between the two kinks in the guidewire is the same as the distance between the ampulla and the entry site. Side holes are created over this span with a standard hole-punching tool.

After catheterization has been completed, the catheter is anchored to the skin with a suture, and the bile is drained externally for 24 to 48 hours. Antegrade drainage is established by capping the hub of the catheter.

To minimize the possibility of bacteremia, broad-spectrum antibiotic therapy is instituted 24 hours before the procedure is begun and continued for the next 3 or 4 days. The patient is discharged from the hospital 4 or 5 days after antegrade drainage has been established. Subsequent maintenance of the catheter is not difficult; in almost all cases it can be done by the patient or his family. The catheter is irrigated every other day by attaching a syringe and removing as much residual bile as possible; 10 cc of sterile saline is then forcefully injected through the catheter. The dressing is changed daily. The skin around the catheter entry site can be kept reasonably dry during showering by taping a plastic bag over the dressing. If an 8.3 French

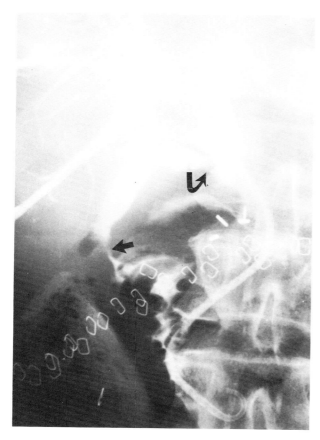

Figure 105-16. Transhepatic biliary drainage for recurrent obstructive jaundice and pancreatic carcinoma. Four months before, this patient had undergone a cholecystoduodenostomy (*curved arrow*) as a palliative operation for pancreatic carcinoma. He developed recurrent jaundice when the tumor extended to obstruct the cystic duct (*straight arrow*). Transhepatic antegrade biliary drainage provides continued palliation without the need for a second operation.

polyethylene catheter is properly cared for, it will generally remain free of obstruction for 4 to 6 months. It is easily exchanged over a guidewire for a new catheter at 3- to 4-month intervals. The exchange, a simple, painless procedure, can be performed on an outpatient basis. Antibiotic coverage is not used nor is analgesia required.

PERCUTANEOUS TRANSHEPATIC BILIARY DRAINAGE FOR MALIGNANT DISEASES

Cholangiocarcinoma
Primary bile duct tumors that originate in the upper common hepatic duct and extend into the right and left ducts (Klatzkin's tumors) are not considered resectable by most authors [16].

These tumors usually grow slowly, however, and extended palliation can be achieved if bile can be drained adequately. Palliation is generally achieved surgically with a permanent drainage tube. Transhepatic catheterization and antegrade drainage provide an attractive alternative to surgery in this setting. Multiple catheters can be introduced to decompress the entire liver. Unlike most surgically implanted tubes, transhepatic catheters are readily replaced and therefore can continue to function indefinitely (Fig. 105-12).

Metastatic Disease in the Porta Hepatis
Metastatic extension to the nodes in the porta hepatis is one of the most common causes of malignant biliary obstruction (Fig. 105-13). This type of obstruction is not usually considered amenable to surgical bypass because the involved segment of duct is in an area that is difficult to reach surgically, and the patients involved are poor operative risks. In most cases, progressive jaundice leads to a highly symptomatic terminal course. Although long-term survival of patients with metastatic tumor is unlikely, intervention is warranted in most cases to relieve pruritus and other symptoms. Furthermore, after biliary decompression has been achieved, a patient's condition may improve sufficiently to permit extensive chemotherapy or radiation therapy. We have seen occasional patients with advanced metastatic tumor who responded dramatically to this type of combined therapy and who were still alive 1 to 2 years later (Fig. 105-14).

Carcinoma of the Pancreas
The incidence of pancreatic carcinoma has increased dramatically in the past 50 years [17]. Despite the advent of imaging techniques that permit more accurate diagnoses, most pancreatic tumors are incurable by the time symptoms develop. Surgical resection of pancreatic carcinoma remains feasible in only 10 to 15 percent of cases [18, 19], and only about 15 percent of the patients who can undergo "curative surgery" live 5 years [20]. The mortality for curative surgery has been considerably reduced in recent years; it is now less than 10 percent [21]. High mortality (16–59%) continues to follow the much simpler palliative operations [22, 23]. It is likely that the high mortality is related to the debilitated condition associated with the widespread malignancy in patients suitable only for palliation. The average length of hospitalization in patients undergoing palliative surgery is 5 to 6 weeks [24]. Such

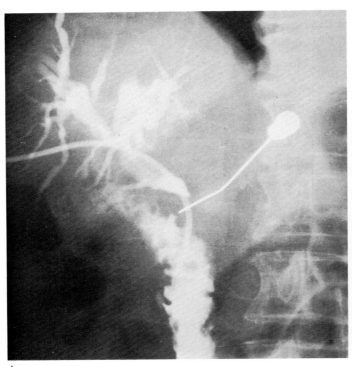
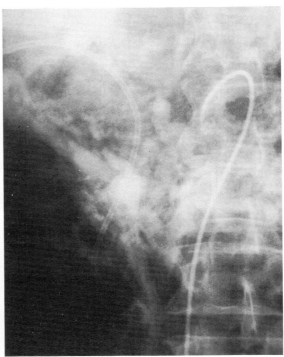

A   *B*

Figure 105-17. Nonoperative management of pancreatic carcinoma. (A) After palliation of the biliary obstruction with a transhepatic catheter, a thin-needle biopsy was performed. It confirmed the diagnosis of adenocarcinoma. (B) The following day, a superior mesenteric arteriogram showed complete occlusion of the mesenteric vein and therefore a nonresectable tumor. The patient was discharged after a total of 4 days' hospitalization.

a prolonged hospitalization assumes great significance for these patients since the mean survival after surgery is only 5.4 months [17].

Percutaneous transhepatic biliary drainage can be useful in the management of biliary obstruction caused by pancreatic carcinoma in the following three settings:

1. *Preoperative decompression* (Fig. 105-15). Patients with marked bilirubinemia are at much greater risk for major surgery. Braasch has shown that the operative mortality for pancreaticoduodenectomy is nearly double when the total serum bilirubin level surpasses 20 mg per 100 cc [21]. He has recommended that surgery be performed in two stages on severely jaundiced patients. An initial surgical drainage procedure, such as a cholecystostomy, is followed by resection when the level of jaundice has diminished. Since percutaneous transhepatic biliary drainage can similarly lead to a prompt reduction in the serum bilirubin levels, it may be used in patients with

resectable tumors as an alternative to the first-stage operation.

2. *After palliative surgery* (Fig. 105-16). Since 80 to 90 percent of patients with pancreatic carcinoma eventually develop biliary obstruction, many surgeons perform a prophylactic biliary anastomosis at the initial laparotomy. If such a bypass is not done and the duct subsequently becomes obstructed, percutaneous transhepatic biliary drainage may be the simplest way to achieve palliation. Similarly, percutaneous transhepatic biliary drainage can be used after cholecystoenterostomy if tumor growth leads to obstruction of the cystic duct orifice.

3. *Tumors that can be shown without exploratory surgery to be unresectable* (Fig. 105-17). Because of the brief anticipated survival and the prolonged hospitalization after surgical bypass, transhepatic drainage may be considered as the primary form of palliation for some patients with advanced tumors. Various staging techniques can be used to show that a tumor is

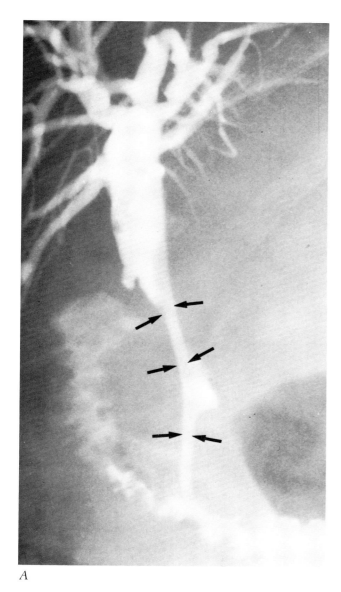

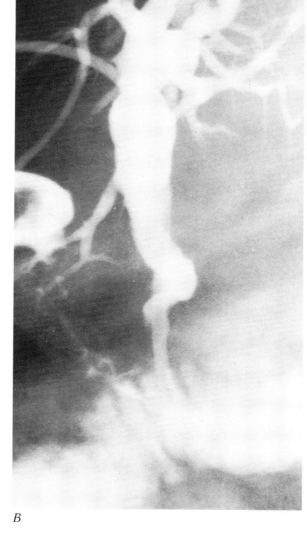

A

B

Figure 105-18. Peripancreatic lymphoma mimicking pancreatic carcinoma. (A) Transhepatic catheterization was performed to relieve obstructive jaundice. An injection after the catheter (*arrows*) had been introduced demonstrates an irregular obstruction of the distal common duct and a mass impressing on the inner margin of the duodenal loop. The appearance is strongly suggestive of carcinoma of the pancreas. (B) Thin-needle biopsy of the mass showed it to be histiocytic lymphoma. Because of the uncertainty of establishing a diagnosis of lymphoma with cytology, an open biopsy was performed. It confirmed the diagnosis. The patient was given radiation therapy with the transhepatic catheter left in place for decompression. A final cholangiogram before removal of the catheter shows resolution of the obstructing mass.

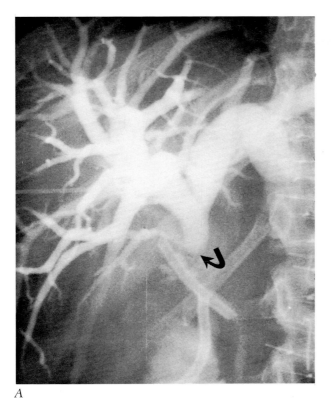

A

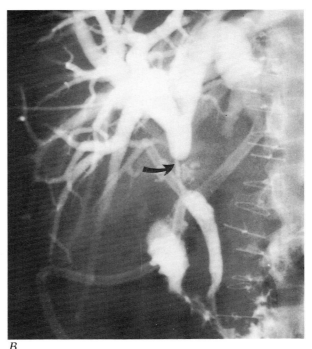

B

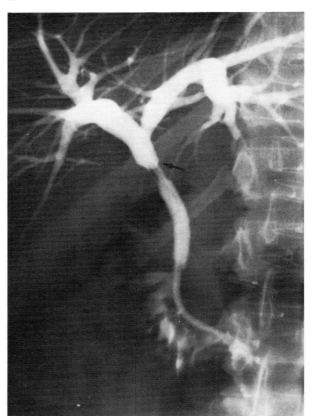

C

D

Figure 105-19. A 21-year-old woman with jaundice following cholecystectomy. Reexploration revealed a stricture. An attempt was made to introduce a T tube through the stricture. (A) A percutaneous transhepatic cholangiogram demonstrates the dilated biliary radicles and the site of obstruction (*arrow*). (B) A catheter was introduced transhepatically and advanced through the obstruction (*arrow*). (C) Antegrade drainage was established with an 8.3 French catheter with multiple side holes (*arrows*). The patient was discharged from the hospital. (D) Periodic cholangiograms done over the next 2½ years revealed progressive shortening of the strictured segment (*arrow*). A second attempt at repair of the stricture was made. At this operation, the adhesions were diminished compared with those seen during the first attempt at repair, and the duct could be identified by palpating the transhepatic catheter. A primary repair of the strictured segment proved to be successful.

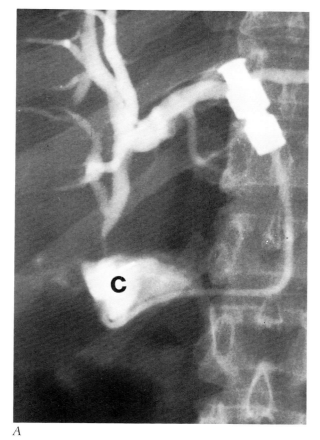

A

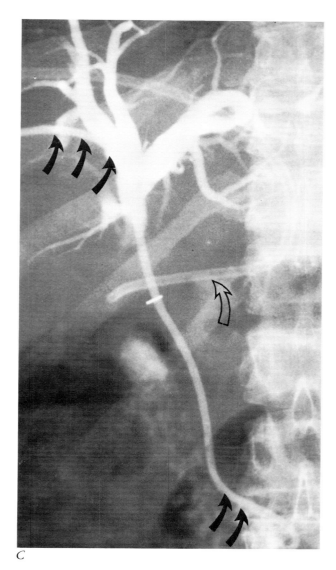

C

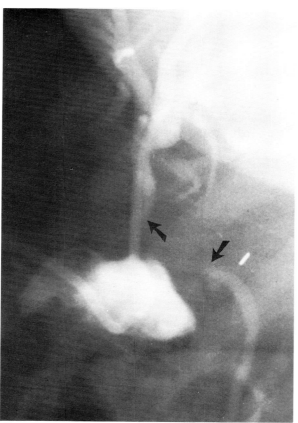

B

Figure 105-20. A 31-year-old woman with a transected common bile duct after cholecystectomy. An attempt to repair the stricture over a T tube was unsuccessful. (A) An injection of contrast material through a rubber catheter introduced through the T-tube tract demonstrated an irregular cavity (*C*). (B) A lateral radiograph opacified the severed ends of the duct above and below the cavity (*arrows*). (C) An 8.3 French catheter was introduced percutaneously and advanced to connect the lumens of the proximal and distal ducts (*solid arrows*). The side holes made in the intrahepatic and duodenal segments of the catheter allowed antegrade drainage of bile. The rubber catheter was left in the cavity for drainage (*open arrow*). Four months later, a choledochoenterostomy was performed.

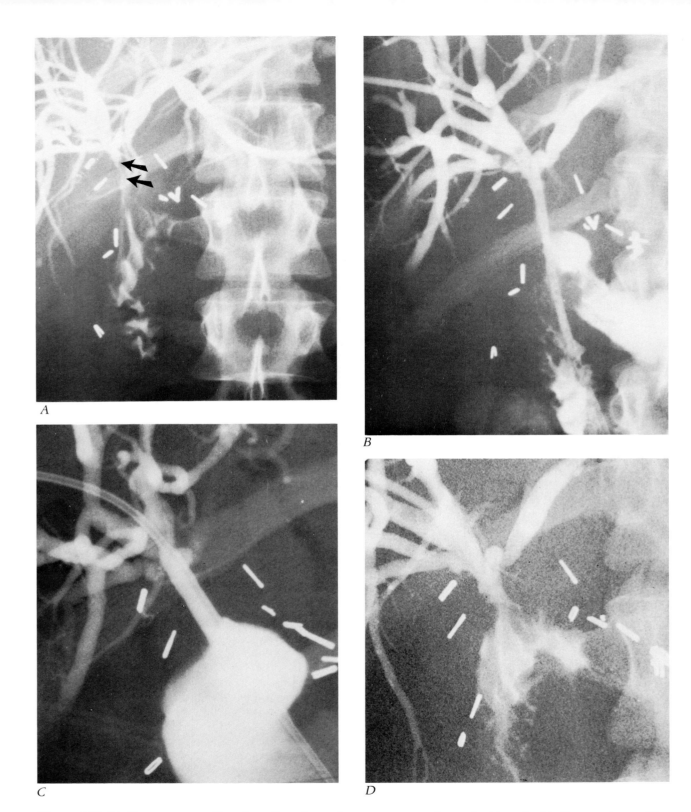

A

B

C

D

Figure 105-21. Percutaneous dilatation of a strictured choledochoenterostomy anastomosis. (A) A transhepatic cholangiogram demonstrated a strictured anastomosis between the duodenum and the common hepatic duct (*arrows*). (B) A transhepatic catheter was introduced and antegrade drainage successfully established. (C) Three months later, dilatation of the stric-

ture was performed with a vinyl balloon catheter. The stricture was progressively enlarged with 4-, 6-, and 8-mm balloons. (D) Six months after the dilatation, the narrowed area remained widely patent. The catheters were removed. Two years later, the patient was still anicteric.

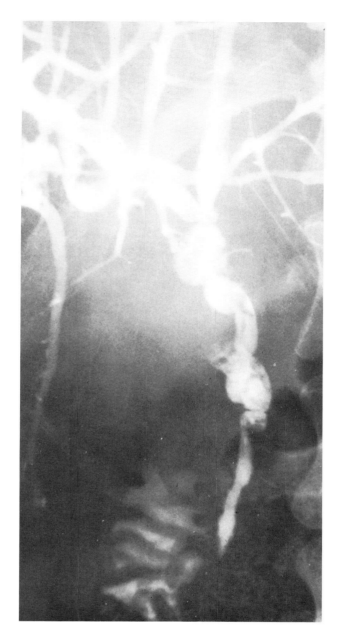

Figure 105-22. Sclerosing cholangitis. A 24-year-old man with ulcerative colitis and jaundice. A thin-needle cholangiogram demonstrated beading and irregularity of the extrahepatic common duct. Multiple small stones were present throughout the biliary tree.

too extensive for resection; radionuclide scans show liver metastasis, computed tomography shows extension into the liver or the retropancreatic nodes, and angiography and percutaneous portography show invasion of the mesenteric vein. For nonoperative therapy to be considered, it is important to do a thin-needle biopsy to confirm that the le-

sion is a carcinoma since biliary obstruction secondary to pancreatitis and lymphoma (Fig. 105-18) appears very similar at cholangiography to biliary obstruction secondary to pancreatic carcinoma.

PERCUTANEOUS TRANSHEPATIC BILIARY DRAINAGE FOR BENIGN DISEASE

Benign Strictures
Approximately 95 percent of benign biliary strictures are related to previous surgery [25]. Operative repair of strictures provides excellent results in only 60 percent of cases. In 1974 Molnar [26] first reported using percutaneous transhepatic biliary drainage in the management of patients with postoperative strictures. He showed that transhepatic antegrade drainage benefited patients who had previously undergone unsuccessful attempts at corrective surgery (Fig. 105-19). To improve the chances of a successful operation, percutaneous transhepatic biliary drainage may also be employed before surgical repair is attempted. By decompressing the bile ducts, transhepatic catheterization may relieve the symptoms of obstruction, allow any infection to clear, and provide time for the patient's nutritional status to be improved. In especially difficult cases, preoperative placement of a transhepatic catheter can allow the surgeon to localize quickly and accurately the course of the common duct intraoperatively (Fig. 105-20).

Successful dilatation of a benign stricture using a balloon catheter was first reported by Burhenne in 1972 [27]. More recently, Molnar [28] successfully used the transhepatic approach to dilate strictured choledochoenterostomy anastomoses. He reported successful dilatations in 8 patients; the dilatations have remained patent after several years of follow-up (Fig. 105-21). The results of balloon dilatation of primary common duct strictures are considerably more variable. While the narrowing at an anastomotic stricture is usually circumferential, primary ductal strictures are most commonly eccentric; attempting balloon dilatation of an eccentric lesion is more likely to displace the softer, noninvolved segments of the duct than to stretch and dilate the rigid scarred area.

Sclerosing Cholangitis
Sclerosing cholangitis is a poorly understood, chronic inflammatory disease of the bile ducts. Its

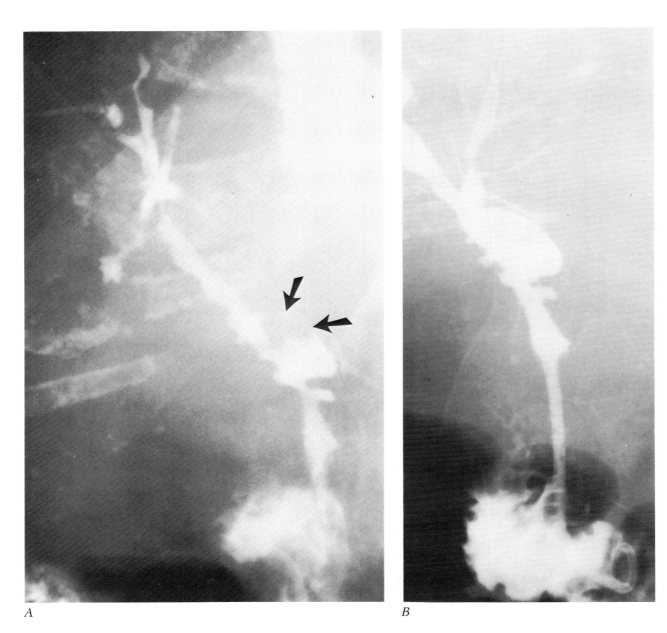

A   *B*

Figure 105-23. Sclerosing cholangitis. A 68-year-old woman with a long history of ulcerative colitis developed fever and jaundice. (A) A thin-needle percutaneous cholangiogram showed a typical appearance of sclerosing cholangitis. There were two stones in the diverticulum of the common bile duct (*arrows*). (B) Because of the patient's poor general condition and a recent stroke, it was elected to attempt percutaneous drainage rather than perform surgery. After antegrade drainage was established, the bilirubin level fell from 12 to 4 mg per 100 cc, and the patient became afebrile. She remained without fever and jaundice but died 7 months later from a massive cerebral vascular accident.

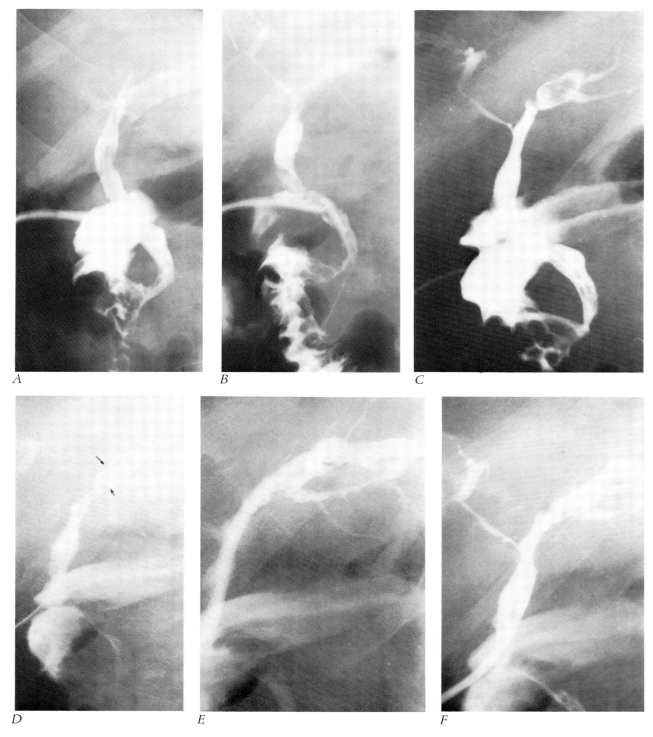

A

B

C

D

E

F

Figure 105- 24. Long-term management of sclerosing cholangitis with intermittent biliary toilet through the T-tube tract. (A) A 47-year-old man with sclerosing cholangitis underwent common duct exploration. A T tube was introduced. Postoperatively, his bilirubin level rose. A T-tube cholangiogram demonstrated that the upper limb of the tube was too long and was wedged in the intrahepatic ducts. There was no flow through the upper limb. (B) The long T tube was removed and a shorter limbed tube introduced. This resulted in rapid clinical improvement. (C) Six months later, the patient returned with recurrent cholangitis. A T-tube cholangiogram demonstrated a new stricture in the left hepatic duct with a stone distal to the stricture. (D) The T tube was removed and the stone was trapped and removed with a Dormia basket (*arrows*). (E) The stricture was then dilated with a coaxial biliary dilator. (F) The T tube was reintroduced. A cholangiogram demonstrated marked improvement of flow through the left duct. The stone was no longer present.

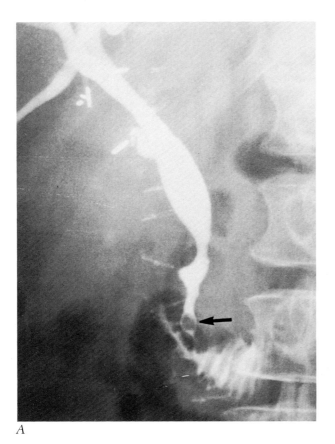

A

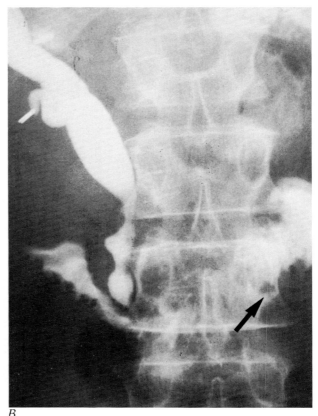

B

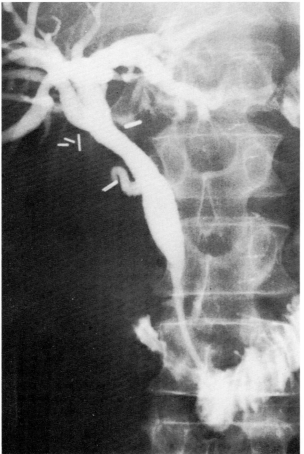

Figure 105-25. Percutaneous transhepatic removal of a retained common duct stone. (A) A debilitated, alcoholic patient underwent emergency cholecystectomy for acute cholecystitis. Ten days later, his serum bilirubin level had risen to 17 mg per 100 cc. A transhepatic cholangiogram demonstrates a stone (*arrow*) in the distal common duct. (B) Because of the patient's poor clinical condition, it was elected to attempt nonoperative therapy. A transhepatic catheter was introduced adjacent to the stone. The stone was trapped in a basket and advanced into the duodenum, where it was released (*arrow*). (C) A transhepatic catheter was left in place for 10 days to decompress the biliary tree.

C

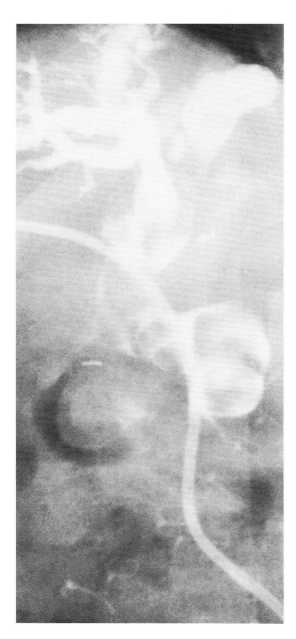

Figure 105-26. Permanent catheter drainage for multiple common duct stones. This elderly patient had been clinically jaundiced for 18 months following an attempt at choledocholithotomy. At surgery, the common duct could not be located because of dense scarring from multiple previous operations. After a transhepatic catheter was introduced through the common duct into the duodenum, the serum bilirubin level rapidly returned to normal. The patient refused attempts at endoscopic stone retrieval and has been maintained on antegrade tube drainage for the past 2 years without jaundice or other symptoms.

etiology is not known. It may occur alone or in association with other diseases, such as ulcerative colitis and granulomatous enterocolitis. Histologically, there is generalized thickening of the submucosal and subserosal layers. The mucosa generally remains intact. Multiple strictures occur in both the intrahepatic and extrahepatic biliary tree, giving rise to a typical appearance at cholangiography (Fig. 105-22).

Surgical therapy may be indicated to relieve extrahepatic obstructions. Generally, a bypass procedure is performed and a T tube is introduced as a stent. In selected patients, percutaneous transhepatic catheters can improve drainage and help resolve episodes of acute cholangitis (Fig. 105-23). However, there are several limitations of percutaneous transhepatic biliary drainage unique to this condition. Because the ducts are generally small and incapable of dilating, percutaneous entry into the biliary tree may be exceedingly difficult. More important, the diffuse narrowing of the ducts can prevent flow through the catheter's side holes. If the outer diameter of the transhepatic catheter is larger than the lumen of the diseased common bile duct, the catheter becomes obturated and acts to worsen the obstruction. Smaller catheters can be used in patients with very small ducts, but their lumens may not be wide enough to permit the flow of viscous bile.

A more appropriate approach to the management of sclerosing cholangitis is to combine the advantages of both radiologic and surgical interventions. After operative repair and T-tube placement, the interventional radiology service maintains functional drainage through the fistulous tract using a combination of the techniques described previously in this chapter. If the tube obstructs, deteriorates, or migrates, it can be disimpacted or replaced; recurrent ductal stones can be extracted, and newly formed strictures can be dilated (Fig. 105-24).

Common Duct Stones

Percutaneous transhepatic drainage catheters are not usually employed in the management of patients with common duct stones. Occasionally, preoperative drainage may be indicated for elderly or especially debilitated patients. Several nonoperative techniques have been used in patients who are considered to be at too great a risk for surgery. Endoscopic cannulation of the ampulla with papillotomy and stone removal is becoming increasingly recognized as a useful clinical

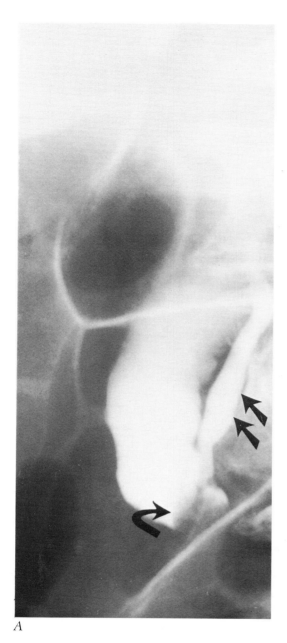

A

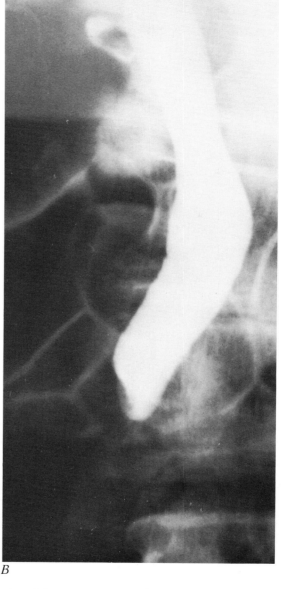

B

Figure 105-27. Percutaneous biliary drainage for acute pancreatitis caused by a stone in the common bile duct. (A) A 52-year-old man with jaundice and severe pancreatitis. A fine-needle transhepatic cholangiogram showed a stone impacted in the ampulla (*curved arrow*) with free reflux into the pancreatic duct (*straight arrows*). (B) A transhepatic catheter was placed above the stone and external drainage was established. Seventeen days later, the patient's condition had improved markedly and the stone was removed surgically.

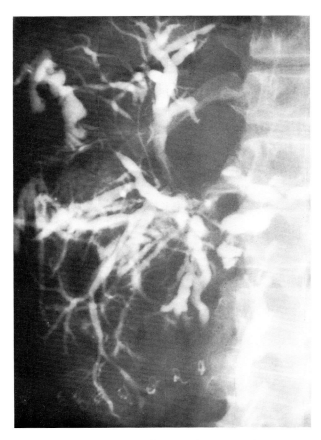

Figure 105-28. Multiple intrahepatic obstructions from cholangiocarcinoma. A thin-needle cholangiogram demonstrated extensive intrahepatic obstruction. Virtually every duct was isolated from every other duct. The obstruction was too extensive for successful transhepatic drainage.

approach in the management of patients with common duct stones [29]. Transhepatic catheters have also been used to advance stones through the ampulla into the duodenum (Fig. 105-25) and to infuse drugs that can dissolve calculi [30]. Permanent transhepatic biliary drainage is indicated for the relief of obstruction caused by stones in only a small group of patients who are not suitable for surgery or some other form of therapy (Fig. 105-26).

Pancreatitis

About 15 percent of patients with acute pancreatitis have associated elevations of the serum bilirubin level [31]. Usually, when there is marked clinical jaundice, the pancreatitis is caused by a biliary calculus impacted in the ampulla of Vater. Percutaneous transhepatic cholangiography can demonstrate the cause of

the obstruction, and percutaneous drainage can provide decompression until the pancreatitis has resolved and the stone can be removed (Fig. 105-27). Because of the theoretic risks of aggravating the pancreatitis by intubating the ampulla, the catheter is not advanced beyond the stone and only external biliary drainage is established.

CONTRAINDICATIONS TO PERCUTANEOUS TRANSHEPATIC BILIARY DRAINAGE

Clinical Contraindications

Bleeding. If the patient has a prolonged prothrombin time, partial thromboplastin time, or a platelet count below 50,000 per cu mm, that problem should be corrected if possible before attempting transhepatic catheterization. Usually, fresh frozen plasma or platelet transfusion can improve coagulation adequately to prevent bleeding during the procedure.

Sepsis. If the patient has overt sepsis, adequate antibiotic coverage must be instituted before instrumentation of the biliary tree. Usually the organism is unknown, and a combination of broad-spectrum antibiotics is employed. If frankly purulent bile is aspirated at catheterization, the biliary tree can be considered a contained abscess. Once the catheter has been introduced and drainage instituted, the fever should rapidly decrease. However, in patients who have sepsis, it is extremely important to minimize the extent of manipulation. The drainage catheter is positioned above the obstruction until the sepsis has completely resolved. Only a minimum volume of contrast material should be added until decompression has been achieved. Although not a constant sequela, septicemia may occur in patients with purulent bile during the procedure. Adequate intravenous hydration must be ensured and vital signs closely monitored for 24 hours following the drainage procedure.

Minimal Symptoms in Terminally Ill Patients. There is a wide variation in the severity of symptoms resulting from obstructive jaundice. Although most patients with serum bilirubin levels greater than 10 mg per 100 cc suffer from severe pruritus and anorexia, these symptoms may be minimal or absent. In patients with incurable tumors, biliary drainage is intended only to relieve symptoms, not to prevent biliary cirrhosis. The procedure should therefore not be employed until the actual need for palliation arises.

Anatomic Contraindications

Satisfactory drainage depends on continuity and interconnections between patent biliary radicles above the level of an obstruction. There are two anatomic settings in which the free flow of bile cannot occur. If either is identified at thin-needle cholangiography, percutaneous biliary drainage should not be considered.

1. *Multiple intrahepatic obstructions.* When a tumor obstructs the ductal system above the level of the porta hepatis and isolates one or two major groups of biliary radicles, total decompression can be achieved with multiple catheters. However, when the level of obstruction is so high that there are innumerable isolated ductal systems, biliary drainage is impractical (Fig. 105-28). A similar situation arises when, after an initially successful trans-

hepatic drainage, the tumor extends intrahepatically and obstructs multiple ducts. Placing additional catheters may help temporarily, but a point is eventually reached when transhepatic drainage is no longer effective.

2. *Intraductal tumor.* There are rare tumors—papillary adenomas, papillary adenocarcinomas, and some metastatic tumors—that grow intraductally and may diffusely fill the biliary tree. Since the tumor-filled ducts have no free lumen to conduct bile into the catheter's side holes, effective biliary drainage is impossible, even if a catheter can be advanced into the duodenum (Fig. 105-29).

ACUTE COMPLICATIONS OF TRANSHEPATIC CATHETERIZATION

The most common and significant complication of transhepatic catheterization is sepsis. Although broad-spectrum antibiotic coverage is routinely instituted before the procedure and maintained

---

Figure 105-29. Intraductal tumor. (A) A thin-needle cholangiogram demonstrated filling defects within the entire biliary tree. Samples were obtained during catheterization and were confirmed histologically to be metastatic lung carcinoma. (B) Despite the fact that the catheter could be advanced through the mass to the duodenum, there was no free lumen to allow bile to flow into the catheter.

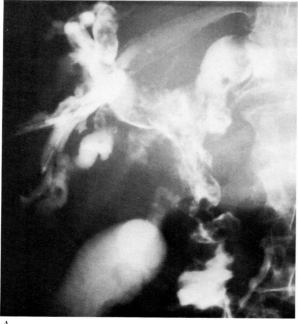

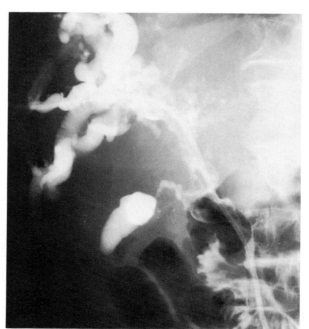

A

B

for several days following catheterization, about 8 percent of patients in our own series developed clinical evidence of sepsis immediately after the procedure. Pneumothorax and hemothorax occur after about 1 percent of transhepatic procedures. Bleeding is a surprisingly infrequent complication. In our series, only 2 of 173 patients had intraabdominal bleeding severe enough to require blood transfusions, and in both patients, bleeding stopped without surgery. In 2 other patients, small subcapsular hematomas surrounding the catheter entry site were noted at surgery. Hemobilia is not uncommon, but it usually develops because a side hole has been positioned in the hepatic parenchyma. Bleeding into the catheter stops when the catheter is exchanged for a drainage catheter that has all the side holes arranged intraductally. Ascites may complicate the procedure considerably. In addition to making it technically more difficult to perform transhepatic drainage, after the catheter has been introduced, the ascitic fluid may shift into the pleural space, collect in the subcutaneous tissue, or leak around the catheter entry site. Fortunately, once biliary decompression has been achieved and the ascitic fluid has been drained, it does not usually reaccumulate.

LONG-TERM COMPLICATIONS

After a transhepatic catheter has been in place for about 1 week, it has the same types of problems as has any permanent indwelling tube. Local infection at the entry site is not uncommon but is easily treated with hot soaks and topical antibiotic ointments. Granulomas that form around the catheter entry site can be cauterized with silver nitrate. If the lumen of the tube becomes obstructed, there is leakage of bile around the entry site, recurrent jaundice, or fever. The obstructed catheter should be replaced and the new catheter placed to external drainage for several days. Late infections, such as subphrenic abscesses and suppurative cholangitis, have not been seen in our own series, but they may occur. Similarly, delayed bleeding from false aneurysms of the hepatic artery have been described [32]. We have seen 1 patient who developed a painful mass at the catheter entry site 2 years after catheter placement for cholangiocarcinoma. The mass was biopsied and found to be a metastatic implant (Fig. 105-30) [33]. This is an extremely unusual complication, and the benefits from the long-term palliation achieved in this patient far outweighed the complication.

Figure 105-30. Metastatic spread along the percutaneous catheter tract. (A) A 54-year-old man with cholangiocarcinoma obstructing the upper common hepatic duct was successfully treated with antegrade biliary drainage. (B) Two and one-half years later, he developed a painful mass around the catheter entry site. The mass was biopsied and confirmed to be adenocarcinoma. A computed tomographic scan demonstrated the mass in the skin and subcutaneous tissues. It was treated with radiation therapy.

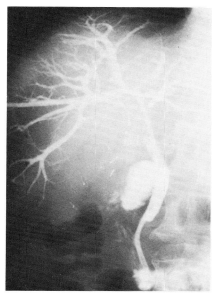

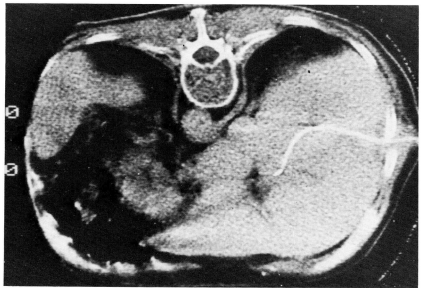

A   *B*

Transhepatic Introduction of a Permanent Indwelling Endoprosthesis

Pereiras has advocated introducing a short segment of Teflon tubing to bridge the obstructed segment [34]. This approach avoids the unwanted psychologic implications of a permanent external catheter segment, the need for catheter maintenance by the patient, and such complications as skin infections and granuloma. On the other hand, once the endoprosthesis has been positioned and the catheter removed, access for tube irrigation and replacement is lost and cholangio-

Figure 105-31. Migration of an endoprosthesis. A 61-year-old man with metastatic carcinoma of the porta hepatis. (A) A transhepatic cholangiogram demonstrated obstruction of the common hepatic duct. (B) A 12 French endoprosthesis was introduced to bridge the obstruction (*arrows*). (C) Two days later the endoprosthesis had migrated through the duct into the duodenum (*arrows*). An 8.3 French biliary drainage catheter was positioned to reestablish drainage.

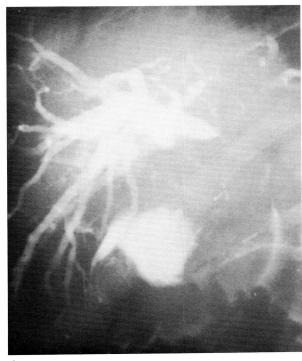

A

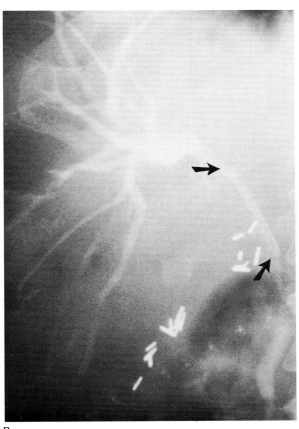

B

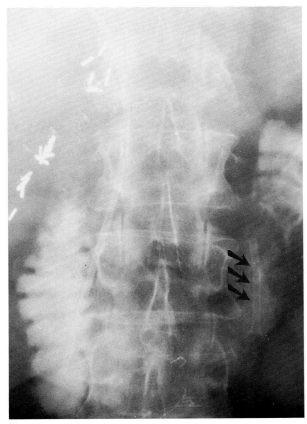

C

graphic examinations cannot be readily performed to determine changes in anatomy.

Because of the tendency of prosthetic devices to obstruct and migrate (Fig. 105-31), we have limited their use to those patients who are incapable of maintaining an external segment of tube.

ACKNOWLEDGMENT

The figures in this chapter appeared in E. J. Ring and G. K. McLean, *Interventional Radiology: Principles and Techniques.* Boston: Little, Brown, 1981. They are used here with the permission of the authors and the publisher.

References

1. Bartlett, M. K., Warshaw, A. L., and Ottinger, L. W. The removal of biliary duct stones. *Surg. Clin. North Am.* 54:599, 1974.
2. Mazzariello, R. M. Removal of residual biliary calculi without reoperation. *Surgery* 67:566, 1970.
3. Caprini, J. A., Crampton, A. R., and Swan, V. M. Nonoperative extraction of retained common duct stones. *Arch. Surg.* 111:445, 1976.
4. Mazzariello, R. M. Residual biliary tract stones: Nonoperative treatment of 570 patients. *Surg. Annu.* 8:113, 1976.
5. Burhenne, H. J. Nonoperative retained biliary tract stone extraction: A new roentgenologic technique. *AJR* 117:388, 1973.
6. Bean, W. J., Smith, S. L., and Calonje, M. T-tube dilatation for removal of large biliary stones. *Radiology* 115:485, 1975.
7. Crummy, A. B., and Turnipseed, W. D. Percutaneous replacement of a biliary T-tube. *AJR* 128:869, 1977.
8. Ring, E. J., Freiman, D. B., Oleaga, J. A., Mackie, J. A., Perez, M. R., and Schiff, D. P. Clinical applications of nonoperative T-tube replacement. *Surg. Gynecol. Obstet.* 148:213, 1979.
9. Warren, K. W., Poulantzas, J. K., and Kune, G. A. Use of a Y-tube splint in the repair of biliary strictures. *Surg. Gynecol. Obstet.* 122:785, 1966.
10. Kaude, J. V., Weidenmier, C. H., and Agee, O. F. Decompression of bile ducts with the percutaneous transhepatic technic. *Radiology* 93:69, 1969.
11. Hoevels, J., Lunderquist, A., and Ihse, I. Percutaneous transhepatic intubation of bile ducts for combined internal-external drainage in preoperative and palliative treatment of obstructive jaundice. *Gastrointest. Radiol.* 3:23, 1978.
12. Ring, E. J., Oleaga, J. A., Freiman, D. B., Husted, J. W., and Lunderquist, A. Therapeutic applications of catheter cholangiography. *Radiology* 128:333, 1978.
13. Mori, K., Misumi, A., Sugiyama, M., Okabe, M., Matsuoka, T., Ishii, J., and Akag, M. Percutaneous transhepatic bile drainage. *Ann. Surg.* 185:111, 1977.
14. Ring, E. J., Husted, J. W., Oleaga, J. A., and Freiman, D. B. A multihole catheter for maintaining longterm percutaneous antegrade biliary drainage. *Radiology* 132:752, 1979.
15. Pollock, T. W., Ring, E. J., Oleaga, J. A., Freiman, D. B., Mullen, J. L., and Rosato, E. F. Percutaneous decompression of benign and malignant biliary obstruction. *Arch. Surg.* 114:148, 1979.
16. Klatskin, G. Adenocarcinoma of the hepatic duct at its bifurcation within the porta hepatis: An unusual tumor with distinct clinical and pathologic features. *Am. J. Med.* 38:241, 1965.
17. Gudjonsson, B., Livstone, E. M., and Spiro, H. M. Cancer of the pancreas: Diagnostic accuracy and survival statistics. *Cancer* 42:2494, 1978.
18. Nakase, A., Matsumoto, Y., Uchida, K., and Honjo, I. Surgical treatment of cancer of the pancreas and the periampullary region: Cumulative results in 57 institutions in Japan. *Ann. Surg.* 185:52, 1977.
19. Lansing, P. B., Blalock, J. B., and Ochsner, J. L. Pancreaticoduodenectomy: A retrospective review 1949–1969. *Am. Surg.* 38:79, 1972.
20. Richards, A. B., Chin, M., and Sosin, H. Cancer of the pancreas. The value of radical and palliative surgery. *Ann. Surg.* 177:325, 1973.
21. Braasch, J. W., and Gray, B. N. Considerations that lower pancreatoduodenectomy mortality. *Am. J. Surg.* 133:480, 1977.
22. Brooks, J. R., and Culebras, J. M. Cancer of the pancreas: Palliative operations for carcinoma of the pancreas. *Arch. Surg.* 103:330, 1971.
23. Buckwalter, J. A., Lawton, R. L., and Tidrick, R. T. Bypass operations for neoplastic biliary tract obstruction. *Am. J. Surg.* 109:100, 1965.
24. Feduska, N. J., Dent, T. L., and Lindenauer, S. M. Results of palliative operations for carcinoma of the pancreas. *Arch. Surg.* 103:330, 1971.
25. Braasch, J. W., Warren, K. W., and Blevins, P. K. Progress in biliary stricture repair. *Am. J. Surg.* 129:34, 1975.
26. Molnar, W., and Stockum, A. E. Relief of obstructive jaundice through percutaneous transhepatic catheter—a new therapeutic method. *AJR* 122:356, 1974.
27. Burhenne, H. J. Nonoperative roentgenologic instrumentation technics of the postoperative biliary tract: Treatment of biliary stricture and retained stones. *Am. J. Surg.* 128:111, 1974.

28. Molnar, W., and Stockum, A. E. Transhepatic dilatation of choledochoenterostomy strictures. *Radiology* 129:59, 1978.

29. Zimmon, D., Falkenstein, D. B., and Kessler, R. E. Endoscopic papillotomy for choledocolithiasis. *N. Engl. J. Med.* 293:1181, 1975.

30. Perez, M. R., Oleaga, J. A., Freiman, D. B., McLean, G. L., and Ring, E. J. Removal of a distal common bile duct stone through percutaneous transhepatic catheterization. *Arch. Surg.* 114:107, 1979.

31. Herlinger, H., and Ring, E. Angiography in Abdominal Visceral Disease. In R. Maingot (ed.), *Abdominal Operations.* New York: Appleton-Century-Crofts, 1980. Vol. 2.

32. Hoevels, J. *Percutaneous Transhepatic Access to Portal Venous and Bile Duct Systems for Diagnostic and Therapeutic Procedures.* Malmö (Sweden): Litos Reprotryck, 1979.

33. Oleaga, J. A., Ring, E. J., Freiman, D. B., McLean, G. K., and Rosen, R. J. Extension of neoplasm along the tract of a transhepatic tube. *AJR* 135:841, 1980.

34. Pereiras, R. V., Jr., Rheingold, O. J., Hutson, D., Mejia, J., Viamonte, M., Chiprut, R. O., and Schiff, E. R. Relief of malignant obstructive jaundice by percutaneous insertion of a permanent prosthesis in the biliary tree. *Ann. Intern. Med.* 89:589, 1978.

Interventional Procedures of the Bile Ducts via the T-Tube Tract

H. J. BURHENNE

Angeion is the Greek word for vessel, borrowed by radiology in the term *angiography* to denote the study of the flow of blood and contrast material in vessels. This definition can be expanded in the context of this chapter to describe the flow of bile and contrast material in the tubular structures of the biliary duct system. During the last decade, interventional radiology of the biliary tract has grown into an essential tool in the treatment of obstructive jaundice. A treatise on special procedures in radiology would be incomplete without a discussion of it.

Access to the Biliary Tract

Nonoperative access to the bile duct system is accomplished by three different routes: the retrograde endoscopic route, the percutaneous transhepatic route, and the route through the sinus tract after T-tube insertion. The first route involves fiberoptic endoscopy for cholangiography or removal of bile duct stones after sphincterotomy [1]. The second, or transhepatic, route is commonly used for cholangiography [2]. It has been used since 1956 for external bile drainage [3] and since 1974 for internal bile drainage in obstructive jaundice [4]. Placement of palliative stents has been accomplished in this fashion [5], and even transhepatic removal of bile duct stones has been reported [6]. The discussion in this chapter is involved with the initial route of drainage and access to the biliary tract, namely instrumentation through the sinus tract after T-tube insertion. By definition, therefore, the T-tube tract approach is used only after choledochotomy.

T Tube and Its Tract

Interventional radiologic procedures via the T-tube tract are accomplished in the postoperative patient with an indwelling T tube. For easier access, the surgeon should bring the T tube in a straight line from the common duct to the outside of the patient through a stab wound in the anterior lateral abdominal wall. T tubes are sometimes placed through anterior abdominal midline incisions. This makes subsequent instrumentation difficult because of a tortuous sinus tract and because it is difficult to keep the radiologist's hands out of the field of radiation. 2381

Catheterization of the T-tube tract is also complicated if a T tube smaller than 14 French was placed by the surgeon. A smaller T tube usually requires initial dilatation of the tract. An even larger T tube can be placed in a small common duct by tailoring the short arms of the tube. The long arm of the T tube should be placed at a right angle to the extrahepatic bile duct. This facilitates easier catheterization from the T-tube tract into both directions of the bile ducts.

We have described the use of a T tube with a large diameter for the long arm to facilitate post-operative T-tube tract instrumentation [7]. This tube is now commercially available [8].

The T tube is left indwelling for 5 weeks after surgery in order to permit a sufficient fibrous reaction around it for the formation of an access channel for biliary tract instrumentation. This fibrous reaction occurs more readily with larger T tubes of rubber. If T tubes smaller than 14 French are in place and if the T tubes are plastic, it is advisable to wait a couple of weeks beyond the usual 5-week period before instrumentation is attempted.

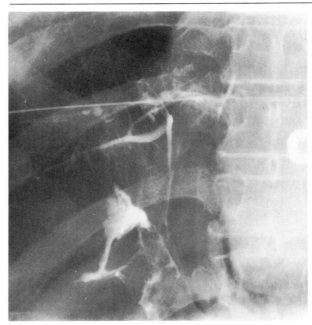

A

Figure 106-1. (A) Transhepatic cholangiogram after a common duct exploration and an iatrogenic injury demonstrating extravasation of contrast material as a result of the attempted duct repair. (B) The steerable catheter was moved through the drainage tract into the distal common duct and was followed by a guidewire. (C) The proximal end of the severed bile duct was visualized with contrast material and was entered with the steerable catheter followed by a guidewire. (D) A T tube was inserted over both guidewires, bridging the common duct injury for internal drainage and palliation. (E) A T tube was seen to provide good drainage 6 weeks after its insertion and before a hepaticojejunostomy procedure was done.

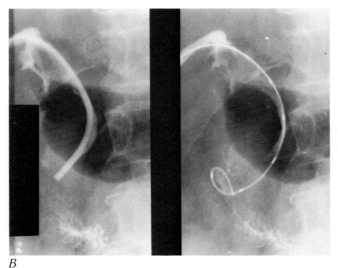

B

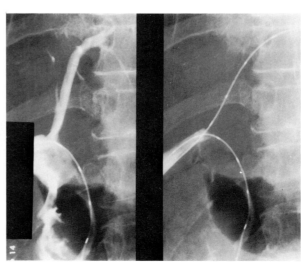

C

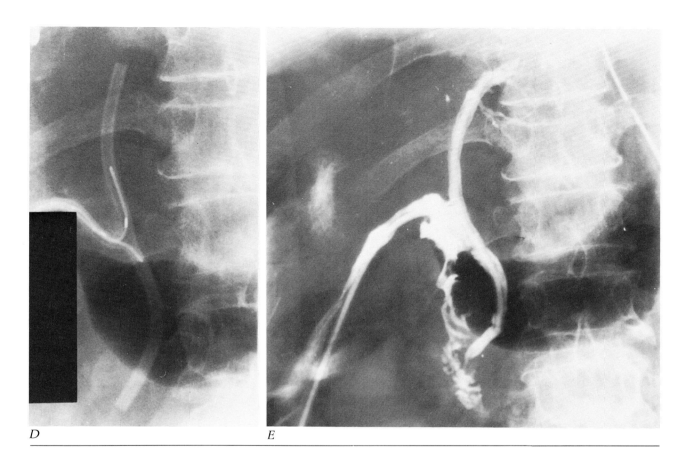

D   E

OBSTRUCTED T TUBES

Indwelling T tubes may become obstructed by encrusted bile. Cholangiography through the T tube will demonstrate partial or complete obstruction of the lumen. This occurs more commonly in the short arms placed in the bile ducts. Obstructed T tubes can be reopened by the radiologist with the use of guidewires under fluoroscopic control [9]. The angle between the long arm and the short arm of the T tube may represent a technical problem for guidewire instrumentation, particularly when a wedge-shaped opening has been placed at the junction of the arms of the T tube by the surgeon. J-shaped guidewires with a retractable core are used to negotiate these turns. The angle at the junction of the arms of the T tube can be rendered more obtuse by slight traction on the T tube. This permits easier manipulation of the guidewire into the short arms for reopening the lumen.

Obstruction of T tubes by encrusted bile, however, is a recurrent problem, and a more satisfactory radiologic intervention consists of T-tube replacement.

T-TUBE REPLACEMENT

Replacement of T tubes through the T-tube tract into the bile ducts is sometimes required after inadvertent extraction or when indwelling tubes become obstructed.

The tract is entered with the steerable catheter, and a guidewire is placed into the duct system. The T tube is inserted over the guidewire. This can be accomplished with a single guidewire [10] or with two guidewires. We place one guidewire in a proximal and one in a distal position in the duct system, inserting the two short arms of the T tube over the guidewires for intraductal placement. Dilatation of the sinus tract may be required in order to replace the tube with another tube of the same French caliber. More T-tube tract diameter is needed because the two parallel short arms of the T tube require more space for insertion through the T-tube tract than does the single long arm of the tube.

T-Tube Replacement After Iatrogenic Duct Injuries

Placement of the T tube after severance of the bile duct can be the palliative procedure of choice to divert bile from the peritoneal cavity to the outside. It may be required if the primary duct repair dehisces and no stenting tube had been placed. Access to the biliary tract in these cases may also be accomplished by catheterization of sinus tracts from Penrose drains. An attempt is made to maneuver the steerable catheter into the duct if contrast material outlines portions of the biliary tract (Fig. 106-1).

Conversion to a U Tube

U tubes are an effective surgical means of palliating strictures in the biliary tract. Long-term maintenance of a U tube is easier than long-term maintenance of a T tube, particularly when inadvertent extraction of the tube can be minimized by connecting the two ends of the U tube on the outside.

In order to convert T tubes into U tubes, a second percutaneous access through the liver to the bile ducts has to be accomplished. This is technically analogous to inserting transhepatic internal drains. A guidewire is moved distally into the common hepatic duct and engaged with a wire basket and pulled through the T-tube tract to the outside [11].

Extraction of Retained Stones

The sinus tract of the postoperative T tube was used for percutaneous retained stone extraction as early as 1955 [12]. Surgeons waited 5 weeks for the establishment of fibrous tracts surrounding the T tube. A semipliable forceps is still the extraction instrument of choice in South America today [13]. The ureteral stone basket developed by Dormia is more ideally suited for this purpose; it was first used in 1969 [14]. We started to use the stone basket (Mueller) in 1971, passing it through the T tube or through a small arterial catheter. This technique was rather time consuming owing to the difficulty in placing the small preshaped arterial catheter into the duct. It was sometimes impossible to negotiate the tip of the stiff catheter around turns in the sinus tract. Our introduction of the steerable catheter in 1972 has made stone extraction technically easier and more practical [15]. This technique is now practiced widely. It can be learned easily by radiologists familiar with arteriography and other special radiographic procedures.

EQUIPMENT

A variety of sizes of steerable catheters and stone extraction baskets are available. Steerable catheters are manufactured in three sizes: 8, 10, and 13 French (Medi-Tech). Sinus tracts from T tubes smaller than 14 French may require dilatation. This is best accomplished with use of the Grüntzig balloon catheter. The 13 French steerable catheter will accept all stone baskets, but the Dormia basket will not pass through a 10 French steerable catheter. It may be used through a 10 French catheter without the catheter sheath, which means that the wire basket has to be inserted open into the end of the 10 French steerable catheter [16].

The Dormia basket comes in one size; Medi-Tech and stone baskets are available in three sizes. Large stones and large ducts require the use of a large basket. Ideally, the open basket touches the walls of the duct during the engagement of retained stones. Even small stones are best engaged by this method with a large basket if the duct diameter is large. The stones will not fall out of the basket if the extraction movement is continuous. We no longer attempt to close the basket once the stone has been engaged. Manipulating the basket often results in fragmentation of the stone or in small stones falling out of the basket.

The pistol-type steering handle from Medi-Tech permits one-finger control and contrast injection through a side port. The wobble plate inside the steering handle may be used for manual operation separately. The four wires of the catheter are attached to the corners of this plate (Fig. 106-2).

Complicated T-tube tract procedures often require the use of guidewires. This applies to small sinus tracts from a T tube smaller than 14 French that requires dilatation. The fibrous reaction surrounding a small indwelling T tube is usually less pronounced than that surrounding larger catheters. This means that perforation of the sinus tract during the extraction of multiple retained stones may occur. The guidewire is left in place through the sinus tract into the duct system during the entire procedure. The steerable catheter and stone extraction baskets are manipulated alongside the guidewire. Reentry of the duct system

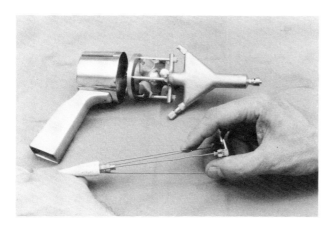

Figure 106-2. The wobble plate is the essential part of the pistol handle. It may be used separately, with the index finger playing on the desired wire for direction inside the sinus tract and bile ducts.

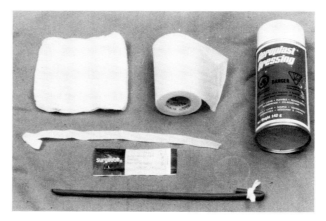

Figure 106-3. The straight catheter used between multiple interventional procedures is bent over on the external catheter and tied with umbilical tape. A dressing is then applied with Aeroplast, 4-×-4 gauze, and wide paper tape.

for the placement of a catheter is always possible in this fashion.

Interventional radiologic procedures of the biliary tract often must be done in multiple sessions. Straight catheters, available in various sizes, are left indwelling in the sinus tract between procedures. We do not employ a skin suture for catheter retention because it often results in minor skin infection, and percutaneous manipulation becomes painful. The indwelling catheter is bent over at the skin level so that it cannot slip inside, and it is kept in place by using an adhesive dressing (Aeroplast; Parke, Davis) (Fig. 106-3).

TECHNIQUE

Stone extraction [7] (Fig. 106-4) involves the following eight essential steps:

1. The ambulatory patient is scheduled for stone extraction 5 weeks after bile duct exploration. If a T tube smaller than 14 French was used, it is preferable to wait an extra 2 weeks for formation of a better sinus tract wall.
2. The extraction procedure is rescheduled if a Penrose drain is in place in addition to the T tube. The Penrose drain is removed, and the patient returns in about 2 weeks for further intervention. We have seen cross-connections between the Penrose drain tract and the T-tube tract, and extravasation may occur.
3. The T tube is extracted and cholangiograms are obtained for localization.

4. The steerable catheter is inserted through the T-tube tract and the bile duct is entered, with the tip of the catheter directed either proximally or distally, depending on the location of the stone.
5. The closed basket is advanced through the steerable catheter alongside the stone and opened distally to it. The wire basket is turned slightly to permit easier stone engagement, and the basket with the stone then is guided through the sinus tract in a continuous extraction movement. If the operator hesitates during withdrawal, the stone may fall out of the side of the basket.
6. Patients with a history of postoperative pancreatitis and patients with "difficult" intrahepatic stones are placed routinely on preinstrumentation antibiotic prophylaxis (Keflex, 250 mg by mouth every six hours). Preinstrumentation bile cultures are recommended.
7. Patients are hospitalized before the procedure only if they have a severe associated medical condition or a history of postoperative sepsis or pancreatitis. We have also taken the precaution of admitting to the hospital patients with cardiac pacemakers.
8. Hand injection of contrast material by syringe is usually adequate for continuous fluoroscopic stone visualization during the manipulation. Contrast drip infusion through a side port is rarely required for continuous cholangiography.

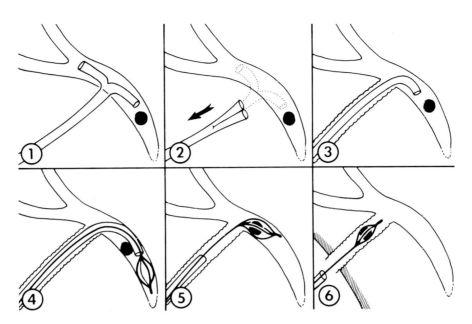

Figure 106-4. Technical steps of percutaneous stone extraction: (1) the stone location is identified, (2) the T tube is extracted, (3) the steerable catheter is maneuvered through the sinus tract close to the retained stone, (4) the wire basket is inserted through the steerable catheter and opened distally to the stone, (5) the stone is engaged in the wire basket, and (6) both are extracted through the sinus tract [7]. (From Burhenne et al. [7]. Reproduced with permission of Charles C Thomas.)

EXTRACTION OF SMALL STONES

If small stones or fragments have not passed spontaneously into the duodenum during the 5-week interval since surgery, they are extracted under fluoroscopic control. Small stones of about 5 mm in size are sometimes difficult to visualize on the television monitor. Good spot-film technique, therefore, is mandatory. We use selective cholangiography, in which the tip of the steerable catheter is placed in the suspected site of the intraductal stone, small amounts of contrast material are injected through the catheter, and collimated spot radiography is conducted in multiple projections. An iodine content of about 25 percent is required for cholangiography with normal-size common bile ducts. Further dilution to about 12.5 percent of iodine content is necessary for ducts distended beyond 10 mm in diameter.

Small stones engaged in the open basket may fall out of the basket if the operator attempts to close the basket before extraction. We have had more success by continuously retracting the open basket after the stone has been engaged.

Small fragments or stones smaller than 4 mm may also be expelled into the duodenum with the use of the steerable catheter [17]. This is attempted only if passage of the catheter through the ampullary portion is first accomplished to measure its diameter. Almost all patients accept a 10 French catheter through the ampullary portion into the duodenum, and about one-third of patients accept a 13 French catheter.

EXTRACTION OF LARGE STONES

Retained biliary stones of up to 8 mm are often extracted intact through the sinus tract of a 14 French T tube. Larger stones must be fragmented. This is best accomplished using traction with the stone wire basket. The thin, sharp wires of the basket are always able to cut the relatively soft retained stones.

In our experience with 661 patients, 91 required stone fragmentation [16]. In this procedure, the stone is maneuvered in the basket to the junction of the bile duct and the sinus tract, where strong resistance to extraction is felt. An increasing and steady pull on the end of the basket wire is then applied for 2 to 4 minutes. A hemostat is clamped to the end of the wire basket for better manual traction. The other hand presses against the abdominal wall over the sinus tract with the wire running between the fingers. A pull of no more than 20 to 25 pounds is indicated and necessary. Sudden jerks are not advisable. The

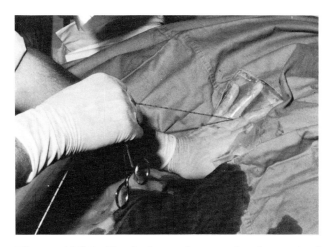

Figure 106-5. Slowly increasing traction is required for the wires of the basket to fragment large retained stones.

steady pull will result in cutting of the stone by the wire basket. We have experienced no common duct injury with this technique (Fig. 106-5).

After fragmentation of large retained stones, the major fragments are extracted during the same session. A straight catheter is then placed, and the patient is discharged to permit spontaneous passage of small fragments into the duodenum. The patient returns a few days later for cholangiography to see if further intervention is required.

If stones or stone fragments become lodged in the sinus tract during extraction, they are pushed back into the bile ducts for reengagement with the stone basket. If the steerable catheter is too soft and unable to displace the stone in the sinus tract, the catheter is stiffened with a stylet or stiff guidewire.

EXTRACTION OF IMPACTED STONES

Stones in the distal common bile duct may become impacted and cause obstruction. Extraction of these distal common duct stones is sometimes difficult and may be the cause of an unsuccessful extraction. We attempt to move the stone into a more proximal position in the duct before basket engagement. This can be accomplished with suction through the catheter or by placing a small steerable catheter distal to the stone and manipulating the stone proximally. If the stone cannot be mobilized, we try to open the basket distally to it or immediately adjacent to it. With rotation of the basket, the stone sometimes enters the wires.

If these maneuvers are not successful, we then proceed to use the Fogarty balloon catheter for stone mobilization. The balloon is inflated with contrast material when it is positioned between the stone and the ampullary portion of the duct. A gentle pull on the catheter should result in mobilization. This is done under direct fluoroscopic supervision, assuring that the balloon is properly positioned above the ampulla and that traction does not result in distortion of the bile duct (Fig. 106-6).

EXTRACTION OF INTRAHEPATIC STONES

The extraction of retained intrahepatic stones is usually more difficult than the extraction of retained extrahepatic stones. The passage of closed stone baskets and Fogarty catheters alongside the retained stones in hepatic radicles can be difficult. The failure rate for extraction procedures is higher for retained intrahepatic stones than for retained extrahepatic stones.

If postoperative T-tube cholangiograms demonstrate retained intrahepatic stones, the radiologist should first ascertain whether the short arm of the T tube prevents stones from passing into extrahepatic ducts. If this is the case, the T tube is replaced by a straight tube, with its tip positioned in the common duct. The patient is then permitted to walk and return in 1 or 2 weeks to allow for distal migration of intrahepatic stones. We have had good success with this method and prefer to use this approach because intrahepatic stone manipulation is more time consuming and difficult (Fig. 106-7).

MULTIPLE SESSIONS

In more than one-third of our patients multiple sessions were required for the nonoperative extraction of retained biliary tract stones [18]. There are a number of situations requiring multiple sessions:

1. If bleeding occurs after T-tube extraction and if blood clots in the bile duct system prevent fluoroscopic identification of stones, a straight catheter is placed and the patient returns for the extraction procedure at a later date, after the blood clots have passed.

2. If a T tube of 12 French or less has been in place, and if dilatation of the sinus tract is indicated as the initial procedure, the patient

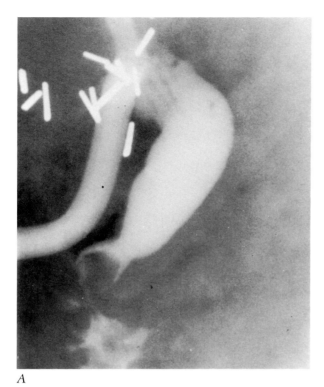

A

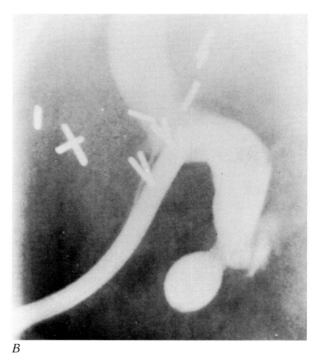

B

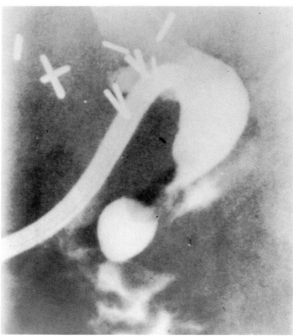

C

Figure 106-6. (A) A large retained distal common duct stone that is partially impacted. (B) A Fogarty balloon in place and distended with contrast material. The oval continuous outline of the Fogarty balloon indicates that it is in an unsatisfactory position. (C) The repositioned inflated Fogarty balloon now shows a deformity by the adjacent stone, indicating good placement for manipulation.

returns for a separate session for stone extraction.

3. If fragmentation of large stones results in multiple small fragments, multiple sessions are indicated to permit spontaneous passage of fragments.

4. If one of the stones escapes into the cystic duct remnant, the patient returns at a later date. The extraction procedure is initiated with the patient in a semierect position on the fluoroscopic table in order to permit maintenance of the stone in the common duct distal to the cystic duct entrance.

5. If dilatation of a bile duct stricture is required as the initial procedure, stones beyond the stricture are removed during the second session, after catheter splinting of the dilated stricture.

6. If extravasation from the sinus tract occurs after stone removal, a second session is scheduled for the extraction of the remaining stones.

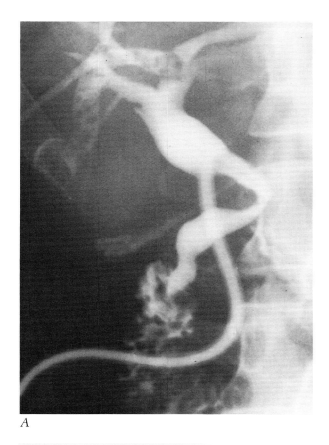

A

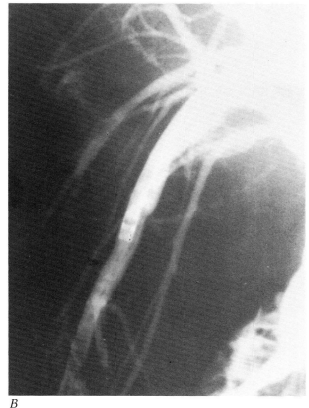

B

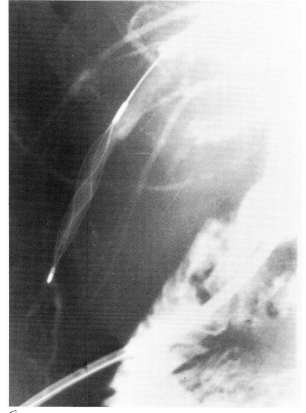

C

Figure 106-7. (A) Multiple retained stones in the dorsocaudal branch of the hepatic ducts. (B) A steerable catheter in place in the same hepatic branch after multiple stone removal. (C) A wire basket in place after the completion of intrahepatic stone removal. (From Burhenne [16]. Reproduced with permission of Charles C Thomas.)

7. If multiple retained stones in an intrahepatic position are present and if the stones do not move distally, the extraction is sometimes accomplished in multiple sessions. As many as 6 extraction procedures have been done in 1 patient with 27 intrahepatic stones.

Nonoperative stone extraction in multiple sessions is easily accomplished in the ambulatory patient. No sinus tract is permitted to close until completion cholangiograms show that the entire duct system is clear of stones. Optimal cholangiograms are sometimes difficult to obtain following instrumentation, particularly if spasm of the ampullary portion is present. It is then best to place a straight catheter through the sinus tract in order to obtain satisfactory completion cholangiograms during a second session.

COMPLICATIONS

Complications occurred in 27 of our 661 patients [16]. The morbidity was 4.1 percent, and no perforation of the biliary tract and no deaths occurred in any of the 661 patients. One death has been reported with acute pancreatitis after radiologic manipulation of a common bile duct stone [19]. This case involved a small distal common duct stone and difficult instrumentation. This patient had a history of acute pancreatitis. The radiologist transferred the patient with instruments in place from one fluoroscopic room to another room that had spot-film facilities as well. We believe that fluoroscopic control alone is insufficient, particularly with small stones. An interventional radiologic procedure should always be done in a room with spot-filming equipment.

In comparing interventional radiologic procedures for treatment of retained stones to the previous method of stone removal, we must remember that reoperation carries a mortality of about 3 percent [20].

SUCCESS AND FAILURE

Our success rate in the removal of retained stones in the biliary tract is 95 percent. (We consider a procedure a success only when the last of several stones has been successfully removed.) This success rate compares favorably with surgical results at reoperation.

Among our 661 patients [16], T-tube tract stone extraction procedures failed in 33. The failures were due to:

1. The inability to catheterize a small tract (in 5 patients).
2. The inability to negotiate the sinus tract for further stone extraction after one stone had been removed (in 7 patients).
3. The inability to extract a cystic duct remnant stone (in 4 patients).
4. The inability to extract an impacted distal common duct stone (in 2 patients).
5. The inability to engage hepatic stones (in 15 patients).

The overall failure rate was 5 percent. It is higher for intrahepatic stones and lower for extrahepatic stones. We have had no extraction failures in patients with large retained duct stones that require fragmentation. We do not believe that mechanical fragmentation devices are necessary for successful intervention [21].

CLINICAL RELEVANCE

Retained ductal stones following cholecystectomy and bile duct operation continue to be an exasperating problem for surgeons. Even the increased use of operative cholangiography and the availability of choledochoscopes have done little to reduce the retained stone rate. The availability, however, of a new nonoperative technique that permits percutaneous removal of retained calculi is a significant advance. Percutaneous stone removal has become safe and practical. Indeed, it is our experience that removal of intrahepatic or distal common duct stones is more easily accomplished by a radiologic interventional procedure done under direct vision than one done during surgery. The use of the Fogarty balloon, for instance, may result in complications when applied without direct vision during surgery [22, 23].

There are other recently described techniques for the nonsurgical removal of retained biliary calculi. Postoperative choledochoscopy via the T-tube tract has been adapted for this purpose [24]. This technique requires that the patient be hospitalized. It is more cumbersome and technically more difficult, because the endoscope is not able to negotiate sharp turns in the sinus tract or turns from the tract into the common duct. Duodenoscopic papillotomy is another endoscopic procedure for the removal of retained stones. It is difficult to learn, has a higher morbidity, and is considerably more expensive. This technique is also associated with complications that end in death [25].

In comparison, our technique of stone removal with the steerable catheter is less costly, more consistently successful, easier to learn, and more simply performed. It is readily learned by radiologists experienced in the performance of special procedures, and it is now used in most major medical centers. Most important, the technique of nonoperative removal through the T-tube tract carries an appreciably lower complication rate than any other technique for the removal of ductal stones or attempts at stone dissolution. At present, it is the therapeutic method of choice [26].

Biopsies

Protruding mucosal lesions in the biliary duct system, such as postoperative iatrogenic mucosal flaps, polyps, or carcinoma, can be biopsied through the T-tube tract with the use of the steerable catheter. This technique was first reported in 1975 [27]. The gastroscopic biopsy wire forceps is best suited for this purpose [28]. Biliary brush biopsy via the percutaneous transhepatic route was reported in 1979. This technique would also be suitable for the T-tube tract approach [29].

Stricture Dilatation

Biliary duct strictures were first dilated via the T-tube tract approach in 1975 [30] and by the percutaneous transhepatic approach in 1978 [31].

We now use the Grüntzig dilatation balloon catheter for this purpose, with manual balloon insufflation of about 4 atmospheres of pressure. This is suitable for both benign and malignant strictures, particularly if internal drainage catheters are placed through carcinomatous lesions.

The steerable catheter is brought through the sinus tract to a point below the stricture. A guidewire is then placed through the stricture and is followed by the balloon dilatation catheter. The balloon is dilated with contrast material in order to permit fluoroscopic control and accurate placement within the stricture. Even long malignant strictures 5-to-6-cm long have been dilated by this method. Stricture dilatation must precede stone extraction. This can be accomplished in

separate sessions. If maintenance of dilated strictures is indicated, catheter stenting through the previous stricture site is required. U tubes are ideally suited for this purpose (Fig. 106-8).

Internal Biliary Drainage

Internal biliary drainage as an interventional radiologic procedure was described first via the percutaneous transhepatic route (in 1974) [4] and then via the T-tube tract route (in 1975) [30].

Internal stenting and drainage of obstructing lesions in the hepatic and common bile ducts is technically easier via the T-tube sinus tract than via the transhepatic route. It is usually possible to insert a larger diameter drainage catheter through the sinus tract and into the duodenum. Catheters of 14 French inserted through the T-tube tract provide more than twice the internal catheter lumen when compared to an 8 French pigtail catheter inserted through the liver. Side holes can be made larger and more accurately for internal bile drainage from the ducts to the gut. Also, transhepatic reinsertion of catheters after inadvertent removal is more cumbersome because the catheter tract between the lateral abdominal wall and the liver capsule is difficult to reenter. There is always the danger of bile leakage and hemorrhage (Fig. 106-9).

Figure 106-8. (A) A dilatation balloon in place in a hepaticojejunostomy stricture. (B) An internal drainage catheter has been positioned with a contrast-inflated balloon in the hepatic duct. The catheter maintained stricture dilatation and provided internal drainage through the side holes in the jejunum. The catheter was closed at the skin.

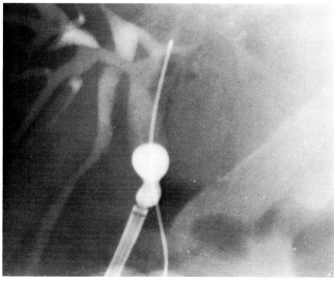
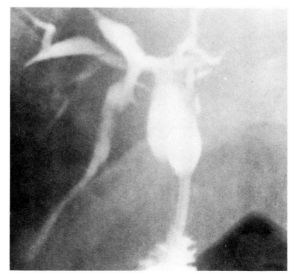

A   B

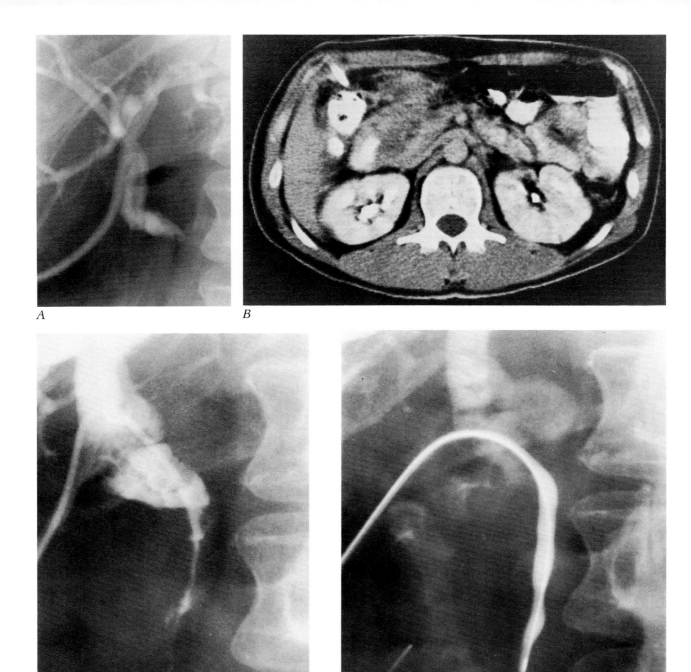

A

B

C

D

Figure 106-9. (A) A malignant distal common duct stricture. (B) Computed tomography scan of the abdomen demonstrated carcinoma of the pancreas. (C) The 8 French steerable catheter had been inserted through the T-tube tract and placed on top of the malignant stricture. Forceful contrast injection now outlined the malignant stricture. (D) A guidewire had been placed through the malignant stricture, which was being dilated with the Grüntzig balloon catheter. (E) An internal 14 French drainage catheter had been placed through the T-tube tract and the dilated malignant stricture, providing drainage through the side holes in the common duct and the end hole in the duodenum. The catheter was closed at the skin.

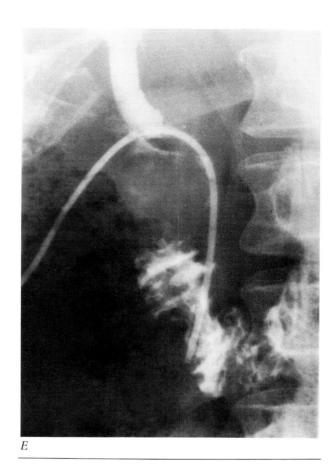

E

Internal drainage catheters used in the T-tube tract can be anchored in the duodenum by contrast inflation of the balloon in Foley catheters. The rubber or Silastic catheter is softer than the stiff transhepatic catheter, a characteristic that permits easier fixation at the skin level and is more comfortable for the patient. The catheter is bent over on itself after it has been cut off close to the skin and is then tied. Anchoring to the skin is not necessary if the Foley balloon in the duodenum and the bent-over catheter on the skin provide only a small amount of internal play by the catheter.

The same is true for internal drainage through the T-tube tract with lesions in the hepatic duct. The balloon is inflated above the stricture, and the indwelling catheter maintaining the dilatation is doubled up at the skin level. Proper end holes and side holes must be constructed to provide for internal drainage from above the obstructing lesion into the duct and into the duodenum. No side holes should be present in the catheter within the sinus tract.

Internal T-tube tract drainage of pancreatic

tumors obstructing the distal common duct of course is applicable only if a T tube has been inserted at the time of exploration. Resectability of small pancreatic carcinomas is best determined at the time of surgical exploration; it is our experience that small masses seen on pancreatic computed tomography and minor arterial abnormalities seen on angiography are often misleading. The pancreatic tumor is usually more extensive when seen at surgery than expected from the radiographic studies alone. At the time of exploration, our surgeons also prefer to provide a gastroenterostomy to palliate future and terminal duodenal obstruction. More recently, we have cooperated with our surgical department and have inserted drainage catheters through a choledochotomy at the time of exploration. This provides for relief of jaundice and pruritus early rather than at a later date, after the T-tube tract has become established.

References

1. Classen, M., and Demling, L. Endoskopische Sphinkterotomie der Papilla Vateri und Steinextraktion aus dem ductus choledochus. *Dtsch. Med. Wochenschr.* 99:496, 1974.
2. Hinde, G. DeB., Smith, P. M., and Craven, J. L. Percutaneous cholangiography with the Okuda needle. *Gut* 18:610, 1977.
3. Remolar, J., Katz, S., Rybak, B., and Pellizari, O. Percutaneous transhepatic cholangiography. *Gastroenterology* 31:39, 1956.
4. Molnar, W., and Stockum, A. E. Relief of obstructive jaundice through percutaneous transhepatic catheter—a new therapeutic method. *AJR* 122:356, 1974.
5. Pereiras, R. V., Jr., Owen, J. R., Hutson, D., Mejia, J., Viamonte, M., Chiprut, R. O., and Schiff, E. R. Relief of malignant obstructive jaundice by percutaneous insertion of a permanent prosthesis in the biliary tree. *Ann. Intern. Med.* 89:589, 1978.
6. Dotter, C. T., Bilbao, M. K., and Katon, R. M. Percutaneous transhepatic gallstone removal by needle tract. *Radiology* 133:242, 1979.
7. Burhenne, H. J. Nonoperative retained biliary tract stone extraction: A new roentgenologic technique. *AJR* 117:388, 1973.
8. Moss, J. P., Whelan, J. G., Powell, R. W., Dedman, T. C., and Oliver, W. J. Postoperative choledochoscopy via the T-tube tract. *J.A.M.A.* 236:2781, 1976.
9. Margulis, A. R., Newton, T. H., and Najarian, J.

S. Removal of plug from T-tube by fluoroscopical controlled catheter: Report of case. *AJR* 93:975, 1965.

10. Russell, E., and Koolpe, H. A. A modified T-tube for use after nonoperative biliary stone removal. *Radiology* 129:237, 1978.

11. Burhenne, H. J., and Peters, H. E. Retained intrahepatic stones. *Arch. Surg.* 113:837, 1978.

12. Del Valle, D. y Colb. *Bol. y Trab. Soc. Arg. de Cirui.* 16:502, 1955.

13. Mazzariello, R. Review of 220 cases of residual biliary tract calculi treated without reoperation: An eight-year study. *Surgery* 73:299, 1972.

14. Lagrave, G., Plessis, J. L., Pougeard-Dulimbert, G., and Passicos, J. Lithiase biliaire résiduelle: Extraction à la sonde de Dormia par le drain de Kehr. *Mém. Acad. Chir.* (Paris) 95:431, 1969.

15. Burhenne, H. J. Extraktion von Residualsteinen der Gallenwege ohne Reoperation. *ROEFO* 117:425, 1972.

16. Burhenne, H. J. Percutaneous extraction of retained biliary tract stones: 661 patients. *AJR* 134:888, 1980.

17. Fennessy, J. J., and You, K. D. Method for expulsion of stones retained in common bile duct. *AJR* 110:256, 1970.

18. Burhenne, H. J., Richards, V., Mathewson, C., Jr., and Westdahl, P. R. Nonoperative extraction of retained biliary tract stones requiring multiple sessions. *Am. J. Surg.* 128:288, 1974.

19. Polack, E. P., Fainsinger, M. H., and Bonnano, S. V. A death following complications of roentgenologic nonoperative manipulation of common bile duct calculi. *Radiology* 123:585, 1977.

20. Smith, H. W., Engel, D., Averbrook, B., and Longmire, W. P., Jr. Problems of retained and recurrent common bile duct stones. *Surgery* 66:291, 1969.

21. Burhenne, H. J. Electrohydrolytic fragmentation of retained common duct stones. *Radiology* 117:721, 1975.

22. Eaton, S. B., Jr., Wirtz, R. D., Ten Eyck, J. R., and Richards, J. C. Iatrogenic liver injury resulting from ductal instrumentation with Fogarty biliary balloon catheter. *Radiology* 100:581, 1971.

23. Burhenne, H. J. Complications of nonoperative extraction of retained common duct stones. *Am. J. Surg.* 131:260, 1976.

24. Yamakawa, T., Mieno, K., Nogucki, T., and Shikata, J. An improved choledochofiberscope and non-surgical removal of retained biliary calculi under direct visual control. *Gastrointest. Endosc.* 22:160, 1976.

25. Safrany, L. Duodenoscopic sphincterotomy and gallstone removal. *Gastroenterology* 72:338, 1977.

26. Classen, M., and Ossenberg, F. W. Progress report: Non-surgical removal of common bile duct stones. *Gut* 18:760, 1977.

27. Burhenne, H. J. Bile duct biopsy with the stone extraction basket. *Radiol. Clin.* 44:178, 1975.

28. Palayew, M. J., and Stein, L. Postoperative biopsy of the common bile duct on the T-tube tract. *AJR* 130:287, 1978.

29. Mendez, G., Jr., Russell, E., Levi, J. U., Koolpe, H., and Cohen, M. Percutaneous brush biopsy and internal drainage of biliary tree through endoprosthesis. *AJR* 134:653, 1980.

30. Burhenne, H. J. Dilatation of biliary tract strictures: A new roentgenologic technique. *Radiol. Clin.* 44:153, 1975.

31. Molnar, W., and Stockum, A. E. Transhepatic dilatation of choledochoenterostomy strictures. *Radiology* 129:59, 1978.

Transluminal Catheter Removal of Foreign Bodies from the Cardiovascular System

CHARLES T. DOTTER
FREDERICK S. KELLER
JOSEF RÖSCH

The first transluminal recovery of an intravascular foreign body, as well as the first such recovery done percutaneously, can be credited to Porstmann [1], in connection with his 1967 catheter technique for ductal closure (see Chap. 98). That Porstmann's foreign body was a guide-spring deliberately passed across the ductus into the right heart and securely held at its other end rather than an accidentally embolized fragment of guidewire or tubing does not detract from his technical accomplishment. As far as is known, all transluminally recovered foreign bodies have gotten into, as well as out of, the vascular system through man's doing. Unlike Porstmann's, however, most of them were turned loose by mishap rather than design; and unlike Porstmann's, they posed a serious risk to their hosts.

This chapter deals specifically with the relatively noninvasive transluminal removal of unwanted errant foreign bodies lodged in the depths of the cardiovascular system. The first such removal was done in 1964 by Thomas, who used bronchoscopic forceps passed through a saphenous vein cutdown [2]. In 1968, Henley accomplished a similar removal percutaneously [3]. In 1971, it was possible to report a total of 29 guided transvascular foreign body retrievals, 6 done percutaneously [4]. By now, there has appeared a seemingly unending series of reports describing a host of methods used to extricate unwanted foreign bodies from various parts of the vascular system. The impulse to publish is understandable, since the presence of such debris poses significant threats to patients, especially the risks of surgical removal or, alternatively, the potential consequences of nonremoval, among which are sepsis and death. Nonremoval or surgical removal is potential grounds for malpractice action and a source of embarrassment to the presumably responsible physician or manufacturer.

The veritable plethora of related reports also reflects the excitement of the actual procedure and the nearly universal patient-doctor feeling of triumph at the moment of success. Thus, editors of scientific journals can expect to continue to receive manuscripts with reviews of the general subject and case reports illustrating minor variations on the many technical wrinkles already described in print. By now, hundreds of foreign bodies have been removed percutaneously from the vascular system, sparing hundreds of patients from surgery or the serious complications of doing nothing. As in dealing with retained bile stones, there is little wonder that image-guided catheter removal has now become the standard therapeutic approach.

Cardiovascular Foreign Bodies—What and Where?

Extensive 1977 reviews on the nonsurgical retrieval of intravascular foreign bodies include the review by Fisher and Ferreyro [5] and Bloomfield's report [6] of an international survey dealing with types and sites of lodgment of some 180 foreign bodies. Of these 180 foreign bodies, 143 were cut-off bits of plastic tubing used for measuring central venous pressure (Fig. 107-1). In addition, Bloomfield reported the recovery of 6 fragments of diagnostic catheters, 6 broken-off guidewires, 7 pacing catheters damaged during pacemaker replacement, 12 errant ventricular-jugular shunt tubes, and 6 other items, ranging from bullets (presumably not iatrogenic) to a Swan-Ganz catheter that had been sewn to the right atrial wall during prior surgery and broken during attempted withdrawal! As detailed in Table 107-1, all but 6 objects came to lie in the veins, right heart chambers, or pulmonary arteries.

Figure 107-1. Detail of a chest film showing an 8-cm fragment of a central venous pressure catheter (*arrowheads*) lodged in the right atrium and extending into the right ventricle of a 3-year-old patient; its radiopacity and position allowed its prompt retrieval with a homemade loop snare.

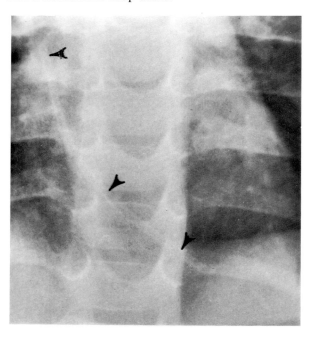

Table 107-1. Distribution of Lodging Sites in the Right Heart of 180 Catheter Fragments

Site	Proximal (Cut) End	Distal (Leading) End
Subclavian vein	11	1
Internal jugular vein	2	1
Superior vena cava	36	6
Right atrium	46	22
Right ventricle	1	38
Pulmonary artery	33	35
Inferior vena cava	9	6
Hepatic vein	—	4
Umbilical vein	1	1

The proximal, most accessible, end of a foreign body fragment can be expected to lie no more central in the circulation than the right atrium unless the entire fragment passes to the pulmonary artery. The only instance of a right ventricular lodging site occurred when a polyethylene catheter doubled over on itself with both ends in the ventricle and the midsection looped in the pulmonary artery. (Adapted from Bloomfield [6].)

teries. The 6 exceptions were guidewire fragments that had lodged in peripheral arteries. If Bloomfield's collection were brought up to date, it would include several instances of Gianturco spring coil occluders being retrieved following their malplacement or subsequent displacement. These and other objects used in the transluminal therapeutic production of vascular —usually arterial—occlusion can get into the wrong places and become the opposite of therapeutic. Fortunately, they are usually susceptible to transluminal, nonoperative disposal. It seems clear that future progress in interventional radiology will bring both the promise of new therapeutic techniques and the problems of unintended, misplaced, or migrant intravascular foreign bodies requiring nonoperative extraction.

Transluminal Retrieval Techniques

There are many ways of finding, visualizing, moving, and, with skill and luck, removing foreign bodies from the heart and blood vessels. Fortunately, surgery is a rarely needed last resort. Though details have varied from one report to the next, in general, angiographers rely upon image guidance—usually fluoroscopy—and the use of the following basic retrievers: (1) loop-snare catheters, (2) hook-tip guidewires or

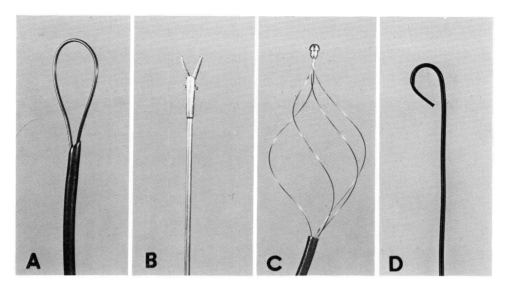

Figure 107-2. Four transluminal retrieval devices used in the cardiovascular system. (A) Loop snare. (B) Grasping forceps. (C) Basket retriever. (D) Hook-tip catheter.

catheters, (3) basket retrievers, and (4) grasping forceps or catheters (Fig. 107-2). Tip deflectors [7] and sheath "introducers" [8] can be useful aids. The tools and techniques must be chosen in accordance with individual circumstances. How to remove the foreign body depends on what is to be removed and on where and how it has come to rest. Loose-ended radiopaque tubing can usually be caught in commercially available (Cook) or improvised loop-snare catheters.

LOOP-SNARE CATHETERS

Loop-snare catheters [9–19] are the catheters through which a flexible, double length of guidewire or thin tubing or monofilament can be passed so as to form a variable loop extending from the central orifice of the introducing catheter. The size, configuration, and orientation of the loop and the introducing catheter are exploited so as to pass the loop over an accessible, free end of the usual embolized length of polyethylene tubing. Naturally, this is greatly facilitated if the foreign body is radiopaque, as is usually the case. Common sense, manipulative skill, and a bit of luck usually result in a successful lassoing. The snare is then drawn into the end of the guiding catheter so as to lock tightly to the foreign body, and both catheter and foreign body are removed together (Fig. 107-3). This approach in one or another of its many reported variations

works equally well with guidewire fragments, provided again that at least one end of the guidewire is free to be snared. Loop-snare catheters have been responsible for most retrievals (Figs. 107-4, 107-5). Porstmann's successful use of the loop-snare method in nearly 200 consecutive patients undergoing transluminal ductal closure offers convincing confirmation of the value of the approach. In accomplishing the fifth and sixth reported percutaneous foreign body retrievals [4], we found that the use of a compound, convoluted loop (see Fig. 107-3C) facilitated fishing for a loose end in the right atrium. Within limits, if one loop could do it, more loops did it sooner, especially when poor visibility impeded precise three-dimensional control of the snaring maneuver. Closed loops are unlikely to be effective when there is no free end to snare.

HOOK-TIP GUIDEWIRES OR CATHETERS

Hook-tip guidewires or catheters [12, 19–24] can be formed ad hoc and used to engage lengths of intravascular debris lacking an accessible free end. Hooked over the offender, they can be used to pull it into a position favorable for snaring; they can be used to twist and thereby engage and withdraw lengths of tubing with ends embedded or otherwise out of reach. Tip-deflector guide systems can be useful, although final removal from the vein of access has usually required a cutdown and venotomy.

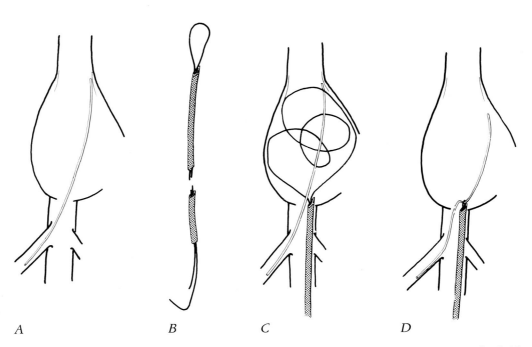

A   B   C   D

Figure 107-3. Mechanics of transluminal retrieval by loop-snare techniques. (A) A fragment of broken central venous pressure catheter in the right atrium and hepatic vein. (B) A homemade loop-snare system with a 12 French Teflon outer catheter and a 4 French Teflon loop. (C) One convolution of a deliberately redundant loop has engaged the foreign body. (D) A fragment securely held and ready to be withdrawn via the inferior vena cava and the femoral vein.

BASKET RETRIEVER CATHETER SYSTEMS

Wire catch baskets similar to those Dormia used for ureteral stones and Burhenne used for retained gallstones work well in the entrapment of tubing lying within such blood vessels as the pulmonary artery or the vena cava [13, 25–29]. In one of our patients, an hour's time was wasted trying to throw a loop snare over a piece of shunt tubing lying within the right pulmonary artery. A basket catheter opened up adjacent to the tubing and rotated slightly before its closure managed the removal on the first try and in less than a minute (Fig. 107-6). A basket retriever system designed for intravascular use is commercially available (Cook). Used and maintained with care, one such catheter can serve several times. For obvious reasons, basket retrievers are used through and in conjunction with larger outer catheters. It is convenient to employ sheaths for their introduction. Since baskets can be expanded to embrace the entire vascular lumen, they necessarily contact and usually can entrap a contained foreign body, be it a bullet or a long length of radiolucent tubing lying flat along the vessel wall. Baskets are best not expanded within cardiac chambers lest trabeculae or valves be unintentionally caught and damaged.

GRASPING FORCEPS OR CATHETERS

Bronchoscopic forceps are of limited value because of their rigidity and short length. They have been used with success in several transluminal retrievals, generally necessitating cutdowns [27, 30–32]. Ranniger [33] devised a flexible catheter with three grasping prongs that successfully recovered a fragment of guidespring from a right ventricle.

BALLOON CATHETERS

Simple balloon-tipped catheters can be used percutaneously to move intravascular foreign bodies into more favorable positions for conventional catheter recovery. Balloons can also be used to prevent undesired distal embolization of foreign bodies during their recovery from pulmonary or systemic arteries. Their planned percutaneous use in removing unwanted material from blood vessels [34] promises to exceed their past value in connection with "blind" surgical embolectomy.

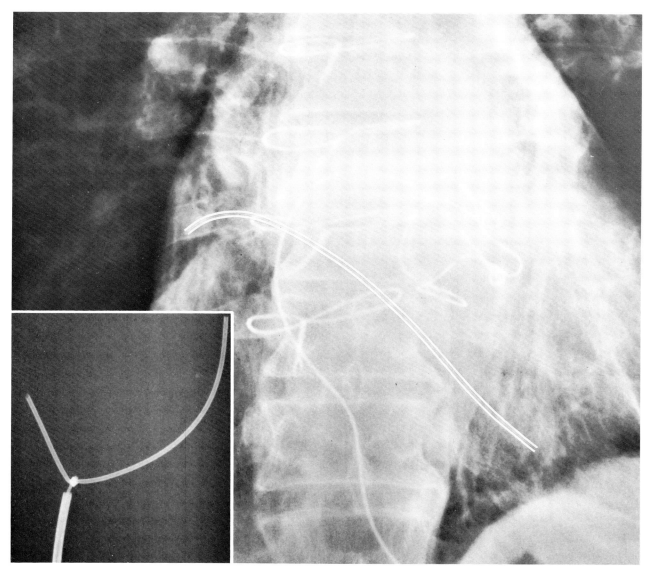

Figure 107-4. Fragment of a broken central venous pressure catheter (retouched) crosses the tricuspid valve with its distal end in the right ventricular apex and its proximal end in the right atrium. Inset at the same scale: a radiograph of 12.5-cm-long central venous pressure catheter fragment after successful retrieval by a loop snare.

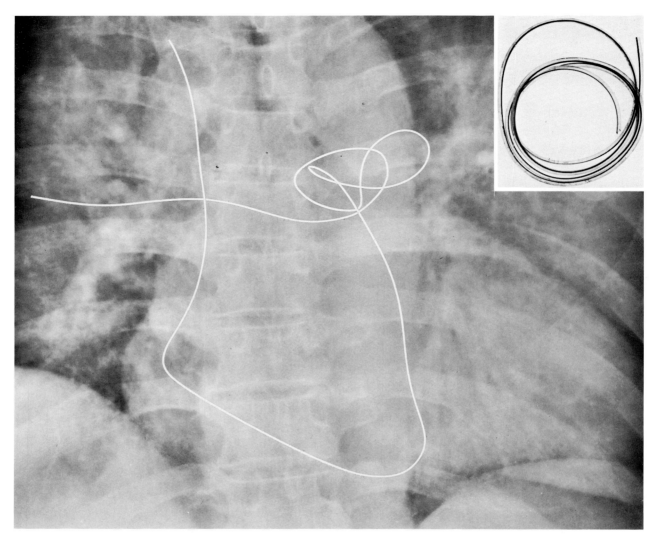

Figure 107-5. Long (5-cm) fragment of a broken central venous pressure catheter (retouched), extending from the superior vena cava through the right atrium, right ventricle, and main pulmonary artery, with its distal end in the right pulmonary artery. Inset at the same scale: a 65-cm-long central venous pressure catheter fragment after successful retrieval with a loop snare.

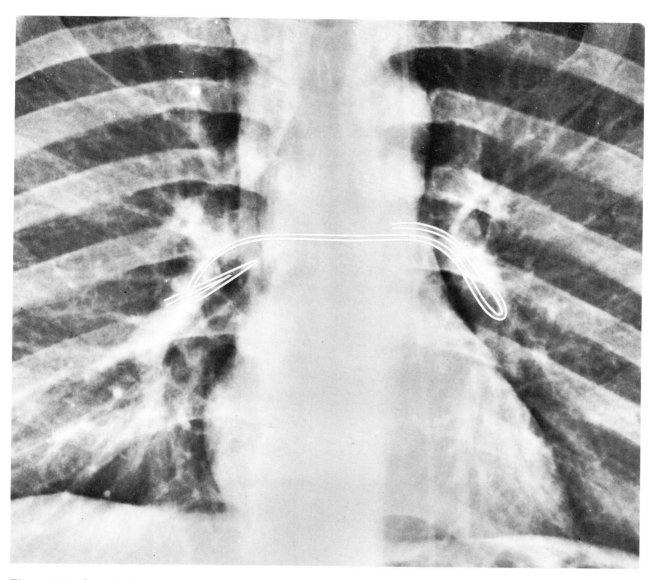

Figure 107-6. Embolized fragment of a ventriculoatrial shunt (retouched) looped across the pulmonary artery confluence with coiled ends in the left and right pulmonary arteries. A new ventriculoperitoneal shunt is already in place. After an hour's failure with loop snares, the shunt was grasped and retrieved within a minute using a basket retriever.

Complications of Percutaneous Transluminal Foreign Body Removal

Considering that most angiographers have learned by actually performing transcatheter retrievals, the complication rate is remarkably low. Katzen reported minor pulmonary embolization after removing a pacemaker wire that had been embedded for 5 years [35]. Two patients experienced transient arrhythmias when the end of a fragment being removed impinged on the right ventricle wall. As far as is known, no one has died as a consequence of attempted catheter recovery of an intravascular foreign body. This cannot be said of the surgical alternative or of nonremoval [6]. In view of its extensive and generally successful use, catheter retrieval is clearly indicated wherever feasible.

Discussion

The percutaneous catheter removal of undesired foreign bodies by techniques selected to suit the individual circumstances is an invaluable aid to modern medical practice. Every facility engaged in vascular catheterization for diagnostic, monitoring, or feeding purposes should have the simple equipment needed to effect transluminal retrievals. The manufacturers of vascular catheters, guidewires, and tubing have done their best to design relatively foolproof products, but their progress in this direction can only reduce, never eliminate, the basic problem. The most carefully prepared instructions and warnings can be overlooked by physician or nurse; the patient, especially when asleep or unconscious, can undo the best of prophylactic efforts. Therapeutically placed vascular occlusive devices can be dislodged, with potentially calamitous results. The prompt transluminal removal of mislodged or displaced spring coil occluders has reportedly been done at least three times [26, 36, 37].

Extrapolation

We can accidentally or intentionally place a variety of foreign bodies within the human cardiovascular system. Surgeons have been installing prosthetic grafts and valves for years. Thus far, when these chanced to become a problem, their removal necessitated further major surgery. As Porstmann has already shown, the radiologist may some day offer alternatives to the surgical placement of prosthetic devices. Although the percutaneous placement of an artificial mitral valve is not just around the corner, it is quite likely that catheters will some day provide a superior transluminal alternative to surgical bypass grafting, endarterectomy, and portosystemic shunting. Such techniques have already been done in experimental animals [38, 39], and it is only a question of time before they will play clinical roles. In the percutaneous transluminal retrieval of unwanted foreign bodies from the cardiovascular, biliary, and gastrointestinal systems, radiologists not only have increased the safety of medicine for many patients but they also have pointed the way for further progress, both in the removal of foreign bodies and in the deliberate therapeutic placement of foreign bodies (perhaps in the latter context the term *prosthetic* is more suitable). We need not and should not confine our thinking to the removal of foreign bodies only. We are on the verge of providing patients with a superior, transluminal means of removing other impediments to normal blood flow. Percutaneous embolectomy offers a good example, one likely to be achieved soon. Transvascular retrieval is an accomplished fact; its success has broad implications for the future of relatively noninvasive image-guided transluminal catheter techniques for accomplishing objectives that today involve the greater pain, risk, cost, and disability inherent in even the most modern surgery. One patient's complication can point the way to another's therapeutic benefit.

References

1. Porstmann, W., Wierny, L., and Warnke, H. Closure of persistent ductus arteriosus without thoracotomy. *German Med. Monthly* 12:1, 1967.
2. Thomas, J., Sinclair-Smith, B., Bloomfield, D., and Davachi, A. Nonsurgical retrieval of broken segment of steel spring guide from right atrium and inferior vena cava. *Circulation* 30:106, 1964.
3. Henley, F. T., and Ballard, J. W. Percutaneous removal of flexible foreign body from the heart. *Radiology* 92:176, 1969.
4. Dotter, C. T., Rösch, J., and Bilbao, M. K. Transluminal extraction of catheter and guide fragments from the heart and great vessels; 29 collected cases. *AJR* 111:467, 1971.
5. Fisher, R. G., and Ferreyro, R. Evaluation of

current techniques for nonsurgical removal of intravascular iatrogenic foreign bodies. *AJR* 130:541, 1978.

6. Bloomfield, D. A. The nonsurgical retrieval of intracardiac foreign bodies—an international survey. *Cathet. Cardiovasc. Diagn.* 4:1, 1978.

7. McSweeney, W. J., and Schwartz, D. C. Retrieval of a catheter foreign body from the right heart using a guide wire deflector system. *Radiology* 100:61, 1971.

8. Soo, C. S., Chuang, V. P., and Wallace, S. Nonsurgical retrieval of a severed catheter from femoral artery using a mylar sheath. *AJR* 135:400, 1980.

9. Bett, J. H. N., and Anderson, S. T. Plastic catheter embolism to the right heart: A technique of non-surgical removal. *Med. J. Australia* 2:854, 1971.

10. Curry, J. L. Recovery of detached intravascular catheter or guide wire fragments: A proposed method. *AJR* 105:894, 1969.

11. Enge, I., and Flatmark, A. Percutaneous removal of intravascular foreign bodies by the snare technique. *Acta Radiol.* 14:747, 1973.

12. Fisher, R. G., and Romero, J. R. Extraction of an embolized central venous catheter using percutaneous technique. *Radiology* 116:735, 1975.

13. Grand, M., Harry, G., Rémy, J., and Doyon, D. Extraction non chirurgicale de corps étrangers iatrogènes intravasculaires. *J. Radiol. Electrol.* 59:479, 1978.

14. Khaja, F., and Lakier, J. Foreign body retrieval from the heart by two catheter technique. *Cathet. Cardiovasc. Diagn.* 5:263, 1979.

15. Massumi, R. A., and Ross, A. M. Atraumatic, nonsurgical technic for removal of broken catheters from cardiac cavities. *Med. Intell.* 277:195, 1967.

16. Miller, R. E., Cockerill, E. M., and Helbig, H. Percutaneous removal of catheter emboli from the pulmonary arteries. *Radiology* 94:151, 1970.

17. Miller, R. E. Internal jugular pulmonary arteriography and removal of catheter emboli. *Radiology* 102:200, 1972.

18. Picard, L., Roland, J., Sigiel, M., Schwartz, J. F., André, J. M., Montaut, J., and Lepoire, J. Transluminal retrieval of ventriculoatrial shunt catheters from the heart and great vessels: A new method. *Neuroradiology* 10:159, 1975.

19. Randall, P. A. Percutaneous removal of iatrogenic intracardiac foreign body. *Radiology* 102:591, 1972.

20. Zollikofer, C., Nath, P. H., Castaneda-Zuniga, W. R., Probst, P., Barreto, A., Tadavarthy, S. M., and Amplatz, K. Nonsurgical removal of intravascular foreign bodies. *ROEFO* 130:590, 1979.

21. Maxwell, D. D., and Anderson, R. E. Transfemoral retrieval of an intracardiac catheter fragment, using a simple hood-shaped catheter. *Radiology* 103:213, 1972.

22. Mullen, J. L., Oleaga, J., and Ring, E. J. Catheter migration during home hyperalimentation. *J.A.M.A.* 238:1946, 1977.

23. Padula, G. Hook and snare technique for intravascular retrieval. *Radiology* 133:529, 1979.

24. Rossi, P. "Hook catheter," technique for transfemoral removal of foreign body from right side of the heart. *AJR* 109:101, 1970.

25. Bessler, V. W. Transvenöse Entfernung embolisierter Katheter. *ROEFO* 127:164, 1977.

26. Chuang, V. P. Nonoperative retrieval of Gianturco coils from abdominal aorta. *AJR* 132:996, 1979.

27. Hasse, J., Burkart, F., and Grädel, E. Behandlung der iatrogenen transvenösen Fremdkörperembolie. *Schweiz. Med. Wochenschr.* 108:1470, 1978.

28. Lassers, B. W., and Pickering, D. Removal of an iatrogenic foreign body from the aorta by means of a ureteric stone catheter. *Am. Heart J.* 73:375, 1967.

29. Ort, V. J., Kolář, J., and Bruthans, J. Erfolgreiche Entfernung eines kurzen Führungsdrahtbruchstückes aus der rechten Herzkammer. *ROEFO* 128:495, 1978.

30. King, J. F., Manley, J. C., Zeft, H. J., and Auer, J. E. Nonsurgical removal of foreign body from right heart. *J. Thorac. Cardiovasc. Surg.* 71:785, 1976.

31. Millan, V. G. Retrieval of intravascular foreign bodies using a modified bronchoscopic forceps. *Radiology* 129:587, 1978.

32. Smyth, N. P. D., Boivin, M. R., and Bacos, J. M. Transjugular removal of foreign body from the right atrium by endoscopic forceps. *J. Thorac. Cardiovasc. Surg.* 55:594, 1968.

33. Ranniger, K. An instrument for retrieval of intravascular foreign bodies. *Radiology* 91:1043, 1968.

34. Dotter, C. T. Interventional radiology—review of an emerging field. *Semin. Roentgenol.* 6:7, 1981.

35. Katzen, B. T. Personal communication, 1980.

36. Radojkóvić, S., Kamenica, S., Jašović, M., and Draganić, M. Catheter-aided extraction of a steel coil accidentally lodged in the right ventricle. *Cardiovasc. Intervent. Radiol.* 3:153, 1980.

37. Weber, J. A complication with the Gianturco coil and its non-surgical management. *Cardiovasc. Intervent. Radiol.* 3:156, 1980.

38. Rösch, J., Hanafee, W. N., and Snow, H. Transjugular portal venography and radiologic portacaval shunt: An experimental study. *Radiology* 92:1112, 1969.

39. Dotter, C. T. Transluminally placed coilspring endarterial tube grafts: Long-term patency in canine popliteal artery. *Invest. Radiol.* 4:329, 1969.

Index

Index

Complications of procedures—*Continued*
in spinal arteriography, 320, 322
spinal cord injuries in, 315, 318, 319, 329–333
in splenoportography, 1574–1575
in thoracic aortography, 345–350
toxic reactions in, 27
in transluminal angioplasty, 2113, 2126–2127
femoropopliteal, 2118, 2120
in upper extremity arteriography, 1924–1925, 1929
in vena cavography, 972
Computed tomography
in abdominal aortic aneurysms, 1079
of abscesses, 1181, 1455, 1567, 2335–2336
for guidance and route planning, 2338–2340, 2346, 2347
signs in, 2336–2338, 2347
of adrenal gland, 1395, 1401
in adenocarcinoma, 1419
in aldosteronism, 1405
in aldosteronomas, 1421
compared to angiography, 1421–1422
in Cushing's disease, 1408
in neuroblastomas, 1418
in nonfunctioning tumors, 1421
in pheochromocytoma, 1411
after aortoiliac surgery, 1828, 1829, 1831
in biopsy guidance, 2080, 2302, 2309
renal, 2321–2322
retroperitoneal, 2313
in bladder tumors, 1758–1760, 1762
in bone tumors, 1952
cerebral angiography compared to, 219–220
in aneurysms, 284–286
in arteriovenous malformations, 295
in cavernous angiomas, 292–293
in head trauma, 305, 310
in tumors, 301, 302, 305
in venous occlusive disease, 281–283
in complications from angiography, 1046
after coronary artery bypass surgery, 703
in dissecting aortic aneurysms, 457, 463–464
in gastrointestinal conditions, 1623, 1655
in gynecology, 1768, 1769
in ovarian and uterine tumors, 1769, 1770
of kidneys, 2321–2322
in abscesses, 1181
in hydronephrosis, 1202, 1213
in inflammatory disease, 1198
in trauma, 1234–1236
in tumors and cysts, 1136, 1153, 1168, 1169, 1171, 1342
veins in, 1335
of lungs, prior to lung biopsy, 2302
lymphangiography compared to, 2080–2082
in lymphoma, 919
of mediastinum, 977
of pancreas, 1427, 1436
in carcinoma, 1443
in cystic neoplasms, 1451, 1455
in pancreatitis, 1452
in pseudocysts and abscesses, 1455
of parathyroid glands, ectopic, 993

Computed tomography—*Continued*
in pelvic lipomatosis, 1768
of retroperitoneal space, 1790, 1796–1797, 2313
in fibrosis, 2034
in tumors of pediatric patients, 1799, 1804
of spinal arteriovenous malformations, 321
of spleen, 1531, 1545, 1568
in abscesses, 1567
in cysts, 1556
in infarction, 1551
posttraumatic, 1561–1562
in tumors, 1560, 1568
in thoracic aortic aneurysms, 418, 436, 457, 463–464
of thoracic duct, 2010, 2020
in thoracic outlet syndrome, 1001
in ureteral obstruction in oliguria, 1301, 1316, 1319
of vena cava, 916, 923, 943, 950, 960–962, 971
in Wilms' tumor, 1125
Computer programmer, cassette changer with, 111
Computerized data analysis, 158, 159, 161
Computerized fluoroscopy, after aortoiliac surgery, 1825–1827, 1828
Concussion, cerebral, 310
Conducting system of heart, 547–551
arterial supply of, 548–550
Confluens sinuum, 260, 307
Congenital anomalies
aneurysms, 283, 1549
aortic, 431–434, 442
coronary artery, 584
upper extremity, 1927
Valsalva sinus, 418, 431–434
aortic stenosis in, 467, 468
arteriovenous malformations. *See* Arteriovenous malformations, congenital
of bladder, 1766
bronchial arteriography in, 846, 853
cerebrovascular, 292–298
coarctation of aorta, 364, 383
coronary arteriography in, 514–515, 531–537, 570, 675–691
ductus arteriosus patency, 372, 2257–2262. *See also* Ductus arteriosus, patency of
of heart
laboratory for study of, 163
x-ray tubes for study of, 135
of kidneys, 1159, 1217–1255, 1229, 1271, 1273
cystic disease, 1165
hydronephrosis in, 1201, 1213
hypoplasia, 1273
renal artery stenosis, 1263
of lymphatic system, 2019, 2023, 2024, 2037
of mesenteric artery, 1641, 1647, 1648
pseudocoarctation of aorta, 479
of pulmonary arteries, 723–740
of pulmonary veins, 739–740, 869–891
of spleen, 1543–1547
splenic artery aneurysms, 1549
subclavian artery compression in, 1002
of testicular vein, 2220–2221

Congenital anomalies—*Continued*
thoracic aortography in, 341, 344–345
of upper extremity arteries, 1927
of vena cava, 947–950, 963–964
Coning, 109, 137, 166
Conray, 17, 19, 58–59. *See also* Iothalamate contrast media
in carotid angiography, 221, 222
chemical composition of, 48
in femoral arteriography, 1847
flow rates of, 197–200
generic names of, 58–59, 75
in jugular venography, 227
in orbital venography, 227
in spinal angiography, 320
in thoracic aortography, 344
usefulness of, 17
in vertebral angiography, 336
viscosity of, 196
Consent to procedures. *See* Informed consent
Contraceptives, oral, disorders from
deep vein thrombosis, 1903
liver tumors, 1491
mesenteric venous thrombosis, 1740
renal hypertension, 1282
upper extremity arterial thrombosis, 1932
Contrast and latitude of film, 146, 148
Contrast media, 15–94, 1043, 1044–1045, 1048
in abdominal aortography, 1030, 1033
in adrenal angiography, 1397, 1398, 1399
allergic reactions to, 27, 1044–1045. *See also* Allergic reactions
in aortoiliac arteriography, postoperative, 1824, 1825, 1828
in balloon occlusion techniques, 2212, 2213, 2215, 2216, 2224, 2225
in biliary interventional procedures, 2385, 2386, 2387
in biopsy procedures, 2308
blood vessel reactions to, 24–25
in bone and soft tissue tumor angiography, 1938, 1939
pooling or laking of, 1939, 1969
staining or blush by, 1939–1940, 1969
in bronchial arteriography, 846
in carotid angiography, 221, 222
catheters and injectors for, 187–203, 1979, 1980
central nervous system reactions to, 20–21
chemical formulas of, 28, 41–76
choice of, 16–19, 30
clinical formulations for, 76
computerized literature retrieval systems for, 76
concentration of, 18, 28–29, 30–31
in coronary angioplasty, 2089
in coronary arteriography, 17, 160, 161, 490, 492, 495, 498
artifacts induced by, 670–672
after bypass surgery, 698, 699
complications from, 511, 514, 515
dose of, 18, 21
flow and pressure changes related to, 670–672
injection rate of, 196, 490, 559
in intramural structures, 554
layering of, 558–559